NNF
Clinical Protocols in
Perinatology

NNF
Clinical Protocols in
Perinatology

Editors-in-Chief

Ashish Jain
Associate Professor
Department of Neonatology
Maulana Azad Medical College and
Associated Lok Nayak Hospital
New Delhi, India

Ballambattu Vishnu Bhat
Director (Medical Research)
Aarupadai Veedu Medical College and Hospital
Vinayaka Mission's Research Foundation—DU
Puducherry, India

Executive Editors

Ranjan Kumar Pejaver
Neonatologist
People Tree Hospitals, Meenakshi Hospital
Bengaluru, Karnataka, India
President
National Neonatology Forum (NNF) of India (2021)
Former Chairperson
Neonatology Chapter of IAP, India

V Shanthakumari
President
Federation of Obstetrics and Gynaecological
Societies of India (FOGSI)

Foreword
Vinod Paul

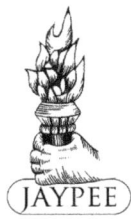

JAYPEE BROTHERS MEDICAL PUBLISHERS
The Health Sciences Publisher
New Delhi | London

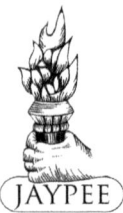 **Jaypee Brothers Medical Publishers (P) Ltd**

Headquarters
Jaypee Brothers Medical Publishers (P) Ltd
EMCA House, 23/23-B
Ansari Road, Daryaganj
New Delhi 110 002, India
Landline: +91-11-23272143, +91-11-23272703
+91-11-23282021, +91-11-23245672
Email: jaypee@jaypeebrothers.com

Corporate Office
Jaypee Brothers Medical Publishers (P) Ltd
4838/24, Ansari Road, Daryaganj
New Delhi 110 002, India
Phone: +91-11-43574357
Fax: +91-11-43574314
Email: jaypee@jaypeebrothers.com

Overseas Office
JP Medical Ltd.
83 Victoria Street, London
SW1H 0HW (UK)
Phone: +44 20 3170 8910
Fax: +44 (0)20 3008 6180
Email: info@jpmedpub.com

Website: www.jaypeebrothers.com
Website: www.jaypeedigital.com

© 2022, Jaypee Brothers Medical Publishers

The views and opinions expressed in this book are solely those of the original contributor(s)/author(s) and do not necessarily represent those of editor(s) of the book.

All rights reserved. No part of this publication may be reproduced, stored or transmitted in any form or by any means, electronic, mechanical, photocopying, recording or otherwise, without the prior permission in writing of the publishers.

All brand names and product names used in this book are trade names, service marks, trademarks or registered trademarks of their respective owners. The publisher is not associated with any product or vendor mentioned in this book.

Medical knowledge and practice change constantly. This book is designed to provide accurate, authoritative information about the subject matter in question. However, readers are advised to check the most current information available on procedures included and check information from the manufacturer of each product to be administered, to verify the recommended dose, formula, method and duration of administration, adverse effects and contraindications. It is the responsibility of the practitioner to take all appropriate safety precautions. Neither the publisher nor the author(s)/editor(s) assume any liability for any injury and/or damage to persons or property arising from or related to use of material in this book.

This book is sold on the understanding that the publisher is not engaged in providing professional medical services. If such advice or services are required, the services of a competent medical professional should be sought.

Every effort has been made where necessary to contact holders of copyright to obtain permission to reproduce copyright material. If any have been inadvertently overlooked, the publisher will be pleased to make the necessary arrangements at the first opportunity. The **CD/DVD-ROM** (if any) provided in the sealed envelope with this book is complimentary and free of cost. **Not meant for sale.**

Inquiries for bulk sales may be solicited at: jaypee@jaypeebrothers.com

NNF Clinical Protocols in Perinatology

First Edition: 2022

ISBN: 978-93-5465-339-1

Dedicated to

All the mothers and their little ones who are in making,
born, lost and are living

Reviewers Panel

Adhisivam B
Professor
Department of Neonatology
Jawaharlal Institute of Postgraduate
Medical Education and Research
Puducherry, India

Amit Upadhyay
Head
Department of Pediatrics and
Neonatology
Nutema Hospital
Meerut, Uttar Pradesh, India

Arjit Mohapatra
Senior Consultant
Department of Pediatrics and
Neonatology
Jagannath Hospital
Bhubaneswar, Odisha, India

Arti Maria
Consultant and Head
Department of Neonatology
PGIMER and Associated Dr RML Hospital
New Delhi, India

Arun Singh
Professor and Former Head
Department of Neonatology
Institute of Post Graduate Medical
Education and Research (IPGMER)
and SSKM Hospitals
Kolkata, West Bengal, India

Bharathi Balachander
Assistant Professor (Neonatology)
St Johns Medical College Hospital
Bengaluru, Karnataka, India

Bijan Saha
Associate Professor
Department of Neonatology
IPGMER and SSKM Hospital
Kolkata, West Bengal, India

Chetan Khare
Assistant Professor
Department of Neonatology
All India Institute of Medical Sciences
Rishikesh, Uttarakhand, India

Deepak Chawla
Professor
Department of Neonatology
Government Medical College and
Hospital
Chandigarh, India

Femitha Pournami
Consultant
Department of Neonatology
Kerala Institute of Medical Sciences
Thiruvananthapuram, Kerala, India

Giridhar Sethuraman
Professor
Department of Neonatology
Chettinad Hospital and Research Institute
Chennai, Tamil Nadu, India

Himanshu Goel
Clinical Lead, Clinical Geneticist
Department of Hunter Genetics
Hunter New England Local Health District
Newcastle, NSW

Jaikrishan Mittal
Director
Department of Neonatology
Neoclinic Children Hospital
Jaipur, Rajasthan, India

Jyotsana Suri
Professor
Department of Obstetrics and
Gynecology
Vardhman Mahavir Medical College and
Safdarjung Hospital
New Delhi, India

Leena Wadhwa
Professor and IVF In-charge
Department of Obstetrics and Gynecology
ESI PGIMSR
Basaidarapur, New Delhi, India

Madhavi M Gupta
Director–Professor
Department of Obstetrics and
Gynecology
Maulana Azad Medical College and
Associated Lok Nayak Hospital
New Delhi, India

Mamta Jajoo
Professor Pediatrics
Head of Office
NICU Incharge
Chacha Nehru Bal Chikitsalaya
New Delhi, India

Mangala Bharathi S
Professor
Department of Neonatology
Madras Medical College
Chennai, Tamil Nadu, India

Manish Kumar
Professor
Department of Neonatology
Christian Medical College and Hospital
Vellore, Tamil Nadu, India

MMA Faridi
Dean, Faculty of Medicine
Era University, Lucknow
Principal, CMS and Professor of Pediatrics
Era's Lucknow Medical College
Lucknow, Uttar Pradesh, India

Monika Kaushal
Consultant Neonatologist and
Head
Department of Neonatology
Emirates Specialty Hospital
Dubai, UAE

Mukul Kumar Mangla
Specialist Neonatology
Department of Neonatology
NMC Royal Hospital
Dubai, UAE

Naveen Jain
Senior Consultant
Department of Neonatology
Kerala Institute of Medical Sciences
Trivandrum, Kerala, India

Nishad Plakkal
Associate Professor
Department of Neonatology
Jawaharlal Institute of Postgraduate
Medical Education and Research
Puducherry, India

Reviewers Panel

Poonam Tara
Senior Consultant
Department of Obstetrics, Gynecology
and Fetal Medicine
Centre for Fetal Maternal Care (CFMC)
New Delhi, India

Pradeep Debta
Professor
Neonatal Division
Department of Pediatrics
Vardhman Mahavir Medical College
and Safdarjung Hospital
New Delhi, India

Pradeep Kumar Sharma
Senior Consultant
Department of Neonatology
SPS Hospitals
Ludhiana, Punjab, India

Ratna Dua Puri
Professor in Genetics
GRIPMER
Chairperson
Institute of Medical Genetics and Genomics
Sir Ganga Ram Hospital
New Delhi, India

Reema Kumar Bhatt
Senior Consultant
Department of Fetal Medicine
Cloudnine Hospitals
New Delhi, India

Sangeeta Gupta
Director Professor
Department of Obstetrics and Gynecology
Maulana Azad Medical College
New Delhi, India

Siddharth Ramji
Director-Professor and Head
Department of Neonatology
Maulana Azad Medical College and
Associated Lok Nayak Hospital
New Delhi, India

Sindhu Sivanandan
Assistant Professor
Department of Neonatology
Jawaharlal Institute of Postgraduate
Medical Education and Research
Puducherry, India

SJ Patil
Senior Consultant Clinical Genetics
Division of Medical Genetics,
Department of Pediatrics
Mazumdar Shaw Medical Centre
Narayana Hrudayalaya Hospitals
Bengaluru, Karnataka, India

Sreeram S
Consultant
Neo BBC children's hospital
Paramitha children's hospital
Hyderabad, Telangana, India

Srinivas Murki
Academic Head
Department of Pediatrics and Neonatology
Paramitha Children's Hospital
Hyderabad, Telangana, India

Sudershan Raj C
Professor and Head
Department of Pediatrics
MediCiti Institute of Medical Sciences
Hyderabad, Telangana, India

Suksham Jain
Professor and Head
Department of Neonatology
Government Medical College and Hospital
Chandigarh, India

Suman Rao
Professor (Neonatology)
St John's Medical College Hospital
Bengaluru, Karnataka, India

Sushma Nangia
Director Professor and Head
Department of Neonatology
Lady Hardinge Medical College and
Kalawati Saran Children's Hospital
New Delhi, India

Tapas Bandyopadhyay
Associate Professor of
Department of Neonatology
(CHS, MOHFW)
ABVIMS and Dr RML Hospital
New Delhi, India

Vijay Gupta
Head
Department of Neonatology
Little Panda NICU
RJN Apollo Spectra Hospital
Gwalior, Madhya Pradesh, India

YM Mala
Director Professor
Department of Obstetrics and
Gynecology
Maulana Azad Medical College
New Delhi, India

Contributors

Abhishek S Aradhya
Consultant Neonatologist
Ovum Woman and Child Speciality Hospital
Bengaluru, Karnataka, India

Aakash Pandita
Consultant
Department of Neonatology
Sanjay Gandhi Postgraduate Institute of
Medical Sciences
Lucknow, Uttar Pradesh, India

Amanpreet Sethi
Assistant Professor (Neonatology)
Department of Pediatrics
Guru Gobind Singh Medical College
Faridkot, Punjab, India

Anahita Chauhan
Consultant
Department of Obstetrics and Gynecology
Saifee Hospital
Mumbai, Maharashtra, India

Anil Kallesh BR
Consultant Neonatologist
Department of Neonatology
Sarji Hospital
Shivamogga, Karnataka, India

Anish Keepanasseril
Additional Professor
Department of Obstetrics and Gynecology
Jawaharlal Institute of Postgraduate
Medical Education and Research
Puducherry, India

Anish Pillai
Consultant Neonatologist
Department of Neonatology
Surya Hospitals
Mumbai, Maharashtra, India

Anita Nyamagoudar
Consultant Neonatologist
Department of Pediatrics
Shanti Hospital
Bagalkot, Karnataka, India

Anu Sachdeva
Associate Professor
Department of Pediatrics
All India Institute of Medical Sciences
New Delhi, India

Anup Thakur
Consultant Neonatologist
Department of Neonatology
Sir Ganga Ram Hospital
New Delhi, India

Aparna Chandrasekaran
Clinical Director (Neonatology) and
Senior Consultant
Krishna Institute of Medical Sciences
(KIMS) Cuddles Mother and
Child Centre
Hyderabad, Telangana, India

Aparna Kulkarni
Senior Consultant
Department of Fetal Medicine
Deenanath Mangeshkar Hospital
Pune, Maharashtra, India

Archana Bilagi
Consultant
Department of Neonatology
St Philomena Hospital
Bengaluru, Karnataka, India

Arjit Mohapatra
Senior Consultant
Department of Pediatrics and Neonatology
Jagannath Hospital
Bhubaneswar, Odisha, India

Ashish Jain
Associate Professor
Department of Neonatology
Maulana Azad Medical College and
Associated Lok Nayak Hospital
New Delhi, India

Ashok Kumar
Professor and Head
Department of Obstetrics and
Gynecology
Atal Bihari Vajpayee Institute of Medical
Sciences and Dr RML Hospital
New Delhi, India

Ashwini RC
Associate Professor
Division of Neonatology
Department of Pediatrics
JJM Medical College and Research Centre
Davangere, Karnataka, India

Avantika Gupta
Associate Professor
Department of Obstetrics and Gynecology
All India Institute of Medical Sciences
Nagpur, Maharashtra, India

Ballambattu Vishnu Bhat
Director (Medical Research)
Aarupadai Veedu Medical College
and Hospital
Vinayaka Mission's Research
Foundation—DU
Puducherry, India

Bhagya Lakshmi
Head
Department of Obstetrics and Gynecology
Mother and Child Unit
Yashoda Multi-specialty Hospital
Hyderabad, Telangana, India

Brajagopal Ray
Associate Professor
Department of Pediatrics and
Neonatology
Vivekananda Institute of Medical Sciences
University of Health Sciences
Kolkata, West Bengal, India

Chanchal Kumar
Consultant Neonatologist
Ankura Hospital for Women and Children
Hyderabad, Telangana, India

Chanchal Singh
Lead Consultant
Department of Fetal Medicine
Madhukar Rainbow Children's Hospital
New Delhi, India

Charu Sharma
Associate Professor
Department of Obstetrics and
Gynecology
All India Institute of Medical Sciences
Jodhpur, Rajasthan, India

Chitra Andrew
Professor
Department of Obstetrics and Gynecology
Sri Ramachandra Institute of Higher
Education and Research Fetal Medicine
Chennai, Tamil Nadu, India

Contributors

Darshan Hosapatna Basavarajappa
Assistant Professor
Department of Obstetrics and Gynecology
Rajarajeshwari Medical College and Hospital
Bengaluru, Karnataka, India

Deepak Chawla
Professor
Department of Neonatology
Government Medical College Hospital
Chandigarh, India

Deepti Gupta
Assistant Professor
Department of Obstetrics and Gynecology
Netaji Subhash Chandra Bose Medical College
Jabalpur, Madhya Pradesh, India
Consultant and Unit Head
Ankur Fertility Clinic and IVF Center
Jabalpur, Madhya Pradesh, India

Deepti Thandaveshwar
Assistant Professor
Department of Pediatrics
JSS Medical College and Hospital
JSS Academy of Higher Education and Research
Mysuru, Karnataka, India

Deviprasadh PM
Resident
Department of Neonatology
Madras Medical College
Chennai, Tamil Nadu, India

Femitha Pournami
Consultant Neonatology
Kerala Institute of Medical Sciences
Thiruvananthapuram, Kerala, India

Girija Wagh
Professor
Department of Obstetrics and Gynecology
Bharati Vidyapeeth University Medical College, Pune, Maharashtra, India
Consultant, Cloudnine Hospitals
Shivajinagar
Apollo Spectra Hospitals
Pune, Maharashtra, India

Gopal Agrawal
Senior Consultant
Department of Pediatrics and Neonatology
Cloudnine Hospital
Gurugram, Haryana, India

Jyothi Unni
Director, Department of Obstetrics and Gynecology, Jehangir Hospital, Pune
Maharashtra, India

K Sankaranarayanan
Senior Consultant Neonatologist
Institute of Reproductive Medicine
Madras Medical Mission
Chennai, Tamil Nadu, India

Kalyan Chakravarthy Balla
Lead Consultant and Neonatologist
Department of Neonatology
Rainbow Children's Hospital
Hyderabad, Telangana, India

Kausik Mandal
Additional Professor
Department of Medical Genetics
Sanjay Gandhi Postgraduate Institute of Medical Sciences
Lucknow, Uttar Pradesh, India

KB Suma
Professor and Head
Department of Obstetrics and Gynecology
JSS Medical College and Hospital
JSS Academy of Higher Education and Research
Mysuru, Karnataka, India

Kirti M Hurakadli
Associate Professor
Department of Obstetrics and Gynecology
SN Medical College
Bagalkot, Karnataka, India

Kumar Ankur
Senior Consultant and Incharge
Department of Neonatology
BLK Max Super Speciality Hospital
New Delhi, India

Lakshmi Shanmugasundaram
Senior Consultant
Institute of Reproductive Medicine and Women's Health
Madras Medical Mission
Chennai, Tamil Nadu, India

Laxman Basani
Chief Neonatologist
Department of Neonatology
Ankura Hospital for Women and Children
Hyderabad, Telangana, India

Madhavi Bahulikar
Consultant
Department of Obstetrics and Gynecology
Deenanath Mangeshkar Hospital
Pune, Maharashtra, India

Madhushree Vijayakumar
Consultant
Department of Obstetrics and Gynecology
Motherhood Hospital
Bengaluru, Karnataka, India

Manikumar S
Neonatologist
Chengalpattu Government Medical College
Chennai, Tamil Nadu, India

Manisha Kumar
Director Professor
Incharge Fetal Medicine Subspeciality
Department of Obstetrics and Gynecology
Lady Hardinge Medical College
New Delhi, India

Manju Gupta
Senior Consultant
Department of Obstetrics and Gynecology
Motherhood Hospital
Noida, Uttar Pradesh, India

Mayur A Thosar
Consultant
Department of Obstetrics and Gynecology
Deenanath Mangeshkar Hospital and Research Center
Pune, Maharashtra, India

Mohini Sinha
Assistant Professor
Department of Obstetrics and Gynecology
Kalinga Institute of Medical Sciences
Bhubaneswar, Odisha, India

Monica Gupta
Assistant Professor
Department of Obstetrics and Gynecology
All India Institute of Medical Sciences
New Delhi, India

Nandita Dimri
Chairperson and Consultant
Fetal Medicine
Department of Fetal Medicine
Sir Ganga Ram Hospital
New Delhi, India

Naveen P Gupta
Senior Consultant
Department of Neonatology
Madhukar Rainbow Children's Hospital
New Delhi, India

Neeraj Gupta
Additional Professor
Department of Neonatology
All India Institute of Medical Sciences
Jodhpur, Rajasthan, India

Neerja Gupta
Associate Professor
Division of Genetics
Department of Pediatrics
All India Institute of Medical Sciences
New Delhi, India

Niharika Allu
Consultant
Department of Obstetrics and Gynecology
Rainbow Children's Hospital and Birthright
Visakhapatnam, Andhra Pradesh, India

Nandkishor Kabra
Consultant Neonatologist and Director of NICU
Surya Hospitals
Mumbai, Maharashtra, India

Parul Chopra Buttan
Senior Consultant
Department of Obstetrics and Gynecology
Cloudnine Hospitals
Gurugram, Haryana, India

Pradip Goswami
Founder Director
Department of Fetal and Maternal Medicine
Fetomat Foundation
Kolkata, West Bengal, India

Prakash V
Assistant Professor
Department of Neonatology
Institute of Obstetrics and Gynecology and Government Hospital for Women and Children
Madras Medical College
Chennai, Tamil Nadu, India

Prasanna Latha
Associate Professor
Department of Obstetrics
Kamineni Academy of Medical Sciences and Research Centre
Hyderabad, Telangana, India

Prathik BH
Associate Professor
Department of Neonatology
Indira Gandhi Institute of Child Health
Bengaluru, Karnataka, India

Pratima Anand
Neonatologist
Department of Pediatrics
Vardhman Mahavir Medical College and Safdarjung Hospital
New Delhi, India

Pravin Singarayar
Consultant
Department of Obstetrics and Gynecology, Tribal Health Initiative
Dharmapuri, Tamil Nadu, India

Princee Sahdev
Consultant
Department of Obstetrics and Gynecology
Sigma Hospital
Jalandhar, Punjab, India

Priyadarshini V
Fetal Medicine Specialist
Department of Obstetrics and Gynecology, Rainbow Children's Hospital and Birthright and Cloudnine Hospitals
Bengaluru, Karnataka, India

Priyanka Karnani
DNB Final Year Resident
Department of Neonatology
Sir Ganga Ram Hospital
New Delhi, India

Pruthvi Raj V
Medical Officer
Department of Obstetrics and Gynecology
Airforce Hospital
Kanpur, Uttar Pradesh, India

Pujitha Devi Suraneni
Senior Consultant
Department of Obstetrics and Gynecology
Krishna Institute of Medical Sciences (KIMS) Cuddles Mother and Child Centre
Hyderabad, Telangana, India

Raja Ashok Koganti
Consultant Neonatologist
Anu My Baby Hospital
Vijayawada, Andhra Pradesh, India

Rajendra Prasad Anne
Assistant Professor
Department of Pediatrics
All India Institute of Medical Sciences
Bibinagar, Telangana, India

Ramani Ranjan
Senior Consultant and HOD
Neonatology and Pediatrics
Apollo Cradle and Children's Hospital
Greater Noida, Uttar Pradesh, India

Ranjan Kumar Pejaver
Neonatologist
People Tree Hospitals, Meenakshi Hospital Bengaluru, Karnataka, India
President
National Neonatology Forum (NNF) of India (2021)
Former Chairperson
Neonatology Chapter of IAP, India

Rema S Nagpal
Associate Professor (Pediatrics)
Department of Pediatrics
BJ Government Medical College and Sassoon General Hospital
Pune, Maharashtra, India

Renu Thosar
Consultant
Department of Obstetrics and Gynecology
Deenanath Mangeshkar Hospital and Research Center
Pune, Maharashtra, India

Rhishikesh Thakre
Director and Chief Neonatologist
Neo Clinic and Hospital
Aurangabad, Maharashtra, India

Ritu Sethi
Consultant
Department of Obstetrics and Gynecology
Cloudnine Hospital
Gurugram, Haryana, India

Rohit Sasidharan
Senior Resident
Department of Neonatology
All India Institute of Medical Sciences
Jodhpur, Rajasthan, India

Ruchi Nimish Nanavati
Professor and Head
Department of Neonatology
Seth GS Medical College and KEM Hospital
Mumbai, Maharashtra, India

Contributors

S Suresh
Director
Mediscan Systems
Honorary Secretary
VHS Hospital
Chennai, Tamil Nadu, India

S Thanigainathan
Assistant Professor
Department of Neonatology
All India Institute of Medical Sciences
Jodhpur, Rajasthan, India

Sakshi Yadav
Fellow in Advanced Ultrasonography
in Obstetrics and Gynecology
Department of Fetal Medicine
MEDISCAN
Chennai, Tamil Nadu, India

Sandeep Kadam
Neonatologist
KEM Hospital
Pune, Maharashtra, India

Sangeeta Gupta
Director Professor
Department of Obstetrics and Gynecology
Maulana Azad Medical College
New Delhi, India

Sanjay Gupte
Director
Gupte Hospital and Center for
Research in Reproduction
Pune, Maharashtra, India

Sanjay Wazir
Director
Department of Pediatrics and
Neonatology
Cloudnine Hospital
Gurugram, Haryana, India

Santosh Kumar Panda
Associate Professor
Department of Pediatrics
Kalinga Institute of Medical Sciences
Bhubaneswar, Odisha, India

Saubhagya Kumar Jena
Professor and Head
Department of Obstetrics and Gynecology
All India Institute of Medical Sciences
Bhubaneswar, Odisha, India

Saudamini Nesargi
Associate Professor
Department of Neonatology
St John's Medical College Hospital
Bengaluru, Karnataka, India

Savita N Kamble
Associate Professor
Department of Obstetrics and Gynecology
BJ Government Medical College and
Sassoon General Hospital
Pune, Maharashtra, India

Seema Grover Bhatti
Professor and Head
Department of Obstetrics and Gynecology
Guru Gobind Singh Medical College
Faridkot, Punjab, India

Seema Thakur
Senior Consultant
Genetic and Fetal Diagnosis
BLK Max Super Speciality Hospital
New Delhi, India

Shikha Rani
Associate Professor
Department of Obstetrics
and Gynecology
Dr BR Ambedkar Institute of Medical
Sciences, Mohali, Punjab, India

Shilpa Kalane
Consultant Neonatologist
Department of Neonatology
Deenanath Mangeshkar Hospital and
Research Center
Pune, Maharashtra, India

Sindhu Sivanandan
Assistant Professor
Department of Neonatology
Jawaharlal Institute of Postgraduate
Medical Education and Research
Puducherry, India

Somalika Pal
Assistant Professor
Department of Neonatology
Lady Hardinge Medical College
New Delhi, India

Srishti Goel
Assistant Professor
Department of Neonatology
Lady Hardinge Medical College
New Delhi, India

Sudarshan Suresh
Consultant Fetal Medicine
Mediscan System
Chennai, Tamil Nadu, India

Sumitra Bachani
Associate Professor and Senior Specialist
Department of Pediatrics
Vardhman Mahavir Medical College
and Safdarjung Hospital
New Delhi, India

Tanushree Sahoo
Assistant Professor
Department of Neonatology
All India Institute of Medical Sciences
Bhubaneswar, Odisha, India

Tapas Som
Associate Professor
Department of Neonatology
All India Institute of Medical Sciences
Bhubaneswar, Odisha, India

Thenmozhi G
Professor
Department of Obstetrics
and Gynecology
Chengalpattu Government Medical College
Chennai, Tamil Nadu, India

Tushar B Parikh
Consultant Neonatologist
Department of Neonatology
KEM Hospital and Motherhood Hospitals
Pune, Maharashtra, India

Umamaheswari Balakrishnan
Professor
Department of Neonatology
Sri Ramachandra Institute of Higher
Education and Research
Fetal Medicine
Chennai, Tamil Nadu, India

Umesh Vaidya
Chief Neonatologist
Department of Neonatology
KEM Hospital and Cloudnine Hospital
Pune, Maharashtra, India

V Shanthakumari
President
Federation of Obstetrics and
Gynaecological Societies of India
(FOGSI), India

Vandana Bansal
Director and Head
Department of Fetal Medicine
Surya Hospital, Mumbai
Associate Professor
Wadia Maternity Hospital
Mumbai, Maharashtra, India

Vandana Hegde
Clinical Director
Department of Obstetrics and Gynecology
Hegde Hospital
Hyderabad, Telangana, India

Venkat Reddy Kallem
Consultant Neonatologist
Department of Neonatology
Paramitha Children's Hospital
Hyderabad, Telangana, India

Vikram Khanna
Associate Professor
Department of Pediatric Surgery
Lady Hardinge Medical College
New Delhi, India

Viraraghavan Vadakkencherry Ramaswamy
Consultant Neonatologist
Department of Neonatology
Ankura Hospital for Women and Children
Hyderabad, Telangana, India

Vishal Vishnu Tewari
Professor
Department of Pediatrics
Command Hospital (SC)
and Armed Forces Medical College
Pune, Maharashtra, India

Yavana Suriya Venkatesh
Assistant Professor
Department of Obstetrics
and Gynecology
Jawaharlal Institute of Postgraduate
Medical Education and Research
Puducherry, India

Foreword

डॉ. विनोद कुमार पॉल
सदस्य
Dr. Vinod K. Paul
MEMBER

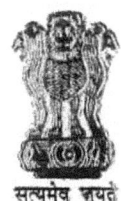

भारत सरकार
नीति आयोग, संसद मार्ग
नई दिल्ली–110 001
Government of India
NATIONAL INSTITUTION FOR TRANSFORMING INDIA
NITI Aayog, Parliament Street
New Delhi-110 001
Tele. : 23096809, 23096820, Fax : 23096810
E-mail : vinodk.paul@gov.in

Perinatal period forms a very critical phase of transition of the fetus to the newborn. It also provides an important window of opportunity for interventions to ensure favorable outcomes of pregnancy, both for the mother and the newborn. This assumes importance for India as it embarks on the journey to achieve single digit neonatal mortality and the goals as enshrined within the SDG framework.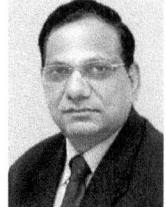

Leveraging this critical perinatal period calls for a coordinated team effort between obstetricians, pediatricians/neonatologists and nurses/midwives for delivery of time-bound actions. More importantly, to assure quality and underline the role of all team members, there is an urgent need for a standard protocol approach which is evidenced based, which is presently a felt gap.

I am happy to note that the National Neonatology Forum (NNF) of India has risen to the occasion by publishing the book, *Clinical Protocols in Perinatology*. The book with 51 chapters covers almost all-important aspects of perinatology highlighting practical aspects with lucid flowcharts. Besides, each chapter has been authored by a team of neonatologists/pediatricians and obstetricians, providing all-round perspectives of clinical management.

I congratulate the editors, authors and the NNF for bringing out this important book, which I am sure in the coming years will stand-out to guide all stakeholders involved in improving newborn health.

Vinod Paul
Honorable Member of the Niti Ayog
Government of India

President's Message

Dear Colleagues,

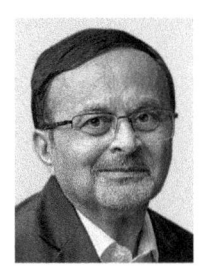

I am extremely happy that the much-awaited book, *NNF Clinical Protocols in Perinatology* is published. This is a unique book. This is a combined effort of leading obstetricians and pediatricians/neonatologists of our country. Each chapter written involves both these professionals. Thanks to all the contributors. I must commend the efforts of the Editors-in-Chief, Dr Ballambattu Vishnu Bhat and Dr Ashish Jain, Section Editors and production team of M/s Jaypee Brothers Medical Publishers (P) Ltd, New Delhi, India.

The book is a testimony to the perinatal approach which should be followed to achieve better outcome of the mother and baby dyad. Newborn is a continuum of fetus. It is very logical that both main specialties of care should be involved right in the beginning and the transfer of care should be smooth. If we have to achieve the India Newborn Action Plan (INAP) goals of single digit neonatal mortality and stillbirths, collaboration between the various specialties (mainly obstetricians and pediatricians) should start in the early antenatal period and in some cases even before conception. Perinatal meetings should be inbuilt into the clinic academic activities of health care. Eventually, every district should have a perinatal center having all the facilities to monitor, investigate and manage the high-risk pregnancies, under one roof.

National Neonatology Forum (NNF) has taken the lead in bringing out this book with more than 100 contributors and 51 chapters. I hope that this book will be a template for designing and implementing perinatal care. Kindly provide your feedback as to enable the process of improvement in the following editions.

With warm regards

Ranjan Kumar Pejaver
FRCP FRCPCH (UK) FIAP FNNF
Neonatologist
People Tree Hospitals, Meenakshi Hospital
Bengaluru, Karnataka, India
President
National Neonatology Forum (NNF) of India (2021)
Former Chairperson
Neonatology Chapter of IAP, India
Executive Editor

Message from the FOGSI President

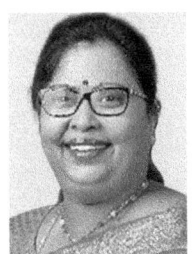

Dear Colleagues,

I am happy to write this message for the book, *Clinical Protocols in Perinatology*, a publication of the National Neonatology Forum (NNF) of India. Perinatal approach is the appropriate way forward, if we have to achieve our goals of mother and child health targets. Mother and baby are a dyad and inseparable. This has to be remembered while providing health care to our mothers and then to our babies. Good and timely antenatal care is the foundation of good outcome of the mother and baby dyad. Cost-effective interventions such as appropriate and adequate nutrition to the pregnant women, safe delivery in an institution with trained personnel supervising the care of the mother and baby is very essential. Delivering the baby on to mother's abdomen, zero separation, Kangaroo mother care and breastfeeding are cornerstones of perinatal care.

It is the responsibility of both the Obstetric and Pediatric teams to liaise right from the antenatal period and at times even before conception. I am happy that Federation of Obstetric and Gynaecological Societies of India (FOGSI) has involved itself intensively in the *Laqshya program* of the Government of India and practices perinatal medicine by including input from the neonatologists too. Recently, the First Perinatal Conference (PERICON) was held with both FOGSI and NNF collaborating with each other. It is proposed to hold these conferences on an annual basis.

NNF Clinical Protocols in Perinatology covers all the important issue of the joint perinatal care. It will go a long way in providing the standards of care and protocols in the practice of perinatology. The contents are nicely planned well written by equal contributions from obstetricians and neonatologists. I am sure that it will prove to be very useful to all those who are involved in managing the mother and baby dyad.

V Shanthakumari
President
Federation of Obstetrics and Gynaecological
Societies of India (FOGSI)
Executive Editor

Preface

"The way I see it, if you want the rainbow, you got to put up with the rain"
— **Dolly Parton**

Knowledge in any medical specialty is expanding rapidly and perinatology is no exception to this phenomenon. Perinatology is unique in itself as it shares commitment and interest from both the obstetricians and neonatologists equally. Perinatology involves the science and discourse of understanding the maternal and fetal dynamics and inter-relation extending from the time the fetus enters the period of viability to end of early neonatal period.

Undoubtedly, this is a crucial period since it covers issues related to fetus and newborn either directly or indirectly influenced by maternal condition. As Albert Einstein put it, "Life is like riding a bicycle and you should keep moving to keep your balance". The practicing primatologists should keep themselves updated with new knowledge and skill in order to give the best of care to the dyad. In this context, it is pertinent to revisit the words, "If one waits for the whole life time for the storm, he will never enjoy sunshine" said by Morris West. Keeping this in mind, and perceiving the long-felt need for the neonatologists and obstetricians to come together seamlessly to put forth best of their experiences for the best of the outcome, the National Neonatology Forum (NNF) of India under the leadership of Ranjan Kumar Pejaver took the initiative to bring out a book on *Clinical Protocols in Perinatology*.

The editorial team thoughtfully after diverse inputs, identified fifty-one common and important topics within the vast field of perinatology and categorized them in seven sections. This was a sincere and unique collaborative effort of the sections editors who were a team of experienced Obstetricians and Neonatologists for each section. Hence, every chapter addresses the perspective of both the Neonatologist and the Obstetricians with special care to provide available information in a comprehensive way. The unique task was possible with the contribution of section editors, viz; Dr Anish Keepanasseril, Dr Archana Bilagi, Dr Arjit Mohapatra, Dr Jyothi Unni, Dr Madhushree Vijayakumar, Dr Princee Sahdev, Dr Sangeeta Gupta, Dr Shilpa Kalane, and Dr Sindhu Sivanandan, who need special mention. We are thankful to the authors of the topics covered under the sections who could draft the contents within a short period. We extend special thanks to Dr Sindhu S for synthesizing such beautiful infographics and pictures, without which this book would have not come up in this picture. We hope that the contents will give the readers the much-required information in a nutshell. As said by Thomas A Edison, "many of life's failures are among people who did not realize how close they were to success when they gave up". If the required knowledge is readily available, it will make clinician's task simpler.

All the topics included are felt needs and faced in day-to-day life. The chapters are written in a lucid and user-friendly way. Each chapter starts with *introduction* and *objectives* and ends with *chapter at a glance* and *key points*. All topics are written by obstetricians and neonatologists to give holistic picture of the available knowledge. Important references are listed at the end for those who want to have more information on the topic. We have also included tables, figures, boxes and flowcharts in order to make the reading easy. We sincerely hope that the contents of this book will help postgraduates, practicing obstetricians, pediatricians and neonatologists.

We also thank National Neonatology Forum of India for giving us this opportunity. We are thankful to M/s Jaypee Brothers Medical Publishers (P) Ltd, New Delhi, India for undertaking the task of bringing out this book within a short period of time. We especially thank Dr Rajul Jain (Development Editor) of M/s Jaypee Brothers Medical Publishers (P) Ltd, New Delhi, India for all the support and help in maintaining all of us active throughout this task.

We end with the advice of spiritual leader Dalai Lama, "The purpose of one's life is to be happy". Let this book help in providing happiness to the parents and future children through you all.

Ashish Jain
Ballambattu Vishnu Bhat

Contents

SECTION 1: Fetal Well-being

Section Editors: *Shilpa Kalane, Jyothi Unni*

1. Prenatal Screening Tests 3
   Sanjay Gupte, Madhavi Bahulikar
2. Assesment of Fetal Well-being 10
   Deepti Gupta, Aparna Kulkarni, Umesh Vaidya
3. Intrapartum Fetal Monitoring 16
   Vishal Vishnu Tewari, Renu Thosar
4. Fetal Therapy 24
   Sudarshan Suresh, S Suresh

SECTION 2: Fetal Disorders

Section Editors: *Ashish Jain, Sangeeta Gupta*

5. A General Approach to Antenatally Detected Birth Defects 35
   Neerja Gupta, Sakshi Yadav
6. Central Nervous System Malformations 40
   Aakash Pandita, Kausik Mandal
7. Fetal Thoracic Malformations 47
   Anup Thakur, Nandita Dimri
8. Fetal Cardiovascular Malformations 54
   Anup Thakur, Priyanka Karnani
9. Genitourinary System Malformation 62
   Kumar Ankur, Seema Thakur
10. Musculoskeletal Malformations 69
    Somalika Pal, Manisha Kumar
11. Gastrointestinal Malformations 78
    Naveen P Gupta, Chanchal Singh
12. Fetal Growth Restriction 86
    Pratima Anand, Sumitra Bachani
13. Hydrops Fetalis 95
    Raja Ashok Koganti, Anu Sachdeva
14. Antenatal Counseling for Fetomaternal Conditions 103
    Umamaheswari Balakrishnan, Chitra Andrew

SECTION 3: Maternal Medical Illness and Fetal Effects

Section Editors: *Arjit Mohapatra, Princee Sahdev*

15. Maternal Endocrine Disorders and Fetal Effects 119
    K Sankaranarayanan, Lakshmi Shanmugasundaram
16. Anemia in Pregnancy 127
    Rhishikesh Thakre

17. **Thrombocytopenia in Pregnancy** 133
    Rhishikesh Thakre, Arjit Mohapatra

18. **Autoimmune Disorders in Pregnancy** 137
    Laxman Basani, Prasanna Latha

19. **Teratogenic Exposure** 147
    Brajagopal Ray, Pradip Goswami

20. **Maternal Medications and Substance Abuse** 153
    Sanjay Wazir, Parul Chopra Buttan

21. **Maternal Systemic Medical Illness and Fetal Effect** 156
    Santosh Kumar Panda, Mohini Sinha

SECTION 4: Obstetric Conditions and Fetal/Neonatal Effects

Section Editors: *Archana Bilagi, Madhushree Vijayakumar*

22. **Preterm Labor and Preterm Prelabor Rupture of Membranes** 163
    Anita Nyamagoudar, Kirti M Hurakadli

23. **Antenatal Steroids** 170
    Viraraghavan Vadakkencherry Ramaswamy, Vandana Hegde, Venkat Reddy Kallem

24. **Prenatal Neuroprotective Strategies** 177
    Rema S Nagpal, Savita N Kamble

25. **Antepartum Hemorrhage** 183
    Ashwini RC, Darshan Hosapatna Basavarajappa

26. **Gestosis in Pregnancy** 187
    Pravin Singarayar, Saudamini Nesargi

27. **Oligohydramnios and Polyhydramnios** 198
    Prathik BH, Ashok Kumar

28. **Multiple Pregnancy** 204
    Anil Kallesh BR, Pruthvi Raj V

29. **Bad Obstetric History** 211
    Kalyan Chakravarthy Balla, Bhagya Lakshmi

30. **Chorioamnionitis** 218
    Deepti Thandaveshwar, KB Suma

SECTION 5: Congenital Infections

Section Editors: *Shilpa Kalane, Ashish Jain*

31. **Approach to a Neonate with Suspected Congenital Infection** 227
    Shilpa Kalane, Ashish Jain

32. **Toxoplasmosis—Perinatal Perspective** 233
    Ruchi Nimish Nanavati, Anahita Chauhan

33. **Rubella—Perinatal Perspective** 239
    Girija Wagh, Sandeep Kadam

34. **Cytomegalovirus—Perinatal Perspective** 244
    Mayur A Thosar, Tushar B Parikh

35. **Herpes Simplex Virus—Perinatal Perspective** 251
    Vandana Bansal, Anish Pillai, Nandkishor Kabra

36. **Syphilis—Perinatal Perspective** 256
    Gopal Agrawal, Ritu Sethi

37. Other Viral Infections such as Zika Virus, Dengue Virus, Chikungunya Virus, Varicella Virus, H1N1 Influenza Virus.. 261
   Amanpreet Sethi, Seema Grover Bhatti
38. Tuberculosis—Perinatal Perspective 271
   Rohit Sasidharan, Neeraj Gupta
39. HIV—Perinatal Perspective... 279
   Prakash V, Deviprasadh PM
40. Viral Hepatitis—Perinatal Perspective 284
   Ramani Ranjan, Manju Gupta
41. SARS-CoV-2 Infection—Perinatal Perspective 289
   Shikha Rani, Deepak Chawla

SECTION 6: Delivery Room Management

Section Editors: *Sindhu Sivanandan, Anish Keepanasseril*

42. Neonatal Resuscitation 299
   Aparna Chandrasekaran, Pujitha Devi Suraneni
43. Umbilical Cord Management.. 309
   Sindhu Sivanandan, Yavana Suriya Venkatesh
44. Perinatal Asphyxia... 314
   Rajendra Prasad Anne, Avantika Gupta
45. Care at Birth 323
   Manikumar S, Thenmozhi G
46. Postnatal Care and Discharge Planning.. 331
   Tanushree Sahoo, Abhishek S Aradhya, Monica Gupta
47. Surgical Conditions Presenting at Birth 337
   Srishti Goel, Vikram Khanna
48. Birth Trauma.. 348
   Chanchal Kumar, S Thanigainathan, Charu Sharma
49. Ethical and Medicolegal Issues in the Perinatal Period 355
   Niharika Allu, Femitha Pournami

SECTION 7: Miscellaneous

Section Editors: *Arjit Mohapatra, Sindhu Sivanandan, Anish Keepanasseril*

50. Stillbirth 365
   Priyadarshini V, Anish Keepanasseril
51. Placental Examination 372
   Saubhagya Kumar Jena, Tapas Som

Index 379

SECTION 1

Fetal Well-being

Shilpa Kalane, Jyothi Unni

- **Prenatal Screening Tests**
  Sanjay Gupte, Madhavi Bahulikar
- **Assessment of Fetal Well-being**
  Deepti Gupta, Aparna Kulkarni, Umesh Vaidya
- **Intrapartum Fetal Monitoring**
  Vishal Vishnu Tewari, Renu Thosar
- **Fetal Therapy**
  Sudarshan Suresh, S Suresh

CHAPTER 1

Prenatal Screening Tests

Sanjay Gupte, Madhavi Bahulikar

INTRODUCTION

Prenatal screening tests are done as a part of universal screening in all pregnant women to detect abnormalities in the fetus as well as comorbidities in the mother which may adversely affect the fetus. Various combinations of tests may be conducted as per local practices, availability of tests, and cost constraints.

Below is a short discussion covering screening for aneuploidies, beta thalassemia, preeclampsia (PE), and gestational diabetes mellitus (GDM).

OBJECTIVES

- To appreciate the need for screening for aneuploidies
- To outline the criteria for providing genetic counseling
- To gain a basic understanding of beta thalassemia, PE, and GDM screening

SCREENING FOR ANEUPLOIDIES

Aneuploidy screening may be divided into first- and second-trimester screening tests which are done as a combination of tests to give the best possible sensitivity. It must be remembered that adequate counseling is required for both pre- and post-testing since a positive screening test entails further invasive diagnostic testing.

First-trimester Screening

This is usually done by the combination of maternal age, fetal nuchal translucency (NT), serum free beta-human chorionic gonadotropin (beta-hCG), and pregnancy-associated plasma protein A (PAPP-A).

- *Maternal age*:
  - The risk of trisomy increases with advanced maternal age.
  - At age 35 years, risk of trisomy-21 is 1 in 250 as compared to age 21 when the risk is 1 in 1,000.
- *NT*:
  - NT is the measurement of the sonographic appearance of a collection of fluid behind the fetal neck in the first trimester of pregnancy. The optimal gestational age for measurement of NT is 11 + 0 to 13 + 6 weeks **(Fig. 1)**. The measurement is taken between crown–rump length (CRL) of 45 and 84 mm.
  - Raised NT is seen in chromosomal abnormalities and also in congenital heart defects. NT may also be increased with structural abnormalities such as exomphalos, diaphragmatic hernia, and fetal infections.
- Serum biochemistry
  - *Beta-hCG and PAPP-A* **(Table 1)**
- *Ultrasound markers*
  - *Nasal bone*:
    - ♦ Absent nasal bone

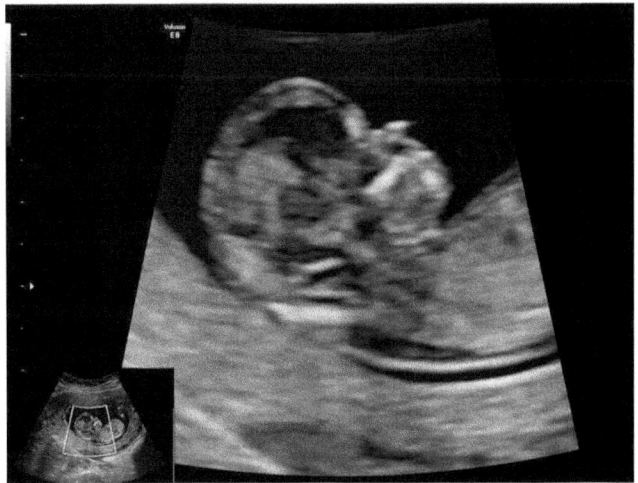

Fig. 1: Measurement of nuchal translucency.

TABLE 1: Beta-hCG and PAPP-A.

	Beta-hCG MoM	PAPP-A MoM
Normal karyotype	1.0	1.0
Trisomy 21	2.0	0.5
Trisomy 18	0.2	0.2
Trisomy 13	0.5	0.3

(beta-hCG: beta-human chorionic gonadotropin; MoM: multiples of the median; PAPP-A: pregnancy-associated plasma protein A)

At 11–13 weeks, the nasal bone is considered to be absent in **(Fig. 2)**:
- Euploid fetuses: 1–3%
- Fetuses with trisomy-21: 60%
- Fetuses with trisomy-18: 50%
- Fetuses with trisomy-13: 40%

- *Ductus venosus flow*:
  - *The ductus venosus* is a short vessel connecting the umbilical vein to the inferior vena cava. It plays an important role in shunting oxygenated blood to the fetal brain.
  - *Blood flow in the ductus* has a characteristic waveform with **(Figs. 3A and B)**:
    - High velocity during ventricular systole (S-wave) and diastole (D-wave)
    - Forward flow during atrial contraction (A-wave)
    - *Reversed A-wave is associated* with an increased risk for:
      - Chromosomal abnormalities
      - Cardiac defects
      - Fetal death

- *If the ductus venosus A-wave is reversed*, it is important that detailed ultrasound examination is carried out to exclude or diagnose major cardiac defects.
- *The risk of miscarriage or fetal death* is high if ductus venosus shows A-wave reversal. Hence, in such cases, frequent monitoring of fetal growth (ultrasound at 20, 28, and 34 weeks) and uterine artery pulsatility index (UAPI) and fetal Doppler is recommended.
  - *Tricuspid flow*:
    - *Tricuspid regurgitation*
    - *At 11–13 weeks*, tricuspid regurgitation is found in about:
      - Euploid fetuses: 1%
      - Fetuses with trisomy-21: 55%
      - Fetuses with trisomy-18: 30%
      - Fetuses with trisomy-13: 30%
  - All women, irrespective of age, who book in the first trimester, should be offered the combined test as screening for Down syndrome. A cutoff of 1 in 250 is considered as screen positive for trisomy-21. Some authors suggest that low risk be taken as <1:1,000, intermediate risk as 1:101 to 1:1,000, and high risk as >1:100. The cutoff for trisomies-18 and -13 is 1:100.
  - Screening in the first trimester gives the couple an opportunity for an early diagnosis in case of a screen positive result.

Second-trimester Screening

Serum Screening

- Screening for aneuploidies in the second trimester should be offered to women who have booked after 13 + 6 weeks.
- The quadruple test can be performed between 15 and 22 weeks but is best performed between 16 and 18 weeks of gestation. It consists of a combination of four

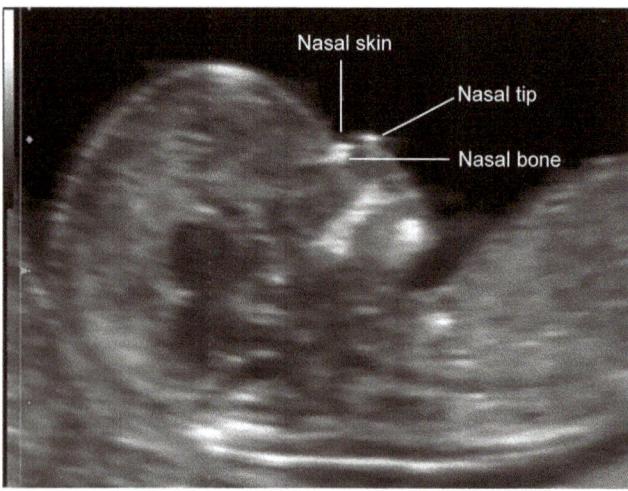

Fig. 2: Nasal bone on ultrasound image.

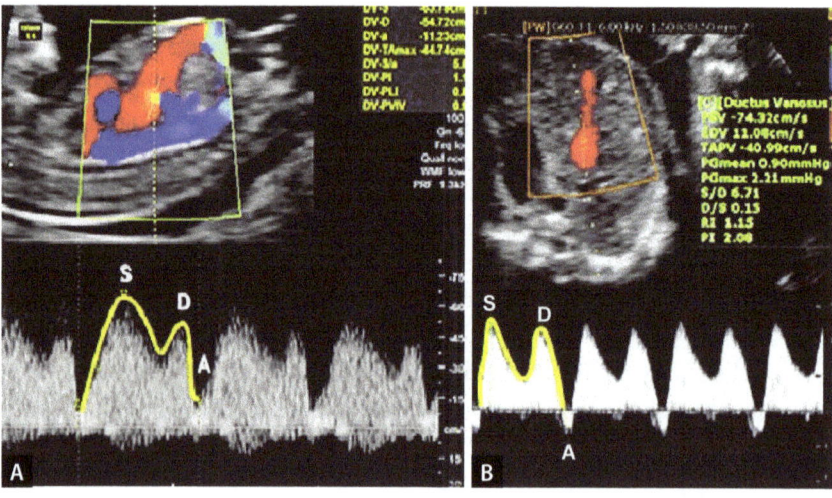

Figs. 3A and B: (A) Normal flow; (B) Reversal of "A" wave (abnormal).

biochemical markers: alpha fetoprotein (AFP), beta-hCG, estriol, and inhibin A. This also screens for neural tube defects.
- The triple test is usually not performed now due to the superior detection rate of the quadruple test.
- The integrated test involves doing the NT scan and PAPP-A in the first trimester. The results are withheld till the second trimester when the quadruple test is performed and a risk is given based on all the tests.
- Sequential screening is a modification of the integrated test, where women who are deemed high risk in the first-trimester screen are offered invasive testing and those who are low risk go on to have the quadruple test and an integrated result is given.

Table 2 compares the efficacy of first- and second-trimester screening tests.

Targeted Anomaly Scan

A comprehensive ultrasound scan or "anomaly scan" is carried out between 18 and 20 weeks to screen for markers suggesting presence of various syndromes as well as a detailed study of each organ system to rule out structural defects.

Markers of chromosomal defects: In the second-trimester scan, each chromosomal defect has its own pattern of detectable abnormalities, such as duodenal atresia and cardiac defects in trisomy -21, Rocker bottom feet in trisomy -18, and holoprosencephaly and microcephaly in trisomy -13.

Major abnormalities: If a major abnormality is detected, even if it appears as an isolated abnormality, it is advisable to recommend fetal karyotyping. If the abnormalities are either lethal or would result in a live birth with severe handicap, counseling should be done informing the parents of the risk of recurrence.

If the abnormality is surgically correctable after birth, such as diaphragmatic hernia, it is important to exclude an underlying aneuploidy. For some conditions, the defect may be associated with trisomy-18 or -13.

Soft markers: Minor fetal abnormalities or soft markers are common. If present as isolated features such as echogenic intracardiac foci or choroid plexus cysts, the parents may be reassured that they do not represent major handicap.

Certain isolated abnormalities are accorded more importance such as nuchal or prenasal edema and hypoplastic nasal bone.

Noninvasive Prenatal Testing (NIPT)

- *Analysis of cell-free fetal DNA (cfDNA) in maternal blood* can be performed after 10 weeks of gestation. It detects about 99% of fetuses with trisomy-21 and 98% of fetuses with trisomy-18 or -13 at a false-positive rate (FPR) of 0.1–0.2%. Therefore, in singleton pregnancies, the performance of screening for these trisomies by cfDNA testing is superior, in terms of both higher detection rate and substantially lower FPR, to that of all other methods combining maternal age, first- or second-trimester ultrasound findings, and first- or second-trimester serum biochemical analysis.

Interpretation of results
- The cfDNA test is a screening rather than a diagnostic test. The results are given in terms of risk, with the majority of companies reporting results for each chromosome as low risk (usually <1 in 10,000) or high risk (>99%).
- *A positive or high-risk cfDNA result should be confirmed by invasive testing.*
- Currently in India, it is being offered in some centers as a primary screening to women over 35 years or to women with an intermediate risk on combined test (**Flowcharts 1 and 2**).

TABLE 2: Detection rates of first- and second-trimester screening tests.			
Screening method	**Gestational age**	**Detection rate (%)**	**False positive rate (%)**
Maternal age		30	5
NT alone	11–13 + 6	77	4.7
Combined test (Maternal age + NT + beta-hCG + PAPP-A)	11–13 + 6	85–90	5
Triple test (AFP + beta-hCG + uE3)	15–22	69	5
Quadruple test (AFP + beta-hCG + E3 + Inhibin A)	15–22	85	5
Integrated test (NT + PAPP-A + Quadruple)	11–13 + 6 and 15–22 weeks	85	1.2

(AFP: alpha fetoprotein; beta-hCG: beta-human chorionic gonadotropin; NT: nuchal translucency; PAPP-A: pregnancy-associated plasma protein A)

Flowchart 1: Routine screening by first-trimester combined test.

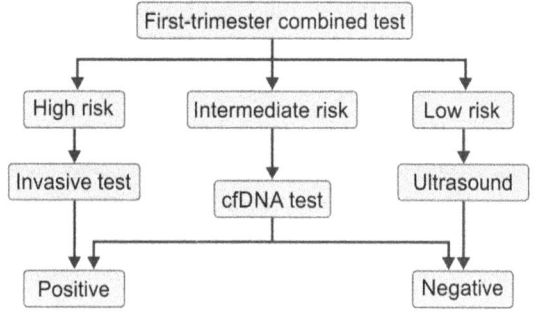

Flowchart 2: Routine screening by cfDNA test.

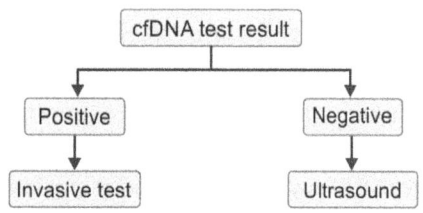

MANAGEMENT OF SCREEN-POSITIVE PREGNANCIES

- Whatever combination of tests is used to screen for aneuploidies, post-test counseling plays an important role. Especially when the test shows a high risk for aneuploidy, the parents need detailed counseling from a fetal medicine expert as well as a geneticist in order to take an informed decision regarding the future course of action.
- If screening tests show a high risk for aneuploidy or ultrasound markers show high possibility of genetic syndromes, the parents should be offered invasive testing for conclusive diagnosis.
- It must be emphasized here that the screening tests are not diagnostic, and hence termination must not be advised solely based on a screen-positive result.
- Further, various ethical and religious considerations play a role in decision regarding continuation versus termination of pregnancy. Adequate facts regarding the condition must be made available to the couple in order to make a decision regarding invasive testing. Some couples may not want to terminate the pregnancy no matter what the test results suggest. In such cases, need for screening tests and invasive testing must be carefully judged.

INVASIVE TESTING

- Couples must be counseled regarding the indication, procedure, and risks of invasive testing. This usually involves either chorion villus sampling or amniocentesis to withdraw a sample of cells which can be further tested by fluorescent in situ hybridization (FISH) or karyotype.
- It is advisable that these tests be carried out by a fetal medicine specialist to reduce risk of complications and ensure best results.

Chorion Villus Sampling

- It is performed between 11 and 14 weeks.
- The procedure may be carried out transabdominally or transvaginally.
- It carries a fetal loss rate of 1–2%.

Amniocentesis

- Amniocentesis is performed after 16 weeks.
- Risk of miscarriage is approximately 1 in 200 to 1 in 300.

Chromosomal Microarray

- One of the newer genetic technologies in the prenatal setting is chromosomal microarray.
- Its advantage is that it can detect submicroscopic abnormalities that are too small to be detected by standard karyotype.
- Chromosomal microarray yields more genetic information because of its higher resolution. As it does not require culturing of the specimen, results are available more quickly than with karyotyping, which requires cultured cells.

PREVENTION OF ECLAMPSIA

Preeclampsia, which affects about 2% of pregnancies, is a major cause of perinatal and maternal morbidity and mortality.

There is an increased risk of perinatal mortality and morbidity in preterm PE and early onset PE (before 26 weeks), rather than term PE.

Screening at 11–13 Weeks

The objective of screening for PE at 11–13 weeks' gestation is to identify the cases that would benefit from prophylactic use of aspirin that reduces the risk of preterm PE by >60%.

Use of aspirin (150 mg/day) from 11 to 14 weeks' gestation until 36 weeks has been associated with a 62% reduction in the incidence of preterm PE and 82% reduction in the incidence of PE at <34 weeks' gestation.

Prediction of Preeclampsia

Maternal Characteristics and History

- *Advancing maternal age:* High BMI
- Afro-Caribbean and South Asian racial origin
- *Maternal medical history*: Chronic hypertension, diabetes mellitus, and systemic lupus erythematosus or antiphospholipid syndrome.
- *In vitro fertilization (IVF) conception*: Family history or personal history of PE (10 times increased risk)

Mean Arterial Pressure

Women with early onset PE have higher mean arterial blood pressure levels at 20 weeks of gestation, compared to normotensive women.

Uterine Artery Pulsatility Index

The UAPI can be measured by either transabdominal or transvaginal sonography.

In normal pregnancies, UAPI is low reflecting low impedance to flow as a consequence of transformation of the spiral arteries from narrow high-resistance vessels to dilated low-resistance channels. In pregnancies with impaired placentation and at high risk of developing preterm PE, the UAPI is high **(Figs. 4 and 5)**.

- *Pregnancy-associated plasma protein-A:* Low PAPP-A levels <0.5 MoMs may be considered as an indicator of development of preeclampsia and fetal growth restriction (FGR) or placental insufficiency.
- *Placental growth factor (PLGF)*: In pregnancies that develop PE, serum PLGF is lower than in normal pregnancies and this decrease is thought to be the consequence of placental hypoxia.
- *Serum-soluble FMS-like tyrosine kinase-1 (sFLT-1)*: In pregnancies with established PE, serum sFLT-1 is high and this increase in level may occur about 5 weeks prior to the development of the disease.
- *Combined screening by maternal factors, mean arterial pressure (MAP), UAPI, and PLGF* predicts about 90% of early PE (<34 weeks), 75% of preterm PE (<37 weeks), and 45% of term PE (≥37 weeks), at a false-positive rate of 10%.

Gestosis Score

Primary clinical assessment for screening and prediction of PE can be objectively performed by "easy-to-use" HDP-Gestosis score.

Process of risk scoring:
- This score involves all the existing and emerging risk factors in the pregnant woman.
- Scores 1, 2, and 3 are allotted to each clinical risk factor as per its severity in the development of PE.
- *Score 1* for age >35 or <19 years, maternal anemia, BMI > 30 kg/m^2, primigravida, short duration of paternity (i.e., cohabitation), woman born small for gestational age, polycystic ovary syndrome (PCOS), interpregnancy interval >10 years, conceived with IVF or intracytoplasmic sperm injection (ICSI), MAP 0.85, chronic vascular diseases including dyslipidemia, and excessive weight gain during pregnancy.
- *Score 2* for maternal hypothyroidism, family history of PE, GDM, BMI > 35 kg/m^2, multiple pregnancy, hypertensive disease during previous pregnancy.
- *Score 3* for pre-GDM, chronic hypertension, mental disorders, inherited/acquired thrombophilia, maternal chronic kidney disease, and autoimmune disease [systemic lupus erythematosus (SLE)/antiphospholipid antibodies (APLA)/rheumatoid arthritis].
- With careful history and assessment of woman, a total score is obtained from time to time.
- When the total score is ≥3, the pregnant woman should be marked as "At risk for preeclampsia".

Indian Scenario

- PLGF and sFLT-1 are not widely available or may not be feasible due to cost constraints.
- UAPI for all at the time of NT scan and MAP measurement at each visit may be the tools easily available for all mothers. Addition of low PAPP-A in estimation of risk may be considered.
- High-risk mothers based on history, UAPI showing diastolic notch, or serum screening showing low PAPP-A can be started on aspirin to reduce the severity of PE and reduce FGR.

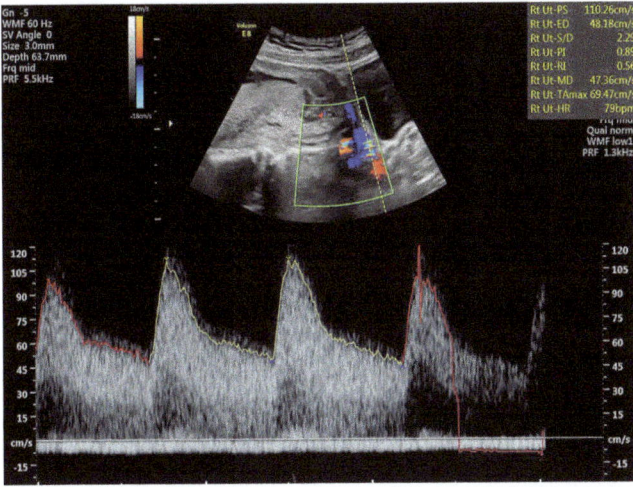

Fig. 4: Normal uterine artery waveform with good end diastolic flow.

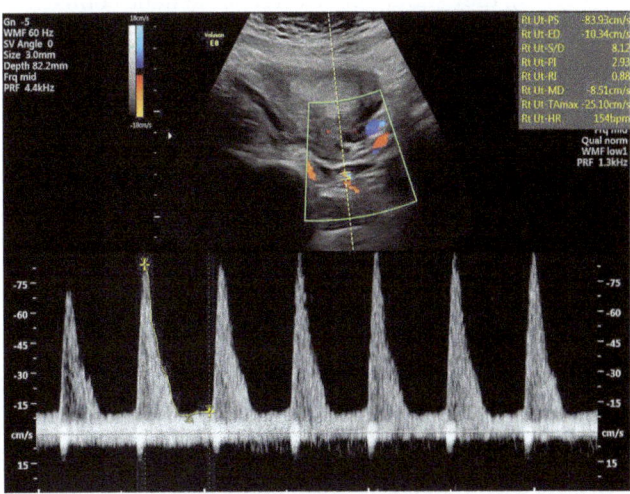

Fig. 5: High-resistance flow in uterine artery.

- In many peripheral areas of India, UAPI and serum screening are not available. In this situation, only MAP and maternal characteristics denoted by Gestosis score are enough to start the patient on low-dose aspirin (75–150 mg).

THALASSEMIA

Prenatal Diagnosis for Thalassemia

- The first step in prevention of a baby affected by thalassemia major is screening of women.
- Often, this is done at first antenatal visit but the best time is premarital or preconceptional.
- The *Nescroft test (or Mentzer's index)* and analysis of red cell indices in hemogram report should give a suspicion of thalassemia minor status.
- Individuals with a mean corpuscular volume (MCV) < 80 fL or mean corpuscular hemoglobin (MCH) < 27 pg can have α- and/or β-thalassemia and/or iron deficiency anemia.
- In general, β thalassemia trait can be reliably diagnosed by hemoglobin electrophoresis or high-performance liquid chromatography (HPLC), with HbA2 and HbF quantification. Patients with β-thalassemia trait have an elevated HbA2, i.e., >3.5%.
- Alternatively, it can be made a routine practice to perform HPLC of all pregnant women in the early first trimester.

Hemoglobin Electrophoresis or HPLC

- *Hemoglobin electrophoresis or HPLC* will allow identification of Hb variants, such as HbS, C, D, and E.
- Testing positive for any of these hemoglobinopathies warrants testing of partner.
- If both partners are found to be carriers of hemoglobin mutations (i.e., any combination of thalassemias and Hb variants), they should be referred for genetic counseling, ideally in the preconception period, or as early as possible in the pregnancy.
- DNA studies must be carried out for the mutation type of both partners. There are 5 common mutations and 12 rare mutations.
- Testing of the fetus can be done by chorionic villus sampling (CVS) or amniocentesis.

Counseling of Couple

If the results of prenatal testing show that the fetus has thalassemia major, the couple should be offered termination. If they choose to continue the pregnancy, they should be referred to a neonatologist and hematologist to be counseled about the expected clinical course.

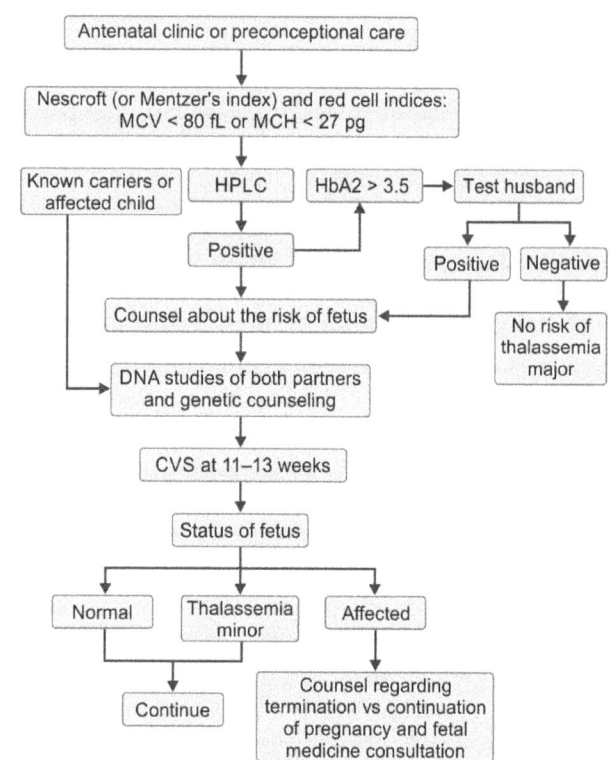

(CVS: chorionic villus sampling; HPLC: high-performance liquid chromatography; MCV: mean corpuscular volume; MCH: mean corpuscular hemoglobin)

GESTATIONAL DIABETES MELLITUS

- Indian population is considered to be ethnically at high risk for development of diabetes. This extends to an increased risk of gestational diabetes and hence requires universal screening for GDM in all mothers. The recommended testing algorithm is shown in **Flowchart 3**.
- The recommended testing in Indian scenario as per diabetes in pregnancy study group of India (DIPSI) guidelines states that fasting blood sugar value is not needed. A single step test after ingestion of 75 g anhydrous glucose in 300 mL water, in a nonfasted state, is followed by blood sugar level 2 hours later and results interpreted as above.

Flowchart 3: Recommended GDM screening algorithm.

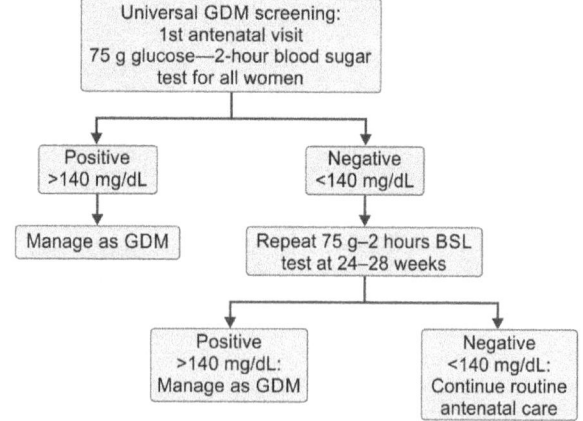

(BSL: blood sugar level; GDM: gestational diabetes mellitus)

CHAPTER AT A GLANCE

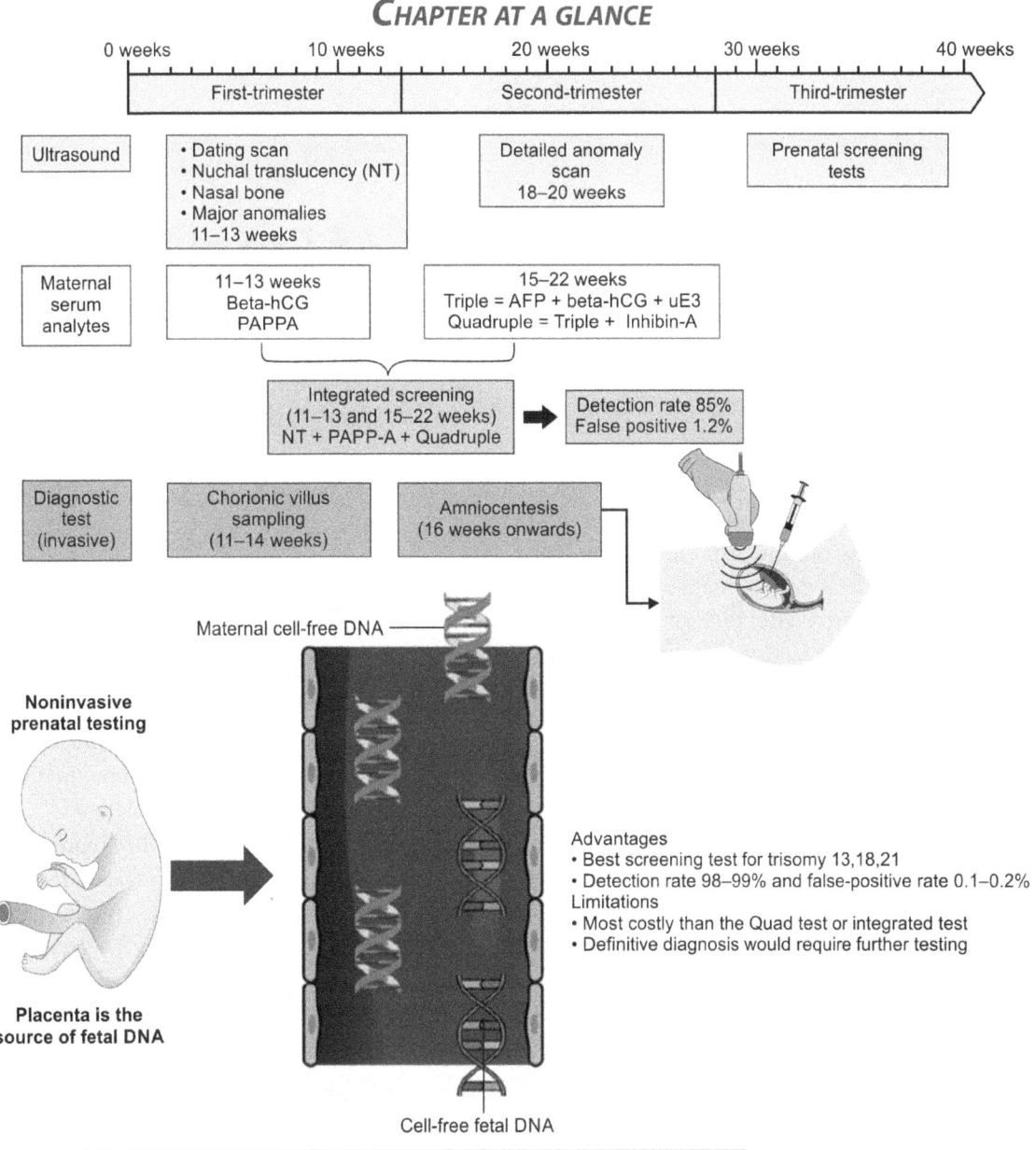

(beta-hCG: beta-human chorionic gonadotropin; PAPP-A: pregnancy-associated plasma protein A)

KEY POINTS

11–13 + 6 weeks:
- First-trimester combined screening (NT scan + beta-hCG + PAPP-A) for aneuploidy screening.
- NIPT if intermediate risk or high risk in combined screen if couple desires.
- Invasive testing if screen positive (CVS or amniocentesis). Options for termination of pregnancy versus continuation to be discussed with couple based on results.
- UAPI, maternal risk assessment, and PAPP-A value for PE screening.
- Aspirin to be started if high risk for PE.

16–20 weeks:
- Quadruple testing (if first-trimester screening has been missed).
- 18–20 weeks' detailed anomaly scan by fetal medicine expert.
- Counseling by fetal medicine specialist and neonatologist in case of major defects detected on sonography.

24–28 weeks: Repeat DIPSI 75 g test for GDM at 24–28 weeks.

SUGGESTED READING

1. Fetal Medicine Foundation. Education resources. [online] Available from https://fetalmedicine.org/.
2. Arias F, Bhide A, Arulkumaran S, Damania K, Daftary SN. Arias' Practical Guide to High Risk Pregnancy and Delivery: A South Asian Perspective. 5th Edition. Elsevier India; 2019.
3. Poon LC, Nicolaides KH. Early prediction of preeclampsia. Obstet Gynecol. Int. 2014;2014:297397.

CHAPTER 2

Assessment of Fetal Well-being

Deepti Gupta, Aparna Kulkarni, Umesh Vaidya

INTRODUCTION

The primary goal of antepartum fetal surveillance is to identify fetuses at risk of intrauterine insult and death. The second goal is to balance fetal and neonatal risks in order to optimize timing of obstetric intervention and prevent progression to stillbirth. The ultimate goal is thus to improve perinatal outcome by decreasing stillbirths and long-term neurologic impairments. An ideal testing protocol should therefore be able to identify the fetus at risk while preventing unnecessary premature delivery with its associated perinatal morbidity/mortality.

OBJECTIVES

- To understand the pathophysiology of fetal compromise
- Know normal fetal wellbeing parameters
- Understand various tests available for fetal surveillance
- Suggest methods for preventing avoidable stillbirths

According to UNICEF (United Nations Children's Fund), globally one stillbirth occurs every 16 seconds which translates to 2 million stillbirths every year. Two-thirds of these are accounted for by 10 countries alone including India. These losses are particularly tragic because majority can be prevented with high quality of care and monitoring in the antenatal period. UNICEF estimates that the Indian subcontinent accounts for 34% of global stillborns with 1 in every 58 children being stillborn.

In a developing country such as India, women of reproductive age group constitute about a fifth of the population. Since 2000, India has shown a 53% reduction in stillbirth rate; however, because of sheer volume of population it ranks first in absolute numbers. India seems to be on the right track and if current trends continue, India is estimated to achieve Every Newborn Action Plan target between 2020 and 2030.

For a long time, the main objective of obstetric practice was prevention of maternal mortality. Over the years with advancement in anesthesia, blood transfusion services, improved surgical techniques, etc., the focus is now shifting to reach the best possible fetal outcomes as well. Approximately 18% of stillbirths are due to congenital anomalies. In about 50% of nonanomalous stillbirths, hypertension, chorioamnionitis, and fetal growth restriction are thought to be the causes. Some of the indirect factors associated with stillbirths are young age, illiteracy, rural residence, missing antenatal visits, more than two pregnancies, assisted vaginal delivery, and pregnancy complications such as anemia, hypertensive disorders of pregnancy, antepartum hemorrhage, and abnormal fetal position.

It seems reasonable to channelize high-risk pregnancies to simple, flexible, and noninvasive fetal monitoring **(Table 1)**.

TABLE 1: Maternal/fetal indications for fetal monitoring.

Medical	*Obstetric*
Anemia	Extremes of maternal age
Chronic hypertension	Preeclampsia
Diabetes mellitus	Rh isoimmunization
Chronic renal disease	Cholestasis of pregnancy
Significant cardiac disease	Multiple pregnancy
Asthma	Fetal growth restriction
Epilepsy	Oligohydramnios
Substance abuse	Preterm prelabor rupture of membranes
Chronic obstructive pulmonary disease	Previous stillbirth/neonatal death/congenital anomaly
Obesity and malnourishment	Decreased fetal movements
Thyroid disorders	Post-term pregnancy
Hemoglobinopathies	Recurrent pregnancy loss
	Bad obstetric history

IMPACT OF SURVEILLANCE ON FETAL/NEONATAL OUTCOMES

Decreasing perinatal mortality requires a continuum of care from preconception to postnatal care and at all levels of healthcare including family and community. Apart from that few interventions have proven benefits. Doppler velocimetry is associated with 29% reduction in stillbirth in growth restricted fetuses.

ROUTINE ANTENATAL CARE

A minimum of four antenatal visits are recommended for all low-risk pregnant women, first as early as possible/in the first trimester, second between 14 and 26 weeks, third between 28 and 32 weeks, and last between 36 weeks to term. However, in high-risk patients, it is advisable to follow World Health Organization (WHO) eight visits schedule or more if needed.

PATHOPHYSIOLOGY OF FETAL COMPROMISE

Fetal hypoxia and acidosis are the final common pathway which lead to fetal compromise and death. Antepartum fetal surveillance relies on the fact that the fetus will respond to developing hypoxemia by a series of detectable physiologic adaptive or decompensatory signs **(Table 2)**.

It is proposed that fetal hypoxia acts by two pathways.
1. Cellular hypoxia of neuronal tissue → central nervous system (CNS) dysfunction → hypotonia, absent breathing and body movements, and nonreactive nonstress test (NST).
2. Chronic hypoxia → response from aortic arch and carotid body chemoreceptors → reflex redistribution of cardiac output → blood diverted to vital organs such as heart, brain, and thymus → poor renal perfusion, decreased fetal urine production, and oligohydramnios.

In response to ongoing fetal hypoxemia usually (can be shown as a flowchart):
- Loss of fetal heart rate (FHR) reactivity and abnormal blood flow in umbilical artery (UA) are earliest changes.
- Then sequential changes in other fetal blood vessels ensue.
- Usually followed by abnormalities in biophysical parameters such as fetal breathing movements, amniotic fluid level, fetal movements, and tone.

Antepartum fetal surveillance should be done when it is possible to follow up results with action, i.e., the obstetrician is in a position to deliver the fetus in case of compromise. This will depend on the neonatal facilities available at the particular center. This would be from 26 to 28 weeks where tertiary level neonatal intensive care facilities are available or 1–2 weeks earlier than timing of stillbirth in previous pregnancy. Where neonatal intensive care unit (NICU) facilities are not available, and it is anticipated that early delivery may be required, in-utero transfer is preferable to transfer of the neonate after delivery.

TESTS FOR ANTEPARTUM FETAL SURVEILLANCE

Biochemical tests: 24-hour estriol and human placental lactogen assays, etc., are not done routinely as they are cumbersome and inconvenient with wide range of variation in laboratory reference values. Besides it only helps in evaluation of placental function primarily, not necessarily fetal reserve and fetal response to hypoxia. Hence, it is obsolete. Mainstay in antepartum fetal surveillance are biophysical tests.
- Score of 8/10-10-10—reassuring
- 6/10 in term fetus—deliver
- 6/10 preterm—give steroids, repeat in 24 hours
- <04/10—delivery warranted

Each variable also has different correlates like absence of fetal movement is a predictor of abnormal FHR in labor, nonreactive (NR) NST for meconium, decreased amniotic fluid volume (AFV) for fetal distress, and poor fetal tone for perinatal death. Biophysical profile (BPP) also correlates well with umbilical vein pH, all having pH > 7.20 when BPP was normal and none when BPP was 0/10 **(Table 3)**.

Relationship between last BPP score and cerebral palsy was shown to be inverse, exponential, and highly significant.

Modified BPP—to reduce testing time, combines amniotic fluid index (index of chronic fetal health), and cardiotocography (CTG) (standard or computerized).

TABLE 2: Underlying pathophysiology and its associated maternal/fetal condition.

Pathophysiologic process	Maternal/fetal condition
Decreased uteroplacental perfusion	• Chronic hypertension • Preeclampsia • Collagen/renal/vascular disease • Most cases of fetal growth restriction <32–34 weeks
Decreased gas exchange	• Postdated pregnancy • Some cases of fetal growth restriction >32–34 weeks
Metabolic disturbances	• Fetal hyperinsulinemia • Fetal hyperglycemia
Fetal infections	• Premature rupture of membranes • Intra-amniotic infection • Maternal febrile illness • Primary subclinical intra-amniotic infection
Fetal anemia	• Fetomaternal hemorrhage • Erythroblastosis fetalis • Parvovirus B19 infection
Fetal heart failure	• Cardiac arrhythmia • Nonimmune hydrops • Placental chorangioma
Umbilical cord accidents	• Umbilical cord entanglement • Velamentous cord insertion • Oligohydramnios

TABLE 3: Biophysical tests for antepartum fetal surveillance.

Name of test	How is it done?	Normal expected findings	Abnormalities	Correlation with outcome	Advantage	Disadvantage
Fetal movement count*	Count to 10, 12-hour method (Cardiff method), Liston count to 6 or Moore count to 2, postmeal method	Mean time interval for 10 movements are 21±18 minutes	If >2 hours for 10 movements, she should report for further evaluation	Count to 10 shown to reduce overall fetal mortality from 8.7/1,000 to 2.1/1,000 and from 44 to 10/1,000 in women with decreased movements	Safe, reliable, simple inexpensive, active participation of patient	Does not predict long-term prognosis of fetus or acute accidents. Perception may be poor in anterior placentation, hydramnios

*Quiet sleep in fetus can range from 20 to 70 minutes. Decreased fetal perfusion, fetal academia/acidosis associated with decreased movements. Fetal activity may be affected by maternal exercise, alcohol intake, and drugs such as narcotics, betamethasone. Unreliable in multiple pregnancies. Neither standardized nor validated.

Name of test	How is it done?	Normal expected findings	Abnormalities	Correlation with outcome	Advantage	Disadvantage
Nonstress test (NST)**	• Done with cardiotocograph • Done for minimum 20 minutes	Normal or reactive basal FHR 110–160 BPM, at least two accelerations of ≥15 beats lasting at least 15 seconds	If not reactive, do extended NST for 40 minutes. If criteria unmet or nonreactive, test for 90 minutes or vibroacoustic stimulation test (VAST) or biophysical profile (BPP)	PPV < 50%, NPV < 90%. Reactive NST more reliable in excluding hypoxia than nonreactive one predicting fetal compromise. Should be done twice weekly	Fairly simple. Inexpensive, easy to perform, can be done on OPD basis, no contraindications	CTG machine not available everywhere. Correlation with gestation important. High inter and intra-observer variation

**Based on principle that well-oxygenated fetus will respond to movement with fetal heart acceleration. Indirectly indicates normal functioning autonomous nervous system and rules out hypoxia.

**Reactivity of test linked with maturity of autonomous nervous system. Premature fetus may give nonreactive trace. 65% reactive trace at 28 weeks, 85% at 32 weeks, 95% at 34 weeks.

**NST patterns consistent with fetal hypoxia are relatively fixed baseline FHR with poor baseline variability, loss of acceleration, and spontaneous deceleration.

Name of test	How is it done?	Normal expected findings	Abnormalities	Correlation with outcome	Advantage	Disadvantage
VAST	Artificial larynx with sound stimulus of 80–100 db placed on maternal abdomen and 2–3 one second stimuli given	Accelerations noted to acoustic stimuli		Same validity as unprovoked reactive NST	Reduces false positive NST	Additional testing equipment
Contraction stress test (CST) or oxytocin challenge test	Idea is to stimulate labor-like conditions using oxytocin infusion or nipple stimulation and monitor fetal response to uterine contractions	Late decelerations with uterine contraction suggestive of placental insufficiency	Called negative test when no decelerations (desirable). Positive when decelerations with at least 50% contractions	Perinatal mortality within a week of Negative CST is 0.4–1.2/1,000	Simulates labor and monitors fetal response	Time consuming and cumbersome, inconvenient, many contraindications, has to be performed in setup with facility for emergency cesarean section
BPP* or manning score (**Table 4**)	Incorporates testing five biophysical parameters, each parameter marked 0 if absent and 2 if present	Score of >8/10 very low false negative rate and adverse perinatal outcome unlikely	Score of 6/10 associated with high (>75%) false positive rate and should be repeated in 24 hours$	Risk of perinatal death within week of normal BPP 0.7–2.3/1,000	Can be used as early as 26–28 weeks of gestation	Time consuming as minimum 30 minutes scanning recommended before assigning abnormal score

*Provides detailed assessment of behavioral state of fetus in utero. It is analogs to neonatal assessment by Apgar score. It can be used as both as backup test or first line test. Normal biophysical variable excludes hypoxia of end-organ generating it. For example:
- Accelerations on CTG suggest good cardiovascular reserve
- Fetal breathing suggests well-oxygenated brainstem
- Fetal tone and movement represent well-oxygenated midbrain and cerebral cortex
- Normal amniotic kidney points to well-perfused kidneys

$Reliability of test depends not just on total score but also on abnormal parameter, especially abnormal amniotic fluid

$Grossly abnormal score of 0–4/10 high probability of fetal hypoxia. With a score of 0, combined morbidity mortality reaches almost 100%

(BPM: beats per minute; CTG: cardiotocography; FHR: fetal heart rate; NPV: negative predictive value; OPD: outpatient department; PPV: positive predictive value)

TABLE 4: Scoring criteria for biophysical profile or Manning score.

Biophysical variable	Normal (score = 2)	Abnormal (score = 0)
Fetal breathing movements	One episode of at least 30 seconds in 30 minutes	Absent or no episode >30 seconds in 30 minutes
Fetal movements	Three discrete body/limb movements in 30 minutes	Two or less in 30 minutes
Fetal tone	One episode of active extension with return to flexion of limbs or trunk	Slow extension with return to partial flexion or movement of limb in full extension or no movement
Amniotic fluid	One pocket measuring at least 2 cm in two perpendicular planes	Either no pocket OR Pocket <2 cm in two perpendicular planes
Nonstress test	Reactive	Nonreactive

TABLE 5: Correlation of vessel studied and information derived.

Vessel examined	Information derived
Uterine artery	Maternal—flow resistance to the uterus
Umbilical artery	Placental—flow resistance to placenta
Arterial circulation (middle cerebral artery)	Fetal adaptation to flow resistance change
Venous circulation (umbilical vein, inferior vena cava, and ductus venosus)	Fetal cardiac function

DOPPLER VELOCIMETRY

Doppler velocimetry is one of the most extensively used techniques that evaluates blood flow in placental/fetal vessels. It is also the only test studied extensively in randomized trials. The information derived depends on the vessel studied.

The routine use of Doppler ultrasound in low risk or unselected pregnancies does not confer any benefit on mother or on fetus. As per the Cochrane review, there is also no difference in incidence in intrapartum fetal distress and caesarean section between Doppler/non-Doppler groups. However, there is definite decrease in perinatal deaths, labor inductions, and hospital admissions in pregnancies managed by Doppler, especially those with hypertension and fetal growth restriction. Doppler velocimetry not only helps in assessment but also guides intensity and frequency of fetal monitoring. It is also useful in identifying small for gestational age fetuses which do not require intensive monitoring unlike fetal growth restriction fetuses which do.

- *UA Doppler:* It is the most common parameter evaluated for assessment of fetal well-being. In normal pregnancy with advancement of pregnancy, the uteroplacental unit resistance decreases, UA diastolic flow increases, and systolic/diastolic (S/D) ratio falls gradually. S/D ratio > 3 is considered abnormal after 30 weeks pregnancy. UA Doppler study is most useful in early-onset growth restriction due to uteroplacental insufficiency. Current American College of Obstetricians and Gynecologists (ACOG) practice guidelines support the use of UA Doppler assessments only in the management of suspected fetal growth restriction.
  It is estimated that >70% placental arteries are obliterated when reversal of end-diastolic flow appears. Reversal of end-diastolic flow is ominous and marker of imminent fetal death. This is preceded by decrease in end-diastolic flow and absent end-diastolic flow.
- *Middle cerebral artery (MCA):* In event of fetal hypoxia, there ensues vasoconstriction in somatic, renal, and hepatic vessels with preferential flow to brain, heart, and adrenals. Hence, a hypoxic fetus would show increased end-diastolic flow in MCA and fall in pulsatility index and resistance index.
- *Fetal venous circulation:* Most commonly studied veins are umbilical vein, inferior vena cava, and ductus venosus. These indices provide additional information and help in deciding time of delivery when UA/MCA Doppler indices are abnormal. In event of persistent fetal hypoxia, first redistribution of blood flow occurs followed by fetal decompensation if uncorrected. A healthy fetus essentially has a nonpulsatile venous circulation. Appearance of pulsatile venous flow is associated with high morbidity and mortality.
- Progressive fetal compromise secondary to placental insufficiency progresses as:
  - Increase in UA resistance without decentralization of blood flow
  - Increased UA resistance with decentralization (brain sparing effect)
  - Absent UA end-diastolic flow
  - Reversed UA diastolic flow
  - Alteration in venous circulation **(Table 5)**.

Emerging methods of fetal surveillance:
- *Fetal actocardiograph:* Electronically records FHR and fetal movement.
- *Fetal magnetoencephalography:* Specialized apparatus which uses ultra-sensitive magnetic field detectors and maps fetal cortical response to visual/auditory stimuli.

SECTION 1 | Fetal Well-being

Indications, frequency, and outcome of antepartum fetal surveillance.

Condition	Estimated stillbirth rate	Gestational age to initiate surveillance	Mode and frequency
Diabetes mellitus on insulin	6–35/1,000	32 weeks	NST/BPP twice/week
Chronic hypertension	6–25/1,000	26 weeks	NST/AFI/MBPP twice/week
Hypertensive disorders of pregnancy mild severe	9–21/1,000 12–29/1,000	At diagnosis At diagnosis	MBPP twice/week NST daily, AFI twice/week
Growth restricted fetus: • Suspected • Confirmed	10–47/1,000		NST, AFI weekly MBPP, umbilical artery Doppler twice/week
Oligohydramnios	14/1,000	At diagnosis	NST/AFI twice/week
Previous stillbirth	9–20/1,000	32 weeks	BPP/CST weekly or MBPP twice/week
Decreased fetal movement	13/1,000	At diagnosis	MBPP

(AFI: amniotic fluid index; BPP: biophysical profile; CST: contraction stress test; NST: nonstress test; MBPP: modified biophysical profile)

CHAPTER AT A GLANCE

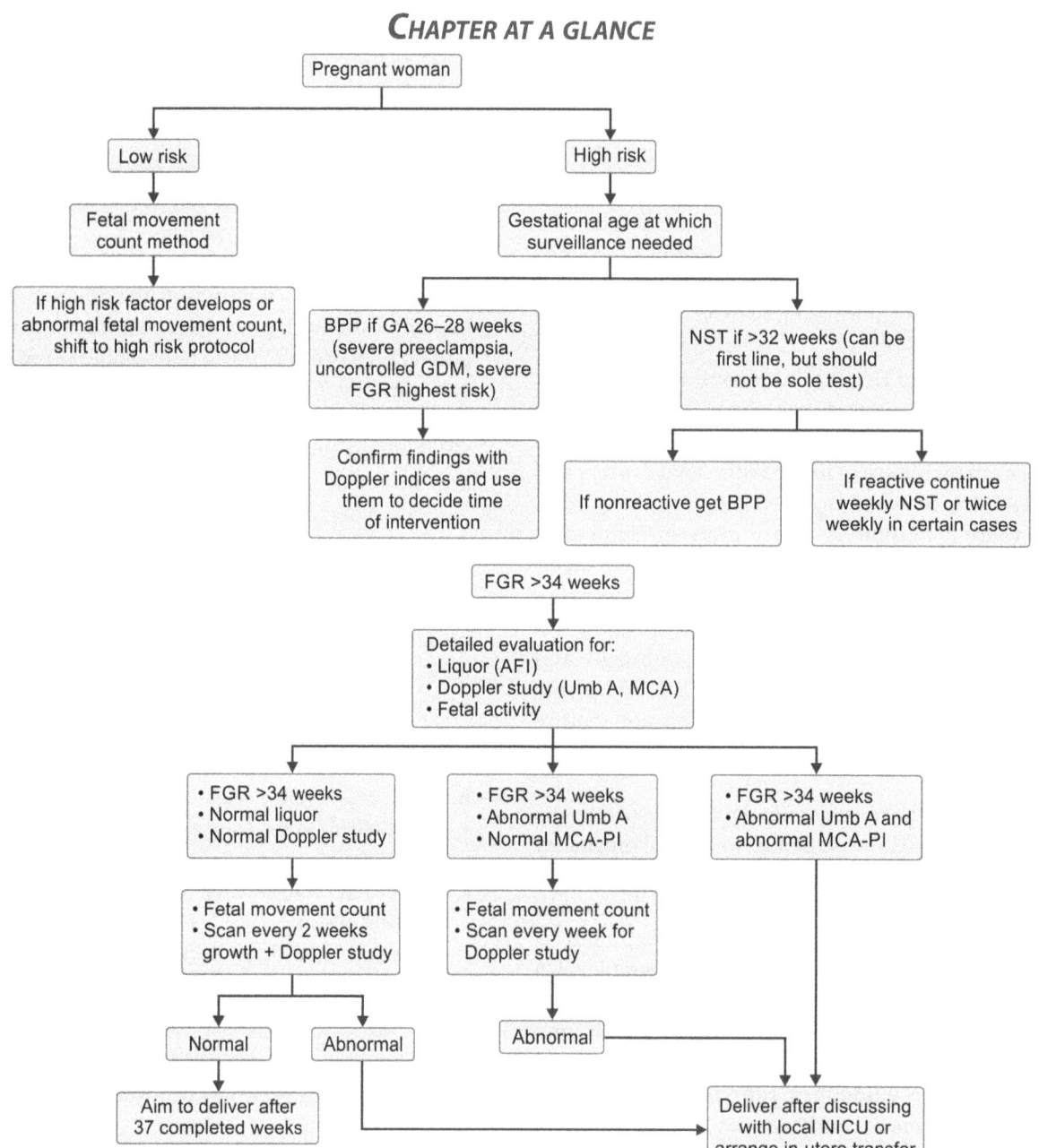

(AFI: amniotic fluid index; BPP: biophysical profile; FGR: fetal growth restriction; GA: gestational age; GDM: gestational diabetes mellitus; MCA-PI: middle cerebral artery pulsatility index; NICU: neonatal intensive care unit; NST: nonstress test)

KEY POINTS

- Fetal testing is based on the hypothesis that the compromised fetus will undergo a series of detectable changes. Some changes such as reduced FHR variability and infrequent breathing are observed in at least 25% normal term fetuses.
- Observational studies have shown 10-fold increase in perinatal mortality in high-risk pregnancies. But the prevalence of high risk pregnancies is low and 30–50% stillbirths occur in "low risk pregnancies."
- Even in a high-risk pregnancy with stillbirth rate of 70/1,000, a test with 99% sensitivity and specificity will give positive predictive value of 88%.
- No known method can prevent sudden events such as cord accident or placental abruption.
- Biophysical profile and Doppler studies are the mainstay of antepartum assessment of fetal well-being.
- It is important to identify those requiring more intensive monitoring so that resources can be used judiciously.

SUGGESTED READING

1. Lees CC, Stampalija T, Baschat A, da Silva Costa F, Ferrazzi E, Figueras F, et al. ISUOG Practice Guidelines: Diagnosis and management of small-for-gestational-age fetus and fetal growth restriction.
2. RCOG. (2013). The investigation and management of small for gestational age fetus. [online] Available from https://www.rcog.org.uk/en/guidelines-research-services/guidelines/gtg31/. [Last accessed November, 2021].
3. Arias F, Bhide AG, Arulkumaran S, Damania K, Daftary SN. Arias' Practical Guide to High Risk Pregnancy and Delivery. Gurugram: Elsevier India; 2015.
4. Misra R. Intrauterine growth restriction. Ian Donald's Practical Obstetric Problems. Delhi: Wolters Kluwer India Pvt. Ltd.; 2020.
5. Signore C, Freeman RK, Spong CY. Antenatal testing-a reevaluation: executive summary of a Eunice Kennedy Shriver National Institute of Child Health and Human Development workshop. Obstet Gynecol. 2009;113(3):687-701.
6. UNICEF. (2020). A Neglected Tragedy The global burden of stillbirths. Report of the UN Inter-agency Group for Child Mortality Estimation. [online] Available from https://data.unicef.org/resources/a-neglected-tragedy-stillbirth-estimates-report/.

CHAPTER 3

Intrapartum Fetal Monitoring

Vishal Vishnu Tewari, Renu Thosar

INTRODUCTION

Normal labor is characterized by regular uterine contractions, which cause repeated transient interruptions of fetal oxygenation. Most fetuses tolerate this process well, but some do not. Fetal heart rate (FHR) pattern is an indirect marker of fetal cardiac and central nervous system (CNS) responses to changes in blood pressure, blood gases, and acid–base status. Although virtually all obstetric societies advise monitoring the FHR during labor, the benefit of this intervention has not been clearly demonstrated. The recommendation is largely based upon expert opinion and previous medicolegal precedent.

OBJECTIVES

- To know about high-risk maternal conditions affecting fetal-neonatal outcomes
- To understand different techniques of intrapartum fetal monitoring (IFM) and its physiological basis
- To understand patterns of variations with cardiotocography (CTG)
- To know correct management of nonreassuring and pathological CTG findings
- To know about IFM and its impact on neonatal outcomes

HIGH-RISK MATERNAL CONDITIONS AFFECTING FETAL-NEONATAL OUTCOMES

Perinatal risk factors including but not restricted to those mentioned in **Table 1** increase the likelihood for neonatal resuscitation and therefore must undergo IFM. A recent systematic review found fetal growth restriction (FGR), nonreassuring CTG, emergency caesarean section, meconium-stained amniotic fluid, and chorioamnionitis to have the highest risk for neonatal hypoxic-ischemic encephalopathy (HIE).

TABLE 1: Maternal-fetal risk factors requiring intrapartum fetal monitoring.

Antenatal risk factors:
- Gestational age <36 0/7 weeks
- Gestational age ≥41 0/7 weeks
- Preeclampsia or eclampsia
- Maternal hypertension
- Polyhydramnios
- Oligohydramnios
- Fresh vaginal bleeding
- Severe chorioamnionitis
- Sepsis or temperature ≥38°C

Intrapartum risk factors:
- Trial of labor in previous cesarean section
- Breech or other abnormal presentation
- Suspicious or pathological cardiotocography
- Maternal general anesthesia
- Maternal magnesium therapy
- Placental abruption
- Oxytocin use
- Intrapartum bleeding
- Narcotics administered to mother within 4 hours of delivery
- Meconium-stained amniotic fluid
- Prolapsed umbilical cord

Fetal factors:
- Fetal macrosomia
- Fetal hydrops
- Fetal growth restriction
- Significant fetal malformations or anomalies
- Multiple gestation
- Fetal anemia
- Fetal hypokinesia

ADAPTED FROM: NEONATAL RESUSCITATION PROTOCOL 8 TH EDITION/TYPES OF INTRAPARTUM FETAL MONITORING

Noninvasive:
- IA (intermittent auscultation)
- CTG (cardiotocography)

Outcomes of interest	Number of studies/total enrolled cases	IA versus CTG; RR (95% CI)	Interpretation
Fetal-neonatal			
Perinatal mortality	13/33,513	0.86 (0.59–1.24)	No difference
Neonatal seizure	9/32,386	0.50 (0.31–0.8)	Favors CTG
Cerebral palsy	2/13,252	1.75 (0.84–3.63)	No difference
Maternal			
Caesarean delivery	11/18,861	1.63 (1.29–2.07)	Increased with CTG
Instrumental vaginal delivery	10/18,615	1.15 (1.01–1.33)	Increased with CTG
Cord blood acidosis	2/2,494	1.16 (0.72–1.89)	No difference

Invasive: CTG with fetal blood sampling (FBS)

Outcomes of interest	Number of studies/total enrolled cases	IA versus CTG; RR (95% CI)	Interpretation
Fetal-neonatal			
Perinatal mortality	7/16,131	0.97 (0.64–1.47)	No difference
Neonatal seizure	5/15,004	0.49 (0.29–0.84)	Favors FBS
Cerebral palsy	2/13,252	1.74 (0.97–3.11)	No difference
Maternal			
Caesarean delivery	7/16,001	1.34 (1.14–1.58)	Increased with FBS
Instrumental vaginal delivery	6/15,755	1.27 (1.16–1.39)	Increased with FBS
Cord blood acidosis	1/1,073	0.45 (0.16–1.29)	Favors FBS

(CI: confidence interval; RR: relative risk)

- *Intermittent auscultation (IA)*: It is an easy as well as effective method for fetal monitoring especially in low-risk pregnancy as well as in low-resource settings. It includes monitoring of FHR by using stethoscope or handheld Doppler device. The FHR is auscultated for duration of 1 minute in between two contractions. The frequency of measurement is generally once in 30 minutes in first stage and once in 15 minutes in second stage of labor.
- *Noninvasive electronic fetal monitoring (EFM)*: External electronic monitors use the principal of Doppler effect to calculate mechanical RR wave interval and create sound patterns. Advantage of EFM includes possible monitoring of heart rate patterns along with maternal parameters, monitoring in twins, monitoring from distant location by wireless signals. Though obesity, polyhydramnios, uterine fibroids, or fetal arrhythmias may produce difficulty in getting reliable trace and in those conditions invasive monitoring is superior.
- *Internal electronic surveillance*: Includes attaching an ECG (electrocardiogram) electrode to fetal scalp and tracing the fetal cardiac electrical activity. Time between two R waves is used to count rate and with each arriving wave rate is changed providing accurate beat-to-beat variability. It is rarely used in India.

FETAL HEART RATE

Baseline Heart Rate

A normal baseline FHR is 110–160 bpm and reflects lack of pathology related to factors that regulate FHR. Baseline bradycardia (FHR < 110 bpm) may be related to maternal β-blocker therapy, hypothermia, hypoglycemia, hypothyroidism, or fetal heart block or interruption of fetal oxygenation. Baseline tachycardia (FHR > 160 bpm) may be related to maternal fever, infection, medications, hyperthyroidism, fetal anemia, arrhythmia, or interruption of fetal oxygenation.

Beat-to-beat Variability

Normal FHR variability is 5–25 bpm. It is the result of integrated activity between sympathetic and parasympathetic autonomic nervous system. Normal variability means oxygenation of CNS is appropriate and absence of hypoxia-induced metabolic acidemia. But minimal or absent variability alone is poor predictor of fetal metabolic academia or CNS hypoxic injury. Minimal or absent variability can be present in fetal metabolic academia, fetal sleep cycle, extreme prematurity as well as in few of congenital anomalies **(Fig. 1)**.

Accelerations

Fetal heart rate accelerations are associated with fetal movements, due to stimulation of peripheral proprioceptors and autonomic stimulation of heart. Presence of accelerations along with variability can reliably rule out fetal hypoxia. However, absence of acceleration alone is also a poor predictor of fetal metabolic academia or hypoxia. Absence of acceleration can be seen in fetal sleep cycle, arrhythmias, prematurity, fetal anemia, and congenital malformations.

Decelerations Unrelated to Hypoxia

Early deceleration: These are decelerations that are shallow, short-lasting with normal variability within the deceleration, and generally coincident with contractions. These are unrelated to fetal oxygenation, represents an autonomic response to changes in intracranial pressure or cerebral blood flow caused by intrapartum compression of the fetal head during uterine contraction and maternal pushing efforts. Early decelerations are clinically benign.

Decelerations due to Compromised Fetal Oxygenation

- *Late deceleration*: Decelerations exhibit a gradual onset and/or a gradual return to the baseline and/or reduced variability within the deceleration. Decelerations typically start >20 seconds after the onset of a contraction, a nadir after the peak of contraction, and a return to the baseline after the end of the contraction. It is a reflex fetal response to transient hypoxemia during uterine contractions. When fetal PO_2 falls below normal range, chemoreceptor initiates an autonomic reflex response, results in decrease in FHR and cardiac output. After the contraction, fetal oxygenation is restored and FHR returns to baseline. Interrupted fetal oxygenation for long results in severe hypoxemia and metabolic academia thereby leading to myocardial depression and late deceleration.
- *Variable deceleration* **(Fig. 2)**: Decelerations of varying size, shape, and varying relationship to uterine contractions that exhibit a rapid drop (onset to nadir in <30 seconds), good variability within the deceleration, rapid recovery to the baseline. It occurs due to baroreceptor-mediated response to increased arterial pressure due to transient mechanical compression of umbilical cord **(Fig. 3)**.

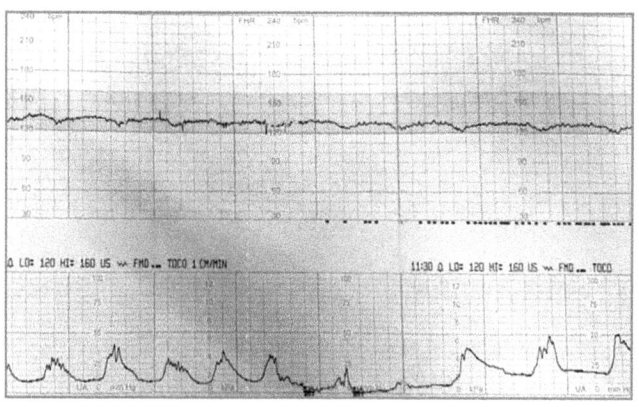

Fig. 1: Cardiotocography trace showing poor beat to beat variability, with no acceleration.

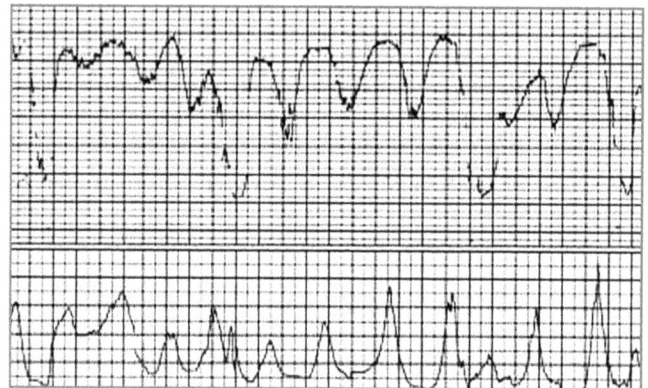

Fig. 2: Late deceleration.

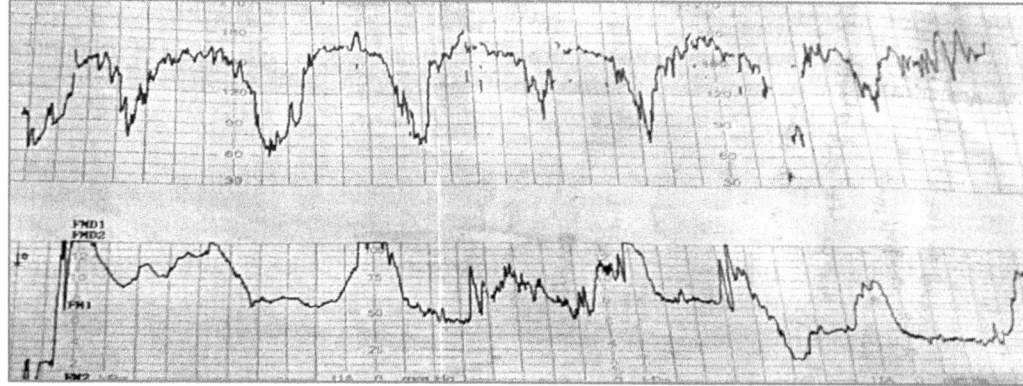

Fig. 3: Recurrent variable deceleration (maintained variability, no relations with contraction, rapid nadir, and rapid recovery).

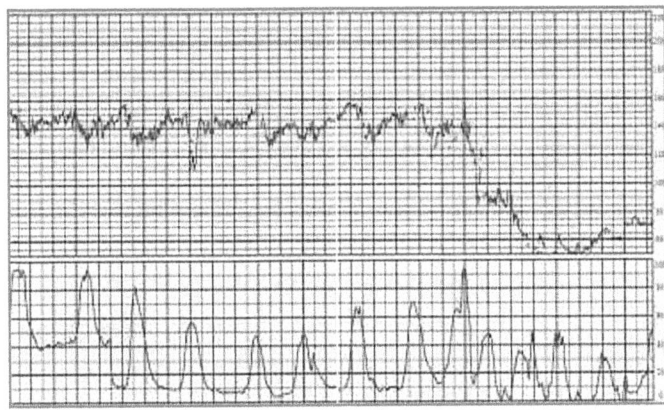

Fig. 4: Prolonged deceleration.

- *Prolonged deceleration*: Fall in FHR by ≥15 bpm, lasting ≥2 minutes but <10 minutes. It is same as deceleration but for a longer period. If fall in FHR lasts ≥10 minutes, it is defined as change in baseline. These are chemoreceptor-induced response to fetal hypoxemia. Prolonged deceleration for >5 minutes with FHR of below 80 bpm is associated with frequent hypoxemia as well as acidosis and requires urgent obstetric interventions **(Fig. 4)**.
- *Sinusoidal pattern*: Smooth, sine wave-like undulating pattern in FHR baseline with a cycle frequency of 3–5 cycles per minute that persists for at least 20 minutes. Though pathophysiology of sinusoidal pattern is not well-established, it is frequently associated with severe fetal anemia. The sinusoidal pattern is typically found in anti-D alloimmunization, fetal-maternal hemorrhage, twin-to-twin transfusion syndrome, and ruptured vasa previa. It has also been described in cases of acute fetal hypoxia, infection, cardiac malformations, hydrocephalus, and gastroschisis.

ACCORDING TO NATIONAL INSTITUTE OF HEALTH AND CARE EXCELLENCE GUIDELINES

- IA to be offered to low-risk women in the first stage of labor. Normal FHR during IA should be between 110 and 160 bpm to be auscultated over 1 minute between contractions.
- If IA shows concern (persistent FHR < 110 or tachycardia >160 bpm), perform continuous CTG for 20 minutes and if tracing is normal, then return back to IA.

PRINCIPLE FOR INTRAPARTUM CARDIOTOCOGRAPHY INTERPRETATION

When reviewing the CTG trace, assessment and documentation of contractions and all four features of FHR (baseline rate; baseline variability; presence or absence of decelerations and concerning characteristics of decelerations if present; presence of accelerations) need to be done.

Once CTG interpretation is done, categorization is done as reassuring, nonreassuring, or pathological CTG. If there is a stable baseline, FHR between 110 and 160 beats/min and normal variability the risk of fetal acidosis is low. In such cases, usual care is to be continued. In case of difficulty to categorize or interpret a CTG trace, a review by a senior obstetrician should be considered **(Table 2)**.

MANAGEMENT DEPENDING ON CARDIOTOCOGRAPHY CATEGORIZATION

- *Normal*: All features are reassuring, managed by either continuous CTG or if no risk factors shift back to IA. Talk to patient and her relatives.
- *Suspicious*: One nonreassuring feature and two reassuring features. Management includes: Correct underlying cause such as:
  - Hypotension
  - Uterine hyperstimulation
  - Perform a full set of maternal observations
  - Start conservative methods such as change in position, intravenous (IV) fluids if hypotension, reduce contraction frequency by stopping oxytocin, or using subcutaneous terbutaline 0.25 mg.
  - To discuss with the woman and her birth companion regarding events on intrapartum monitoring and to take her preferences into account.
- *Pathological*: One abnormal or two nonreassuring features. Management includes:
  - To exclude acute events (cord prolapse, suspected placental abruption, or suspected uterine rupture)
  - Correct any underlying causes, such as hypotension or uterine hyperstimulation
  - Start one or more conservative measures
  - If the CTG trace is still pathological after implementing conservative measures—offer digital fetal scalp stimulation and document the outcome.
  - *If the CTG trace is still pathological after fetal scalp stimulation*: Consider fetal blood sampling (FBS) or consider expediting the birth.
- *Need for urgent intervention*: Acute bradycardia or single prolonged deceleration for 3 minutes or more. Management includes:
  - Expediting birth in case of an acute event (e.g., cord prolapse, suspected placental abruption, or suspected uterine rupture).
  - Correct any underlying causes, such as hypotension or uterine hyperstimulation
  - Start one or more conservative measures
  - Make preparations for an urgent birth
  - Talk to the woman and her relatives about what is happening and take her preferences into account.
  - Expedite the birth if the acute bradycardia persists for 9 minutes.

TABLE 2: Description of cardiotocograph trace features (NICE guidelines CG190 2017).

	Baseline (beats/min)	Baseline variability (beats/min)	Decelerations
Reassuring	110–160	5–25	• No decelerations OR • Early variable decelerations with no concerning characteristics* for <90 minutes
Non-reassuring	100–109 OR 161–180	<5 for 30–50 minutes OR >25 for 15–25 minutes	• Variable decelerations with no concerning characteristics* for 90 minutes or more OR • Variable decelerations with any concerning characteristics* in up to 50% of contractions for 30 minutes or more OR • Variable decelerations with any concerning characteristics* in over 50% of contractions for <30 minutes OR • Late decelerations in over 50% of contractions for <30 minutes, with no maternal or fetal clinical risk factors such as vaginal bleeding or significant meconium
Abnormal	Below 100 OR Above 180	<5 for >50 minutes OR >25 for >25 minutes OR Sinusoidal	• Variable decelerations with any concerning characteristics* in over 50% of contractions for 30 minutes [or less if any maternal or fetal clinical risk factors (see above)] OR • Late decelerations for 30 minutes (or less if any maternal or fetal clinical risk factors) OR • Acute bradycardia, or a single prolonged deceleration lasting 3 minutes or more

*Concerning characteristics in variable deceleration includes biphasic W shape, no shouldering, failure to return to baseline, reduced baseline variability within deceleration, lasting >60 seconds.
(NICE: National Institute of Health and Care Excellence)

- If the FHR recovers at any time up to 9 minutes, reassess any decision to expedite the birth, in discussion with the woman.
- *3-6-9-12 rule*:
  - If deceleration up to 3 minutes—call for help
  - 6 minutes—shift to theater for intervention
  - 9 minutes prepare for delivery
  - 12 minutes baby should be delivered
- *Role of conservative management*: Nonreassuring pattern on EFM may point toward varied etiologies which may cause reduced oxygen delivery or blood circulation to fetus. The mode of treatment needs to be directed toward suspected cause. Recurrent late or variable decelerations may suggest cord compression or pressure on aorta by gravid uterus. Giving left lateral position or putting a wedge on one side may reduce pressure on cord or improve blood circulation preventing hypoxia. Similarly in case of poor hydration or hypotension administration of IV fluids may revert back the changes of nonreassuring type.
- *Tocolysis*: Proper uterine relaxation in between contractions is one of most important factor to maintain adequate placental perfusion. In case of tachysystole, i.e., more than five contractions over 10 minutes over the duration of 30 minutes is associated with significant reduction in relaxation time causing abnormalities on EFM. Stopping or reducing dose of oxytocin augmentation or administration of terbutaline should be considered in case of tachysystole.
- *Maternal oxygen therapy*: Improved maternal oxygen saturation was hypothesized to reduce fetal hypoxia and improve outcomes. Though oxygen therapy helps to revert nonreassuring changes in the CTG and has also demonstrated improved oxygenation in umbilical vessels, it has not been shown to improve neonatal outcomes. Rather intrauterine hyperoxemia along with acidosis can cause increase in free radical injury and cause increased neonatal morbidity.

INTRAPARTUM FETAL MONITORING AND ITS IMPACT ON NEONATAL OUTCOMES

The notion of monitoring FHR in labor is based on the fact that changes in fetal cardiac rhythm/rate are corroborated as CNS response to fetal hypoxia. IFM aims at early identification of fetal acidemia and hypoxemia based on fetal neurological and cardiovascular responses. Although some evidence suggests that compared to IA, EFM is associated with a reduction in intrapartum death and early neonatal seizures but there is no reduction in neurodevelopment impairment on long-term follow-up. Rather EFM is found to be associated with high false positive rate resulting in increased numbers of operative deliveries. Even though no statistical difference was found in two techniques (IA vs. EFM) in respect to acidemia, low Apgar score, neonatal intensive care unit (NICU) admission, HIE, perinatal mortality, cerebral palsy, and neurodevelopment impairment; noninvasive electronic fetal heart monitoring is most common modality of intrapartum monitoring in most developed countries. Recent high-quality evidence evaluating 33 studies for IA, CTG, computerized cardiotocography (cCTG), fetal scalp pH, fetal scalp lactate, fetal pulse oximetry, and fetal electrocardiogram for ST segment analysis in combination with CTG found that IA reduced emergency lower segment caesarean section (LSCS) deliveries without increasing adverse fetal outcomes. Increased uterine activity has been found to be a nonspecific predictor of neonatal depression at birth. Presence of tachysystole defined as >5 contractions in 10 minutes averaged over 30 minutes increased the risk of neonatal encephalopathy at birth. In low-middle income countries (LMIC) setting, use of a partograph and IA resulted in improved perinatal outcomes while use of CTG resulted in higher LSCS rates without any additional benefit in perinatal outcomes. Doppler is superior to the stethoscope for detection of intrapartum FHR abnormalities in LMIC setting. Oxygenation status of the fetal myocardium assessed using fetal ECG analysis of the ST segment (STAN) has been shown to reduce fetal acidosis by 36%. However, this technique is limited by its availability in our centers.

ROLE OF OTHER ADJUNCT TESTS

Fetal Scalp Stimulation

If the cardiotocograph trace is pathological, fetal scalp stimulation is an easy test to offer. Fetal scalp is stimulated by vaginal examination or by use of vibroacoustic stimulation device kept on maternal abdomen. Stimulation should be done when FHR is at baseline and not during decelerations. Induction of accelerations with stimulation is equally sensitive to diagnose fetal acidosis as of spontaneous accelerations. Absence of acceleration with stimulation may suggest ongoing acidosis with pH <7.2 in up to 50% of the cases.

Fetal Blood Sampling (Rarely Performed in India)

Nonreassuring CTG or no acceleration with fetal scalp stimulation raises suspicion of fetal hypoxia and acidosis.

TABLE 3: Fetal blood sampling (FBS) result and recommendations.

FBS result pH lactate	Recommendation
Normal: pH (7.25 or above) Lactate (≤4.1)	• FBS should be repeated in 1 hour if FHR abnormality persists or sooner if there are further abnormalities • If result remains stable after second test, a third/further sample may be deferred unless there are further abnormalities of the CTG
Borderline: pH = 7.21–7.24 Lactate = 4.2–4.8	• Repeat FBS within 30 minutes if the FHR remains pathological or sooner if there are further abnormalities • If the third sample is indicated, a consultant obstetric opinion should be sought
Abnormal: pH ≤ 7.20 Lactate ≥ 4.9	• Consultant obstetric advice should be sought • Urgent delivery within 30 minutes

Source: Adapted from suggested actions if CTG pathological (PROMPT Course Manual 2008)
(CTG: cardiotocography; FHR: fetal heart rate)

FBS helps to confirm the pH as well as rule out hypoxia. A sample of blood is collected from the baby's head by making a small scratch on the baby's scalp. The scratch heals quickly after birth, but there remains a small risk of infection. The blood sample collected is used to measure the pH of blood which helps to understand fetal oxygenation during labor stress. Results of FBS and recommended actions are as given in **Table 3**.

Contraindications to FBS include:
- Evidence of serious and sustained fetal compromise
- Risk of fetal bleeding disorders (e.g., fetal thrombocytopenia and hemophilia)
- Nonvertex presentation
- Maternal infection [e.g., human immunodeficiency virus (HIV), hepatitis B, hepatitis C, active primary herpes, and suspected fetal sepsis].

ADDITIONAL FACTORS

- *Fetal growth restriction*—is considered a state of chronic placental insufficiency as well as state of redistribution of blood flow in fetus. A fetus with growth restriction is more likely to have late decelerations and less likely to have reassuring accelerations compared to an appropriate to gestation grown fetus. The beneficial effect of conservative treatment in these fetus is doubtful with nonreassuring EFM pattern.
- *Meconium-stained liquor*: Meconium-stained liquor is present in up to 10–12% of pregnancies while the incidence is much higher in group with nonreassuring finding on EFM. Prolonged deceleration, severe

TABLE 4: Salient points about neonatal resuscitation in asphyxiated neonates.

Resuscitation step	Guidance
Team composition	A pediatrician or neonatologist skilled in NRP must be present
Cord management	Optimal cord management strategy to be followed—delayed clamping, milking, or intact cord resuscitation is not clear
Umbilical cord blood acid–base status	Umbilical vessel pH ≤ 7 and base deficit of −16 mmol/L indicates hypoxic ischemic injury and is strongly associated with neonatal mortality, neurological morbidity including HIE, IVH, and PVL and long-term neurological disability including cerebral palsy
Heart rate assessment	Auscultation for initial assessment; pulse oximetry and ECG for continuous assessment
Respiratory support	Mask ventilation using self-inflating bag or T-piece resuscitator
Oxygen	Room-air resuscitation to be done during ventilation alone; increase to FiO_2 1.0 if chest compressions are needed
Adrenaline	Injection adrenaline (1:10,000) in a dose of 0.02 mg/kg (0.2 mL/kg) followed by 3 mL normal saline flush
Meconium-stained amniotic fluid and nonvigorous infant	Endotracheal suction is not recommended as a routine. However, if thick viscous meconium is seen obstructing the airway suctioning to be done
Temperature management	Passive hypothermia is recommended in NRP. However, due to conflicting evidence on benefit of therapeutic hypothermia in our setting, adoption of this strategy should be done with caution
Parent counseling	Prenatal counseling of the parents and family members must be done as a team along with the obstetrician and due informed written consent must be obtained

(HIE: hypoxic-ischemic encephalopathy; IVH: intraventricular hemorrhage; NRP: neonatal resuscitation protocol; PVL: periventricular leukomalacia)

recurrent variable decelerations as well as bradycardia are common findings in this group. As amnioinfusion in this group has not been found very useful, meconium-stained liquor, especially thick meconium should be used for risk stratification to decide further treatment plan.

- *Magnesium sulfate treatment*: Magnesium sulfate ($MgSO_4$) treatment is considered for seizure prophylaxis as well as fetal neuroprotection in impending preterm birth. Magnesium freely crosses placenta and being antagonist of calcium may cause fall in baseline FHR as well as reduced variability. Possible changes with Mg should be considered before categorizing trace as nonreassuring.
- *Neuraxial anesthesia*: Maternal spinal epidural analgesia may cause hypotension in up to 10% of cases. It is also hypothesized that sudden neuraxial analgesia or anesthesia causes sudden imbalance of maternal adrenaline–noradrenalin causing uterine hypertonia. EFM should be offered before and after neuraxial anesthesia to look for signs to intervene. Correction of hypotension with IV fluids or administration of ephedrine can be considered.

INVESTIGATIONAL TREATMENTS

Sildenafil citrate, a selective inhibitor of phosphodiesterase-5 (PDE5), is considered to have vasodilatory action on placental circulation due to abundance of PDE5 receptors on placental vessels. Due to its expected vasodilatation, it is expected to reduce fetal hypoxia, reduce need of LSCS, or operative vaginal delivery associated with nonreassuring or pathological trace of EFM. A recent trial in a small group of patients suggested positive outcomes with 41% reduction of pathological findings on EFM and 51% reduction in emergency operative deliveries with no consequential increase in neonatal or maternal morbidity. Further studies are required before sildenafil can be used for pathological EFM or routine use in labor.

NEONATAL RESUSCITATION

Anticipation and preparedness are the cornerstones of successful resuscitation of an asphyxiated neonate at birth by the team attending the delivery. Salient features of the neonatal resuscitation protocol (NRP) which elucidates the guiding principles and algorithm for resuscitation of an asphyxiated neonate is given below as **Table 4**.

CHAPTER 3 | Intrapartum Fetal Monitoring

CHAPTER AT A GLANCE

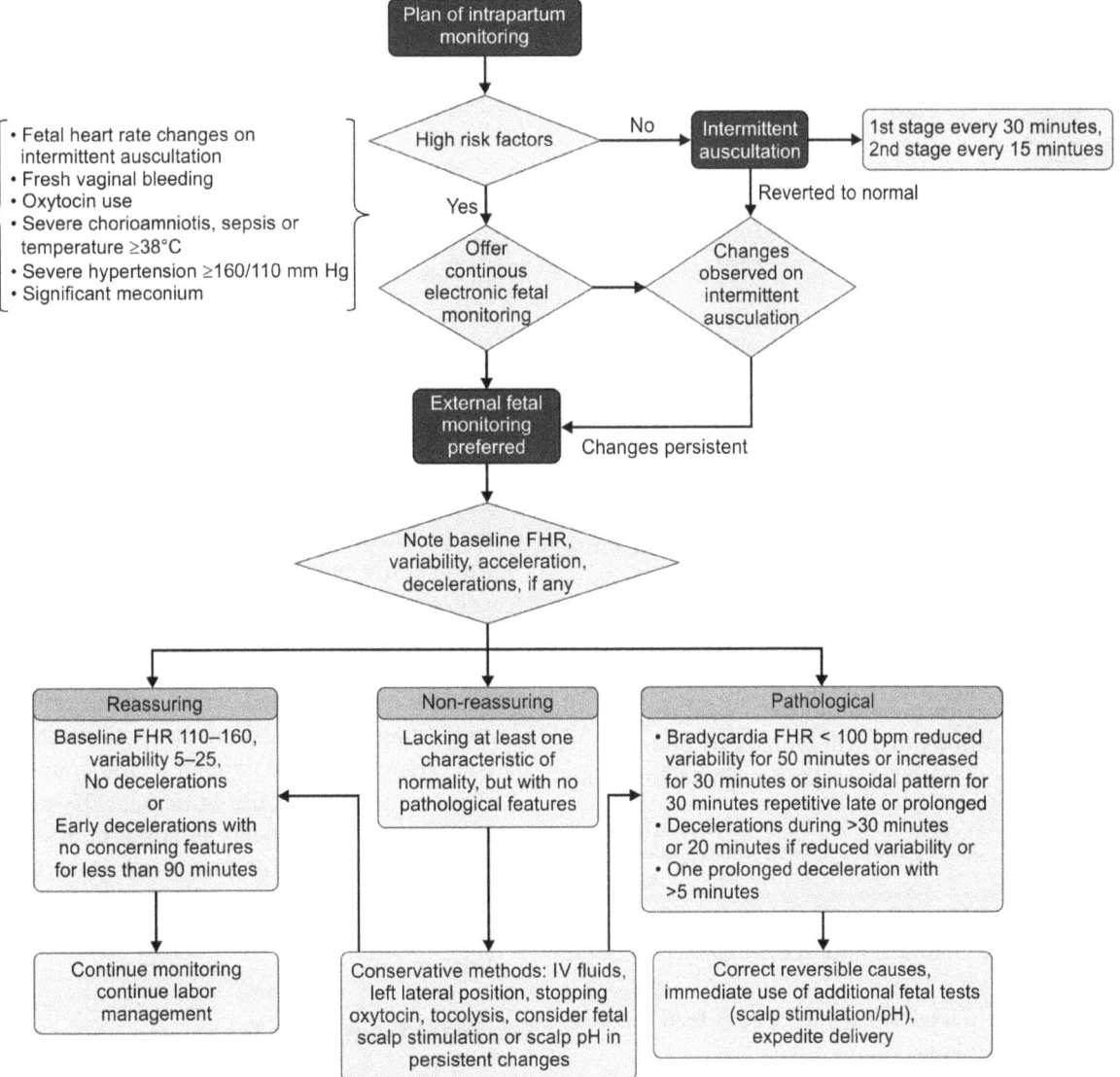

(FHR: fetal heart rate)

KEY POINTS

- IFM aims to identify compromise or deoxygenation before neurological injury in the fetus.
- IFM using IA and partograph reduces adverse perinatal outcomes in LMIC setting.
- Normal EFM trace suggests very low risk of intrapartum hypoxia, while abnormal trace needs further evaluation.
- The FHR tracing can be affected by many physiological and pathological factors other than hypoxia.
- Three-tier categorization of EFM trace corroborates well with risk of hypoxia and helps to decide the management.
- Potential for development of true hypoxia with nonreassuring pattern is variable.
- Pathological pattern on EFM needs expedited delivery due to high risk of developing fetal hypoxia.

SUGGESTED READING

1. Alfirevic Z, Devane D, Gyte GM, Cuthbert A; Cochrane Pregnancy and Childbirth Group. Continuous cardiotocography (CTG) as a form of electronic fetal monitoring (EFM) for fetal assessment during labour. Cochrane Database Syst Rev. 2017;2017(2):CD006066.
2. Ayres-de-Campos D, Spong CY, Chandraharan E. FIGO consensus guidelines on intrapartum fetal monitoring: Cardiotocography. Int J Gynecol Obstet. 2015;131:13-24.
3. Bruckner M, Lista G, Saugstad OD, Schmolzer GM. Delivery room management of asphyxiated term and near-term infants. Neonatology. 2021;118(4):487-99.
4. Cristina Rossi A, Prefumo F. Antepartum and intrapartum risk factors for neonatal hypoxic–ischemic encephalopathy: a systematic review with meta-analysis. Curr Opin Obstet Gynecol. 2019;31(6):410-7.
5. National Collaborating Centre for Women's and Children's Health (UK). Intrapartum Care: Care of Healthy Women and Their Babies During Childbirth. London: National Institute for Health and Care Excellence (UK); 2017 (NICE Clinical Guidelines, No. 190.)
6. Raghuraman N, Cahill AG. Update on fetal monitoring: Overview of approaches and management of category II tracings. Obstet Gynecol Clin North Am. 2017;44(4):615-24.

4

Fetal Therapy

Sudarshan Suresh, S Suresh

INTRODUCTION
- The fetus developing in the womb was considered inaccessible during its antenatal journey till Liley in 1962 demonstrated that an Rh isoimmunized fetus could be treated in utero by intraperitoneal transfusions therapy. Today, several fetal conditions can be treated percutaneously with acceptable success rates.
- The International Society for Prenatal Diagnosis in its consensus statement mentioned that "fetal therapy is offered for conditions that will worsen in utero if left untreated and will result in increased perinatal mortality or morbidity."

OBJECTIVES
- To learn the importance of fetal medicine
- To understand the clinical and ethical aspects of fetal therapy
- To learn the role of fetal therapy in various fetal medical and surgical conditions

WHAT IS FETAL THERAPY?
- Fetal therapy, also known as fetal treatment, offers an intervention before birth for the purpose of correcting, treating, or diminishing the deleterious effects of a fetal condition.
- It includes medical interventions—such as medications given to the mother to cross the placenta and reach the fetus—and surgical interventions to help an unborn baby that might die or be disabled if no action was taken. The objective is to maximize gestational age prior to delivery and minimize the consequences of the defect and improve fetal outcome.

Types of Fetal Therapy (Box 1)
Fetal therapy may be broadly classified into four headings:
1. Medical therapy
2. Percutaneous needle-based therapy
3. Fetoscopic surgical therapy
4. Open fetal surgery

Ethics of Fetal Therapy
- Management of a fetus with an anomaly by fetal treatment has significant ethical constraints. In many conditions, adequate information on the long-term outcomes of a procedure may not be available due to a dearth of well-controlled randomized controlled trials (RCTs) in evaluating the benefits of fetal therapy for prenatal conditions. Ethical dilemmas are complicated further by the presence of the laws of the land and religious beliefs.
- Counseling for prenatal therapy poses many challenges. The operator should explain to the couple clearly, in simple understandable language, the nature of the procedure and its benefits and risks, both short term and long term. The decision to undergo the procedure must be taken by the patient and a detailed consent form must be obtained. The costs of the procedure should also be discussed.

The Fetal Treatment Team

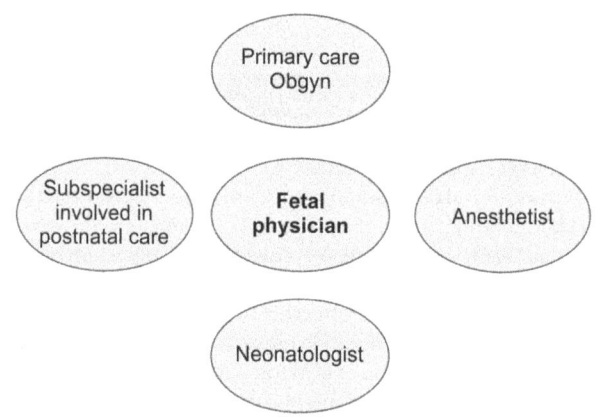

FETAL THERAPY

Fetal Arrhythmias
- Fetal arrhythmias are seen in about 2% of the population and most often are detected during a routine obstetric exam. The most common arrhythmia is atrial ectopics which often run a benign course.

BOX 1: An overview of fetal therapy.

Prevention of birth defects:
- Folic acid
- Periconceptual glucose control in diabetes

Hormonal therapy:
- Thyroid hormone
- Antenatal corticosteroids for acceleration of pulmonary maturation
- Corticosteroids for congenital adrenal hyperplasia

Prevention and treatment of anemia:
- Anti-D globulin (Rhogam) at 28 weeks' gestation to prevent erythroblastosis
- Intrauterine transfusion with ultrasound guidance for severe fetal anemia

Treatment and prevention of infection:
- Spiramycin for toxoplasmosis
- Zidovudine or other agents for human immunodeficiency virus
- Antibiotics for premature rupture of membranes
- Intrapartum penicillin for group B streptococcal disease

Treatment of cardiac arrhythmias: Agents administered to mother, injected into amniotic fluid or directly into the fetus

Fetal surgery—highly selected cases: Percutaneous ultrasound-guided laser for vascular occlusion under direct vision:
- TTTS recipient fetal hydrops
- TRAP acardiac twin
- Placental chorioangioma
- Solid CPAM with attempt at occlusion of a feeding vessel (after corticosteroid use)

Radiofrequency ablation (RFA):
- TRAP
- Bronchopulmonary sequestration
- Sacrococcygeal or mediastinal teratoma (feed vessel size dependent)

Percutaneous ultrasound-guided pig-tailed shunt:
- Macrocystic CPAM (after percutaneous drainage and corticosteroid use)
- Pleural effusions (pleurodesis or thoracoamniotic shunt)
- *Lower urinary tract obstruction:* Posterior urethral valves, urethral stenosis, urethral atresia

Percutaneous ultrasound-guided fetal cardiac balloon valvuloplasty: Aortic stenosis with possible development of hypoplasia left heart syndrome, prematurely closed foramen ovale

Open maternal fetal therapy:
- CPAM solid or cystic
- Sacrococcygeal or mediastinal teratoma

EXIT delivery:
- Cervical teratoma with hydrops and polyhydramnios secondary to esophageal compression
- CHAOS caused by laryngeal obstruction

(CHAOS: congenital high airway obstruction; CPAM: congenital pulmonary adenomatoid malformation; EXIT: ex utero intrapartum treatment; TRAP: twin-reversed arterial perfusion; TTTS: twin-to-twin transfusion syndrome)

- The incidence of structural or functional heart disease is 50% in bradyarrhythmias versus 10% in tachyarrhythmias **(Table 1)**.

Management of fetal tachyarrhythmia: Sustained tachycardia at >200–220 bpm, noted over 50% of time monitored, is an indication for prenatal therapy. Management depends upon the gestational age, presence of hydrops, maternal conditions, or risk factors that may impact therapy. Transplacental therapy with oral antiarrhythmic agents are the first line for management, except for fetuses with hydrops when a combination of direct fetal treatment concomitantly is considered. Maternal risks are rare; however, close monitoring of calcium, magnesium, electrolytes, and ECG (to look for long QT syndromes), and if feasible drug level, to reduce the risks, is advised **(Table 2)**.

Management of fetal bradyarrhythmia: Treatment of fetal bradyarrhythmias is not warranted at most times. Fetuses tolerate heart rate above 60 bpm well. If there is sustained bradycardia of <55 bpm, risk of hydrops exists and may necessitate delivery or neonatal therapy. Structural assessment [to rule out heterotaxy atrioventricular septal defect (AVSD), congenitally corrected transposition of the great arteries (cc-TGA)] and evaluation of autoimmune causes [Anti-Ro, Ant-LA, maternal IgG and IgM for TORCH (toxoplasmosis, rubella, cytomegalovirus, herpes simplex, and HIV)] is essential. Treatment with dexamethasone is considered primarily for immune-mediated fetal bradycardia to prevent hydrops.

Fetal Goiter (Fig. 1)

- Fetal goiter is suspected when the thyroid circumference or diameter >95th percentile for gestational age. It is usually noticed after 22 weeks with normal or increased liquor.
- Fetal goiters could be due to maternal hyper- or hypothyroidism or can happen in a euthyroid mother. Transplacental passage of antithyroid drugs given to the mother is the most common cause of fetal hypothyroidism.
- Confirmation of the diagnosis of fetal hypothyroidism is done by demonstration of increased levels of thyroid stimulating hormone (TSH) levels in the fetal blood.
- The treatment is to ensure that maternal thyroid values are kept at the upper limit of normal. Direct fetal treatment is done by injecting intra-amniotic L thyroxine at a dose of 100–200 µg/kg and this is repeated at 1–2 weekly intervals until delivery at term.

Fetal Anemia: Intrauterine Fetal Blood Transfusion

- Fetal hemoglobin concentration increases with gestational age with median values ranging from 10.6 at 18 weeks to

TABLE 1: Summary of fetal arrhythmias.

Fetal heart rate (beats/min)	Fetal heart rate pattern	Fetal echocardiography findings	Probable diagnosis
100–160	Variable	1:1 conduction, normal atrioventricular (AV) interval	Sinus rhythm
<80	Fixed	• AV dissociation • Normal atrial rate	Complete heart block
50–180	• Irregular • Possibly abrupt drops in heart rate	• 1:1 conduction with early atrial signals • Blocked atrial ectopics	• Atrial or ventricular premature beats • Blocked atrial beats (most common) • Blocked atrial bigeminy • Possibly "low-grade" ectopic atrial tachycardia
180–200	• Minimal variability • Smooth increases	• 1:1 conduction • Normal AV intervals	Sinus tachycardia
180–220	• Essentially normal • Abrupt drops to normal	• 1:1 conduction • Normal AV intervals	Persistent or permanent junctional reciprocating tachycardia type supraventricular tachycardia
200–220	Fixed	2:1 atrial to ventricular conduction	Atrial flutter
>240	• Fixed • Episodic break to 100–160 beats/min	1:1 conduction	Supraventricular tachycardia

TABLE 2: Maternal medical administration.

Drug	Dosage	Indication	Therapeutic range
Digoxin	• *Loading dose*: 1,200–1,500 µg/day, Q8H • *Maintenance dose*: 375–750 µg/day, Q8H PO • Direct IM Rx to the fetus in severely hydropic status, with low BPP	First line in SVT without hydrops	0.7–2 ng/mL
Flecainide	100–300 mg/day 8–12 hours PO	• First line in SVT with hydrops • Second line in SVT without hydrops nonresponsive to Rx	0.2–1 µg/mL
Sotalol	160–480 mg/day Q8–12 hours PO	First line Rx in atrial flutter	Levels not monitored

(BPP: biophysical profile; IM: intramuscular; SVT: supraventricular tachycardia)

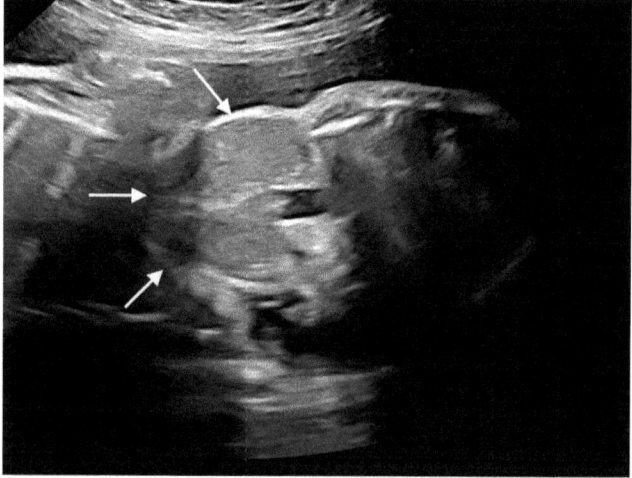

Fig. 1: *Fetal goiter*: Coronal section of the fetal neck showing an enlarged thyroid gland (arrows). Note the tracheal compression in the middle.

13.8 at 40 weeks. Fetal anemia can result from immune and nonimmune causes. Maternal red cell alloimmunization due to RhD antigen is the most common cause of immune anemia The etiology for nonimmune anemia includes infections like parvovirus, cytomegalovirus (CMV), toxoplasmosis, inherited genetic disorders like lysosomal storage disorders, alpha thalassemia, Fanconi anemia, G6PD deficiency, and pyruvate kinase deficiency. Other causes include fetomaternal hemorrhage and twin-to-twin transfusion syndrome (TTTS).

- Irrespective of the etiology, an accurate noninvasive diagnosis of fetal anemia is made by measuring the peak systolic velocity of the middle cerebral artery and calculating the multiples of median (MoM) for that gestation. A middle cerebral arterial peak systolic velocity (MCA PSV) of >1.5 MoM for gestational age, if used as a screening test for moderate-to-severe fetal anemia, has a

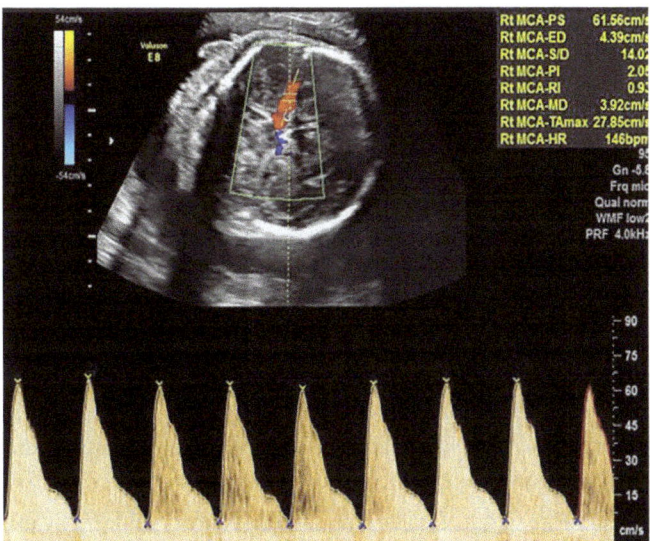

Fig. 2: Doppler of the middle cerebral artery in a 28-week fetus showing high-peak systolic velocity (61 cm/sec >1.5 MoM), which indicates severe fetal anemia.

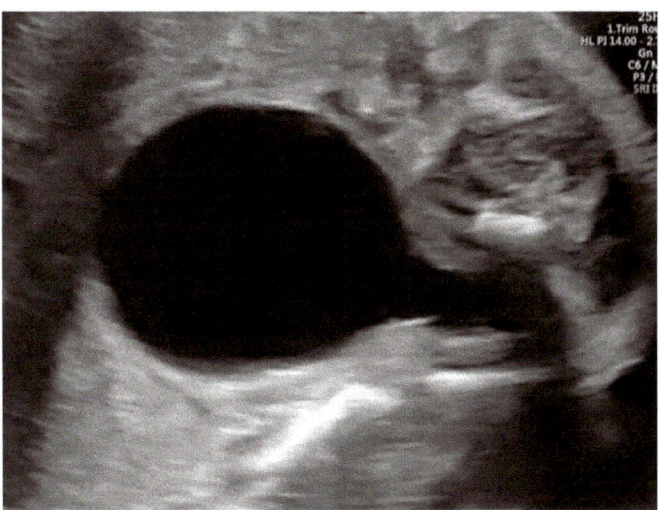

Fig. 3: Distended bladder with dilated posterior urethra in a case of posterior urethral valve.

sensitivity of >95% with a false-positive rate of 12%. False-positive rates can be reduced to 5% if serial measurements are taken which show an increasing trend.

Management of Rh isoimmunization: Rh isoimmunization is diagnosed in a pregnant woman by a positive indirect Coombs test and estimating the Rh antibody titers in her serum. A titer of >1:16 is considered to be an indication for serial MCA monitoring and a titer increasing from 1:16 to 1:64 or 1:64 to 1:256 is considered significant. However, the decision to intervene is done by MCA PSV MoM and not by serial titers. A pregnant woman previously diagnosed to have a fetus with severe anemia should have serial MCA Dopplers, starting at least 8–10 weeks prior to the time of diagnosis in the previous pregnancy. If the MCA PSV is >1.5 MoM, an intrauterine transfusion is planned **(Fig. 2)**.

Intrauterine Transfusion

- The routes of intrauterine transfusion include intraperitoneal, intravascular, and intracardiac routes. Of these, intravascular route is the most preferred. The donor blood which is O negative leukodepleted, washed, and packed cells with a hematocrit of 75–80% is transfused. The final desired hematocrit could be decided as per the gestational age or having a fixed target of 45–50 for nonhydropic fetuses. In the author's own experience, a high-volume transfusion helps to prolong the interval between transfusions.
  Fetoplacental volume (mL) is calculated by the formula: 1.046 + fetal weight (g) × 0.14.
  Volume to be transfused = Fetoplacental blood volume × (Final hct – Initial hct)/Donor hct
- During the transfusion, the fetal hematocrit is checked to ensure that the transfusion is stopped after an adequate volume has been given. Subsequent transfusions are based on fetal MCA PSV. Survival rates of over 95% are reported and our own experience of over 220 transfusions provides a similar picture.

Bladder Outlet Obstruction

- Fetal lower urinary tract obstructions can be due to urethral atresia or posterior urethral valve. It can be associated with severe oligohydramnios, pulmonary hypoplasia, neonatal death, end-stage renal disease in 25–30% needing renal transplant or dialysis by 5 years of age.
- Treatment of posterior urethral valves is either by vesicoamniotic shunting or fetal cystoscopic fulguration of the posterior urethral valves. Both these procedures help to improve survival at birth but have not been shown to improve long-term renal function **(Fig. 3)**.

Vesicoamniotic shunting:

- The procedure involves placing of a double pigtail shunt between the bladder and the amniotic fluid. Fetal paralysis and analgesia are achieved by an intramuscular injection of fentanyl and pancuronium or vecuronium. A double pigtail shunt is introduced with the fetal end in the bladder and the other end in the amniotic cavity. Urine will be seen spurting out of the shunt into the amniotic cavity. The specific complications of this procedure include improper placement, displacement of the shunt, and urinary ascites due to leak from the bladder. If the shunt is retained, it is removed after the baby is delivered and fulguration of the valves is done.
- The PLUTO (Percutaneous shunting in Lower Urinary Tract Obstruction) trial concluded that while vesicoamniotic shunting improved survival rates, it did not significantly improve long-term fetal renal function. Case selection and parent choices need to be considered.

Pleural Effusion

- Fetal hydrothorax or pleural effusion occurs in 1:10,000 to 1:15,000 pregnancies. This can be primary or secondary [congenital pulmonary airway malformation (CPAM), chromosomal abnormality, anemia, congenital heart disease]. It may regress in 20% of cases. However, it can result in hydrops and mortality varies between 22 and 55%. Evaluation includes a detailed anatomical assessment to rule out associated malformations, infection screen, and karyotyping/chromosomal microarray.
- Expectant management is a reasonable option for isolated effusions without hydrops but would need close monitoring. Serial thoracocentesis can be tried and in many cases, the fluid accumulation may reduce as gestational age advances. In cases of impending hydrops, and if the gestational age is <32 weeks, a thoracoamniotic shunt is placed between the thoracic cavity and the amniotic fluid. The procedure is similar to that described for vesicoamniotic shunting. The overall survival rate in nonhydropic cases with any form of therapy is about 65%.

Congenital Diaphragmatic Hernia

- Congenital diaphragmatic hernia has a prevalence of 1–14/10,000 births and in 86% of cases is left sided. An isolated congenital diaphragmatic hernia (CDH) needs definitive postnatal surgical correction, but the greater concern is of in-utero pulmonary hypoplasia, which results in significant mortality and morbidity postnatally due to respiratory insufficiency and persistent pulmonary artery hypertension despite the surgical therapy. Fetuses with associated malformations and syndromic causes have a poor prognosis. Prenatal therapy hence is restricted to isolated cases with no known genetic etiology diagnosable prenatally. An observed-to-expected lung-to-head ratio (o/e LHR) and location of fetal liver in thoracic cavity are used to classify the severity of the lesion. Outcomes in severe CDH have poor prognosis with survival rate in expectant management in severe cases (o/e LHR <25%) 15% and moderate cases (o/e LHR 25–35%) 40–50%.
- Fetoscopic endoluminal tracheal occlusion (FETO) to improve the lung development is the current accepted prenatal therapeutic option for cases of CDH. Tracheal occlusion prevents egress of lung fluid, enables lung stretch, and accelerates lung growth forming the basis of the treatment. The risk of premature rupture of membranes (PROM) and preterm birth is close to 40%. The procedure needs to be in a setting with significant expertise in fetoscopy and the ability to remove the balloon by USG or fetoscopically prior to birth.

Complications of Monochorionic Twins

All monozygotic twins are monochorionic and share a common placenta. Two important aspects of these placentae which influence outcome are (1) placental vascular anastomoses between the twins and (2) cord insertion sites in the placenta which may be central, marginal, velamentous, or membranous, and this decides the degree of placental territory sharing between the placentae and influences the fetal size. In almost 80–85% of pregnancies, the flow is "balanced" between the twins. In about 9–10%, there is an imbalance of flow with one fetus becoming the donor and the other becoming the recipient and leads to TTTS. In about 9%, the placental territory sharing is inequal and leads to growth restriction of one twin and is called selective fetal growth restriction (sFGR). The other complications are twin anemia polycythemia sequence, twin reversed arterial perfusion sequence (TRAP), and structural anomaly which may be concordant or discordant.

Twin-to-twin Transfusion Syndrome

- In TTTS, one twin (recipient) receives more blood flow from the cotwin resulting in volume overload, more cardiac output, and increased urine production resulting in polyhydramnios. The cotwin (donor) shows oligohydramnios due to reduced blood flow and reduced urine production. The diagnosis of TTTS is made when the single deepest pool of amniotic fluid is <2 cm in the donor sac and >8 cm in the recipient sac between 18 and 20 weeks and more than 10 cm after 20 weeks. Once the diagnosis is made, the staging of TTTS (Quintero) is done as follows:
  - *Stage I*: The bladder of the donor twin is seen.
  - *Stage II*: The bladder of the donor twin is not seen. There is usually a large bladder in the recipient twin.
  - *Stage III*: Critically abnormal Doppler studies in either twin.
  - *Stage IV*: Fetal hydrops (mostly in the recipient twin).
- It is also essential to monitor the cardiac function of the recipient twin and sometimes the cardiac changes due to overload may be very pronounced.
- Untreated severe TTTS can result in extreme preterm delivery, cardiac failure, or demise of one or both twins. If a single fetal demise occurs, it can result in severe neurological sequelae for the cotwin.

Management of TTTS: Fetoscopic laser photocoagulation:

- The treatment of TTTS from stage 2 to 4, between 16 and 26 weeks, is fetoscopic laser photocoagulation of the anastomotic vessels, which ensures that the placenta behaves like that of a dichorionic twin with each fetus having its own circulation. Following this, the excess fluid in the recipient sac is drained. Subsequently, the fetuses

are closely monitored for bladder, liquor, Doppler, and growth.
- The complications of the procedure include preterm premature rupture of the membranes (PPROM), preterm labor, intrauterine demise of one or both the members, twin anemia polycythemia sequence, and rarely placental abruption.
- Management of stage 1 TTTS between 16 and 26 weeks has been a subject of debate for a long time and the present consensus is as follows:
    - *Group 1*: Stage 1 with no maternal discomfort from uterine distension and cervical length > 2.5 cm with weekly assessment of amniotic fluid, Dopplers every 2 weeks, and growth every 3–4 weeks.
    - *Group 2*: Where there is maternal distress and cervical length < 2.5 cm, selective laser photocoagulation can be offered. The optimal management is still in "equipoise."
- Beyond 26 weeks for stage 1, close monitoring and serial amnioreduction, if required, can be performed to gain gestational age.
- The outcomes after laser depend on the center, better outcomes being reported from more experienced centers. Overall, there is a 76% survival of at least 1 twin and about 50% survival of both twins after laser. Long-term neurological sequelae may be seen in about 5% of survivors which is significantly lower than when amnioreduction alone is performed. Hence, selective laser photocoagulation is a definitive treatment and should be considered as standard of care **(Fig. 4)**.

Serial amnioreduction: Amniodrainage is considered if the gestational age is >26 weeks and if the amniotic fluid index is greater than 40 cm and/or there is significant maternal discomfort, a clinically tense uterus, or cervical shortening. It is not a primary treatment of choice when TTTS is diagnosed prior to 26 weeks. While amnioreduction can improve outcome by reducing preterm delivery secondary to polyhydramnios, 25% of survivors may have long-term neurological sequelae.

Selective fetal reduction: Selective fetal reduction can be offered where one fetus is deemed to be preterminal (stage 3/4 TTTS) as an alternative to laser ablation because some parents may feel that a better prognosis for one twin is preferable to a guarded prognosis for both. This can be done either by bipolar cord occlusion or by radiofrequency ablation.

Selective Fetal Growth Restriction

- Selective fetal growth restriction is diagnosed when there is significant discordance in size between the twins. Velamentous cord insertions are often associated with sFGR.
- *The criteria for diagnosis are as follows*:
    - Estimated fetal weight (EFW) of one twin <3rd centile OR
    - Combination of three of the four following criteria:
        - EFW < 10th centile
        - Abdominal circumference (AC) <10th centile
        - EFW discordance of ≥25%
        - Umbilical artery pulsatility index (PI) smaller twin >95th centile
- *According to Gratacos, sFGR is classified into three groups*:
    - *Type 1*: Both twins have normal end-diastolic flow (EDF) in the umbilical arteries. This is seen in 40% of the cases and has a 97% good outcome with expectant management. Risk of intrauterine demise is around 3%. This can be managed expectantly with weekly Dopplers and delivery is effected by about 34 weeks.
    - *Type 2*: Persistent and consistent absent/reversed EDF in the umbilical arteries of the smaller twin. This is seen in 40% of cases and carries the risk of sudden fetal demise in about 17%. Selective fetal reduction can be offered if the gestational age is previable and Dopplers are deteriorating. If Dopplers are stable, then elective delivery can be done by 32 weeks.
    - *Type 3*: Intermittently absent/reversed EDF in the umbilical arteries of the smaller twin. This is seen in 20% of cases. It is preferable to offer selective reduction due to unpredictability of the natural history and sudden intrauterine demise. If it is expectantly managed, delivery should be done by 30–32 weeks.
- The risk of intrauterine demise is between 15 and 20% and in the survivors there is a 15–30% risk of neurological sequelae. Selective fetal reduction can be done by either bipolar cord coagulation or radiofrequency ablation. Both the procedures done in experienced centers have a successful outcome in about 80–85%. Selective laser photocoagulation is also being done for sFGR but poses many challenges.

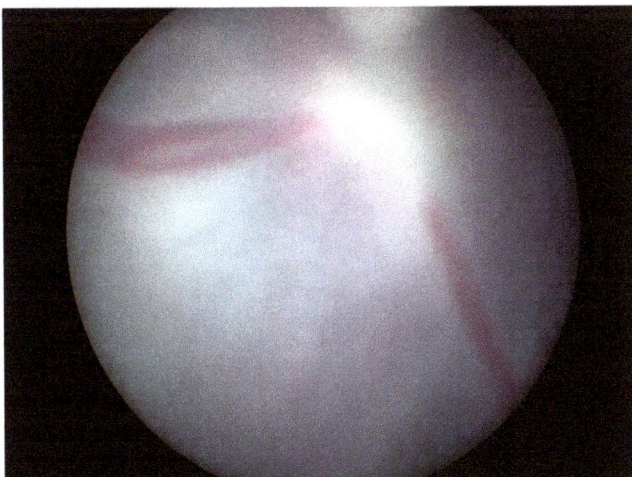

Fig. 4: Fetoscopic selective laser photocoagulation. The blanched area is one of the anastomoses that is being lasered.

Twin-reversed Arterial Perfusion

- TRAP sequence occurs in monochorionic twins wherein one fetus is an acardiac acephalic twin and the other fetus is normal. They share an artery-to-artery anastomosis through which reversal of blood flow happens in the umbilical artery of the acardiac fetus.
- The definitive diagnosis of acardiac twin is established with color flow imaging by demonstrating the presence of blood flow in the reverse direction in the umbilical artery and vein within the abnormal fetus.
- *Treatment options*: Expectant management is recommended in cases where there is spontaneous cessation of flow in the acardiac twin in the first or very early second trimester. The current opinion is to treat the acardiac twin by either bipolar cord occlusion, radiofrequency ablation or interstitial laser. Successful outcome has been reported in about 70–80% of the treated cases.

Meningomyelocele

- Spina bifida—meningomyelocele (MMC) is a congenital anomaly with an incidence of 3–4/10,000 live births. This can occur anywhere along the spine but most commonly occurs at the lumbar or cervical vertebral levels. The primary manifestations include neurologic deficits with motor and somatosensory abnormalities that correspond to the level of the spinal defect, autonomic nervous system injury resulting in impaired bowel and bladder function, and the Chiari II malformation of the hindbrain leading to hydrocephalus and the need for ventriculoperitoneal (VP) shunting.
- The rationale for fetal intervention in MMC is based on a "two-hit" hypothesis for morbidity development, in which the first hit is the original neural tube defect that results in an open spinal canal and the second hit is trauma to the exposed neural elements while the fetus is in utero. Through fetal repair, secondary trauma to the exposed neural elements can be reduced. It was hypothesized that neurologic outcomes for MMC could be improved.
- Currently, advances are being made in terms of research into both refinement of techniques for fetal surgery, using placenta-derived mesenchymal stem cells to augment the repair, and usage of tissue engineering methods. In India, fetal MMC repair has not taken off yet, in part due to the difficulty/support for post care and the risk of maternal complications and procedure costs, thus making patients choose termination of pregnancy over prenatal surgery.

CHAPTER AT A GLANCE

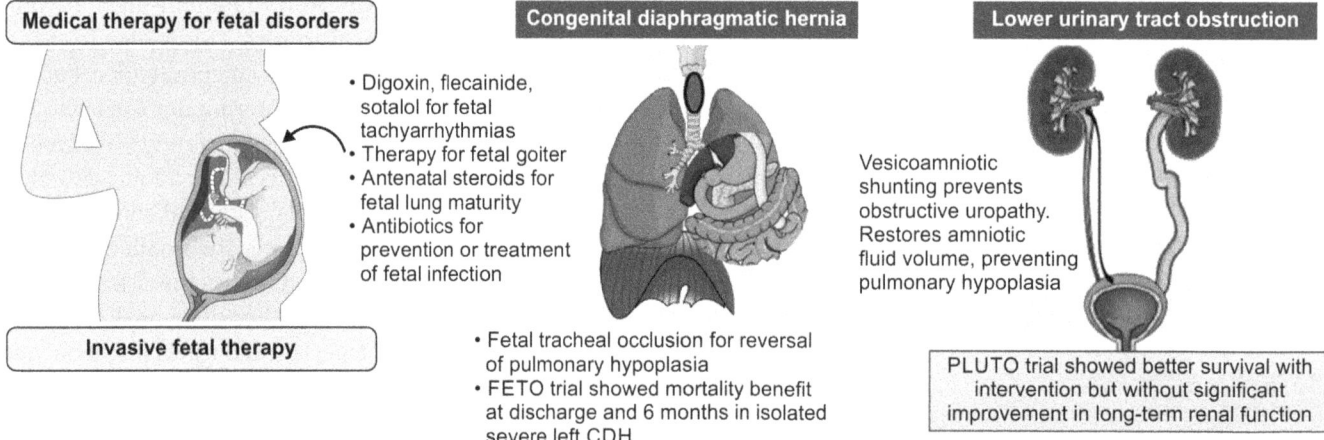

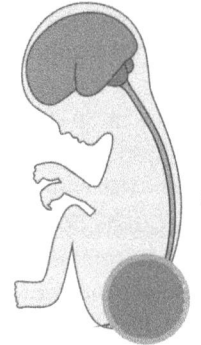

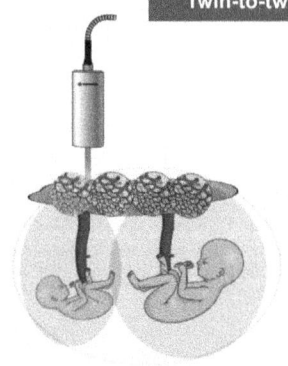

(CDH: congenital diaphragmatic hernia; FETO: fetoscopic endoluminal tracheal occlusion; MOMS: Management of Myelomeningocele Study; PLUTO: Percutaneous shunting in Lower Urinary Tract Obstruction)

KEY POINTS

- Fetal medicine is still a developing field, with many scientific, clinical, and ethical problems to be answered and innovations to be forged.
- When making treatment decisions, the well-being of the expectant mother must take precedence.
- Any fetal intervention carries substantial risk of obstetric complications, including preterm labor, PPROM, membrane separation, and chorioamnionitis; open hysterotomy necessitates eventual delivery by cesarean section.
- Innovation in surgical instrumentation and technique has led to effective percutaneous and fetoscopic minimally invasive therapies for most conditions amenable to prenatal intervention.

SUGGESTED READING

1. Deprest J, Brady P, Nicolaides K, Benachi A, Berg C, Vermeesch J, et al. Prenatal management of the fetus with isolated congenital diaphragmatic hernia in the era of the TOTAL trial. Semin Fetal Neonatal Med. 2014;19(6):338-48.
2. Gratacós E, Lewi L, Muñoz B, Acosta-Rojas R, Hernandez-Andrade E, Martinez JM, et al. A classification system for selective intrauterine growth restriction in monochorionic pregnancies according to umbilical artery Doppler flow in the smaller twin. Ultrasound Obstet Gynecol. 2007;30(1):28-34.
3. Johnson MP, Bennett KA, Rand L, Pamela K, Thom EA. MOMS: obstetrical outcomes and risk factors for obstetrical complications following prenatal surgery. Am J Obstet Gynecol. 2018;215(6):1-16.
4. Lindenburg ITM, Van Kamp IL, Oepkes D. Intrauterine blood transfusion: Current indications and associated risks. Fetal Diagn Ther. 2014;36(4):263-71.
5. Pandya VM, Stirnemann J, Colmant C, Ville Y. Current practice and protocols: endoscopic laser therapy for twin-twin transfusion syndrome. 2020;2(1):34-47.
6. Peranteau WH, Adzick NS, Boelig MM, Flake AW, Hedrick HL, Howell LJ, et al. Thoracoamniotic shunts for the management of fetal lung lesions and pleural effusions: a single-institution review and predictors of survival in 75 cases. J Pediatr Surg. 2015;50(2):301-5.
7. Polak M, Van Vliet G. Therapeutic approach of fetal thyroid disorders. Horm Res Paediatr. 2010;74:1-5.
8. Prefumo F, Fichera A, Fratelli N, Sartori E. Fetal anemia: diagnosis and management. Best Pract Res Clin Obstet Gynaecol. 2019;58:2-14.
9. Ruano R, Sananes N, Wilson C, Au J, Koh CJ, Gargollo P, et al. Fetal lower urinary tract obstruction: proposal for standardized multidisciplinary prenatal management based on disease severity. Ultrasound Obstet Gynecol. 2016;48(4):476-82.
10. Seshadri S, Shinde RR, Ram U. Intrafetal laser for midtrimester TRAP sequence-experience from a single center. Prenat Diagn. 2020;40(7):885-91.

SECTION 2

Fetal Disorders

Ashish Jain, Sangeeta Gupta

- **A General Approach to Antenatally Detected Birth Defects**
  Neerja Gupta, Sakshi Yadav
- **Central Nervous System Malformations**
  Aakash Pandita, Kausik Mandal
- **Fetal Thoracic Malformations**
  Anup Thakur, Nandita Dimri
- **Fetal Cardiovascular Malformations**
  Anup Thakur, Priyanka Karnani
- **Genitourinary System Malformation**
  Kumar Ankur, Seema Thakur
- **Musculoskeletal Malformations**
  Somalika Pal, Manisha Kumar
- **Gastrointestinal Malformations**
  Naveen P Gupta, Chanchal Singh
- **Fetal Growth Restriction**
  Pratima Anand, Sumitra Bachani
- **Hydrops Fetalis**
  Raja Ashok Koganti, Anu Sachdeva
- **Antenatal Counseling for Fetomaternal Conditions**
  Umamaheswari Balakrishnan, Chitra Andrew

CHAPTER 5

A General Approach to Antenatally Detected Birth Defects

Neerja Gupta, Sakshi Yadav

INTRODUCTION

Birth defects (also referred to as congenital anomalies/congenital malformations) are defined as abnormalities of body structure and function that occur during intrauterine life, which can be identified prenatally, at birth, or later in life. Globally, 7.9 million births occur annually with serious birth defects and about 2.95 lakhs of neonates die every year due to these. More than 90% of these births occur in middle- and low-income countries. The prevalence of birth defects in India is 6–7% which translates to around 1.7 million birth defects annually. Birth defects lead to long-term morbidities and thus may impose a huge burden on society, families and, the healthcare system.

With advancements in technology and expertise, most birth defects are detected antenatally. Appropriate counseling and planning the management would greatly alleviate the stress and psychological trauma for parents.

This chapter provides a general approach to antenatally detected malformations.

OBJECTIVES

- To review various types of birth defects identified antenatally and their etiological spectrum
- To discuss the general approach of multidisciplinary planning and management

Types of Birth Defects and Etiology

Birth defects can be categorized either as major or minor according to its impact on an individual.

Major birth defects have significant medical, functional, or cosmetic impact on an individual and require either surgical or medical intervention. Around 2–3% of all live births and 15–20% of stillbirths have at least one major birth defect. Examples include neural tube defects, cleft lip/palate, abdominal wall defects, and hydronephrosis.

Minor birth defects although more prevalent (4% of the general population) have little cosmetic or functional consequences. Some examples include clinodactyly, simian crease, ear tag, tongue-tie, and polydactyly. The presence of two or more minor defects and their particular pattern may be suggestive of a syndrome.

Birth defects can involve a single structure (isolated) or developmental abnormality of two or more systems (multiple malformation syndrome).

Based upon the morphogenesis, the defects may be classified as malformation, deformation, disruption, or dysplasia (**Flowchart 1**).

Etiologically, birth defects may have chromosomal (10–15%), monogenic (15–20%), and environmental (including maternal illness and infection, drugs, physical agents) (10%) causes. The cause remains unidentified in about 40–50%. Isolated abnormalities with varying prevalence of chromosomal abnormalities are listed in **Table 1**.

Flowchart 1: Classification of malformation based on morphogenesis.

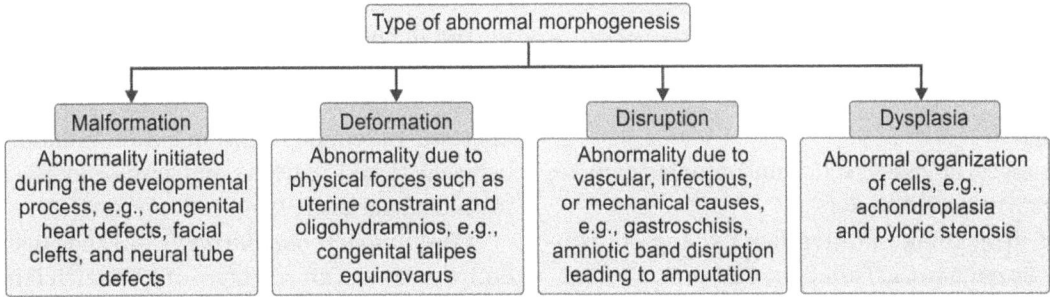

TABLE 1: Frequency of chromosomal abnormalities in common birth defects.

Type of fetal birth defect	Percentage of chromosomal abnormality
Hydrocephalus/ventriculomegaly	10–16%
Holoprosencephaly	55%
Dandy–Walker malformation	35%
Cleft lip, +/− palate	21%
Tracheoesophageal fistula/esophageal atresia	6–10%
Cardiac structural anomalies*	40%
Congenital diaphragmatic hernia	5–15%
Omphalocele	4.5–35%
Gastroschisis	0–2%
Duodenal atresia	20–50%
Club foot (b/l)	3–5%
Hydronephrosis/multicystic kidneys	10–12%

*About 4% of fetuses with cardiac defects (especially conotruncal anomalies) have 22q11.2 deletion on chromosomal microarray.

For the majority of isolated localized defects, the outcome after surgical intervention is generally excellent. A multifactorial recurrence risk of about 2–5% may be given to the unaffected parents. However, for the multiple malformation syndromes where the causes may be chromosomal, monogenic, or environmental, a precise diagnosis using chromosomal analysis or DNA testing is needed for accurate recurrence risk assessment.

Approach

Whenever a fetus is detected to have a birth defect, the following steps of evaluation are recommended. It includes a detailed history, ultrasound examination to look for other associated abnormalities, need assessment for invasive testing, subsequent antenatal, and postnatal follow-up for further management. Fetal autopsy is offered in cases of medical termination of pregnancy due to fetal abnormalities or stillbirths.

Maternal History

A detailed maternal and family history should be taken including:
- Maternal age
- Maternal medical illnesses such as uncontrolled diabetes and connective tissue disorders
- History of drug intake [antiepileptics, angiotensin-converting enzyme (ACEs) inhibitors, lithium, retinoids, etc.], alcohol/smoking/any drug abuse.
- History of maternal fever with or without rash or exposure to zika virus.
- Pregnancy complications such as oligohydramnios, polyhydramnios, and decreased fetal movements.
- History of periconceptional folic acid intake in case of neural tube defects.
- History of any recurrent abortions/stillbirth/baby with congenital malformation/s in the earlier conception or the family.
- History of consanguinity
- Three-generation pedigree chart

Fetal Ultrasonography

The presence of any major anomaly on antenatal ultrasound anomaly scan should prompt the fetal medicine expert to look for additional abnormalities. The presence of multiple malformations points toward an underlying genetic etiology which may be either chromosomal or single-gene disorders. With the routine use of antenatal ultrasound in the first and second trimesters, the majority of the major birth defects can be detected during the pregnancy. Still, some of the evolving birth defects can be missed during earlier antenatal scans and are better diagnosed in later gestation such as cortical malformations and sulci-gyri patterns in the brain. **Table 2** gives the list of commonly encountered fetal abnormalities, their possible etiologies, and the test required.

Fetal Magnetic Resonance Imaging

With the advent of three-dimensional (3D)/four-dimensional (4D) technology in ultrasound and high-resolution imaging, very few cases require fetal magnetic resonance imaging (MRI). It is mostly used as an adjunct imaging technique mainly for the central nervous system and thoracic abnormalities. It is also useful in cases associated with oligoamnios where ultrasound evaluation is suboptimal. It is generally performed in the late second or third trimester depending on the indication. Common indications for antenatal fetal MRI include brain malformations such as ventriculomegaly, cortical malformation, intracranial hemorrhage, corpus-related abnormalities, congenital cystic adenoid malformation (CCAM), neural tube defects, and abdominal masses.

Fetal Genetic Testing

In case of antenatally detected structural birth defects with a possible underlying genetic etiology, an option of invasive testing (amniocentesis/chorionic villous sampling) is offered to the couple. Chorionic villus sampling is performed between 11 and 14 weeks and amniocentesis after 16 weeks to obtain fetal tissue for genetic tests.

Chromosomal microarray (CMA) has been recommended by American College of Obstetricians and Gynecologists (ACOG) for multiple structural birth defects as

TABLE 2: List of commonly encountered fetal birth defects, their possible etiologies, and the test required.

Fetal birth defect	Etiology	Associated fetal abnormalities to be looked for	Genetic testing
Holoprosencephaly	• Trisomy 13 • Single gene defect	Polydactyly, heart, kidney, diaphragm, and cleft lip/palate	Karyotype ± CMA ES#
Microcephaly	• Cytomegalovirus • Zika virus • Chromosomal • Monogenic	• Other CNS anomalies such as lissencephaly, agenesis of the corpus callosum • Features of TORCH infections like echogenic bowel, periventricular calcification, and early-onset IUGR	Karyotype ± CMA TORCH serology ES#
Hydrocephalus	• Chromosomal • A single gene (L1CAM gene*, ciliopathies) (including Joubert and Meckel–Gruber syndrome, Walker–Warburg syndrome)	Adducted thumbs, corpus callosum, and cerebellar peduncles	CMA ES#
Dandy–Walker malformation	Chromosomal abnormalities, microdeletions, genetic syndromes including Joubert and Meckel–Gruber syndrome, Walker–Warburg syndrome, congenital infection, or teratogens	Gyri/sulci abnormalities (lissencephaly), polydactyly, and microphthalmia	CMA ES#
Microretrognathia	• Single gene defect • Treacher Collins syndrome or hemifacial microsomia	• Cleft palate • Ear anomalies	ES# if associated anomalies**
Esophageal atresia with tracheoesophageal fistula (TEF)	• Chromosomal • VACTERL association (vertebral, anal atresia, cardiac, TEF, renal, and limb abnormalities)	Spine, limbs, kidneys, genitourinary system, and cardiovascular	Karyotype ± CMA
• Cardiac defects • Atrioventricular defect • Conotruncal abnormalities	Chromosomal	Size of the thymus in conotruncal malformation	Karyotype ± CMA
Congenital diaphragmatic hernia	Chromosomal/single gene	Cardiac defects, renal, and CNS malformations	Karyotype ± CMA ES#: In case of familial recurrence
Omphalocele	Isolated/OEIS/limb body wall complex/Beckwith–Wiedemann syndrome (BWS)	Spine, foot, limbs, and craniofacial abnormalities like macroglossia	Karyotype ± CMA MLPA: If features of BWS
Spina bifida	Chromosomal if associated with other abnormalities	Thorough evaluation for structural abnormalities	Karyotype ± CMA
Occipital encephalocele	• Chromosomal • Single gene	Bilateral polycystic kidneys, and postaxial polydactyly (rule out Meckel–Gruber syndrome)	Karyotype ± CMA ES#
Large echogenic kidneys	ARPKD/ADPKD/Meckel Gruber	To check for parental kidneys	ES#
Limb reduction defects	Isolated/single gene/chromosomal		Karyotype; ES#
Skeletal dysplasia	Single gene	Polydactyly	ES#

*Check family history #if phenotype suggestive.
**Extensive genetic counseling is needed because of nonlethal nature # only when a monogenic etiology is suspected.
(Whole/clinical exome as per provisional diagnosis). Whole ES is preferred to clinical exome for nonspecific fetal malformations.
(ARPKD: autosomal recessive polycystic kidney disease; ADPKD: autosomal dominant polycystic kidney disease; CMA: chromosomal microarray; CNS: central nervous system; ES: exome sequencing; IUGR: intrauterine growth restriction; MLPA: multiplex-ligation dependent probe amplification; OEIS: omphalocele, exstrophy, imperforate anus, spinal defect; TORCH: toxoplasmosis, other (syphilis, varicella-zoster, parvovirus b19), rubella, cytomegalovirus, and herpes)

the yield of CMA is higher than the karyotype by 4–5%. In routine practice, if there is a suspicion of common chromosomal aneuploidies, rapid testing using quantitative fluorescent polymerase chain reaction/fluorescent in situ hybridization (QFPCR/FISH) is performed first, followed by CMA. CMA-negative fetuses can be subjected to exome sequencing (ES) if there is a high possibility of genetic etiology.

Exome sequencing can also be performed directly in case of highly suspected monogenic etiology based on pedigree and the fetal phenotype such as skeletal dysplasia and Noonan syndrome. One of the largest cohorts studied by Lord et al. [as a part of Prenatal Assessment of Genomes and Exomes (PAGE) study], revealed an overall yield of 8.5% and maximum yield of 15% in fetuses with multiple malformations.

It is prudent to provide adequate pre-test and post-test counseling as these genomic tests (CMA and ES) can result in variants of unknown significance and incidental findings. The turnaround time for the test results is varying from 2 to 6 weeks. Maternal cell contamination needs to be ruled out before conducting genomic testing. It is important to remember that the results of such testing may have their limitations as fetal phenotype might not have evolved fully to interpret the results correctly. Fetal samples for DNA and RNA studies must be stored for further validation studies.

Evaluate Fetus by Fetal Autopsy

As per the current prenatal diagnostic act, if any lethal abnormality/multiple malformations are detected before 20 weeks, an option of termination followed by conventional autopsy (CA) or minimally invasive autopsy (MIA) should be given to the couple. Performing postnatal autopsy may help in confirming the antenatal findings and additional abnormalities may be detected which have been missed on ultrasonography. MIA involves performing radiological investigations such as computed tomography (CT), MRI, and USG along with guided biopsies of organs involved in the fetus postabortion. Many researchers have focused on evaluating the role of MIA in fetuses as compared to CA. In 2019, Votino et al. studied the feasibility of doing MIA (USG-based) and found that there was high sensitivity of MIA in detecting abnormalities as compared to CA and can be performed as early as 11 weeks. The detection rate of brain abnormalities was ~90% with a specificity of 85%. Overall, autopsy provides additional information in around 30–40% of cases that contributed to the diagnosis or assisted in parental counseling.

POSTNATAL EXAMINATION

Postnatal Evaluation

Fetuses with major congenital malformations should be delivered in a tertiary care hospital and require a multidisciplinary approach for appropriate management. Late detection of some of the congenital malformation requires a close follow-up during pregnancy and also postnatally. For example, antenatal detection of mild urinary tract dilatation requires the pregnancy to be followed up in the third trimester and postnatally to look for progression of dilatation. Postnatal detailed renal sonography is performed to look for the degree of dilatation and to decipher the etiology and initiate proper management. Expert opinion from a pediatric urologist/nephrologist may be sought accordingly.

A comprehensive head-to-toe and front-to-back clinical screening of the newborn as listed below is required to find minor anomalies and rule out associated internal malformations. A thorough history and maternal risk factors assessment and family history are helpful.

Comprehensive head-to-toe and front-to-back clinical screening of the newborn includes the following:

- *Head*: Microcephaly, macrocephaly, and scalp defects
- *Face*: Dysmorphic facies, facial asymmetry, epicanthal folds, cataract, external ear malformations, retrognathia, and orofacial clefts.
- Nose abnormalities
- Ear abnormalities
- *Eye abnormalities*: Aniridia/coloboma
- *Chest*: Pectus excavatum/carinatum
- *Cardiac*: Congenital heart defects
- *Upper and lower limbs*: Polydactyly, syndactyly, clinodactyly, oligodactyly, brachydactyly, limb length discrepancy, joint contracture/laxity, and club foot.
- *Abdomen*: Umbilical hernia
- *Spine*: Kyphosis/scoliosis/tuft of hair
- Urogenital abnormality
- Anorectal malformation
- Neurological assessment for floppiness
- Presence of any skin hemangiomas, skin tags, pigmentation, and café-au-lait spots.

The diagnostic approach for the postnatal detection of multiple malformations includes karyotype with or without CMA. In the case of strongly suspected Mendelian etiology, either single-gene sequencing (if the diagnosis is certain and the gene is small or has a hot spot mutation) or ES (for a nonspecific or genetically heterogenous condition) is performed. Genetic testing should be performed with pretest and post-test counseling about the nature of the report, variant of unknown significance, limitations, turn around time, cost, and further implications.

To conclude, antenatal detection of fetal malformation initiates a battery of tests including eliciting specific maternal and family history. It is important to seek a clinical genetics consultation to rule out underlying genetic etiology and to make a precise diagnosis and provide adequate genetic counseling to prevent the recurrences in the subsequent pregnancies.

CHAPTER AT A GLANCE

```
Antenatally detected fetal malformation
    │
    │  • Detailed maternal history
    │  • Family history
    │  • Three-generation pedigree charting
    ▼
Detailed ultrasonography and echocardiography
    │
    ├─────────────────────────┬─────────────────────────┐
    ▼                                                   ▼
Isolated malformation                       Multiple fetal malformations
    │                                                   │
    • Prenatal counseling                               • Genetic counseling
    • Prognostication and genetic testing               • Invasive testing for genetic testing
      depending upon the type of abnormality              (karyotyping chromosomal microarray and/or
    │                                                     whole-exome sequencing and targeted gene panels)
    ▼
    • Pregnancy follow-up
    • Postnatal evaluation, multidisciplinary care,     • Malformations with poor outcomes—offer termination
      and follow-up abnormality                           and autopsy if detected before 20 weeks
                                                        • Postnatal evaluation in case of late detection
```

KEY POINTS

Steps in the evaluation of antenatally detected malformation:
- Perform a detailed anomaly scan to rule out multiple malformations.
- Classify as isolated or multiple; major or minor; lethal versus nonlethal.
- Clinical genetics opinion and genetic counseling.
- Perform appropriate invasive testing if genetic testing is opted for with adequate pretest and post-test counseling.
- Seek individual specialty opinion especially for the nonlethal malformations.
- Discuss about termination of pregnancy and fetal autopsy in case of timely detection of lethal and severe malformations.
- Thorough postnatal genetic evaluation of the fetus (fetal autopsy)/live born to exclude syndromic association and genetic counseling.

SUGGESTED READING

1. American College of Obstetricians and Gynecologists. Committee Opinion No. 581. The use of chromosomal microarray analysis in prenatal diagnosis. Obstet Gynecol. 2013;122(6):1374-7.
2. Christianson AL, Howson CP, Modell B. March of dimes global report on birth defects: The hidden toll of dying and disabled children. White Plains. New York, USA: March of Dimes Birth Defects Foundation; 2006.
3. Lewis C, Hutchinson JC, Riddington M, Hill M, Arthurs OJ, Fisher J, et al. Minimally invasive autopsy for fetuses and children based on a combination of post-mortem MRI and endoscopic examination: a feasibility study. Health Technol Assess. 2019;23(46):1-104.
4. Lord J, McMullan DJ, Eberhardt RY, Rinck G, Maher ER, Hamilton SJ, et al. Prenatal Assessment of Genomes and Exomes Consortium. Prenatal exome sequencing analysis in fetal structural anomalies detected by ultrasonography (PAGE): a cohort study. Lancet. 2019;393(10173):747-57.
5. Milunsky A, Jeff M. Milunsky JM. Genetic Disorders and the Fetus: Diagnosis, Prevention, and Treatment. 8th edition. Hoboken: Wiley Blackwell; 2021.
6. National Health Portal. Congenital anomalies (birth defects). [online] Available from https://www.nhp.gov.in/disease/gynaecology-and-obstetrics/congenital-anomalies-birth-defects. [Last accessed November, 2021].
7. Paladini D, Volpe P. Ultrasound of Congenital Fetal Anomalies (Differential Diagnosis and Prognostic Indicators), 2nd edition. Boca Raton: CRC Press; 2007.
8. Votino C, Cos Sanchez T, Bessieres B, Segers V, Kadhim H, Razavi F, et al. Minimally invasive fetal autopsy using ultrasound: A feasibility study. Ultrasound Obstet Gynecol. 2018;52(6):776-83.
9. World Health Organization. Congenital anomalies. [online] Available from https://www.who.int/health-topics/congenital-anomalies#tab=tab_1. [Last accessed November, 2021].
10. World Health Organization. Management of Birth Defects and Haemoglobin Disorders: Report of a Joint WHO-March of Dimes Meeting. Geneva: WHO; 2006.

Central Nervous System Malformations

Aakash Pandita, Kausik Mandal

INTRODUCTION

Central nervous system (CNS) malformations are one of the most common major malformations found in a fetus or a neonate and represent an important cause of morbidity and mortality in children. The incidence varies from 0.1 to 0.2% and 3 to 6% in live births and stillbirths, respectively.

Various environmental factors including folic acid deficiency and teratogens are implicated in the genesis of malformations of the CNS. On the other hand, there are various chromosomal and single-gene disorders which give rise to specific patterns of malformations; recognition of such genetic disorders is necessary for management, prognostication, diagnostic genetic testing, and prenatal diagnosis to prevent recurrences. Routine antenatal screening with ultrasound at 18–22 weeks of gestation has improved the antenatal diagnosis of fetal CNS malformations. Magnetic resonance imaging (MRI) may be required only in select cases with uncertainty of diagnosis. Ultrasound has a diagnostic accuracy of 68% compared to 93% with MRI.

OBJECTIVES

- To review the normal CNS development
- To discuss the various congenital CNS malformations
- To discuss antenatal diagnosis of various CNS malformations
- To discuss the role of genetic counseling

NORMAL CENTRAL NERVOUS SYSTEM DEVELOPMENT

The process of CNS development consists of five basic stages. These include:

1. *Induction*: The underlying mesoderm signals the overlying ectoderm to develop into neural tissue.
2. *Neural tube formation*: The neural ectoderm folds to form neural tube and runs for most of the length of the embryo. Fusion of neural tube occurs by 18–26 days after conception. Failure of closure of neural tube leads to neural tube defects (NTDs).
3. *Regionalization and specification*: Specification occurs in both the rostral/caudal and dorsal/ventral axes of the neural tube. The forebrain, midbrain, and hindbrain develop at the rostral end of the tube, while the spinal cord develops more caudally.
4. *Proliferation and migration*: The most dorsal cells of the tube, known as neural crest, migrate away to form the peripheral nervous system. The germinal matrix, an area adjacent to the lumen of the neural tube, provides stem cells which act as precursors for the neurons, oligodendrocytes, and astrocytes. These precursor cells migrate along specialized cells known as radial glial cells between 3rd and 5th months of gestation, to reach their final and specific locations among one of the six layers of the cerebral cortex. Any disturbance of the migration results in schizencephaly and lissencephaly.
5. *Connection and selection*: After cells are specified and are at their appropriate locations, axon outgrowth and synapse formation occur. However, failure to establish the correct connections leads to apoptosis of some of the cells due to lack of survival factors produced by the target cells.

CLINICAL CLASSIFICATIONS OF CENTRAL NERVOUS SYSTEM MALFORMATIONS

- Ventricular system (ventriculomegaly, aqueduct stenosis)
- NTDs (encephalocele, anencephaly, myelomeningocele)
- Midline abnormalities [holoprosencephaly (HPE), agenesis of corpus callosum, absent cavum septum]
- Cortical formation abnormalities (schizencephaly, lissencephaly, heterotopia, microcephaly)
- Abnormalities of posterior fossa (mega cisterna magna, Dandy–Walker, Blake's pouch cyst, vermian hypoplasia)
- Destructive lesions (cysts, periventricular leukomalacia, infections, hydranencephaly, dysplasias, tumors/mass lesions, and other lesions)
- Vascular abnormalities (hemorrhage, hematoma, dural fistula, aneurysms)

Covering all the above malformations is beyond the scope of this chapter; however, we will be covering some of the most common malformations in this chapter.

Ventricular System

Ventriculomegaly (VM) is the most common CNS condition diagnosed in utero and is also the most common indication for fetal MRI. Severity of ventriculomegaly is based on the measurement of width of the atrium of the lateral ventricle. It is classified as mild, moderate, or severe based on the atrial widths of 10-12, 12-15, and >15 mm, respectively.

Outcome of Fetal Ventriculomegaly

In order to recognize other anomalies associated with ventriculomegaly, the use of MRI has been advocated.

The outcome of fetuses with VM depends on the severity of the associated anomaly. However, counseling is difficult in patients with isolated VM. Isolated severe VM carries the worst prognosis. However, the outcome of patients with isolated borderline VM is variable in different studies. Another factor which should be taken into account before counseling the parents is the progression of the VM. A progressing VM caries the worst prognosis.

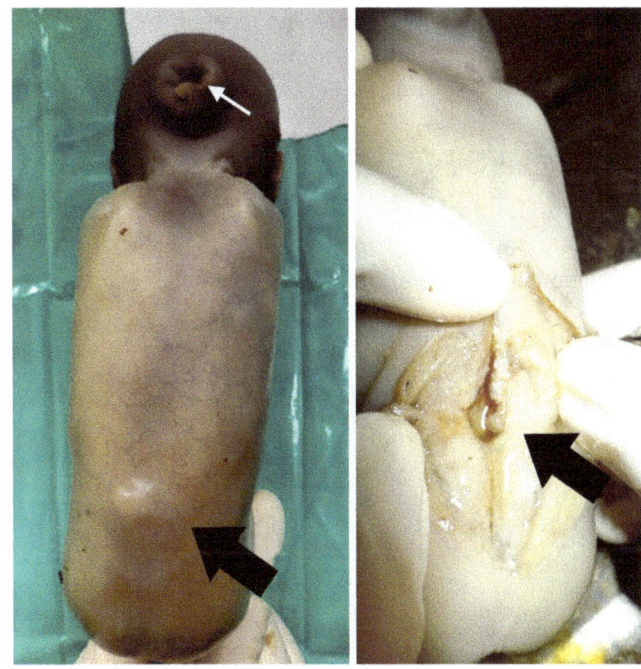

Fig. 1: More than one defect in the neural tube in the same fetus; occipital encephalocele (arrow) and lumbar meningomyelocele (broad arrow).

Neural Tube Defects

Neural tube defects are a result of defect in formation of the primary neural tube. Failure of closure of neural tube may result in encephalocele, anencephaly, spina bifida, or spina bifida occulta. Though the molecular basis of neural tube closure defects is likely to be quite heterogeneous, periconceptional folic acid supplementation has been found to reduce the risk by around 70%. Since the process of neurulation occurs at the fourth week of gestation, the requirement of folic acid is much early in the development. It is recommended that a woman should start taking folic acid as soon as she plans a pregnancy (at least 3 months prior to pregnancy) to prevent NTDs in the fetus. The common practice of starting folic acid after a positive pregnancy test offers limited protection.

Prenatal diagnosis: The common screening test of maternal serum alpha-feto-protein (AFP) (16-18 weeks) and subsequent amniotic fluid AFP lacks both sensitivity and specificity and will only detect the open NTD. Ultrasonography is recommended for women with positive serum AFP screening, history of intake of drugs associated with NTD, and previously affected child. Anencephaly can be detected as early as 12 weeks of gestation and ultrasonography can detect spina bifida from 16 weeks onwards. However, spina bifida in lumbosacral region (particularly L5-S2) may be missed **(Figs. 1 to 3)**.

Management and Outcome

Individuals with spina bifida with optimal medical and surgical treatment can survive; however, craniorachischisis and anencephaly are lethal conditions. Based on available

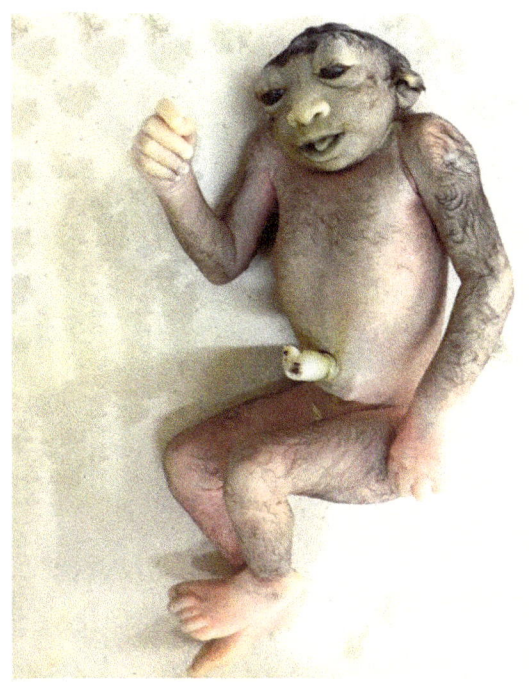

Fig. 2: Anencephaly.

data, fetal surgery appears to decrease the need for postnatal shunting and improves motor development and function. However, expertise required for such procedures is not always available. The children with spina bifida are at risk of hydrocephalus, complications of Chiari II malformations, sensory loss, lower limb paralysis, bowel and bladder dysfunction, club foot, and spinal deformities. Although majority of children treated adequately have normal intelligence, some cognitive and learning problems are common in such children. The level of the lesion is an important determinant of neurological outcome; the more proximal the lesion, the poorer the outcome.

Genetic Counseling

The couple must be counseled about the possibility of chromosomal abnormality, single-gene disorder or teratogenic exposure in a small percentage of such babies.

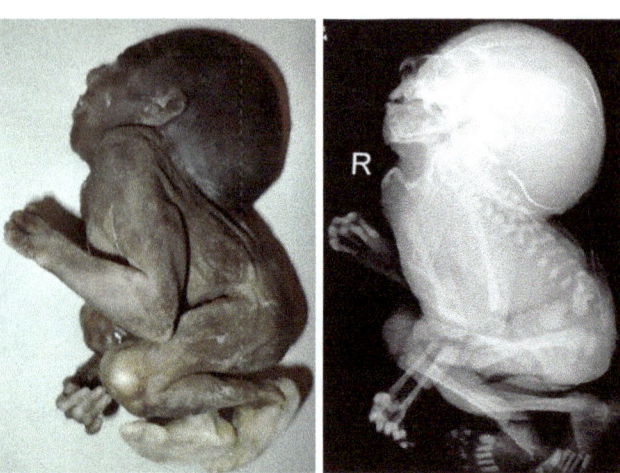
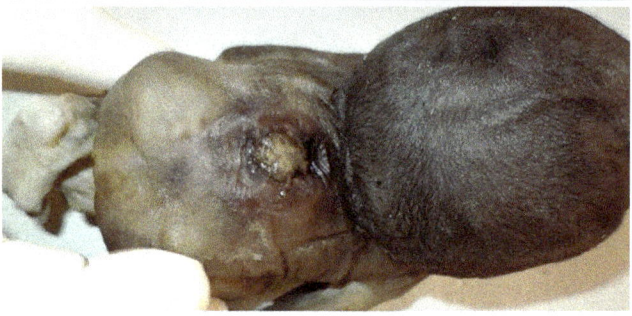

Fig. 3: Fetus with inencephaly showing extreme retroflexion (backward bending) of the head and a open spina bifida.

Prenatal testing for chromosomes and probable single-gene disorders should be offered to all couples. Those who opt for termination with or without prenatal testing should be offered postmortem examination. Such testing and examination are essential for effective genetic counseling which helps couples to take future decisions. Recurrence risk depends on the underlying cause, if any. When a chromosomal and single-gene disorder is not identified, the recurrence risk is around 3–5% with one affected sibling and the risk is approximately 10% with two affected siblings.

Special care should be taken during counseling of women, where there is a probable teratogenic cause. Women on antiepileptic drugs need to be counseled about possible teratogenic effects including NTD. As a rule, possible monotherapy at possibly the lowest dose for effective control of seizures needs to be adjusted in prepregnancy period. Valproate use should be avoided in pregnant women by all possible means.

Midline Malformations of the Forebrain

Holoprosencephaly results from incomplete or failed separation of the forebrain early in gestation.

Classification of Holoprosencephaly

Classic HPE includes a continuum of brain malformations **(Table 1)** and can be classified in order of decreasing severity as **(Fig. 4)**:

- *Alobar HPE*: There is a single monoventricle with no separation of the cerebral hemispheres making it the most severe form of HPE.
- *Other types include semilobar, lobar, middle interhemispheric, septopreoptic, and microforms of HPE* which have mild craniofacial anomalies without any obvious neurologic findings on conventional neuroimaging.

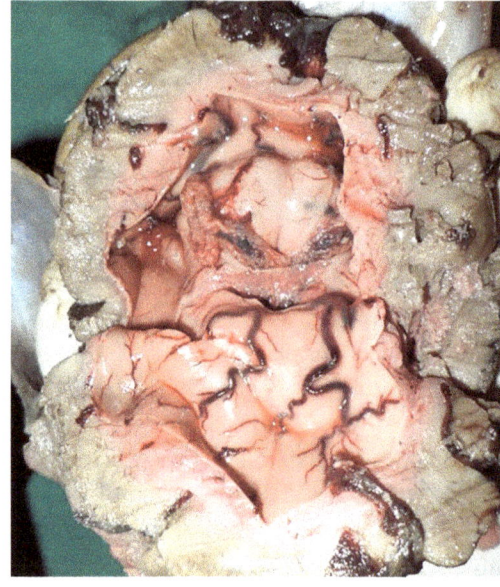
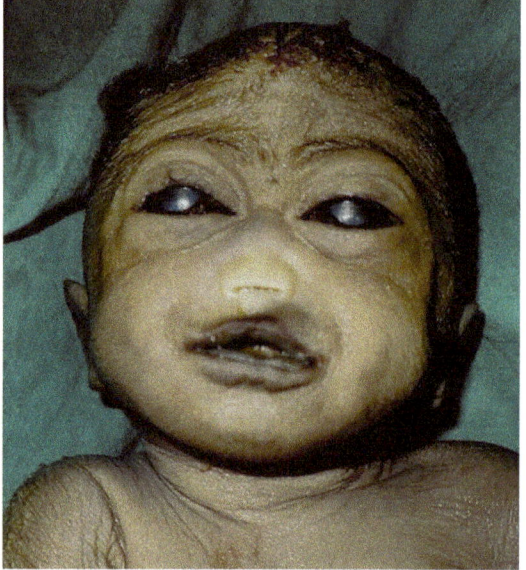

Fig. 4: *Semilobar holoprosencephaly, in brain:* Left and right frontal and parietal lobes are fused and the interhemispheric fissure is only present posteriorly. Note the closely spaced eyes with single-nostril in nose (cebocephaly) in the fetus.

TABLE 1: Common brain malformations and their clinical manifestations.

Developmental stage	Malformation	Clinical features
Abnormal neurogenesis	• Microcephaly • Hemimegalencephaly	• Mental retardation, epilepsy rare • Mental retardation, early onset seizures, and intractable epilepsy
	Focal cortical dysplasia	Focal and generalized seizures
Abnormal neuronal migration	Subcortical band heterotopia	Mental retardation, epilepsy
	Periventricular heterotopia	Normal intelligence, late-onset (adolescence) seizures
Abnormal arrest in neuronal migration	Cobblestone lissencephaly	• Fukuyama congenital muscular dystrophy • Muscle–eye–brain disease • Walker–Warburg syndrome
Abnormal neuronal organization	Polymicrogyria	Epilepsy

Etiology of Holoprosencephaly

Environmental causes

Cholesterol-lowering agents: Use of statins by mother has been associated with HPE.

Infants of diabetic mothers: Women who are diabetic before pregnancy have a 200-fold increase for delivering a neonate with HPE.

Chromosomal anomalies: Around 25–50% babies with HPE have a chromosomal abnormality. Trisomy 13, trisomy 18, and triploidy (total 69 chromosomes) are the most common numerical chromosomal anomalies associated with HPE. Structural chromosomal abnormalities associated with HPE have been commonly reported with deletions and duplications involving chromosomes 13q, 18p, 7q, 3p, 2p, 21q, etc., probably denoting the areas of genome harboring the various genes associated with HPE.

Single-gene disorders: Mutation in single genes can cause syndromic and nonsyndromic forms of HPE.

Outcome of Holoprosencephaly

Most fetuses affected with HPE do not survive, and mostly die in utero. Mildly manifesting individuals with "microform" HPE survive till adulthood and produce children.

Diagnosis of Holoprosencephaly

- MRI of brain can be used for confirmation of HPE and also to identify other associated CNS anomalies.
- Approximately half of HPE patients have chromosomal abnormality which can be detected with karyotype or chromosomal microarray.
- Similarly around 25% of monogenic HPE patients are syndromic. Furthermore, cholesterol biosynthesis defect can be seen in 10% of individuals with HPE. Molecular genetic testing of putative genes is indicated either by Sanger sequencing or by next-generation sequencing (NGS) techniques, which is indicated in all monogenic forms of HPE.

Management

Treatment should be preferably by a multidisciplinary team. The various components of treatment are:
- Antiepileptic drugs for management of seizures
- Hormone replacement therapy for pituitary dysfunction
- Surgical treatments for feeding difficulties and gastro-esophageal reflux, like gastrostomy tube and Nissen fundoplication.
- Special feeding bottles and surgical repair of cleft lip and/or palate
- Ventriculoperitoneal shunt placement for hydrocephalus
- Physiotherapy, occupational therapy, and special education for developmental disabilities.
- Parental support and counseling

Genetic Counseling

Counseling and risk assessment depend on the specific cause of HPE. Mutation testing can be offered for prenatal testing if mutation is detected in the affected child. Prenatal ultrasonography is likely to detect most major brain anomalies and aid in prenatal diagnosis of HPE.

Dysgenesis of the Corpus Callosum

The defect may be partial (hypoplasia) or complete (agenesis).

Patients with isolated hypoplasia of the corpus callosum are often asymptomatic. However, in a patient with agenesis, the associated abnormalities are seen in 20–90% of cases, which dictate the prognosis. Agenesis of corpus callosum may be associated with intrauterine infectious, genetic, toxic (alcohol), or vascular etiology.

Antenatal Diagnosis

Antenatal ultrasonography can be useful for the diagnosis based on the following signs:
- *Racing car sign*: Widely spaced lateral ventricles like parallel bodies
- *Tear drop sign*: Colpocephaly with small frontal horns

- A dilated third ventricle may be elevated or dorsally displaced.
- Absent septum pellucidum

Aicardi Syndrome

Aicardi syndrome, an X-linked dominant disorder, is characterized by a triad of infantile spasms, brain malformation, and chorioretinopathy. Affected males die in utero. Affected females develop partial seizures by 3 months followed by infantile spasms.

Disorders of Cortical Development

Disorders of Proliferation and Differentiation

Microcephaly: A small head size of <3 SD on occipitofrontal head circumference charts is known as microcephaly. The usual implication of this important clinical sign is abnormal brain growth. The causes may be broadly divided into genetic and nongenetic causes.

Megalencephaly: It indicates increased brain size. This can be familial, but inherited megalencephaly may be associated with significant learning difficulties, neurological impairment, and seizures. Hemimegalencephaly refers to unilateral enlargement of the brain and may be restricted to the hemisphere only. Patients may present with developmental delay, intractable seizures, and hemiparesis.

Disorders of Migration

Failure of neurons to leave the ventricular zone results in periventricular heterotopias whereas affection of only a subpopulation of neurons results in subcortical heterotopias (nodular or band heterotopias). If the neurons fail to complete their migration in the cortex, lissencephaly occurs.

Periventricular heterotopias may be part of a syndrome or they may be isolated. The clinical manifestations are protean and vary from an asymptomatic state to being associated with seizures and developmental problems. Nodular heterotopias are associated with other migration disorders and may manifest as partial seizures.

Agyria (Lissencephaly)

Agyria (lissencephaly) is characterized by complete absence of gyri. Pachygyria is used for a reduced number of gyri with less folding of the cortex than normal. Both agyria/pachygyria may occur in the same brain.

Type 1/classical lissencephaly: The brain is small having mainly the primary and rarely a few secondary gyri. Patients with type I lissencephaly can be subdivided into two groups. The dysmorphic features of the Miller-Dieker syndrome (MDS) associated with deletions of *LIS1* gene is observed in only few. The majority have no dysmorphic features known as the isolated lissencephaly sequence (ILS). Patients with classical lissencephaly often have intellectual disability and profound developmental delay, and many patients die during infancy or early childhood. Furthermore, these children often have early onset seizures, during the first 6 months of life.

On MRI, the cerebral hemispheres show lack of gyri or broadening of gyri or both. The absence of frontal and temporal opercula leads to "figure-of-eight" appearance of the brain on axial images with bitemporal hollowing. Corpus callosum agenesis and small midline calcifications near septum pellucidum may also be seen in children with MDS.

Type II lissencephaly or cobblestone lissencephaly or Walker-Warburg syndrome: The cortex appears granular covered with thickened meninges occurring as a result of mesenchymal proliferation.

Both the nervous system and muscle abnormalities are seen. The infants have anterior segment anomalies and microphthalmia with retinal dysplasia. Hydrocephalus may be seen but microcephaly is rare. Similar to muscular dystrophy, there is necrosis of fibers in all muscles, leading to elevation of serum creatine kinase.

Schizencephaly

The "schizencephaly" is characterized by abnormal cleft in the cerebral hemispheres. Schizencephaly may be closed-lip schizencephaly or open-lip schizencephaly. In open-lip schizencephaly, the space between the two walls is filled with cerebrospinal fluid (CSF). The clinical presentation includes seizures and developmental delay. On examination, the patient may have microcephaly, hydrocephalus, paralysis, and hypotonia. Severity depends on extent of clefts and associated CNS malformations.

Abnormalities of Posterior Fossa

Mega Cisterna Magna

The space between the inferior margin of the vermis and the posterior rim of the foramen magnum is known as cisterna magna. An enlarged cisterna magna, of >10 mm, is known as Mega cisterna magna. It is a diagnosis of exclusion and can be differentiated from Dandy–Walker malformation (DWM) by absence of dilation of the fourth ventricle, presence of normal cerebellar vermis, and normal posterior fossa. Mega cisterna magna has been associated with trisomy 18 and cytomegalovirus (CMV) infection. Prognosis depends upon associated malformations. Isolated mega cisterna magna usually has a favorable prognosis.

Dandy–Walker Malformation

In DWM, there is abnormal closure of the fourth ventricle leading to dilatation of the fourth ventricle and enlargement of the posterior fossa. There is associated hypoplasia or agenesis of the cerebellar vermis and communication of the cisterna magna with the fourth ventricle. DWM may be associated with certain genetic syndromes, especially trisomy of chromosome 13 or 18. Diagnosis is usually made after 18 weeks of gestation by antenatal ultrasonography. Isolated DWM with normal vermis has been shown to be associated with a good neurodevelopmental outcome. In the remaining cases, prognosis depends on the severity of ventriculomegaly in antenatal scans and subsequent postnatal MRI of brain.

Vascular Abnormalities

Vein of Galen (VOG) malformation is an AV malformation and is the most common vascular anomaly of fetal brain. VOG is seen as a midline anechoic cystic mass posterior to the thalamus and third ventricle. Doppler imaging study demonstrates a turbulent waveform and presence of low-resistance flow. VOG may present as high-output cardiac failure leading to fetal hydrops. Hydrocephalus may result from obstruction of the aqueduct of Sylvius from mass effect. A neonate with VOG may present with enlarged head circumference, pulmonary hypertension, or congestive heart failure. Treatment includes early embolization and is associated with good outcome in majority of patients.

Investigations

- MRI to delineate the extent and associated anatomical abnormalities
- If CNS malformation is associated with developmental delay or learning difficulties, consider chromosome analysis, especially if there is a positive family history and consanguinity.
- Mutation analysis of specific genes should be used to confirm a clinical diagnosis.
- Fluorescent in situ hybridization (FISH) studies can be used for diagnosing microdeletion syndromes, such as MDS.
- If no diagnosis can be reached, one should extract and store DNA, especially if life expectancy is short.

Risk Assessment

- A three-generation family tree should always be plotted, and one may need to order examination and investigate close relatives for evidence of a disorder with subtle expression or for carrier state.
- If there is absence of precise etiology, an empiric recurrence risk estimation can be done following thorough examination of the parents.

Prenatal Diagnosis

- Prenatal diagnosis and termination of affected pregnancies may be considered in conditions which are incompatible with life or associated with a poor neurodevelopmental outcome.
- Preimplantation genetic diagnosis is not yet feasible for the majority of developmental disorders of the CNS.
- For conditions with Mendelian inheritance, donor gametes may be considered.
- For conditions associated with environmental exposure, measures should be taken to minimize the exposure in future pregnancies.
- In cases with chromosomal anomaly, genetic mutation or biochemical defect prenatal diagnosis by chorion villus sampling at 11 weeks' gestation is possible in future pregnancies.

CHAPTER AT A GLANCE

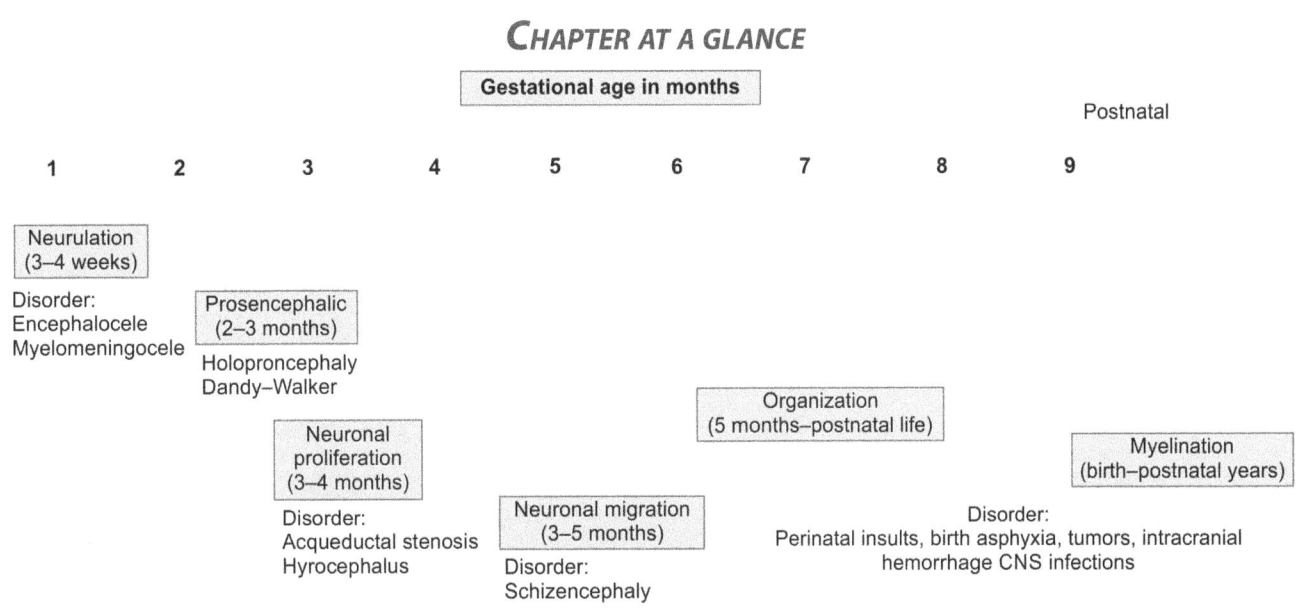

(CNS: central nerous system)

> **KEY POINTS**
> - Recent improvement in ultrasound technology has led to improved diagnosis of congenital CNS malformations.
> - All women of childbearing age should take folate supplements before conception.
> - Head circumference is one of the simplest and important clinical signs and should be measured at birth and subsequently at each visit and should be plotted on a centile chart.
> - Combined malformations may be found in infants with malformation of any one system and therefore a complete survey to look for all possible malformations should be done.

SUGGESTED READING

1. Guibaud L, Lacalm A. Etiological diagnostic tools to elucidate 'isolated' ventriculomegaly. Ultrasound Obstet Gynecol. 2015;46(1):1-11.
2. Masselli G, Vaccaro Notte MR, Zacharzewska-Gondek A, Laghi F, Manganaro L, Brunelli R. Fetal MRI of CNS abnormalities. Clin Radiol. 2020;75(8):640.e1-e11.
3. Mitchell LA, Simon EM, Filly RA, Barkovich AJ. Antenatal diagnosis of subependymal heterotopia. Am J Neuroradiol. 2000;21:296-300.
4. Şorop-Florea M, Ciurea RN, Ioana M, Stepan AE, Stoica GA, Tănase F, et al. The importance of perinatal autopsy. Review of the literature and series of cases. Romanian J. Morphol. Embryol. 2017;58(2):323-37.
5. Stutterd CA, Leventer RJ. Polymicrogyria: a common and heterogeneous malformation of cortical development. Am J Med Genet C Semin Med Genet. 2014;166C:227-39.

CHAPTER 7

Fetal Thoracic Malformations

Anup Thakur, Nandita Dimri

INTRODUCTION

Fetal lung malformations or congenital thoracic malformations (CTMs) include a group of disorders affecting fetal pulmonary parenchyma, airways, or vasculature. Some of these malformations are known to regress during pregnancy. As a result, the diagnosis is usually confirmed in postnatal life on imaging or autopsy findings. CTMs rarely pose problems in intrauterine life; however, large intrauterine cystic lesions may lead to hydrops due to pressure effect and may need fetal interventions to improve survival.

OBJECTIVES

- To review stages of fetal lung development
- To discuss the classification of CTMs
- To discuss fetal and postnatal management of CTMs

CONGENITAL THORACIC MALFROMATIONS

Stages of Fetal Lung Development

Fetal lung development starts in the 4th week of embryonic life and proceeds through five stages of lung development: (1) Embryonic, (2) Pseudoglandular, (3) Canalicular, (4) Saccular, and (5) Alveolar stage. The major events in each stage and the potential risk for lung malformations are discussed in **Table 1**.

Classification of CTMs

Congenital thoracic malformations are broadly classified into three groups: (1) Lung parenchymal malformations, (2) Thoracic vascular malformations, and (3) Hybrid lesions. Most common amongst these are the lung parenchymal malformations.

TABLE 1: Development of lung and fetal malformations.

Stage of lung development	Major events	Fetal lung malformations
Embryonic (4–6 weeks)	• Formation of lung bud from ventral esophagus • Branching into two major bronchi and subsequent lobar and segmental bronchi	• Pulmonary agenesis/hypoplasia • Extralobar bronchopulmonary sequestration • Bronchogenic cysts • Pulmonary vascular malformations
Pseudoglandular (6–16 weeks)	• 15–20 generations of terminal bronchi branching • Maturation of lung mesenchyme and pulmonary vasculature • Cartilage and smooth muscle development	• Intralobar bronchopulmonary sequestration • Cystic pulmonary airway malformation • Pulmonary hypoplasia/congenital diaphragmatic hernia • Pulmonary hypoplasia/renal agenesis with oligohydramnios
Canalicular (17–26 weeks)	• Formation of acinus • Epithelial differentiation • Formation of air–blood barrier (alveolar capillary membrane)	Pulmonary hypoplasia/oligohydramnios
Saccular (26–36 weeks)	• Maturation of type 2 pneumocytes and surfactant formation • Maturation of alveolar capillary membrane	Pulmonary hypoplasia/oligohydramnios
Alveolar (36 weeks to beyond term)	• Appearance of alveolar septa containing capillaries, elastin, and collagen fibers • Microvascular maturation	Pulmonary hypertension

- *Lung parenchymal malformations*: Congenital diaphragmatic hernia (CDH), congenital pulmonary airway malformations [CPAMs, previously known as congenital cystic adenomatoid malformation (CCAM)], congenital large hyperlucent lobe (CLHL, previously known as congenital lobar emphysema), bronchopulmonary sequestration (BPS), pulmonary hypoplasia, and bronchogenic cysts.
- *Thoracic vascular malformations*: Absent main pulmonary artery, anomalous origin of right or left pulmonary artery, and anomalous pulmonary venous drainage.
- *Mixed or hybrid lesions*: CPAM with pulmonary sequestrations or CPAM with systemic arterial supply.

Common Lung Malformations and their Management

Congenital Diaphragmatic Hernia

Congenital diaphragmatic hernia is one of the most common lung malformations with an incidence of 1/3,500 live births. Diaphragmatic hernias are classified based on their anatomical location. The most common location is posterolateral (Bochdalek hernia—70-90%) followed by anteromedial (Morgagni hernia—25-30%), and very rarely central (2-3%). CDH is left sided in 85%, right sided 13%, and 2% of cases have bilateral involvement.

Development of diaphragm is completed by 9th week of fetal life with closure of right side preceding the left. If embryogenic defect in pleuroperitoneal membrane persists at 10 weeks, the physiologically herniated intestine may enter into the defect instead of being retained in the abdominal cavity as the contents return at 10 weeks of pregnancy. In left-sided CDH, the stomach is often involved, while the liver commonly herniates in right-sided defects. Both types involve herniation of bowels into the thoracic cavity. The resultant herniation and proposed a priori maldevelopment of the lung (double hit theory) lead to decrease in bronchoalveolar development and resultant pulmonary hypoplasia. Associated truncation and overmuscularization of pulmonary arteries lead to pulmonary hypertension. Abnormal lung development also leads to poor surfactant synthesis. CDH can occur sporadically as an isolated defect or may be associated with a syndrome. The cause is not known in up to 70% cases and 10-30% cases have associated chromosomal defects. Structural defects are seen in up to 25-55% of cases with CDH. Commonly seen structural defects include cardiac malformations most commonly ventricular septal defects, gut malrotation, omphalocele, neural tube defects, and limb deformities.

Prenatal diagnosis of CDH is usually done on antenatal ultrasound during routine anomaly scan at a mean gestation of 22-24 weeks **(Fig. 1)**. Large defects may be diagnosed even in the first trimester and is associated with poor prognosis. The diagnosis is made on ultrasonography (USG) with findings of a fluid-filled stomach near the heart and mediastinal shift. Liver herniation may be present and appears as homogenous mass adjacent to the heart. Polyhydramnios may be present due to esophageal compression or fetal hydrops secondary to compression of great vessels. Both the conditions are associated with poor prognosis. Fetal magnetic resonance imaging (MRI) is used in advanced referral centers for confirming the diagnosis, visualization of liver herniation, detection of other structural defects, and volumetric assessment of fetal lung.

Prenatal prognostic markers on imaging have been used to assess disease severity in isolated CDH. In addition to prognostic markers mentioned above, the most commonly used accepted parameter is the amount or volume of fetal lung tissue. It is calculated by measuring the area of the contralateral lung at the level of four chambers of heart divided by the head circumference as visualized on antenatal USG (lung area to head circumference ratio—LHR). LHR < 1 is associated with poor prognosis. However, LHR varies with gestational age as lung growth is more in early gestation than head growth. Therefore, LHR is expressed as a percentage of normal expected LHR corrected for gestation called observed-to-expected lung head ratio (O/E LHR). Currently O/E LHR is the most preferred surrogate marker for assessment of fetal lung on USG. O/E ratio < 25% on the left and <45% on the right side is suggestive of severe pulmonary hypoplasia. Two other important markers assessed on fetal MRI are observed/expected total fetal lung volume (O/E TFLV) and percentage of liver herniation. O/E TFLV < 25% and liver herniation >21% are good predictors of neonatal mortality in CDH.

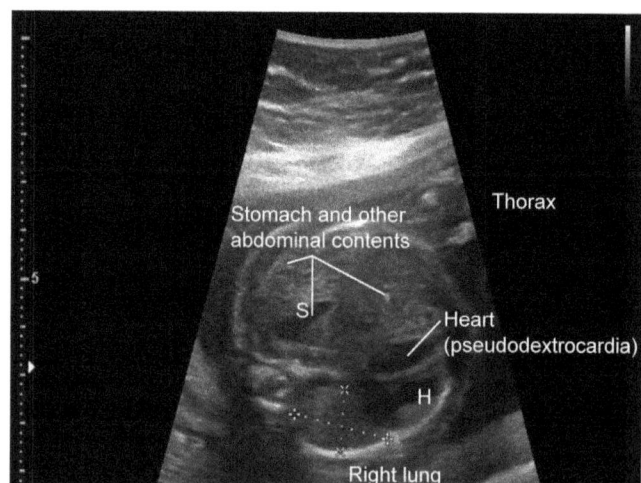

Fig. 1: *Congenital diaphragmatic hernia (CDH)*: Prenatal ultrasound at 22 weeks with transverse section of fetal thorax showing a left-sided space-occupying lesion (left CDH), with stomach (S) and other abdominal organs as its contents herniating into thorax and heart pushed to extreme right (called as pseudodextrocardia). Lung head ratio is measured on the contralateral lung (right lung) as the product of two perpendicular maximum diameters divided by head circumference.

Prenatal interventions used in severe CDH involve tracheal occlusion with plug unplug sequence called fetal endoscopic tracheal occlusion (FETO). The plausibility is that tracheal occlusion leads to impediment of lung fluid egress and promotes lung growth. FETO is usually performed between 26 and 29 weeks of intrauterine life. Indications for FETO include isolated CDH with severe forms with O/E LHR < 25%, O/E TFLV < 25%, and liver herniation > 21%. Currently reversal of FETO is done at 34 weeks of intrauterine life to allow growth of type II pneumocytes. A meta-analysis included five studies that used LHR ≤ 1 to define severe CDH. It reported that survival was better after FETO (OR 13.32; 95% CI, 5.40-32.87) as compared to control group. A recently published randomized controlled trial (RCT)—Tracheal Occlusion To Accelerate Lung Growth (TOTAL trial)—failed to show any benefit of fetal intervention with FETO in moderate left-sided CDH at 30-32 weeks of gestation. However, in fetus with isolated left-sided severe CDH, fetal intervention with FETO at 27-29 weeks of gestation resulted in improved survival at discharge and 6 months follow-up. Current recommendation for FETO outside clinical trial is not warranted. Use of corticosteroids in CDH was another fetal intervention thought to improve outcomes by promoting growth of type II pneumocytes with resultant increased surfactant production and decreased medial hypertrophy of pulmonary arterioles. However, in studies, use of corticosteroids in CDH has not shown to decrease need for mechanical ventilation or shorten duration of hospital stay.

Postnatal diagnosis can be suspected in a neonate with severe respiratory distress at birth with scaphoid abdomen. Resuscitation involves immediate intubation with avoidance of bag and mask ventilation and abdominal decompression through orogastric tube. *Postnatal management* focuses on gentle ventilation strategies with permissive hypercapnia and back up extracorporeal membrane oxygenation (ECMO). High-frequency oscillatory ventilation was not found to be superior to conventional ventilation in the care of neonates with CDH. Ventilation in infants with CDH: an international RCT (VICI trial) showed similar rates of mortality and bronchopulmonary dysplasia with the two modes of ventilation. Shorter duration of ventilation and reduced need for ECMO was seen in conventional ventilation group. Use of inhaled nitric oxide (NO) in treatment of persistent pulmonary hypertension of neonates (PPHN) in neonates with CDH is associated with worse outcomes. Surgical treatment involves either a primary repair or patch repair and is usually delayed until physiological stabilization and improvement in PPHN. Primary predictor of mortality is severity of pulmonary hypertension and lung hypoplasia.

Congenital Pulmonary Airway Malformation

Congenital pulmonary airway malformation previously also known as congenital cystic adenomatoid malformation is the most common cystic lung lesion, accounting for 95% of all congenital cystic lung disease. It is a rare malformation with 1 in 25,000-35,000 live births.

Stocker classified CPAM into five classes based on clinical, macroscopic, and microscopic features and also renamed it from CCAM to CPAM since the lesions are not always cystic or adenomatous. *Type 0 CPAM* occurs in 1-3% of cases and is characterized by acinar dysplasia with a maximum cysts size of 0.5 cm. It is the most severe variant involving all the lobes of the lung and is lethal at birth. *Type I* is the most common variant seen in 65% of cases and is characterized by multiple large cysts measuring up to 10 cm in diameter or a single dominant cyst. It is associated with risk of malignant transformation to bronchioalveolar carcinoma later in life. *Type II CPAM* is characterized by a sponge-like appearance due to presence of multiple evenly spaced cysts with maximum cyst size of 2.5 cm. *Type III* is a bulky firm mass (adenomatous appearance), which affects the entire lobe or lung at the level of bronchiolar or alveolar duct. *Type IV CPAM* is characterized by peripheral cysts, occurs in 10-15% of cases, and affects usually one lobe at the level of distal acinus.

Prenatal diagnosis of CPAM is usually done on prenatal ultrasound at 18-20 weeks of gestation. These lesions may progress to life-threatening hydrops fetalis or may undergo complete regression in utero during mid third trimester at 32-34 weeks of gestation. On fetal USG, CPAMs appear as hyperechoic heterogenic tissue with multicystic lesions with cysts of different size and number **(Fig. 2)**. Color Doppler can help in differentiating CPAM from BPS as CPAMs derive their blood supply from pulmonary circulation, whereas BPS has a systemic arterial supply **(Figs. 3 and 4)**. Fetal MRI can be done in doubtful cases. Prognosis of CPAM depends on

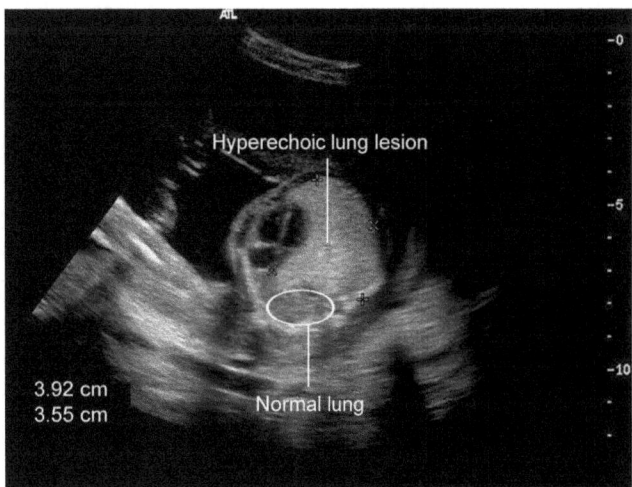

Fig. 2: *Congenital pulmonary airway malformation*: Prenatal ultrasound at 23 weeks with transverse section of thorax showing hyperechoic lung lesion appearing as solid mass occupying one hemithorax with normal contralateral lung and heart pushed to other side.

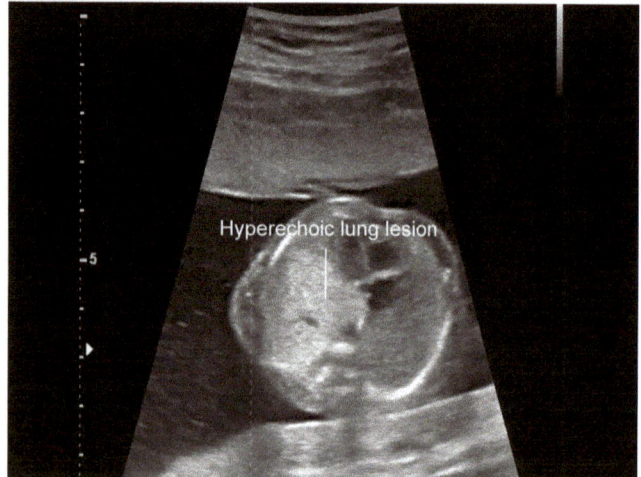

Fig. 3: *Bronchopulmonary sequestration (BPS):* Prenatal ultrasound at 19 weeks with transverse section showing hyperechoic lung lesion likely BPS as solid appearing mass.

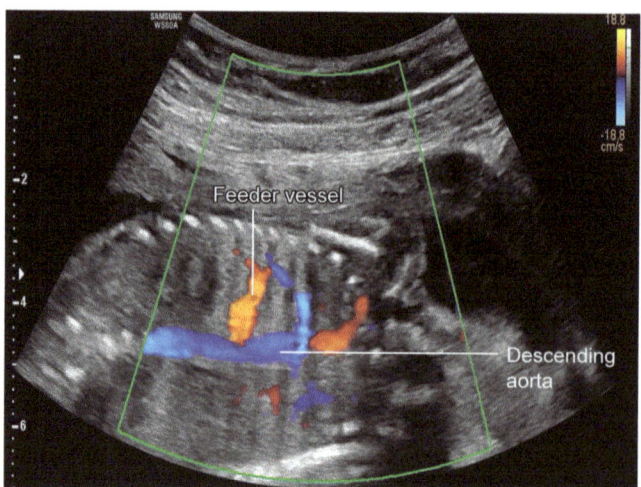

Fig. 4: The diagnosis of bronchopulmonary sequestration is confirmed by Doppler scan showing a feeder vessel arising from splanchnic circulation as seen in coronal section of thorax.

various factors such as the presence or absence of hydrops, presence or absence of other congenital anomalies, size of lesion, and its secondary effects such as mediastinal shift, polyhydramnios, extent of pulmonary hypoplasia, and cardiovascular compromise. Presence or absence of hydrops is the strongest predictor of survival and death occurs in 95% of such cases with expectant management. Ultrasound measurement of CPAM volume ratio (CVR—defined as ratio of CPAM volume to head circumference) is another important predictor of outcome. A CVR > 1.6 predicts increased risk for hydrops fetalis, whereas the risk is <3% with a CVR of ≤1.6 in the absence of a dominant cyst.

Prenatal management of CPAM is based on gestational age, type of lesion (macrocytic/microcytic), presence or absence of hydrops, CVR, and associated anomalies. Betamethasone administration may cause resolution of large macrocystic CPAM (CVR > 1.6) with associated hydrops, albeit with unknown mechanism of action and remains a reasonable first choice. Thoracoamniotic shunt (TAS) may be required in selected cases of CPAM with gestation 20–32 weeks for large macrocytic lesions causing mediastinal shift and polyhydramnios, fetal hydrops, unilateral or bilateral effusions with suspected pulmonary hypoplasia, and macrocystic CPAM with a dominant cyst (CVR > 1.6). Open fetal surgery is reserved for refractory cases with no improvement in CVR or worsening of hydrops after TAS. In advanced pregnancies >32 weeks, the presence of a large fetal lung mass with severe mediastinal shift or hydrops associated with persistently elevated CVR > 2.2 is an indication to perform ex-utero intrapartum (EXIT) procedure allowing large fetal lung resections, while the neonate is maintained on placental circulation.

Postnatal management of CPAM depends on clinical presentation. In symptomatic neonates with severe respiratory distress at birth, initial stabilization should be done to manage PPHN and optimize ventilation and oxygenation. Computed tomography (CT) scan of chest is recommended in all cases as postnatal thin-walled cyst may be missed on plain radiographs. Surgical options following stabilization include thoracoscopic/open lobectomy or parenchyma sparing resection. However, total lobectomy is the usual procedure of choice as CPAM can rarely lead to neoplastic transformations into bronchioalveolar carcinoma or pleuropulmonary blastoma and infection in remnant tissue. In asymptomatic neonates, optimal timing of surgery is controversial. The initial evaluation at birth involves screening chest X-ray to confirm the findings followed by a follow-up CT scan at 3 months of age. Surgery in asymptomatic neonates is usually performed at 6–12 months of age as early lobectomy provides opportunity for compensatory lung growth and possibly decreases chances of malignant transformation of CPAM.

Bronchopulmonary Sequestration

Bronchopulmonary sequestration is characterized by a portion of lung not in connection with remaining lung parenchyma and having its own systemic arterial supply, usually from thoracic or abdominal aorta. The differentiating features between CPAM and BPS are mentioned in **Table 2**. BPS is of two types—extralobar or intralobar sequestration. Extralobar sequestration is characterized by presence of its own pleural covering and a separate systemic venous drainage, whereas intralobar is usually believed to develop from a supernumerary lung bud and therefore shares the pleural covering with normal lung and drains into the normal pulmonary venous drainage. Extralobar sequestrations are associated with other congenital anomalies such as CPAM, CDH, foregut duplication cysts, or cardiovascular malformations. Occasionally, it may be located below the

TABLE 2: Differentiating features between congenital pulmonary airway malformation (CPAM) and pulmonary sequestration.

CPAM	Pulmonary sequestration
Classified into five types (0–4)	Classified as intralobar or extralobar
Connection to tracheobronchial tree is present	No connection to tracheobronchial tree
Pulmonary blood supply	Systemic blood supply
Associated malformations are common specially with type 2	Less common
Located usually in either lower lobe	Left lower lobe
Spontaneous antenatal regression seen in 15%	Spontaneous antenatal regression seen in 75% cases
Modified	

diaphragm and appear like a neuroblastoma or adrenal hemorrhage.

On prenatal USG evaluation, extralobar pulmonary sequestration appears as homogeneous hyperechoic paraspinal mass with a feeding artery originating from abdominal aorta as seen on color Doppler. However, extralobar sequestration may also present as hybrid lesions along with microcystic CPAM. Fetal interventions are usually not required except in cases with large sequestrations affecting venous return and resulting in hydrops. Feeding vessels in both types of sequestration should be ligated. In case of a single well-defined arterial connection with concerns of high cardiac output failure, embolization may be considered.

Postnatally, extralobar may present in the neonatal period, whereas intralobar may present in late childhood or adulthood. Recurrent pneumonia responding inadequately to antibiotics may be a presenting feature. Symptomatic patients may require prompt surgical correction postnatally. Even in asymptomatic cases, elective surgical resection is performed due to risk of infection, bleeding, and probable malignancy.

Bronchogenic Cysts

Bronchogenic cysts are part of spectrum of fore-gut duplication cysts formed as a result of abnormal development of tracheobronchial tree during 26th–40th day of fetal life. *Prenatal diagnosis* is made on antenatal USG by findings of a presence of unilocular fluid-filled cystic structure in middle or posterior mediastinum near the carina. *Postnatal diagnosis* is done on CT scan which shows cysts as hypoattenuating lesions with smooth, imperceptible walls. Most newborns are asymptomatic, and diagnosis is usually incidental. The most common presentation involves symptoms secondary to compression of structures adjacent to cysts such as trachea or esophagus presenting with wheeze, stridor, and dysphagia. These cysts may also present with recurrent infections. Symptomatic cases require complete surgical resection.

Congenital Large Hyperlucent Lobe

Congenital large hyperlucent lobe is usually characterized by progressive lobar emphysema leading to compression of ipsilateral lung. It may occur either secondary to intrinsic obstruction as a result of weak cartilage or extrinsic compression due to bronchogenic cyst or an aberrant artery. The compression acts as a ball valve mechanism causing trapping of air and resultant emphysema. The most common lobe involved is left upper followed by right middle lobe. In severe cases, it may lead to mediastinal shift, impaired venous return due to increase in preload and subsequent hydrops. *Prenatal diagnosis* is made on USG findings showing a large homogenously hyperechoic mass.

Postnatal management depends on clinical presentation. Expansion of emphysema may lead to mediastinal shift, widening of ribs, depression of hemidiaphragm, and compressive atelectasis. On radiograph, this is often confused with pneumothorax or pulmonary cyst but can be identified by presence of organized pulmonary markings over the distended lung. In neonates with mild respiratory distress, treatment may vary from conservative approach to low pressure ventilatory support. Those neonates presenting with severe respiratory distress may require emergent surgical resection of the affected lobe.

Pulmonary Agenesis, Aplasia, and Hypoplasia

Pulmonary underdevelopment is a congenital lung malformation characterized by impaired development of lung tissue. It is classified into three types: (1) Pulmonary agenesis: Complete absence of lung parenchyma, bronchus, and pulmonary vasculature, (2) Pulmonary aplasia: No lung parenchyma or vasculature but presence of rudimentary blind ending bronchus, and (3) Pulmonary hypoplasia: Presence of variable amount of lung parenchyma with bronchus present, with decreased number of alveoli, airways, and pulmonary vessels.

Pulmonary agenesis is hypothesized to occur during the 4th week of gestation due to abnormal blood flow from dorsal arch. More than half of affected fetus have other associated anomalies such as tracheoesophageal fistula, imperforate anus, renal, cardiovascular, or skeletal abnormalities. Postnatal radiography shows diffuse opacification of the hemithorax with mediastinal shift to the ipsilateral side. CT scan helps to confirm the diagnosis.

Pulmonary hypoplasia on the other hand may be primary due to maturational arrest in pseudoglandular stage of development or secondary due to an imbalance in mechanical forces between intraluminal airways and extraluminal space resulting in compression of airways and resultant hypoplastic lungs. Secondary pulmonary hypoplasia may be caused due to intrathoracic or extrathoracic factors. Intrathoracic causes include CDH, CPAM, BPS, cardiac or mediastinal mass, lymphatic malformation, and agenesis of diaphragm. The most common extrathoracic cause is severe oligohydramnios before 25 weeks of gestation secondary to genitourinary abnormalities such as renal agenesis or prolonged rupture of membrane. A hypoplastic chest in skeletal dysplasia can also lead to pulmonary hypoplasia. Postnatal clinical presentation of pulmonary hypoplasia may vary from severe respiratory insufficiency at birth to chronic lung disease and recurrent infections in adulthood.

Other Congenital Thoracic Malformations

Other CTMs that may manifest clinically include congenital high airway obstruction syndromes, bronchial atresia, and Scimitar syndrome.

Congenital high airway obstruction syndrome is a rare entity caused by laryngeal or tracheal atresia, tracheal stenosis, or web or rarely due to compression by double aortic arch. Due to obstruction to egress of fetal lung fluid, there is pulmonary hyperplasia seen on prenatal USG as B/L symmetrical echogenic lungs, fluid-filled trachea and bronchi, and inverted hemidiaphragm. EXIT procedure and establishment of functional airway is the only hope for survival in these fatal cases.

Bronchial atresia is another rare anomaly that occurs due to focal obliteration of a bronchus at segmental, subsegmental, or lobar level. Bronchial atresia is usually an incidental finding in adults and do not present in neonatal period unlike congenital hyperlucent lung. On prenatal USG, echogenic mass of fluid-filled lung distal to obstruction may be seen. CT scan done postnatally shows mucus filled bronchus with distal air trapping. Recurrent infection is the only major indication for surgery in these patients.

Scimitar syndrome or pulmonary venolobar syndrome is characterized by ipsilateral anomalous pulmonary drainage from all or part of right lung usually to inferior vena cava below the right hemidiaphragm. It is associated with hypoplasia of right lung and dextroposition of heart. The right bronchial tree may be abnormal and mirror the left side. The abnormal pulmonary venous return manifests as left-to-right shunt. Prenatal USG shows dextrocardia, mildly narrowed right pulmonary artery, and polyhydramnios. Postnatal radiograph may outline a curvilinear density in right lower lobe directed toward the right diaphragm. A small shunt may be asymptomatic and manifest later with recurrent infection or exertional dyspnea. A large shunt may manifest in infancy with signs of volume overload, congestive cardiac failure, and pulmonary hypertension.

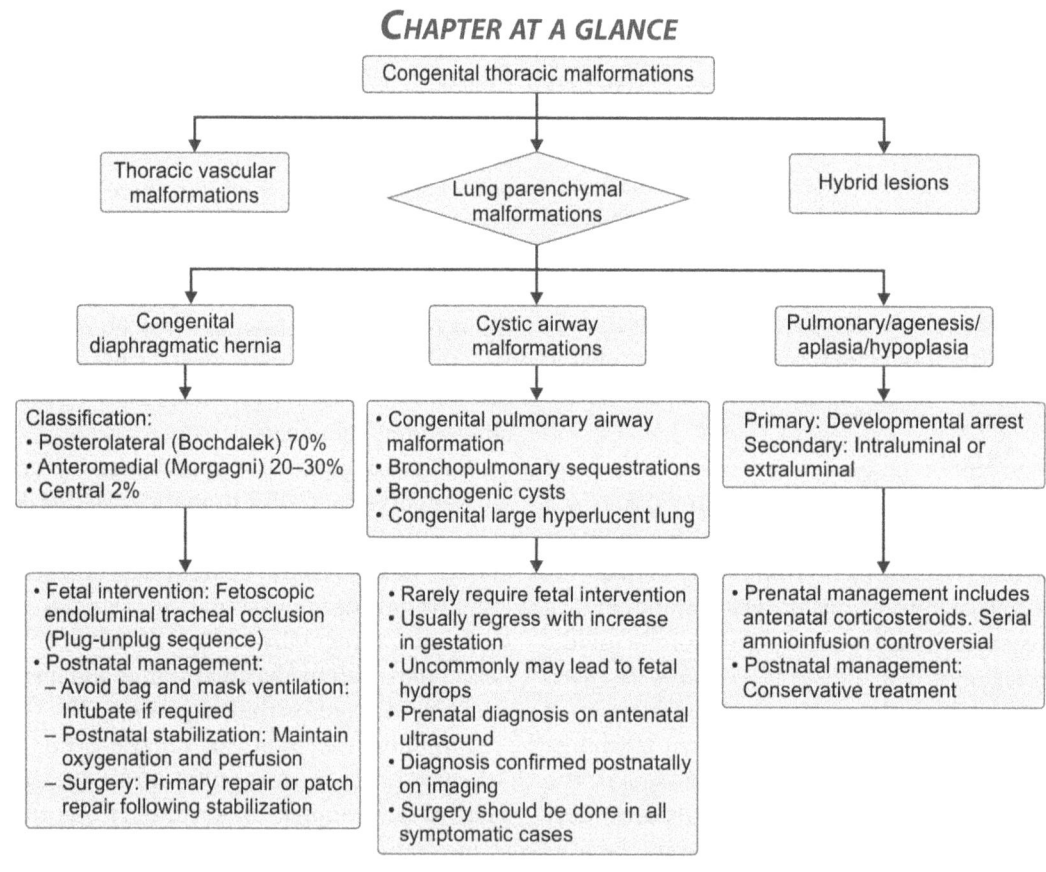

KEY POINTS

- CTMs are rare malformations. While some are known to regress during pregnancy, very few require emergent neonatal care.
- Observed to expected lung area and head circumference ratio and observed to expected total fetal lung volume ratio are important prenatal indices which help predict disease severity in CDH and decide timing for fetal interventions.
- CPAM volume ratio also known as CVR ratio is important fetal index to assess CPAM severity and timing for intervention.
- Pulmonary sequestrations are second most common congenital lung cystic lesions and can be differentiated from CPAMs by systemic arterial supply.
- Surgery is indicated in all cases of symptomatic CTMs. The exact management and timing for surgery in asymptomatic CTMs is still controversial.

SUGGESTED READING

1. Annunziata F, Bush A, Borgia F, Raimondi F, Montella S, Poeta M, et al. Congenital lung malformations: Unresolved issues and unanswered questions. Front Pediatr. 2019; 7:239.
2. Biyyam DR, Chapman T, Ferguson MR, Deutsch G, Dighe MK. Congenital lung abnormalities: embryologic features, prenatal diagnosis, and postnatal radiologic-pathologic correlation. Radiographics. 2010;30(6):1721-38.
3. Kosiński P, Wielgoś M. Congenital diaphragmatic hernia: pathogenesis, prenatal diagnosis and management – literature review. Ginekol Pol. 2017;88(1):24-30.

CHAPTER 8

Fetal Cardiovascular Malformations

Anup Thakur, Priyanka Karnani

INTRODUCTION

Development of fetal cardiovascular system starts between 3 and 4 weeks of intrauterine life. Malformations of fetal heart are the most common congenital malformations occurring in 1% of neonates. Some of these conditions may require urgent fetal intervention. Prenatal diagnosis of fetal cardiac malformations helps in timely transfer of expectant mothers to tertiary care centers. Some critical cardiac malformations may require immediate delivery room (DR) support and early cardiorespiratory interventions for survival and improved outcomes.

OBJECTIVES

- To briefly review development of heart
- To discuss recommendations for screening of congenital heart disease (CHD) in pregnancies at risk
- To discuss imaging modalities to diagnose fetal cardiac malformations
- To discuss briefly fetal intervention, DR support, and neonatal management of CHDs

CARDIAC DEVELOPMENT AND MALFROMATIONS

Development of Fetal Heart

Formation of fetal heart is a result of complex in-utero interactions and folding of heart tube to form the four cardiac chambers **(Fig. 1)**. It begins with migration of precardiac epiblast cells on either side of primitive streak in between the two primitive layers—ectoderm and endoderm. These cells eventually give rise to cardiac myoblasts and form horseshoe-shaped first and second heart fields on the sides

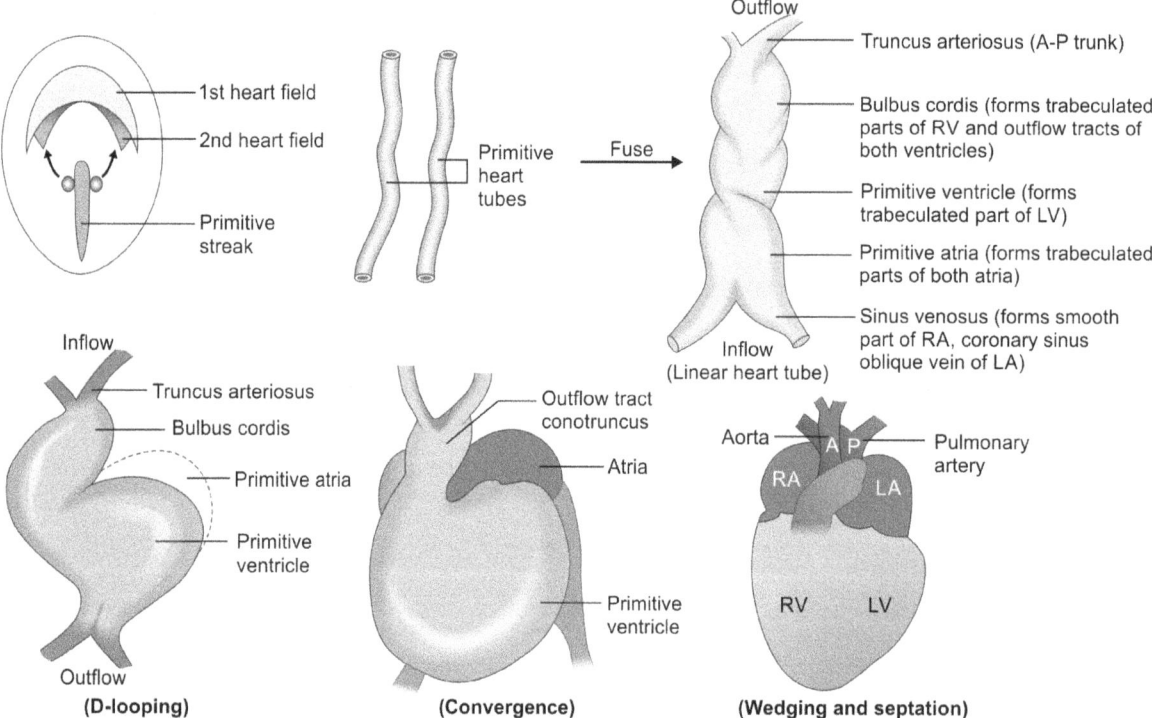

Fig. 1: Development of heart.
(AP: aortopulmonary; LA: left atrium; LV: left ventricle; RA: right atrium; RV: right ventricle)

of primitive streak. The cranial lateral plate mesoderm then initiates vasculogenesis within these cardiac fields eventually forming two endocardial tubes. The endocardial tubes with surrounding mesoderm come close in the thoracic region with lateral body folding. These two tubes with surrounding myocardium fuse to form primitive heart tube which is divided into chambers by the sulci.

The three connected steps namely, looping, convergence, and wedging in primitive heart tube lead to normal cardiac septation. The cranial end of heart tube directs blood into dorsal aorta, whereas the caudal end receives blood from systemic venous return. *Looping* begins at days 22-23 and is completed in 5 days. The cranial aspect bends ventrocaudally and to the right and caudal end bends dorsocranially and toward the left. *Convergence* results in proper orientation of outflow tracts. The first heart fields forming primitive heart tube give rise to left ventricle (LV) and portions of atrioventricular (AV) canal. The addition of second heart fields invaded by neural crest cells leads to elongation of primitive heart tubes and eventually gives rise to outflow tracts, right ventricle (RV), and atria. The neural crest cells contribute to proximal aorta, proximal coronary arteries, and sympathetic and parasympathetic innervations of heart. *Wedging* occurs in parallel to convergence and is characterized by counterclockwise rotation of outflow tracts by 45° resulting in aorta lying posterior to pulmonary artery. Septation of cardiac chambers occurs between 27 and 37 days of fetal life due to swelling of extracellular matrix between endocardium and myocardium. These tissues called endocardium cushions give rise to AV septa, valves, canals, and aortic and pulmonary vessels. Formation of aorticopulmonary septum occurs during the 5th week of intrauterine life with appearance of right superior and left inferior swellings in the wall of truncus, which rotate around each other and eventually fuse. The swellings divide septum into two parts namely aortic channel and pulmonary channel. This is followed by swellings in wall of conus which divide the primitive ventricular outflow tract into anterolateral outflow tract of the RV and posteromedial outflow tract of the LV. Abnormal cardiovascular morphogenesis can give rise to various CHDs **(Table 1)**.

Recommendations for Screening Pregnancies at Risk for Congenital Heart Diseases

According to American Heart Association (AHA) recommendations, pregnancies which exceed 3% risk for CHD based on history of previous child with CHD, either or both parent with CHD, maternal medical conditions and high risk for CHD based on prenatal screening tests should be evaluated with fetal echocardiography, whereas in pregnancies with >2-3% of CHDs, it is reasonable to screen based on additional risk factors. The common indications for referral for fetal echocardiography are mentioned in **Box 1**.

TABLE 1: Etiology of congenital heart diseases (CHDs).

Stages of heart development	Defect in development	CHD
Formation of cardiac axis	Failure of development of left-right axis	Heterotaxy and situs inversus
Primitive heart tube and normal D-looping	Abnormal looping (L-loop or A-loop)	Dextrocardia and crisscross heart
Development of ventricles from first heart field	Failure to form RV and LV	HLHS, HRHS, and single ventricle
Formation of inflow tract	Defects in formation of AV valves and septum	Endocardial cushion defects
Formation of outflow tract	Rightward shift of outflow tract	TA and PA/IVS
Convergence, wedging, and formation of spiral aorticopulmonary (AP) septum	Malalignment ± abnormal septation	TGA (straight AP septum), TOF (anteriorly deviated AP septum), PTA (no septation), DORV (leftward shift of conus ostium or incomplete spiral AP septum)
Interatrial and interventricular septum formation	Abnormal atrial and ventricular septum formation	ASD and VSD
Pulmonary venous drainage into left atrium	Anomalous drainage of pulmonary venous flow into systemic veins	TAPVR and PAPVR
Aortic arch formation	Abnormal aortic arch development from pharyngeal arches	IAA and vascular ring

(ASD: atrial septal defect; DORV: double outlet right ventricle; HLHS: hypoplastic left heart syndrome; HRHS: hypoplastic right heart syndrome; IAA: interrupted aortic arch; LV: left ventricle; PA/IVS: pulmonary atresia with intact interventricular septum; PAPVR: partial anomalous pulmonary venous return; PTA: persistent truncus arteriosus; RV: right ventricle; TA: truncus arteriosus; TAPVR: total anomalous pulmonary venous return; TGA: transposition of great arteries; TOF: tetralogy of Fallot; VSD: ventricular septal defect)

SECTION 2: Fetal Disorders

BOX 1: Pregnancies at risk for fetal congenital heart disease (CHD).

Indications for referral for fetal echocardiography

Pregnancies with estimated risk >2%:
- Pregestational diabetes mellitus or diabetes mellitus diagnosed in the first trimester
- Uncontrolled maternal phenylketonuria (preconceptual serum phenylalanine level >10 mg/dL)
- Anti-Ro/SSA or anti-La/SSB antibody positivity especially with previous affected sibling
- *Maternal intake of medications*: ACE inhibitors, retinoic acid, or NSAIDs
- Maternal first trimester infection with rubella
- Any maternal viral infection with suspicion of fetal myocarditis
- Assisted reproductive technology
- CHD in first-degree relative of fetus or a relative with a disorder of Mendelian inheritance with CHD association
- Suspected cardiac or extracardiac major anomaly on obstetric ultrasound
- Fetal karyotype abnormality
- Fetal tachycardia or bradycardia or frequent persistent irregular heart rhythm
- Increased nuchal translucency >95 percentile
- Monochorionic twin gestation
- Any evidence of fetal hydrops or effusions

Pregnancies with estimated risk of 1–2%:
- *Maternal medications*: Anticonvulsants, lithium, vitamin A, paroxetine, etc.
- Maternal alcohol intake
- CHD in second-degree relative
- Abnormality of umbilical cord or placenta

Pregnancies with risk <1% (fetal echocardiography not indicated):
- Maternal gestational diabetes with HbA1c ≤ 6%
- Isolated CHD in third-degree relative
- *Maternal medications*: Vitamin K antagonist and SSRI (other than paroxetine)

(ACE: angiotensin converting enzyme; HbA1c: hemoglobin A1c; NSAID: nonsteroidal anti-inflammatory drug; SSRI: selective serotonin reuptake inhibitor)
Modified from American Heart Association Recommendations for Fetal Cardiac Diseases, 2014.

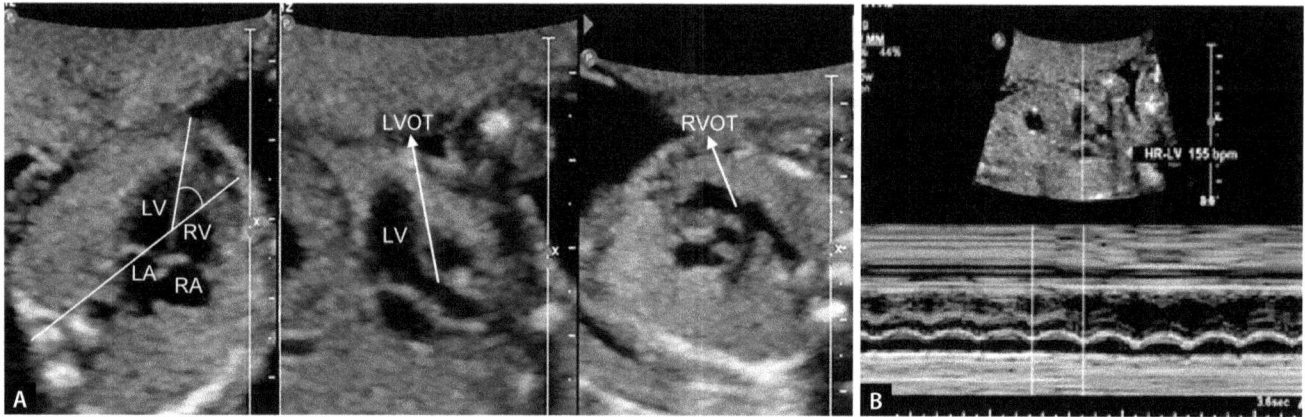

Figs. 2A and B: Fetal echocardiography normal views: (A) Transverse section of fetal thorax with fetal heart occupying roughly one-third area of thorax, showing cardiac axis, parasternal long axis, and short axis views showing left ventricular outflow tract and right ventricular outflow tract; (B) Cardiac rhythm assessment seen on M mode echocardiography.
(HR: heart rate; LA: left atrium; LV: left ventricle; LVOT: left ventricular outflow tract; RA: right atrium; RV: right ventricle; RVOT: right ventricular outflow tract)

Fetal Echocardiography

Fetal echocardiography is the most widely used primary tool to diagnose and evaluate cardiovascular malformations. For screening CHDs in high-risk pregnancies, fetal echocardiography should be performed at 18–22 weeks of gestation. It should involve all the standard views including still frame and moving clips of four-chamber view with sweeps through outflow tracts, short axis, long axis views, three vessels and trachea views with sweeps through the mediastinum, superior and inferior vena cava view, and ductal and aortic arch view. The standard four-chamber image is obtained through apical or long axis view **(Figs. 2A and B)**. The fetal heart should roughly occupy one-third area of the chest. The RV lies anterior most, while the left atrium is the most posterior chamber. The normal fetal cardiac axis is 45°. Any deviation in axis should arouse a suspicion of outflow tract anomalies. A segmental approach should be applied that includes assessment of systemic and pulmonary venous connections, AV connections and morphology, AV and semilunar valve continuity, ventricular arterial connections, great artery, and ductal and aortic arch assessments. Cardiac biometry should be evaluated. In the fetus, left and right ventricle lengths are equal in four-chamber view and right-sided valves are slightly larger than left. Any discrepancy in size of cardiac chambers or vessels should raise suspicion of a structural malformation and should be assessed quantitatively. Color and pulse wave Doppler should include interrogation of patency and anatomy of all inflow and outflow tracts including AV, semilunar valves, superior and inferior vena cava, and systemic and pulmonary veins. Detailed rhythm assessment should include evaluation of heart rate and AV relationship/rhythm. In addition, it is important to assess the ventricular function of the fetal heart with at least exclusion of hydrops, cardiomegaly, and qualitative assessment of ventricular contractibility. Additional elements of functional assessment include parameters such as ventricular shortening fraction, myocardial performance index, cardiac output, and isovolumic contraction and relaxation time. **Figures 3 and 4** show fetal echocardiography suggestive of Ebstein anomaly with hypoplastic RV and critical pulmonary stenosis (PS) with a gradient of 63 mm Hg across the pulmonary valve, respectively.

Despite being an excellent tool, the limitations of fetal echocardiography should be understood. With suboptimal image resolution due to smaller fetal cardiac structures, maternal habitus, and fetal lie, certain cardiac abnormalities might be missed. A small size ventricular septal defect (VSD)/atrial septal defect (ASD), minor valve lesions, and coronary artery abnormalities are some examples. In addition, cardiac lesions including obstructive lesions and tumors may progress in late gestation.

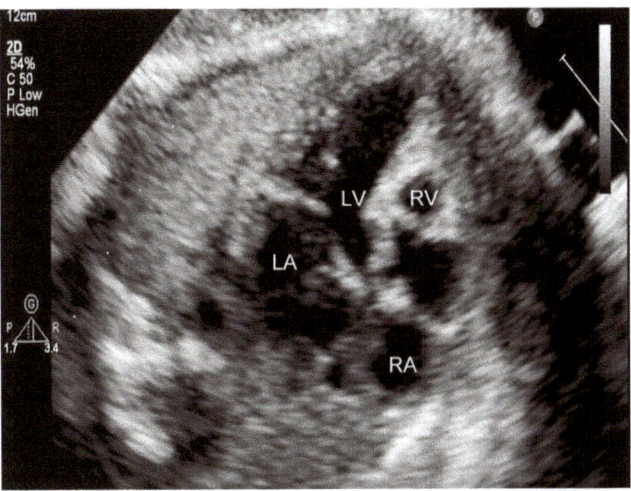

Fig. 3: Fetal echocardiographic showing Ebstein anomaly with hypoplastic right ventricle.
(LA: left atrium; LV: left ventricle; RA: right atrium; RV: right ventricle)

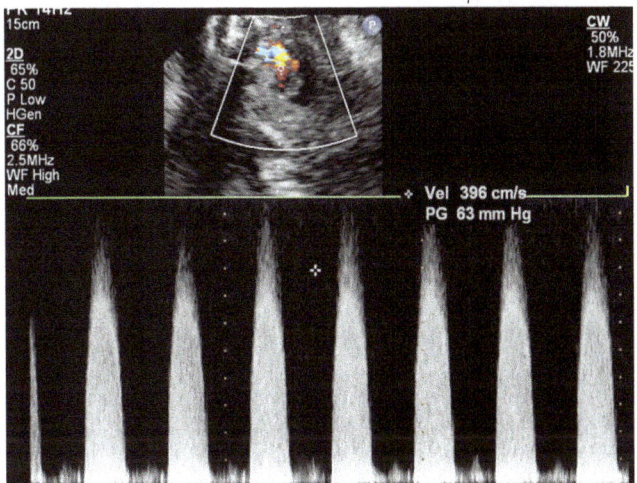

Fig. 4: Fetal echocardiogram showing critical pulmonary stenosis with a gradient of 63 mm Hg across pulmonary valve.

Fetal Interventions for Congenital Heart Disease

Fetal cardiac interventions (FCIs) are considered in CHDs where postnatal intervention is deemed palliative or when the disease is known to progress with gestation, therefore posing risk of fetal demise and/or severe life-threatening presentation at birth. Cardiac lesions amenable to fetal interventions are discussed below.

- *Hypoplastic left heart syndrome (HLHS) with restrictive or intact interventricular septum*: HLHS is a spectrum of disease characterized by the varying degree of hypoplasia of left heart structures namely aorta, aortic valve, LV, mitral valve, and left atrium. The rationale for FCI is to prevent chronic in utero pulmonary venous hypertension and pulmonary vasculopathy. Selection for FCI depends on assessment of Doppler profile of pulmonary vein to evaluate degree of impediment to left atrium egress. Fetal procedure involves opening up of atrial septum and is usually performed at 24–30 weeks of gestation.

- *Aortic stenosis (AS) with evolving HLHS*: In HLHS, left-sided structure is unable to support systemic circulation because of inadequate size, function, or both. Severe AS in early or mid-gestation may progress to HLHS. The defect in AS may arise due to annulus hypoplasia or fusion of cusps/dysplasia or secondary to thickening of leaflets. The objective of fetal intervention is to open up the aortic valve to promote antegrade flow and growth of left heart structures. This may prevent disease progression to HLHS and improve postnatal chances of biventricular repair. Prenatal aortic balloon valvuloplasty may be considered in cases of severe valvular restriction in midtrimester with a salvageable LV.

- *Pulmonary atresia (PA) with intact interventricular septum and PS*: It is characterized by imperforate pulmonary valve with duct-dependent pulmonary circulation. Pulmonary valve atresia may develop during early or during late period in embryogenesis and as a result, RV caliber may vary depending on the timing of defect. Fetal intervention is likely to promote the growth of right heart structures therefore increasing the chances of postnatal biventricular repair. In addition, associated tricuspid valve anomalies such as atresia or stenosis, severe tricuspid regurgitation may lead to hydrops fetalis and impending fetal demise. In such cases, prenatal interventions may be life-saving. The limited retrospective data suggests tricuspid valve size is the most important ultrasonographic marker predicting outcome in cases with PA/PS. The intervention of balloon dilatation of PV may be considered only when the tricuspid valve annulus is between –2.5 and –4 SD with quantitative RV hypoplasia.

- *Mitral valve dysplasia syndrome with mitral regurgitation (MR) and AS*: This cardiac anomaly is characterized by aortic atresia or stenosis, dilated LV, and severe MR. Structural abnormality in mitral valve arcade along with restrictive or intact atrial septum leads to left atrial dilatation. Severe dilatation of left-sided structure may compress the right heart leading to fetal hydrops and demise. Suggested fetal cardiac interventions are to open up the aortic valve to improve forward flow or opening the left atrial septum for decompression. However, due to presence of LV dysfunction and mitral valve abnormality, biventricular repair may still not be feasible after birth and a strategy of single ventricle physiology may be required.

Delivery Room Management of Critical Congenital Heart Diseases

Critical CHDs refer to heart defects with highest risk of cardiovascular compromise in DR requiring surgery or catheter-based interventions within first year of life. The basic principles in most cases are to maintain oxygen saturation (SPO_2), consider early elective intubation, secure vascular access/umbilical venous access to start prostaglandin E1 (PGE1) infusion, consider nitric oxide for CHDs with associated pulmonary hypertension, and extracorporeal membrane oxygenation (ECMO) as back up. The critical CHDs which may require DR intervention based on fetal echocardiographic findings are outlined in **Table 2**.

Postnatal Management of Congenital Heart Disease

Postnatal management of CHDs should emphasize on adequate respiratory and cardiovascular support followed by timely correction or palliation of the lesion as indicated. A detailed discussion on postnatal management of CHDs is beyond the scope of this chapter. Lesions can be broadly classified into duct-dependent systemic circulation, duct-dependent pulmonary circulation and some life-threatening cardiac lesions which are neither duct-dependent systemic or pulmonary circulation such as total anomalous pulmonary venous return (TAPVR) with obstructed pulmonary blood flow. A brief outline of postnatal management of specific CHDs is outlined in **Tables 3 and 4**.

ACKNOWLEDGEMENT

We acknowledge Dr Neeraj Agarwal, Senior Consultant, Department of Pediatric Cardiology for providing us with echocardiographic images of **Figures 3 and 4**.

TABLE 2: Fetal echocardiographic parameters to suggest need for specialized DR interventions.

CHD	Fetal echocardiographic parameters	DR interventions
D-TGA with restrictive atrial septum	<ul><li>Angle of septum primum <30° to the atrial septum</li><li>Bowing of septum primum into the left atrium >50%</li><li>Lack of normal swinging motion of septum primum</li><li>Hypermobile septum primum</li></ul>	<ul><li>Intubation and MV (SPO_2 target 75–85%)</li><li>Initiate PGE1 in DR after establishing vascular access</li><li>Consider NO/ECMO in severe PAH</li><li>Plan for urgent BAS in DR or transfer to catheterization laboratory</li></ul>
HLHS with restrictive/intact interatrial septum	*Ratio of pulmonary vein antegrade*: Retrograde velocity-time integral <3	<ul><li>Intubation and MV (SPO_2 target 75–85%)</li><li>Initiate PGE1 in DR after establishing vascular access</li><li>Plan for urgent intervention to decompress left atrium—(catheterization-balloon, stent; surgery)</li></ul>
Obstructed TAPVR	<ul><li>Decompressing vein below the diaphragm</li><li>Accelerated flow in decompressing vein</li></ul>	<ul><li>Intubation and MV (SPO_2 target 75–85%)</li><li>Initiate PGE1 in DR after establishing vascular access—maintain patency of ductus venosus in infracardiac TAPVR and patency of ductus arteriosus in setting of pulmonary hypertension to allow right-to-left shunt to maintain systemic flow</li><li>Transfer to OT for surgery</li><li>Consider ECMO if neonate is hypoxic pending surgery</li></ul>
TOF with absent pulmonary valve	Lung finding suggestive of lobar emphysema (fluid trapping) on MRI	<ul><li>Consider 100% oxygen—(target SPO_2 > 90%)</li><li>Prone positioning</li><li>Avoid intubation if possible</li><li>If intubated and mechanically ventilated-consider high PEEP</li></ul>

Contd...

Contd...

CHD	Fetal echocardiographic parameters	DR interventions
Severe Ebstein anomaly with hydrops	• Hydrops fetalis • Uncontrolled arrhythmia (SVT)	• Consider early delivery • Consider PGE1 in cases of severe RV dysfunction to ensure pulmonary flow via PDA • Consider 100% oxygen—(target SPO_2 > 90%) to decrease PVR • Treat arrhythmias • Consider inhaled nitric oxide to decrease PVR • Consider ECMO

(BAS: balloon atrial septostomy; DR: delivery room; ECMO: extracorporeal membrane oxygenation; MV: mechanical ventilation; NO: nitric oxide; OT: operation theater; PAH: pulmonary artery hypertension; PDA: patent ductus arteriosus; PEEP: positive end expiratory pressure; PGE1: prostaglandin E1; PVR: pulmonary vascular resistance; SVT: supraventricular tachycardia; HLHS: hypoplastic left heart syndrome; TAPVR: total anomalous pulmonary venous return; TOF: tetralogy of Fallot; CHD: congenital heart disease)

TABLE 3: Specific management of defects with duct-dependent systemic circulation.

Cardiac defect	Clinical presentation	Specific management/surgery
Critical coarctation of aorta (COA): Narrowing of descending aorta typically located at insertion of ductus arteriosus	• Asymptomatic in-utero • After birth, depending on severity may present with mild systolic hypertension, differential cyanosis, cardiac failure, and/or shock	• Corrective intervention (surgery or transcatheter) indicated in cases of critical COA (risk of CHF/death as DA closes), coarctation gradient >20 mm Hg, radiological evidence of clinically significant collateral flow and systemic hypertension or heart failure attributable to COA • In infants <4 months of age, surgical repair is preferred over balloon angioplasty as risk of reintervention is low • It is usually performed toward the end of the first week
Interrupted aortic arch: Interruption can occur at various sites: After all arch vessels arise (type A), before left subclavian artery (type B) or before left carotid artery (type C)	Differential cyanosis (pattern of cyanosis depends on type of defect)	Surgery in neonatal period
Critical aortic valve stenosis: Severe stenosis rendering systemic circulation duct-dependent	May present as heart failure or shock after DA closes	• Balloon valvuloplasty is the treatment of choice in neonatal period • Surgical treatment with valve repair reserved for cases developing severe AR following balloon dilatation

Hypoplastic left heart syndrome	• *Without restrictive ASD (90%):* Late presentation usually at the end of the first week
	• *With restrictive ASD (10%):* Present shortly after birth with severe cyanosis and respiratory distress
		• Transcatheter balloon atrial septostomy or surgical atrial septoplasty at birth in HLHS with restrictive ASD
		• Staged palliative repair:
		  – *Stage 1:* Norwood in the first week of life
		  – *Stage 2:* Bidirectional Glen procedure at 4–6 months
		  – *Stage 3:* Fontan procedure at 2–5 years of age
		• Definite treatment is cardiac transplantation

(ASD: atrial septal defect; CHF: congestive heart failure; DA: ductus arteriosus; HLHS: hypoplastic left heart syndrome)

TABLE 4: Specific management of defects with duct-dependent pulmonary circulation.

Cardiac defect	Clinical presentation	Specific management/surgery
Pulmonary atresia (PA) with intact interventricular septum: Complete RV outflow obstruction with varying degrees of RV and tricuspid valve atresia	• Cyanosis due to right-to-left shunt at atria • Mild tachypnea • Life-threatening presentation with DA closure	Based on the size of RV, tricuspid valve, and right ventricular dependent coronary circulation (RVDCC): • *Biventricular repair (BVR)*: TV z-score >−3, membranous PA, no RVDCC. BVR involves surgical or catheter-based RVOT decompression followed by stabilization on PG1 for 4–6 weeks • *Univentricular repair (UVR)*: Severe muscular PA, TV severely hypoplastic, TV z-score >−4, RVDCC. UVR involves first stage formation of systemic-to-pulmonary shunt in neonatal period followed by staged univentricular palliation
Tetralogy of Fallot and pulmonary atresia with VSD	• Depends on pulmonary blood flow to systemic blood flow (Qp:Qs ratio) • Cyanosis due to right-to-left intracardiac shunt (VSD)	*Surgery*: Steps include unifocalization (detachment of collateral vessels from their aortic origin and anastomosis to central pulmonary arteries), RVOT reconstruction, and VSD closure • Large caliber MAPCAs without stenosis—single-staged neonatal repair • Small caliber MAPCAs without stenosis—need staged repair. BT shunt in neonatal period followed by VSD closure and RVOT reconstruction in second stage at 1–2 years

Tricuspid atresia:
• Type I (most common 70–80%) with normal anatomy of great vessels
• Type II (12–25%) associated with TGA
• Type III (3–6%) malposition defects of great vessels (e.g., DORV and truncus arteriosus)
	• Tricuspid atresia usually has a VSD. If VSD is small, it can present as duct-dependent pulmonary (duct-dependent systemic if TGA associated) circulation
	• Cyanosis on day 1 of life (50% cases)
		• Staged palliative repair:
		  – Stage 1: Norwood in first week of life
		  – Stage 2: Bidirectional Glen procedure at 4–6 months
		  – Stage 3: Fontan procedure at 2–5 years of age
		• *Definite*: Cardiac transplantation

Ebstein anomaly: Severity depends on degree of tricuspid valve displacement, presence of interatrial communication, and severity of right ventricular dilatation and dysfunction	• Signs of heart failure and cyanosis in cases with severe TR with duct-dependent pulmonary flow (shunting across ASD) • May present with severe hypoxia and respiratory distress secondary to lung hypoplasia (due to massive cardiomegaly)	• Depends on functional versus anatomical pulmonary valve atresia • Surgery is done in neonatal period if there is difficulty to wean from ventilator or severe persistent metabolic abnormalities, severe persistent cyanosis, cardiomegaly with CT ratio >80% or severe TR with persistent right heart failure • Surgical repair includes tricuspid valvuloplasty or replacement, closure of intracardiac shunts, selective plication of the atrialized right ventricle, and any indicated arrhythmia procedures
Transposition of great arteries: Aorta arising from right ventricle and pulmonary artery from left ventricle	• Cyanosis (degree depends on the amount of intracardiac mixing) • With intact interventricular septum presents with severe cyanosis in neonatal period	• In neonates with inadequate mixing and severe hypoxemia, balloon atrial septostomy can be done • *Definite repair*: Arterial switch performed within first 2 weeks of life
Total anomalous pulmonary venous return with obstruction to pulmonary blood flow	Cyanosis, respiratory failure, and shock in immediate newborn period	Emergency open heart corrective surgery after stabilization to connect pulmonary veins to left atrium

(ASD: atrial septal defect; BT shunt: Blalock–Taussig shunt; BVR: biventricular repair; DA: ductus arteriosus; DORV: double-outlet right ventricle; MAPCAs: major aortopulmonary collateral arteries; RV: right ventricle; RVDCC: right ventricle dependent coronary circulation; RVOT: right ventricular outflow tract; TGA: transposition of great arteries; TR: tricuspid regurgitation; TV: tricuspid valve; UVR: univentricular repair; VSD: ventricular septal defect)

CHAPTER AT A GLANCE

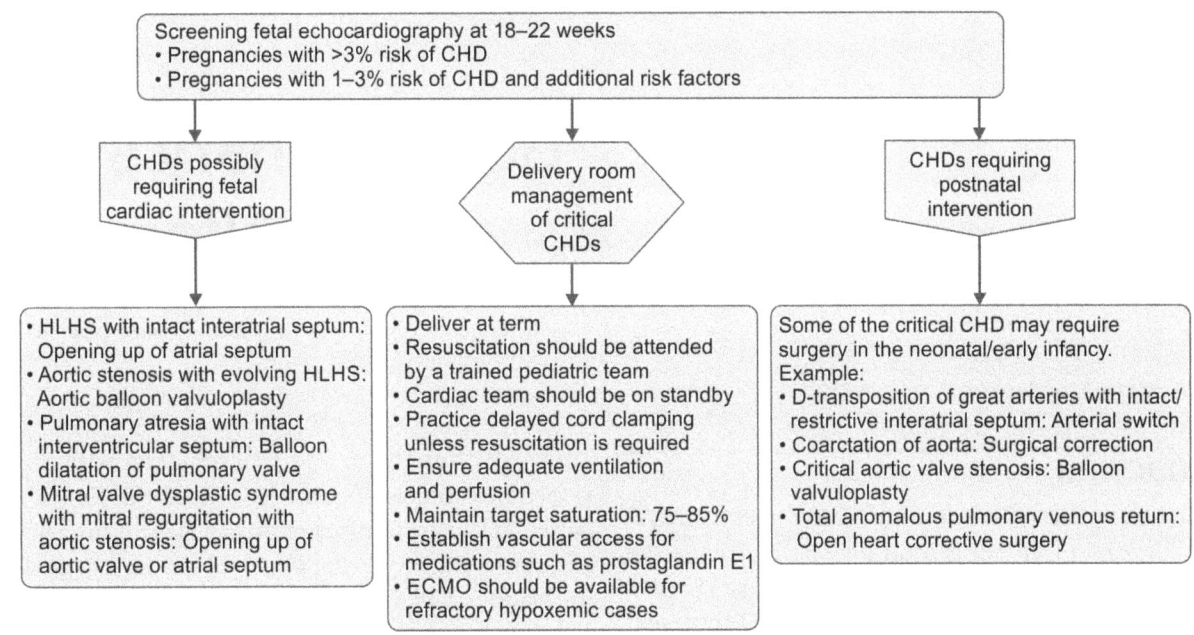

(CHD: congenital heart disease; HLHS: hypoplastic left heart syndrome; ECMO: extracorporeal membrane oxygenation)

KEY POINTS

- Fetal echocardiography is recommended in high-risk pregnancies.
- Ultrasound-guided, catheter-based percutaneous fetal cardiac interventions can help improve perinatal care in selective fetal cardiac malformations.
- Specific DR preparation and early intervention can improve neonatal outcomes in critical CHDs.

SUGGESTED READING

1. Donofrio MT, Moon-Grady AJ, Hornberger LK, Copel JA, Sklansky MS, Abuhamad A, et al. Diagnosis and treatment of fetal cardiac disease: a scientific statement from the American Heart Association. Circulation. 2014;129(21): 2183-242.
2. Mellander M. Diagnosis and management of life-threatening cardiac malformations in the newborn. Semin Fetal Neonatal Med. 2013;18(5):302-10.
3. Pruetz JD, Wang SS, Noori S. Delivery room emergencies in critical congenital heart diseases. Semin Fetal Neonatal Med. 2019;24(6):101034.

CHAPTER 9

Genitourinary System Malformation

Kumar Ankur, Seema Thakur

INTRODUCTION

Congenital anomalies of kidney and urinary tract (CAKUT) account for 20% of all congenital defects and have the potential to eventuate in end-stage renal disease (ESRD). The incidence is about 1 in 500 live births. CAKUT represent a broad spectrum of disorders which include asymptomatic to lethal anomalies and include mainly obstruction of the urinary tract, agenesis of kidneys, or cystic dysplasia. The current classification of malformations is based on a genetic/nongenetic basis.

OBJECTIVES

- To review the embryonic development of the genitourinary system
- To discuss the various malformations affecting the genitourinary system
- To discuss the role of antenatal/prenatal diagnostic features
- To discuss clinical presentation, various intervention strategies, and prognostication

EMBRYOLOGY OF UROGENITAL SYSTEM

Urinary and genital systems together form the two elements of urogenital system.

Fetal Kidney and Urinary Tract

Kidneys develop from intermediate mesoderm. There are three stages or segments of embryonic kidneys: (1) the pronephros and pronephric duct, (2) the mesonephros and mesonephric duct, and (3) the metanephros and metanephric duct. Pronephros and mesonephros involute while the metanephros develops into the ultimate kidney which is detectable between 5th and 6th week of gestational age. Ureteric bud originates from the mesonephric duct that invades the metanephric mesoderm and undergoes a series of divisions to form the nephrons, renal pelvis, and ureters. The development of the bladder begins during 4th week of gestation and process starts with division of cloaca by urorectal septum. It divides the cloaca into two parts—(1) the rectum posteriorly and (2) the urogenital sinus anteriorly. The urogenital sinus will continue to grow to form the bladder with the inferior end forming the urethra. As the mesonephric duct fuses with the cloaca, part of the duct gets incorporated into the posterior wall of the bladder. Although the ureteric bud is an outgrowth from the mesonephric duct, it opens separately into the urinary bladder. As the kidneys ascend, the ureters elongate and open into the bladder superiorly, while the roots of the mesonephric ducts are carried inferiorly before fusing to form the trigone region.

Fetal Genital Differentiation

The genital differentiation, which determines the gender of the fetus, commences at 7–8 weeks of pregnancy and finalizes by 12–13 weeks.

Prenatal Diagnosis

An anomaly scan at 18–20 weeks of pregnancy is a standard of care nowadays. So, many of these anomalies can be diagnosed antenatally. The common anomalies include pelviuretric junction obstruction, posterior urethral valves (PUV), polycystic kidneys, or renal agenesis. A thorough anatomic survey is suggested so as to detect any associated anomalies. Current recommendations suggest genetic counseling and genetic testing by microarray. Next-generation sequencing (NGS)-based analysis is advised if a monogenic syndrome is suspected.

ANOMALIES OF THE KIDNEY

Cystic Kidney Disease

Polycystic Kidney Disease

Polycystic kidney disease (PKD) is the most common inherited renal disease. Autosomal dominant polycystic kidney disease (ADPKD) is common as compared to the rare autosomal recessive polycystic kidney disease (ARPKD).

Autosomal Dominant Polycystic Kidney Disease

The incidence of ADPKD is 1 in 500 to 1 in 1,000 live births. ADPKD accounts for 5-10% of ESRD. They usually present around the fifth decade. Fetal presentation is also reported. Fetal ultrasonography (USG) findings include bilateral, enlarged kidneys with cysts, and may include increased or poor corticomedullary differentiation. ADPKD generally presents during the late second or third trimester. In the case where ADPKD is suspected, renal ultrasound of the parents followed by genetic counseling is recommended. Prenatally manifesting ADPKD has a poorer prognosis than the late-onset disease. ADPKD is caused by two genes—*PKD1* and *PKD2* genes. Recurrence risk is 50% in affected persons; prenatal diagnosis is possible if the mutation is identified.

Autosomal Recessive Polycystic Kidney Disease

Autosomal recessive polycystic kidney disease is a cystic renal disease involving kidneys and the biliary tract. The incidence is 1 in 20,000 live births with varying time of presentation and severity. USG findings include presence of bilateral, large, hyperechogenic kidneys usually at >24 weeks. The reniform shape is maintained and oligohydramnios may be present. The disease is caused by mutations in the *PKHD1* gene on chromosome 6p21. The risk of recurrence is 25% that makes prenatal diagnosis in families at risk by first-trimester chorion villous sampling necessary.

Children who are diagnosed with ADPKD usually have maintained renal functions until fourth decade of life; however, a small subset of children do get symptomatic early that progresses to end-stage kidney disease (ESKD) requiring renal replacement therapy. Almost half of the patients with ARPKD diagnosed during neonatal period will have respiratory distress due to pulmonary hypoplasia. They have massively enlarged kidneys and a subset will also have features of Potter syndrome.

Multicystic Dysplastic Kidney

Multicystic dysplastic kidney (MCDK) is one of the most frequent occurring CAKUT abnormalities, with an incidence of 1 in 3,640 births. USG shows multiple irregular cysts of variable size with intervening hyperechogenic stroma and nonvisualization of renal pelvis. Mostly single kidney is affected however both kidneys can get affected in 20% cases leading to oligohydramnios. Abnormalities of the contralateral kidney are seen in 25% and include duplex system, pelvic-ureteric obstruction, agenesis, ectopic, or affected by vesicoureteric reflux. Antenatal counseling depends upon the presence of associated anomalies, either renal or extrarenal origin. Association with trisomy 18 has been found in 3 and 15% of unilateral and bilateral cases, respectively. Other syndromes such as branchiootorenal syndrome, Meckel-Gruber syndrome, and short rib polydactyly are also found be associated in 10% of cases. Counseling regarding prognosis is based upon following:

- *Bilateral*: Fatal either in utero or in the neonatal period due to pulmonary hypoplasia.
- *Unilateral*: Favorable prognosis if isolated MCDK. Postnatally, most urologists follow an expectant approach as the kidney gradually shrinks and may disappear.
- Prognosis is poor in case of associated anomalies.
- *Recurrence risk*: 1-2%

Multicystic dysplastic kidney usually does not require treatment. If it is unilateral, then the affected kidney will regress and eventually disappear, leaving the child with one healthy kidney. If the MCDK does not disappear or is growing larger, surgery may be necessary.

Renal Ciliopathies

Defect in genes encoding components of the primary cilium can lead to a diverse group of multisystem diseases, known as ciliopathies. In kidney, ciliopathies include nephronophthisis, cystic kidneys, or renal cystic dysplasia and are associated with renal cyst formation, ultimately leading to renal failure. Extrarenal features are often associated with frequent involvement of brain and retina. Currently, no curative treatment is available for renal ciliopathy syndromes and patients depend on renal replacement therapies.

Renal Agenesis and Ectopia

Renal Agenesis

Renal agenesis can be either unilateral or bilateral. While bilateral renal agenesis occurs in 0.1-0.3 of 1,000 births but unilateral renal agenesis can be seen in 1 of 1,000 pregnancies. Bilateral renal agenesis is diagnosed by ultrasound findings of hydramnios, absent bladder, absence of renal tissue, and absence of color Doppler flow from renal arteries which arise from the aorta. Diagnosis of unilateral agenesis is difficult on antenatal ultrasound and is diagnosed by absent renal tissue and absent renal artery with normal amniotic fluid and urinary bladder. If renal agenesis (unilateral or bilateral) is identified, a detailed ultrasound to view all organ systems is recommended. In the majority of cases, renal agenesis is a sporadic and isolated abnormality. Chromosomal anomaly such as trisomy 18 is associated with 1-2% of cases. Other associated syndromes such as Fraser syndrome, VACTERL association, MURCS association (sporadic; hypoplastic or bicornuate uterus, renal agenesis or dysplasia, vertebral and rib abnormalities) are found in 10% of cases. Prognosis of unilateral agenesis is good if the contralateral kidney is normal while poor prognosis is associated with bilateral agenesis due to which termination is advised. Recurrence risks are 3% with isolated abnormalities.

Renal Ectopia

Renal ectopia refers to the abnormal location of the kidney. The incidence of renal ectopy is reported as 1 in 1,000 autopsies. The majority of patients with renal ectopy is asymptomatic. The diagnosis is often made coincidentally during routine antenatal or postnatal USG. To rule out other urological abnormalities, radiological testing is recommended. Prognosis is generally good if isolated.

ANOMALIES OF THE URETER AND BLADDER

Vesicoureteral Reflux

Retrograde flow of urine from the bladder to the kidneys is known as vesicoureteral reflux (VUR). The incidence of VUR is between 8 and 50. It is often diagnosed when a prenatal ultrasound shows pyelectasis. Postnatal diagnosis of grades of VUR is made by MCU (micturating cystourethrogram). International Reflux Study has categorized it from grade I to V **(Fig. 1)**. The sensitivity of ultrasound for the detection of VUR is low, though it can reveal ureteral or renal pelvis dilation in high grades of VUR. Diagnosis of VUR is essential as a neonate with a severe grade of VUR may benefit from daily antibiotic urinary tract infection (UTI) prophylaxis. Management of VUR can be medical or surgical. Medical management is based on the observation that low-grade VUR will resolve spontaneously. Selected patients may benefit from daily antibiotic UTI prophylaxis. Surgical management may be considered with coexisting upper or lower urinary tract anomalies or recurrent UTI.

Pelviuretric Junction Obstruction

Pelviuretric junction (PUJ) obstruction is the most common cause for antenatally detected hydronephrosis at around 80% of all causes. Its incidence is 1 in 500 live births at fetal anomaly scan. Males are affected more commonly than females, and left side lesions are found more frequently than on the right side. Bilateral involvement is approximately 10%. Intrinsic stenosis is the more common cause of PUJ as compared to extrinsic compression (accessory renal artery) of the PUJ. Most cases of PUJ obstruction are detected as a result of antenatal hydronephrosis at anomaly scan. The diagnosis is confirmed after birth by diuretic renography.

For mild-to-moderate hydronephrosis in asymptomatic patients, observation is advisable. These patients should be followed up with ultrasound examination every 4–6 months in the first year of life followed by every 12–18 months thereafter. If there is an increase in the degree of hydronephrosis, diuretic renography should be performed. If the affected kidney has <40% of split renal function or there is a serial loss >10% from a previous study, surgical intervention is recommended.

Posterior Urethral Valve

The PUV is one of the most common causes leading to ESRD in children, with an incidence of 1:5,000 live male births. Antenatal ultrasound findings **(Fig. 2)** suggesting PUV are bilateral hydroureteronephrosis, dilated prostatic urethra (keyhole sign), and a distended bladder with bladder wall thickness >3 mm with poor emptying. The presence of cyst in the kidney demonstrates renal dysplasia. In the first trimester, the condition presents as megacystis (longitudinal bladder diameter of ≥7 mm). 90% of the cases resolve spontaneously if the bladder diameter is 7–15 mm. If the bladder diameter is ≥15 mm, the condition is invariably associated with progressive obstructive uropathy leading to renal damage. Trisomy 21, 18, or 13 are reported in about 10% of cases that makes the basis for performing amniocentesis or cell-free fetal DNA extraction from maternal blood.

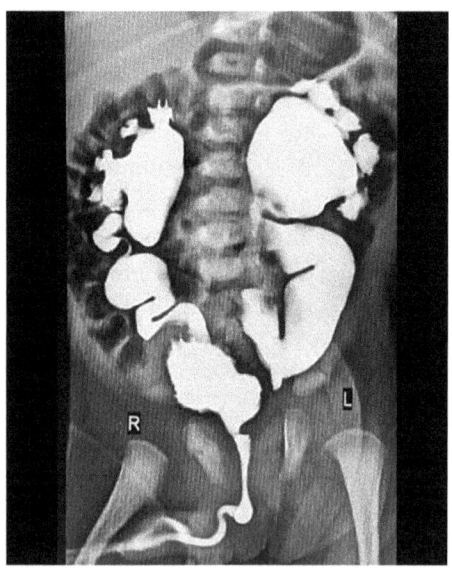

Fig. 1: Vesicoureteral reflux (VUR) (Bilateral grade V primary VUR).

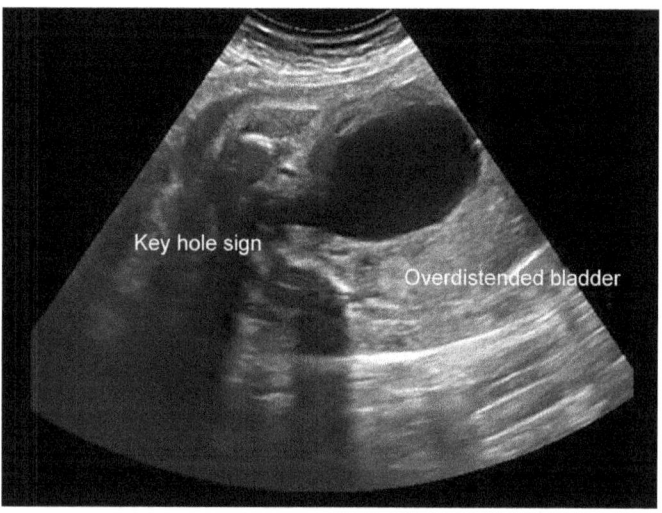

Fig. 2: Ultrasonography at 30 weeks showing overdistended bladder with dilated urethra with "*keyhole*" sign.

Severe cases have a poor prognosis for survival, and if they survive, 30% may have poor renal function requiring dialysis or transplantation. Isolated PUVs have no increased risk of recurrence.

Fetal procedure such as vesicoamniotic shunting is known to improve perinatal survival but long-term; however, parents should be counseled about the risks of pregnancy loss with or without shunt insertion. Other fetal intervention such as fetoscopic laser ablation is an alternate option as bladder decompression therapy in selected cases with anhydramnios; however, risk of renal failure would be still there.

GENITAL ANOMALIES

Congenital Cryptorchidism (Undescended Testes)

Cryptorchidism is one of the most common congenital anomalies in boys. Among boys with birth weight >2,500 g, prevalence is between 1.8 and 8.4%, but in preterm/low birth weight boys, prevalence increases and lies between 1.1 and 45.3%. One or both testes fail to descend into the scrotum **(Fig. 3)**; rather, it is found at a location along the route of testicular descent. It may have an intra-abdominal, inguinal, suprascrotal, or high scrotal position. Due to future risk for developing testicular germ cell tumors, early orchiopexy is recommended. Usually, it is an isolated condition, and specific underlying causes in the majority of cryptorchidism cases cannot be identified.

As probability of spontaneous descent of testes beyond corrected 6 months of age is very unlikely that is why infants should be referred to pediatric surgeon to prevent from further damage to testes.

Hypospadias

Hypospadias is the second most common anomaly after undescended testis, with an incidence of nearly 18.6 per 10,000 births with a higher prevalence amongst small for gestational age infants. The etiology of hypospadias is multifactorial in general. The association of severe hypospadias with maternal hypertension and oligohydramnios is possibly due to placental insufficiency. One should always rule out a disorder of sexual development (DSD) in the case of concomitant unilateral or bilateral undescended testis. Postnatal USG should be done in proximal and complex hypospadias to detect other associated issues. American Academy of Pediatrics recommends that operative intervention should be considered between 6 and 18 months to limit psychological stress and subsequent behavioral problems seen in toddlers undergoing genital surgery.

Disorder of Sexual Development

Disorder of sexual development is considered when genitalia cannot be clearly differentiated between male or female phenotype **(Fig. 4)**. DSD can be classified into three broad categories: 46, XX DSD, 46, XY DSD, and sex chromosome DSD. Various physical features that suggest possibility of DSD include apparent female genitalia with clitoromegaly, inguinal or labial mass, or posterior labial fusion; micropenis with bilateral nonpalpable testes, hypospadias with undescended testes, isolated penoscrotal, or perineoscrotal hypospadias. Clitoral length >9 mm or width >6 mm is defined as clitoromegaly and if the stretched penile length is −2.5 SD below the mean for age, then it is considered as micropenis **(Fig. 5)**. Complete assessment of a newborn with ambiguous genitalia requires detailed clinical examination, biochemical investigations, and various imaging. A family history of ambiguous genitalia, urologic anomalies, or female infertility/amenorrhea should also be obtained. Routine chromosome analysis should be performed as early as possible for early sex assignment and to allay the anxiety of parents.

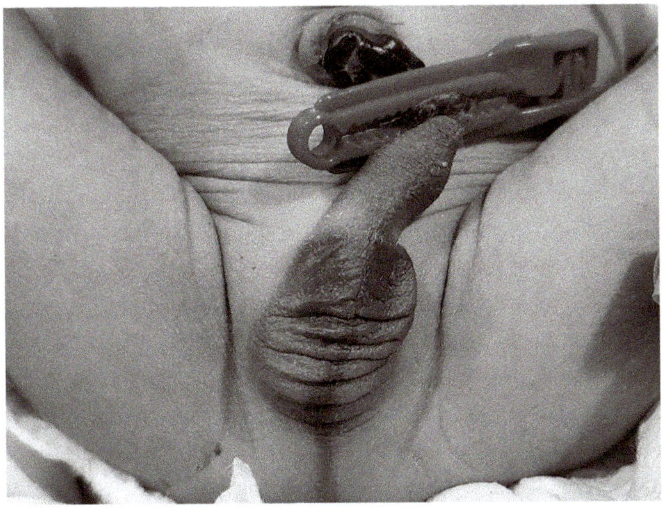

Fig. 3: Cryptorchidism (undescended testes).

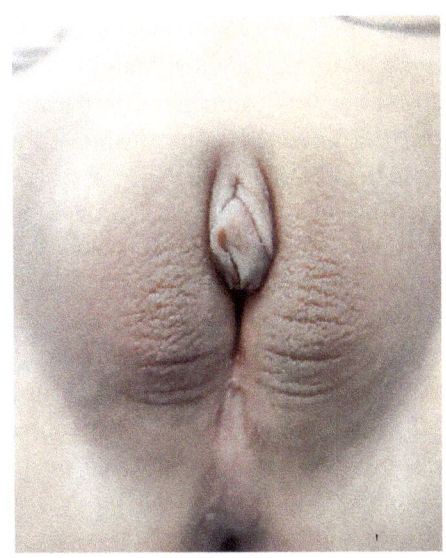

Fig. 4: Disorder of sexual development.

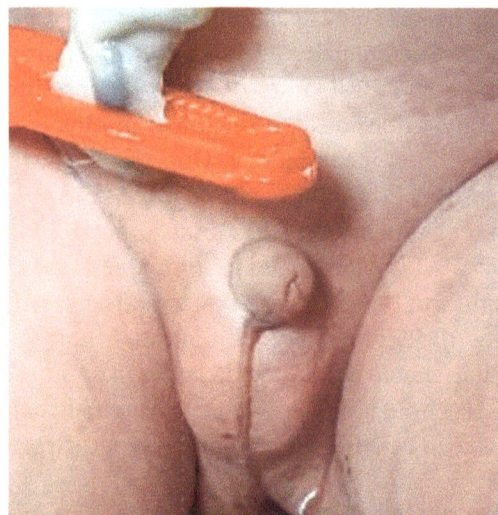

Fig. 5: Micropenis.

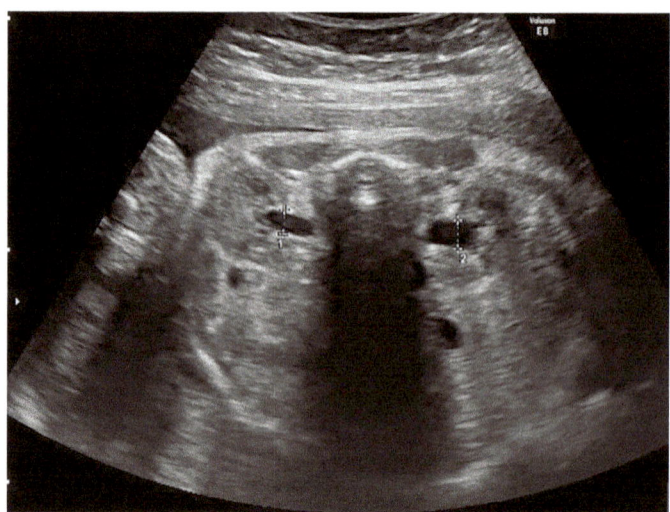

Fig. 6: Hydronephrosis in ultrasonography.

PRUNE BELLY SYNDROME

Prune belly syndrome is also called as Eagle-Barrett syndrome and is characterized by deficient or absent abdominal wall musculature, bilateral intra-abdominal cryptorchidism, and urinary tract anomalies, including megalourethra, megacystis, hydroureteronephrosis, and renal dysplasia. It affects boys and is associated with multisystem anomalies with an incidence of 3.8 per 100,000 live births. During an antenatal scan, it sometimes creates confusion with PUVs due to presence of distended bladders and hydronephrosis.

RENAL PELVIS DILATATION/ANTENATAL HYDRONEPHROSIS

Renal pelvic dilatation **(Fig. 6)** is common finding seen during antenatal ultrasound examinations. Severity of hydronephrosis is categorized on the basis of the anteroposterior diameter of the pelvis.

- *Mild (only renal pelvis)*: About 4-7 mm in the second trimester (7-9 mm in the third trimester)
- *Moderate (pelvis and calyces)*: About 8-10 mm in the second trimester (10-15 mm in the third trimester)
- *Severe (cortical thinning)*: >10 mm in the second trimester (>15 mm in the third trimester).

Abnormalities of contralateral kidneys, multicystic kidneys, and renal ectopia can be associated findings. The risk of chromosomal anomalies is low and karyotyping is advised only in cases of associated anomalies. There is no increased risk of recurrence in cases of isolated anomaly. Serial ultrasound every 4 weeks is advised for follow-up. Most cases, either remains stable or resolves during neonatal period. Ureteropelvic junction obstruction or VUR constitutes 20% of cases causing moderate antenatal hydronephrosis which would require serial postnatal follow-up or surgery **(Flowchart 1)**.

PRENATAL ULTRASONOGRAPHY

Ultrasound remains the mainstay to diagnose fetal CAKUT. The fetal kidney is usually seen in. The fetal kidney is usually seen by 13 weeks of gestation. During early gestation, the kidneys appear echogenic, and gradually they become hypoechoic. With pregnancy, the kidney size increases proportionately, and adrenal glands can be seen on the superior pole. Persistent nonvisualization of the bladder should be considered abnormal from 15 weeks as it can be easily seen in the pelvis from 11 to 12 weeks. Normally fetal ureters are not visible in antenatal scans unless they are dilated. Between 8 and 10 weeks of gestation fetal urine production begins. Genitalia can be differentiated in approximately 60% of fetuses at 14–18 weeks of gestational age and it can be better visualized with the use of three/four-dimensional USG.

INTRAUTERINE INTERVENTIONS AND DELIVERY ROOM MANAGEMENT

The fetal intervention (vesicoamniotic shunting) in lower urinary tract obstruction is considered only to bypass the urethral blockage which would actually improve pulmonary development by preventing chronic oligohydramnios. However, decision to proceed with surgery or terminate the pregnancy will be based upon the results of fetal imaging and of amniotic fluid analysis. Due to limited sensitivity and specificity to predict long-term renal outcomes, it has been difficult to select cases that would really benefit from intervention. Rarely fetal ascites due to obstructive uropathy or hydrops would require immediate ascites fluid drainage with bladder catheterization to improve lung compliance at the time of resuscitation in the delivery room.

Flowchart 1: Algorithm for evaluation and management of antenatal hydronephrosis.

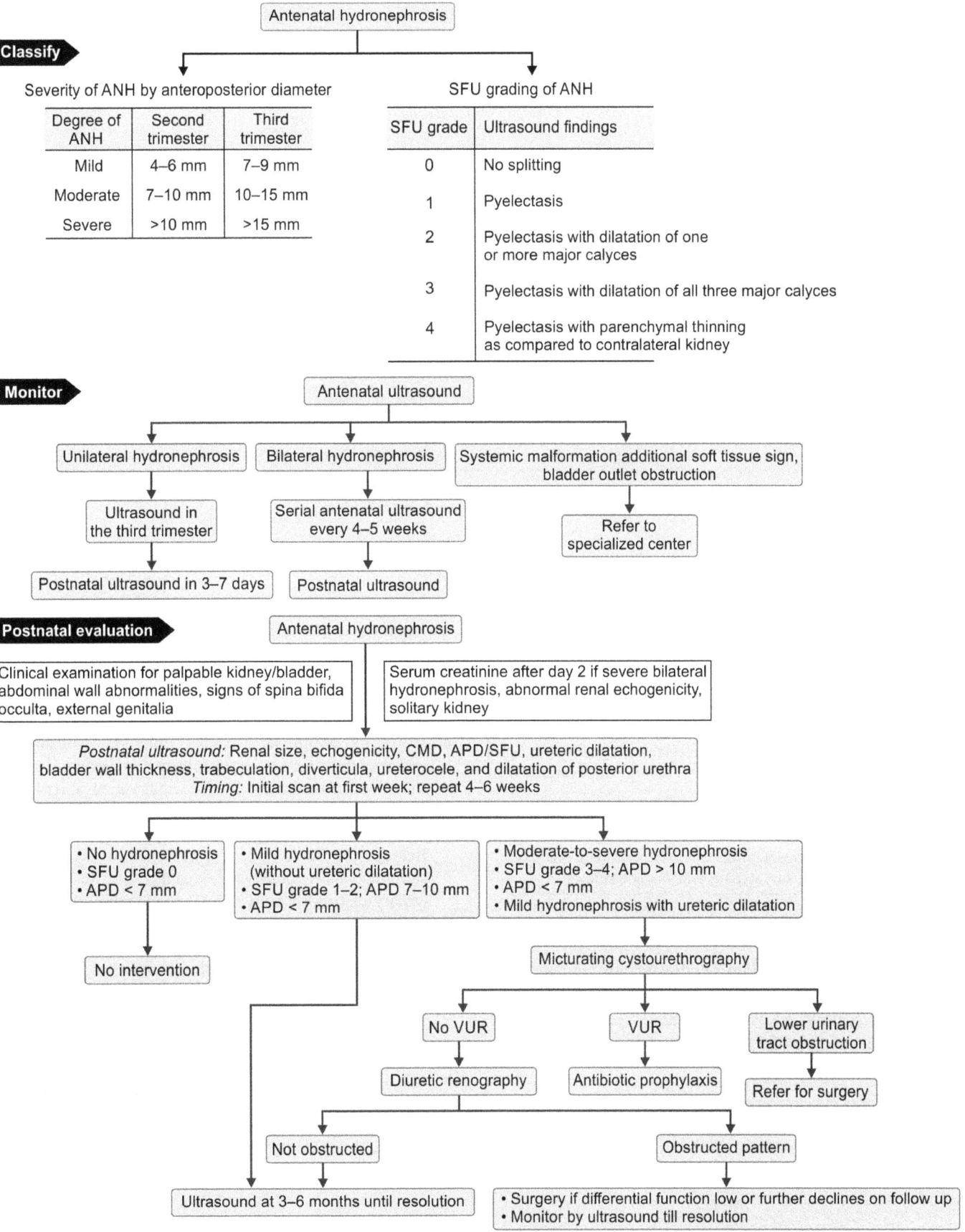

(APD: anteroposterior diameter; ANH: antenatal hydronephrosis; CMD: corticomedullary differentiation; SFU: Society of Fetal Urology; VUR: vesicoureteric reflux)

CHAPTER AT A GLANCE

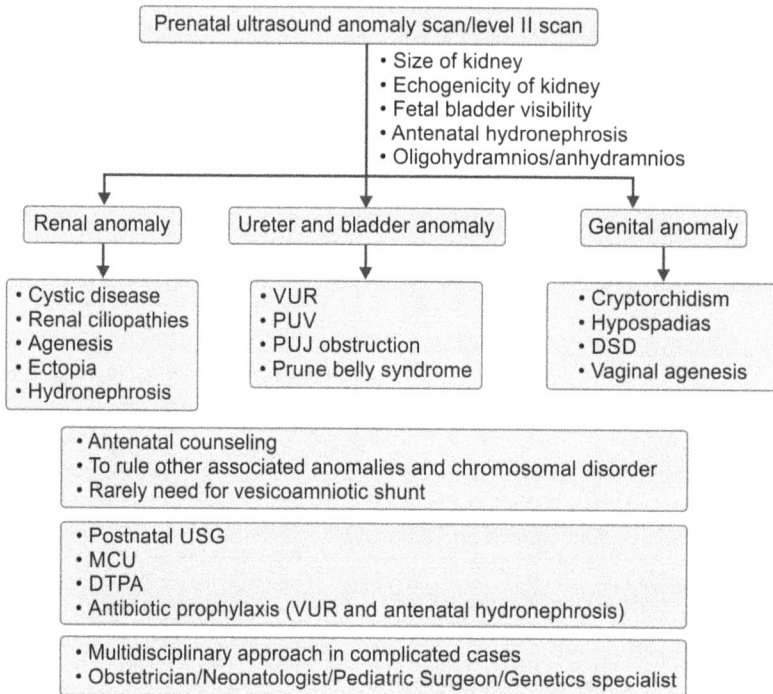

(DSD: disorder of sexual development; DTPA: diethylene-triamine-pentaacetate; PUV: posterior urethral valve; PUJ: pelviuretric junction; MCU: micturating cystourethrogram; USG: ultrasonography; VUR: vesicoureteric reflux)

KEY POINTS

- The diagnosis of most CAKUT is generally suspected when imaging studies are done during anomaly scans.
- Antenatal counseling by the perinatal team is required to allay the anxiety of the expecting mother.
- Every aim should be made to delay the pregnancy till full-term gestation except in the case of severe oligohydramnios/anhydramnios.
- Most of the time, prenatal intervention or early delivery of fetuses is not required.
- Ambiguous genitalia require a detailed history, clinical evaluation, biochemical testing, karyotyping, and imaging studies.

ACKNOWLEDGMENT

We thank Dr Prashant Jain (Pediatric Surgeon at BLK-MAX Super Speciality Hospital, Delhi); Dr Swati Bhardwaj (Pediatric Nephrologist, FMRI Gurgaon), and Dr Anita Kaul (Fetal Medicine at Apollo Hospitals Indraprastha, Delhi) for providing us the figures.

SUGGESTED READING

1. Devlin LA, Sayer JA. Renal ciliopathies. Curr Opin Genet Dev. 2019;56:49-60.
2. Martínez JM, Masoller N, Devlieger R, Passchyn E, Gómez O, Rodo J, et al. Laser ablation of posterior urethral valves by fetal cystoscopy. Fetal Diagn Ther. 2015;37(4):267-73.
3. McCann-Crosby B. Ambiguous genitalia: Evaluation and management in the newborn. NeoReviews. 2016;17(3):e144-53.
4. Morris RK, Malin GL, Khan KS, Kilby MD. A systematic review of the effectiveness of antenatal intervention for the treatment of congenital lower urinary tract obstruction. BJOG. 2010;117(4):382-90.
5. Morris RK, Malin GL, Quinlan-Jones E, Middleton LJ, Hemming K, Burke D, et al. Percutaneous vesicoamniotic shunting versus conservative management for fetal lower urinary tract obstruction (PLUTO): a randomised trial. Lancet. 2013;382(9903):1496-506.
6. Sinha A, Bagga A, Krishna A, Bajpai M, Srinivas M, Uppal R, et al. Revised guidelines on management of antenatal hydronephrosis. Indian J Nephrol. 2013;23(2):83-97.
7. Stonebrook E, Hoff M, Spencer JD. Congenital anomalies of the kidney and urinary tract: A clinical review. Curr Treat Options Pediatr. 2019;5(3):223-35.
8. Talati AN, Webster CM, Vora NL. Prenatal genetic considerations of congenital anomalies of the kidney and urinary tract (CAKUT). Prenat Diagn. 2019;39(9):679-92.
9. Vricella GJ, Coplen DE. Neonatal urogenital issues: Evaluation and management. NeoReviews. 2017;18(6):e372-85.

CHAPTER 10

Musculoskeletal Malformations

Somalika Pal, Manisha Kumar

INTRODUCTION

Musculoskeletal (MS) malformations in the fetus are detected in about 0.02% of fetuses. Most such malformations (around 80%) occur in pregnancies with no prior obstetric history of skeletal defects. These may range from simple deformities of hands and feet easily amenable to treatment to some of the most lethal skeletal dysplasias. Early prenatal detection is thus important as it helps with prognostication of the family, and decisions pertaining to need of invasive genetic testing or presence of skilled resuscitation team at birth. These disorders may be sporadic or genetic. Antenatal ultrasonography (USG) is the most popular and cost-effective imaging modality for diagnosis usually followed by biochemical and genetic workups wherever required and available. Early prenatal recognition of MS anomalies also allows for the early involvement of a multidisciplinary team for management which should preferably include a pediatric orthopedic surgeon and medical geneticist along with obstetrician, fetal medicine expert, and neonatologist for a comprehensive prenatal parental counseling. Early diagnosis may help in enabling fetal surgery if available, but its role for nonlethal malformations remains controversial.

OBJECTIVES

- To understand the heterogeneous spectrum of conditions encompassed under the broad heading of MS malformations of the fetus and hence their variable prognosis.
- To understand the investigational modalities available for antenatal diagnosis and the approach to ultrasound assessment of the fetus for MS malformations.
- To provide a brief classification and diagnostic overview of some common MS malformations.
- To propose a simple diagnostic approach to be followed during antenatal surveillance in low-risk and high-risk pregnancies for identification of MS fetal anomalies.
- To provide a simple diagnostic approach toward skeletal dysplasia.
- Parental genetic, obstetric, and orthopedic counseling.

NORMAL EMBRYOLOGY AND PATHWAYS OF MUSCULOSKELETAL MALFORMATIONS

Musculoskeletal malformations are mainly congenital, making an understanding of the basic concepts of MS embryology essential. The development of the MS system can be understood in terms of development in two stages—embryonic and fetal. The embryonic stage is marked by differentiation and organogenesis, whereas the fetal stages are mainly periods for further growth and development. Hence malformations, deformations, and disruptions are all possible in the MS system of the developing fetus depending on the timing of the insult.

Embryonic Development of the Musculoskeletal System

Collections of mesoderm on either side of the developing notochord and neural crest are called somites. Entire bony skeleton, muscle, and dermal elements of body develop from these somites and are hence mesodermal in origin.

Differentiation of spine starts around the 4th week (embryonic period), first in the occipital region and extends simultaneously cranially and caudally between 4 and 6 weeks. Migrations of mesoderm from the somites give rise to connective tissue which form the trunk, vertebral bodies, ribs, and limbs. Chondrification in the mesoderm forming vertebral bodies starts at 6 weeks. Ossification of cartilage occurs subsequently in second and third trimesters, whereas ossification of neural arches and their coalescing with the vertebral body begins during the second trimester, and continues during the first 3 years of life after birth.

Limb buds (mesodermal) develop into upper and lower extremities starting around the 4th week of embryonic life. Further growth and development occurs in proximal to distal direction over subsequent 4 weeks. The upper limbs development is earlier and faster than the lower limb development. Dermatomes (mesodermal) form skin, myotomes (mesodermal) form muscle, and sclerotomes (mesodermal) form bone and cartilage. Hand and digits appear by 5th and 6th weeks respectively and notches between digits during the 7th week. The landmark during this time is the rotation of upper and lower limbs in opposite directions by 90°, i.e., externally and internally respectively to finally position the thumb laterally and the great toes in the midline.

Fetal Development of the Musculoskeletal System

The axial and appendicular skeletons arise from ossifications of cartilage. Primary ossification centers are fully developed by the end of the first trimester and the long bones continue to grow in length by endochondral growth at the ends till the growth plate eventually closes and fuses with the epiphyses around puberty.

An Ultrasonographic Timeline of the Developing Musculoskeletal System of the Fetus

The sonographic appearance of bones in the human fetus changes due to changing mineralization with changing gestation. Most anomalies are detectable at mid trimesters but lethal dysplasias may be suspected earlier with routine measurements of the long bones.

It is possible to visualize limbs on USG by 9 weeks of gestation and the length of long bones can be measured by 10 weeks. Skull, spine, and thorax anomalies may be detected by 10-12 weeks, whereas hip joint anatomy can be delineated only in the third trimester.

Implications

It is possible to detect most (up to 90-95%) of fetal MS anomalies on USG before 17 weeks. USG assessment of fetal MS system calls for a global approach to assessment of fetal skeletal and other organs due to presence of associated malformations in other regions and systems, except in certain cases of distinct regional disorders such as limb reduction defects or amniotic band syndromes. Early detailed systematic transvaginal sonography (TVS) screening in early pregnancy (14-15 weeks) is essential as some soft markers of chromosomal syndromes may not be evident at advanced gestations, followed by a late transabdominal sonography (TAS) at 20-23 weeks of gestation which is helpful for some additional information or for follow-up of disorders detected in the earlier scan. An even earlier evaluation of the fetal skeleton (as early as 9th week) has been advocated by some incases of high-risk pregnancies. Three-dimensional (3D) USG may provide multiplanar imaging and surface-rendering reconstructions for easier delineation of anomalies and in some cases may have advantages over conventional two-dimensional (2D) sonography.

Genetic tests and counseling should be rapidly sought where abnormal findings are suspected and genetic mutations and inheritance patterns are known.

Pathways of Fetal Musculoskeletal Malformations

Adverse teratogenic and genetic factors especially during embryonic period may result in malformations of MS system. Also other susceptible differentiating organ systems are simultaneously affected, leading to clustering of malformations in the form of syndromes or associations, e.g., cardiac and genitourinary system anomalies with congenital spinal deformities.

Teratogenic Abnormalities

Teratogens account for around 5% of all malformations. Common teratogens are certain maternal infections, e.g., varicella and cytomegalovirus, some therapeutic (e.g., lithium and thalidomide) and substances of abuse (e.g., alcohol), irradiation, and industrial chemicals.

Genetic Disorders

Some MS disorders have a genetic basis such as Mendelian (e.g., achondroplasia and diastrophic dwarfism), chromosomal (e.g., trisomies), or multifactorial (e.g., talipes equinovarus).

ROLE OF IMAGING STUDIES AND INVESTIGATIONS IN PRENATAL DIAGNOSIS

The prenatal diagnosis of MS malformations largely relies on USG. With TVS and 3D ultrasounds widely available, magnetic resonance imaging (MRI) and plain radiographs have been replaced by improved USG. With a wide and diverse spectra of disorders under MS system anomalies (>400) imaging studies require a holistic but sequential approach for evaluation of fetal MS system. In high-risk conditions or in cases with high suspicion of fetal MS malformations, additional early investigations (genetic studies) should be undertaken.

Ultrasonography

- Its availability, low cost, safety, accuracy in expert hands, and real-time imaging ability makes this the imaging modality of choice. Both 2D and 3D USG may be used.
- TVS is superior to TAS, especially in early pregnancy since it can visualize structures around 4 weeks earlier and is unaffected by factors such as obesity, scars, or uterine myomas in the mother. It is best if performed between the end of first to beginning of second trimester. However, TVS has a short focal distance and is not reliable after around 17 weeks of gestation, when TAS is preferable.

CHAPTER 10 | Musculoskeletal Malformations

TABLE 1: Information to be sought during sonographic evaluation of the skeleton.

Structure	What to look for on ultrasonography
Upper and lower limbs	• Degree of limb shortening (expressed in centiles. <5th centile suggests severe shortening, <2.5th centile suggests strong suspicion of skeletal dysplasia) • Pattern of limb shortening (regional, e.g., acromelia, mesomelia, or rhizomelia vs. generalized, i.e., micromelia) • Degree of mineralization best appreciated in the calvarium (look reduced acoustic shadow and long bone fractures) • Presence of fractures, bowing, or angulation • Limb-reduction anomalies
Spine	• Degree and pattern of demineralization • Continuity (scoliosis, kyphosis, diastematomyelia, and spina bifida) • Perispinal soft tissue masses • Hemivertebrae, fused vertebrae, etc.
Thorax	Hypoplastic versus normal (by cardiothoracic ratio or thoracic circumference or area)
Hands and feet	• Postural deformities • Abnormal number of digits
Skull	• Shape of skull (e.g., clover leaf, acrocephaly, etc.) • Craniosynostosis • Degree of mineralization • "Banana sign"
Bone mineralization	• Best visualized in calvarium—by checking compressibility (by pressing with transducer) or reduced acoustic shadow and hence better visualized brain • Presence of fractures of long bones
Joints and soft tissue	Contractures

- 3D USG has a role where multiplanar imaging of skeletal structures is required which is not readily visualized by 2D USG (e.g., syndactyly, skull sutures, and ribs), or surface-rendering reconstructions are required (e.g., in joint contractures in cases of fetuses with abnormal postures), for detection of anomalies not otherwise detectable on 2D USG (e.g., delayed or abnormal ossification of cranial sutures, additional ribs or fusion of ribs, vertebral body fusion or hemivertebrae, facial anomalies, e.g., cleft palate and lip). Additionally by better and clearer display of structures it improves the diagnostic accuracy and confidence of the sonographer.
- Color Doppler USG is useful for assessing blood flow, for example, in a limb with constriction band.
- **Table 1** describes the sonographic details to be collected for detection of MS anomalies.

Genetic Screening

- Genetic analysis of sample collected by invasive prenatal tests such as chorionic villus sampling and amniocentesis and more recently from cell free fetal DNA in maternal circulation should be used wherever mutations are known (e.g., FGFR3 mutations in achondroplasia and chromosomal aberrations in trisomies).
- Indications for genetic screening may include ultrasonographic suspicion of a major malformation or syndrome with or without risk factors such as advanced maternal age, either parents suffering from skeletal dysplasia or imaging study suggesting an anomaly or syndrome in an otherwise low-risk pregnancy with an available genetic test.
- Specific tests are unavailable for most skeletal anomalies.
- The genetic mutations identified may then be used to evaluate either parent for such mutations based on risk assessment in subsequent pregnancy depending on the mode of transmission of identified disorders.
- It is important to realize that genetic defects identified on genetic screening may have been inherited from either/both parents or may have arisen de novo.

SOME COMMON MUSCULOSKELETAL MALFORMATIONS

Benign MS malformations are quite frequently encountered, whereas lethal ones are rare. A detailed and systemic evaluation by an experienced sonologist is of extreme importance to understand the severity of the malformations and associated anomalies in other organ systems, so that appropriate counseling pertaining to survival, prognosis for functionality of limb/joint, and extent of orthopedic (and other) interventions required can be done. The commonly encountered MS malformations along with their key diagnostic and prognostic points are discussed in **Table 2**.

TABLE 2: Some common musculoskeletal malformations diagnosed prenatally.

Anatomical region	Relevant and important points about antenatal diagnosis and prognosis
Upper and lower extremity: • Failure of formation of part or whole limb and limb reduction defects (LRDs): – 30–45% of LRD cases are associated with other malformations, Most common (MC) ones are: • Phocomelia • Absent radius or radial clubhand • Absent fibula or fibular hemimelia • Amelia is less common but most severe	• LRDs may occasionally be regional. However, if antenatal USG detects LRD or fetal finger anomalies, a thorough search for associated malformations is mandatory • Prognosis is variable, isolated cases have better prognosis
• *Syndactyly*: May be (a) isolated or (b) associated with genetic syndromes	• Not easily detected in conventional 2D USGs: – 59–60% cases of fetal finger abnormalities are associated with other malformations and/or chromosomal disorders • *If antenatal USG detects fetal finger anomalies*: A thorough search for associated malformations is mandatory. Prognosis is variable, isolated cases have better prognosis

• Polydactyly:
     – Isolated form, usually detected in fetuses with a normal karyotype
     – With associated abnormalities
 • Chromosomal disorders in 59–60% cases (e.g., trisomy 13, Meckel–Gruber, Ellis–van Creveld, and short rib polydactyly)
	If antenatal USG detects fetal finger anomalies: A thorough search for associated malformations is mandatory. Prognosis is variable, isolated cases have better prognosis

• Long-bone abnormalities:
     – *Severe shortening of long bones*: Usually associated with lethal skeletal dysplasia, e.g., achondrogenesis, osteogenesis imperfecta type II, and thanatophoric dwarfism
     – *Moderate shortening of long bones*: MC is proximal femoral deficiency/hypoplasia
 	
     – *Mild shortening*: MC is proximal femoral deficiency/hypoplasia
	• *On antenatal USG*: Detected by delay of >3–4 weeks in bone length in early pregnancy
	 • Almost always lethal
	 • *On antenatal USG*: A delay of 2–3 weeks in the size of bones, diagnosis possible as early as the 12th week of gestation
	 • Follow-up USG scans are mandatory in order to exclude a false positive diagnosis of bone dysplasias
	 • Prognosis variable
	 • *On antenatal USG*: Bones appear within the normal range in early pregnancy and their shortening is only obvious after 23 weeks of gestation
	 • Prognosis variable

• Clubfoot:
     – Prevalence ranges from 0.09% in newborn to 0.43% when detected by USG in the intrauterine phase
     – Bilateral in 40–50% cases
     – Usually idiopathic, but may be associated with other structural anomalies such as hydrocephalus, neural tube defects, cleft lip/palate and heart defects, and/or chromosomal abnormalities
	• *On antenatal USG*: 45% identified by week 17, 45% detected between 18 and 24 weeks, and 10% recognized between 25 and 32 weeks
	 • It is important to look for any associated malformations.
	 • Prognosis depends on severity, presence, and nature of associated anomaly

Vertebrae and spine:
 • Congenital malformation of vertebrae:
     – Failure of formation—hemivertebra and absence of vertebrae (as in caudal regression syndrome)
     – Failure of segmentation, such as fused vertebrae and unsegmented bar, which causes congenital scoliosis or kyphosis
	• Ossification centers of each parallel vertebrae should be visualized in a single line to rule out hemivertebra, fused vertebra, absence of vertebra, widening of the spinal canal, or kyphoscoliosis
	 • Earliest reported age of detection of abnormal spinal curvatures is 14th week of gestation
	 • Prognosis variable

• Disorders of continuity of vertebral column
 • May be sporadic, genetic, or teratogenic
 • Most notable ones are:
     – Spina bifida
 	
     – *Caudal regression syndrome (CRS)*: Rare fetal complication of diabetic pregnancy:
	• Antenatal USG may show skin defects posterior to the vertebral column, a cystic lesion protruding from the spinal canal, a U-shaped appearance of the vertebra, or the "banana sign"
	 • >90% of these signs can be seen at 12–17 weeks of gestation
	 • Prognosis variable
	 • TVS may diagnose caudal regression syndrome even by 9th or 11th week gestation, but most cases are diagnosed during the second trimester
	 • Prognosis poor

Contd...

Contd...

Anatomical region	Relevant and important points about antenatal diagnosis and prognosis
– Presents as mild incomplete development of the sacrum to severe agenesis of the lumbosacral spine, including disruption of the distal spinal cord and lack of growth of the caudal region – Associated anomalies include neurologic, urologic, and orthopedic manifestations	
– Scoliosis, kyphosis, and diastematomyelia – Diastematomyelia is a rare expression of spinal dysraphism that can be associated with other spinal anomalies, such as spina bifida, hemivertebra and butterfly vertebra	• Antenatal sonographic detection of diastematomyelia is possible mostly in the third trimester • Extensive USG scanning and/or MRI in order to exclude more serious neural tube defects is warranted • Prognosis variable
Skull: • Craniosynostosis: – *Inheritance*: Autosomal dominant or sporadic – A heterogeneous condition in which cranial sutures close prematurely → early fusion of the skull-plates → expansion of brain parenchyma in available planes → Abnormal head shape – Incidence 1 per 2,000/2,500 live births – Usually isolated defect (85%), or part of syndrome in 15% (e.g., Apert syndrome, Crouzon syndrome, or Pfeiffer syndrome) – MC: Sagittal synostosis → skull is longer and narrower posteriorly (dolico/scaphocephaly)	• Prenatal diagnosis by USG (findings include: Long and narrow head, brachycephaly, frontal bossing, midfacial hypoplasia, and hypertelorism) possible as early as 12 weeks • Both 2D and 3D USG can be used, but 3D superior to 2D to visualize sutural fusion • Further thorough investigation is possible using MRI • *Prognosis:* Termination advisable, if detected early during pregnancy
Joints: • Congenital multiple arthrogryposis: – Multiple joint contractures of variable and heterogeneous etiologies with a prenatal onset – Contractures may be of isolated multiple joints (classic), or associated with other malformations and syndromes Examples: • Pterigia • Fetal akinesia syndromes	• Prenatal USG detects arthrogryposis mainly during early second trimester (findings include persistently reduced/absent fetal movements, deformed long bones, joint contractures, clubhand) (severe flexed hands), absent muscles or markedly reduced soft tissue, clubfoot, subcutaneous edema with skin creases, abnormal joint positioning and the "Buddha" position (in as many as 95% cases) • Prognosis mostly poor
Miscellaneous: • *Constriction band syndrome (or amniotic band syndrome)*: Presents as constriction and amputation of fingers, toes, and limbs: – May be associated with a wider spectrum of craniofacial, visceral, and limb anomalie – Sporadic and rare	• May be detected as early as 18 weeks by antenatal USG • Prognosis variable

Generalized skeleton:
• Skeletal dysplasia:
– Includes around 436 disorders classified within 42 groups, with around 364 identified genetic defects
– Birth incidence of 1 per 5,000, prevalence 5 per 10,000 births
– Spectrum of presentation variable ranging from lethal to nonlethal phenotypes with varying grades of functional impairments
  - *Common lethal skeletal dysplasia*: Thanatophoric dysplasia (most common lethal), achondrogenesis, campomelic dysplasia, osteogenesis imperfecta type II, Jeune thoracic dystrophy
  - *Common nonlethal skeletal dysplasias*: Achondroplasia (most common nonlethal), club and rocker-bottom feet (vertical talus), diastrophic dysplasia, and osteogenesis imperfecta type I, III, and VI, radial ray aplasia/hypoplasia
	• Intrauterine diagnosis should focus on early identification of lethal forms for purposes of counseling regarding termination of pregnancy, or the more severe disorders expected to require skilled resuscitation at birth and involvement of multidisciplinary teams for management
	• Lethal forms can be diagnosed toward the end of the first trimester whereas the nonlethal forms can be diagnosed between 22 and 23 weeks of gestation
	• The accuracy of prenatal diagnosis using routine USG is merely 40%, hence all cases of prenatally diagnosed skeletal dysplasias should have a final diagnosis made by expert clinical and radiologic evaluation

(2D: two-dimensional; 3D: three-dimensional; MRI: magnetic resonance imaging; TVS: transvaginal sonography; USG: ultrasonography)

FETAL SCREENING FOR DIAGNOSIS OF MUSCULOSKELETAL MALFORMATIONS

Approach to a pregnancy to evaluate for MS malformations should include the following in a systematic and sequential manner:

- *History*: Family history (e.g., in achondroplasia and osteogenesis imperfect type I) and antenatal history (including exposure to teratogenic medications such as lithium and warfarin, perception of fetal movements—reduced in generalized arthrogryposis, e.g., fetal akinesia syndrome, history of gestational diabetes, e.g., in proximal femoral deficiency), past obstetric history (e.g., for neural tube defects and skeletal dysplasias).
- *Clinical examination of the pregnant woman*: May yield markers of skeletal dysplasia in the mother (e.g., blue sclera in osteogenesis imperfecta type I, characteristic short stature and body proportions in achondroplasia), clinical examination for liquor status.
- Fetal screening by USG for diagnosis of MS malformations:
  - *Timing*: Consensus supports early systematic and detailed USG screening at 14th and 15th weeks of gestation followed by a late scan at 20 or more weeks for the detection of MS anomalies. Some defects may be visualized as early as 10–12 weeks and may be considered in high-risk cases.
  - In experienced hands simple 2D USG is usually adequate, 3D USG is important for detection of some MS disorders, e.g., delayed or abnormal ossification of cranial sutures, additional ribs or fusion of ribs, vertebral body fusion or hemivertebrae, facial anomalies, e.g., cleft palate and lip, and also for better multiplanar visualization which improves diagnostic accuracy.
  - Fetal skeletal parameters that are measured on USG should be compared against normative values. Measures include head circumference and biparietal diameter, chest/thoracic circumference, cardiothoracic ratio, fetal long bones, etc., as mentioned above.
  - On suspicion of significant MS malformation, e.g., identification of long bone length <5th centile in <24 weeks of gestation, patient should be referred to a center that has expertise in evaluating the entire fetal skeleton and has the ability to provide genetic counseling and immediate neonatal management of such neonates.
- MRI has negligible yield in the diagnosis of MS disorders in modern-day obstetrics, as the disadvantages associated with it far outweigh the advantages.
- Genetics work-up and genetic counseling wherever available should be offered. If antenatal diagnosis is not possible, all attempts should be made to identify genetic defects in postnatal life.
- **Flowchart 1** presents a flowchart to help guide screening of fetuses for MS malformations.

APPROACH TO A CASE WITH SUSPECTED SKELETAL DYSPLASIA

Approach to a Pregnancy at High Risk of Skeletal Dysplasia

A pregnancy at high risk of skeletal dysplasia is one where either/both parents suffer from skeletal dysplasia, or a previous pregnancy was affected by skeletal dysplasia with or without a genetic mutation identified. Genetic diagnosis and counseling should be offered in all pregnancies at-risk for homozygous or compound heterozygous mutations (e.g., genetic tests for FGFR3 mutation is easily available and should be ordered if one or both parents have achondroplasia and fetus is detected to have limb shortening with preserved head circumference). Ideally, mutations in both parents should be evaluated before pregnancy. Mode of delivery may need to be discussed due to maternal stature.

Approach to a Pregnancy with Skeletal Dysplasia Detected During Antenatal Surveillance

A systematic algorithmic approach should be used. Prenatal USG diagnosis involves measuring and identifying degree, distribution and pattern of shortening in bones involved (In micromelia, all segments of the limb are abnormally shortened, whereas rhizomelia refers to disproportionate shortening of proximal limbs, mesomelia refers to shortened middle parts of the limbs and acromelia to disproportionately shortened distal limb regions), presence of bowing of bones (campomelia refers to bowing of the long bones), along with degree of mineralization (best detected in calvarium by overtly well visualized fetal brain or presence of multiple fractures visualized by abnormal bowing/angulation and/or beaded ribs appearance), and other systems involvement, e.g., cardiovascular, spine, face, and kidneys **(Flowchart 2)**. Suspicion of lethal forms is usually triggered by early scans (end of the first trimester), whereas nonlethal forms are detectable later (usually between 22 and 23 weeks of gestation).

A systematic approach involves assessment of lethality as the first step. Pointers suggesting lethality on antenatal USG are heart-to-chest circumference ratio (HrC/CC ratio > 50% suggesting lethality), thoracic circumference to abdominal circumference ratio (TC/AC ratio < 0.7 suggesting lethality), and the femur length to abdominal circumference ratio (FL/AC ratio of <0.16 suggesting lethality). Disorders with severe degrees of hypomineralization and multiple fractures on early scans are lethal too, as are those with severe thoracic constriction (pulmonary hypoplasia).

As many skeletal dysplasias are associated with a significant recurrence risk a thorough clinical and radiologic

Flowchart 1: The approach toward screening for musculoskeletal (MS) malformations.

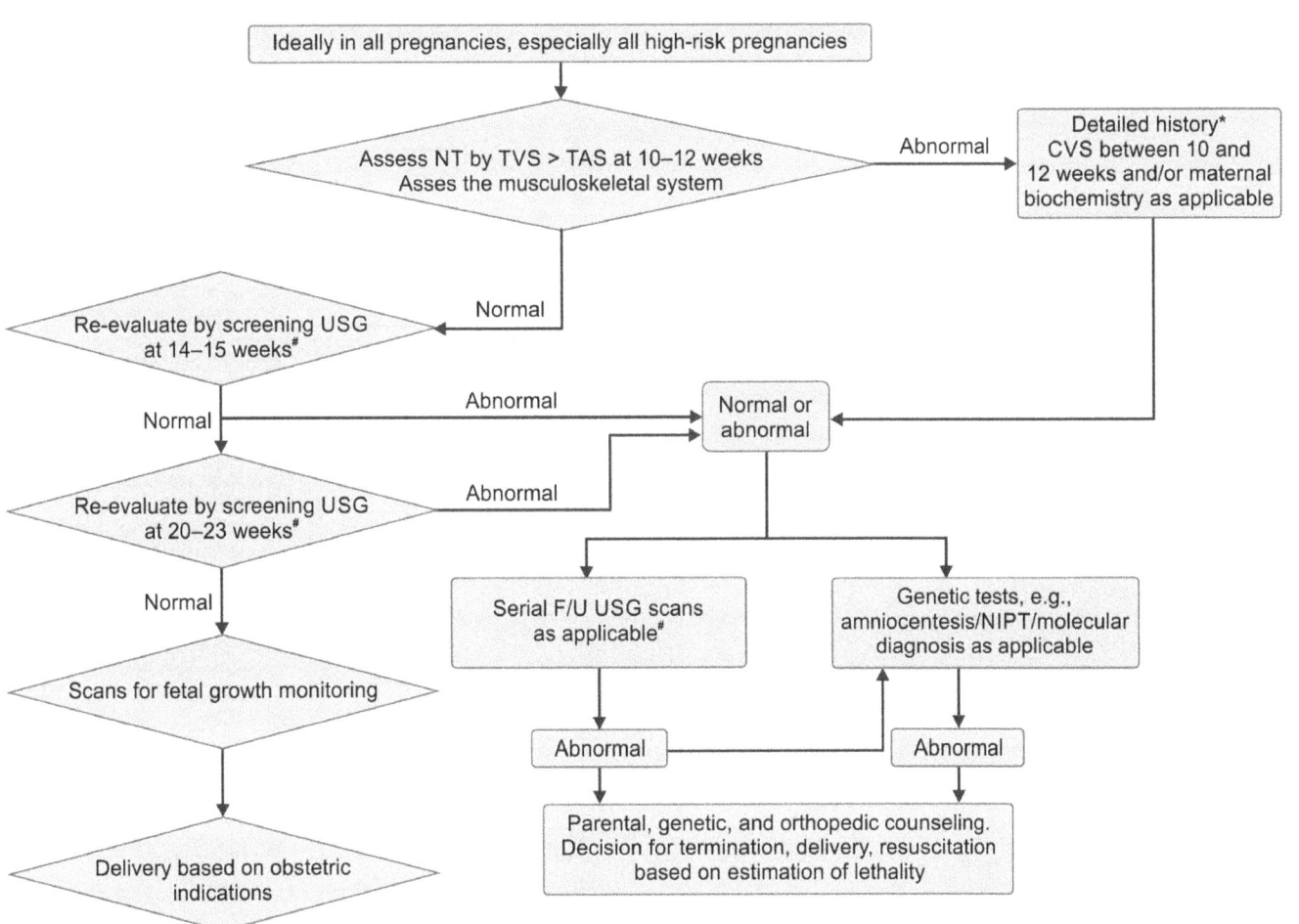

(CVS: chorionic villus sampling; NIPT: noninvasive prenatal test; NT: nuchal translucency; TAS: transabdominal sonography; TVS: transvaginal sonography; USG: ultrasonography)
*History should include family history of MS disorders, antenatal history (e.g., exposure to teratogenic medications, diabetes, perception of fetal movements, and past obstetric history).
#USG should focus on detailed skeletal survey which must include measurements of long bones, degree of mineralization and thoracic hypoplasia for assessment of lethality, assessment of calvarial shape and suture, fetal fingers and toes, facial structures, and other system involvement.
NIPT for free fetal DNA in maternal circulation.

evaluation should ideally be done in all fetuses suspected of having a skeletal dysplasia postdelivery and/or postmortem. This evaluation should include X-rays anterior–posterior (AP) views of axial and appendicular skeleton including hands and feet with lateral views of skull and vertebral column as well (infantogram or babygram), clinical photographs of the baby, tissue, or blood samples for genetic tests and pathological autopsies wherever possible for detailed assessment and genetic diagnosis.

An algorithmic approach to diagnosis of skeletal dysplasia has been presented in **Flowchart 2**.

ANTENATAL COUNSELING

Antenatal Counseling in Cases of Presumed Lethal Skeletal Dysplasias

The counseling of such cases should ideally be done by a medical geneticist. The poor prognosis for survival should be explained. The options available to parents are termination of pregnancy (if detected early) or continuation. The high likelihood of in-utero fetal demise in the latter case should be explained. If born alive, the extent of neonatal resuscitation and life support to be offered needs to be discussed, documented, and communicated to the delivery team. The risk of recurrence in future pregnancies and the benefits and limitations of a genetic and molecular diagnosis needs to be discussed. Consent for preservation of DNA/tissue sample needs to be taken.

If parents do not wish for advanced life support, comfort care needs to be provided. In case of in-utero or early neonatal demise, autopsy should be offered. After due consent, 2–5 mL cord/baby blood in ethylenediaminetetraacetic acid (EDTA) tube for DNA extraction, a babygram, and clinical photographs should be taken.

Parental DNA evaluation by linkage studies may be undertaken if mutation can be identified.

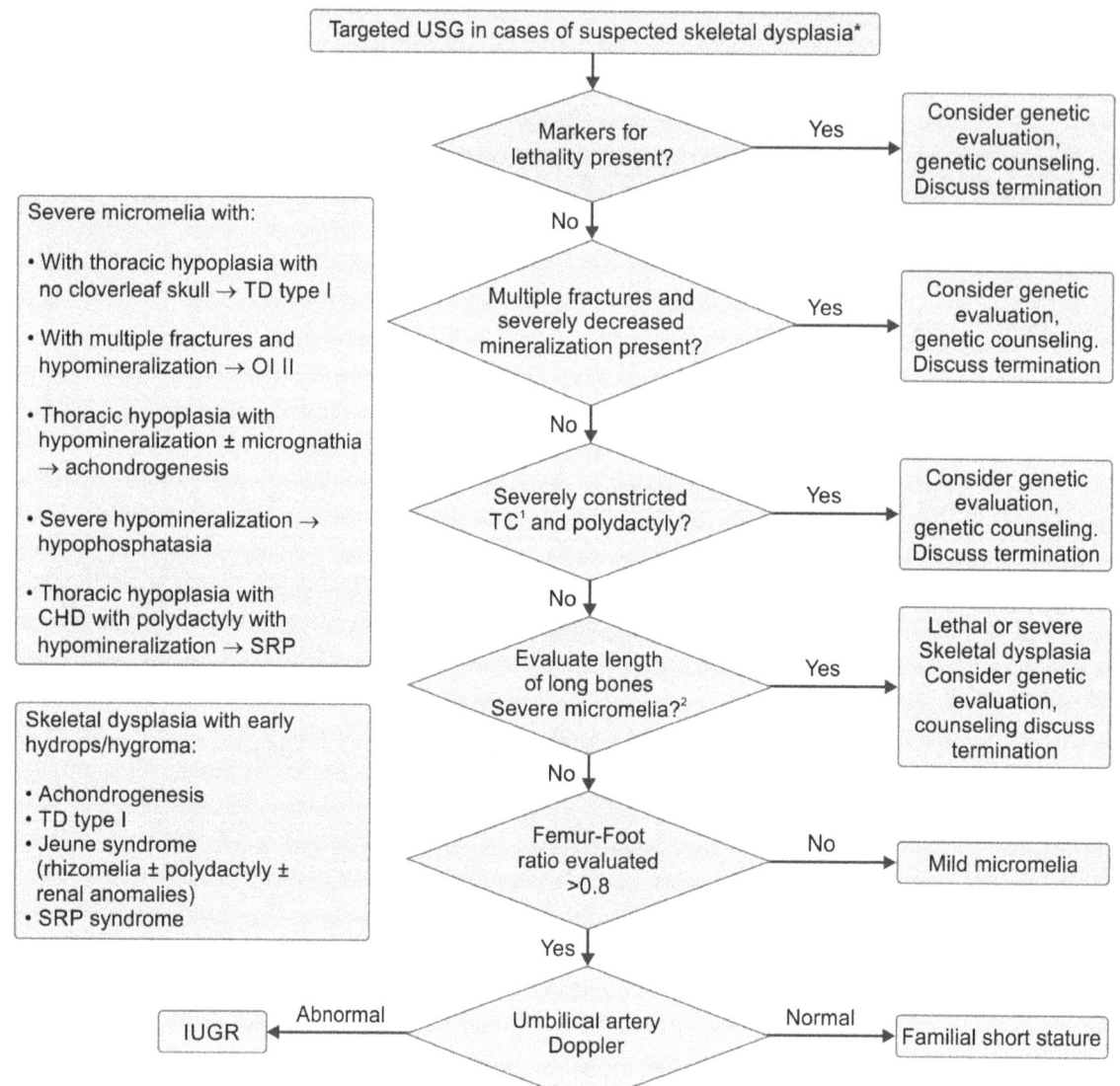

Flowchart 2: Algorithmic approach to a case of suspected skeletal dysplasia.

(CHD: congenital heart disease; IUGR: intrauterine growth restriction; OI: osteogenesis imperfecta; SRP: short rib polydactyly syndrome; TC: thoracic circumference; TD: thanatophoric dysplasia)
*Suspect skeletal dysplasia if screening USG reveals suggestive markers, e.g., long bone length <5th centile or <2 SD.
[1]TC is thoracic circumference measured at the level of the four-chamber view of the heart in axial section, and a value of <2.5th centile suggests severe constriction.
[2]FL (femur length) of <4 SD or <3 SD or <2.5 centile has been considered as severe micromelia.

Antenatal Counseling in Cases of Presumed Nonlethal Skeletal Malformation

The counseling of such cases should ideally be done by a medical geneticist or neonatologist. A pediatric orthopedic surgeon may be involved if needed. The parents need to be counseled about the functional and/or cosmetic impairments based on the likely presumed phenotype as understood on prenatal USG. The mode of delivery may need to be discussed in the presence of an obstetrician in case either/both parents suffer from skeletal dysplasia [most common (MC) nonlethal types are achondroplasia and osteogenesis imperfecta type I]. Delivery should be undertaken at a site equipped for advanced resuscitation in the lactated Ringer (LR) and advanced life support in neonatal intensive care unit (NICU), in case antenatal findings suggest small thoracic circumference or associated other system malformations. After delivery, a babygram, imaging for associated malformations, and blood for genetic diagnosis should be drawn.

CHAPTER 10 | Musculoskeletal Malformations

CHAPTER AT A GLANCE

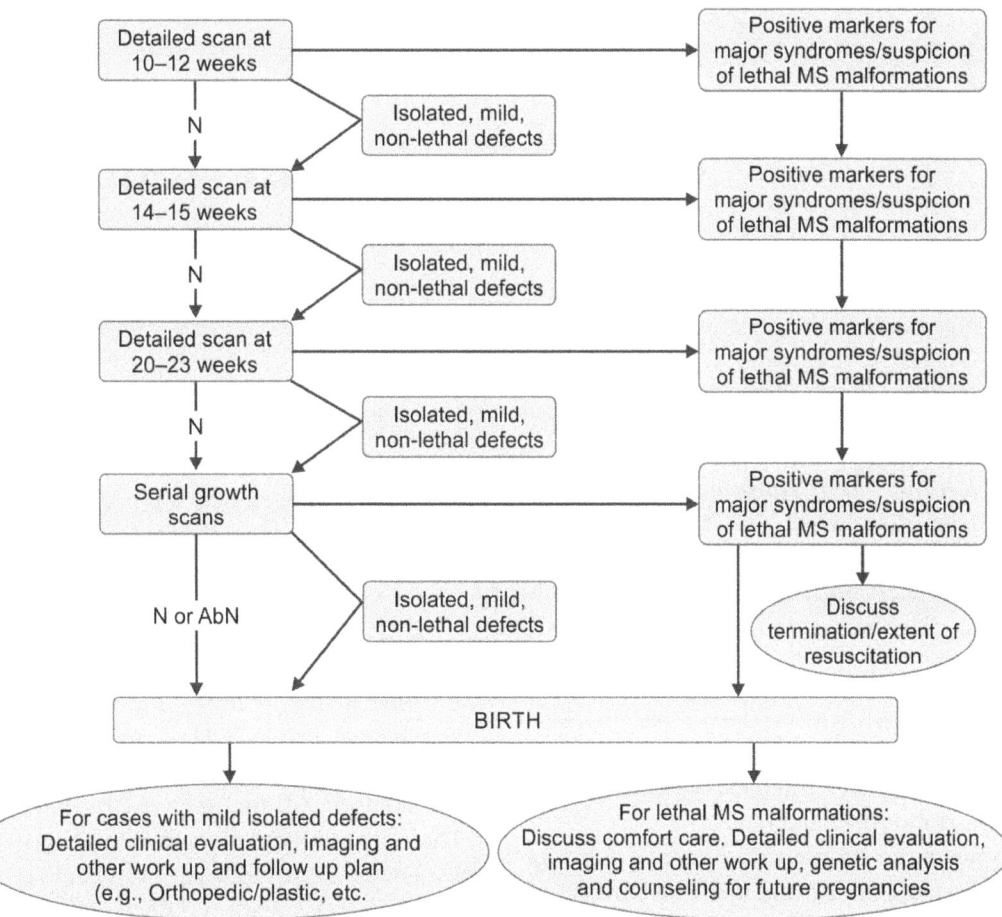

KEY POINTS

- As a group, MS malformations are not uncommon.
- USG remains the mainstay for antenatal diagnosis with TVS useful in early diagnosis and TAS in later gestations.
- A systematic evaluation of the skeleton at 14–15 weeks in every pregnancy and then again at 20–23 weeks is important for detection of major skeletal malformations.
- Antenatal diagnosis of skeletal dysplasias is complex due to the heterogenous nature of conditions within this broad entity. An algorithmic approach to diagnosis at a center with expertise in imaging the fetal skeleton and facilities for genetic and molecular diagnosis can help in knowing the exact disorder and aid in parental counseling for present or subsequent pregnancies. Identification of lethal conditions separate from nonlethal ones with reasonable accuracy is the key to this diagnostic algorithm.

SUGGESTED READING

1. Dighe M, Fligner C, Cheng E, Warren B, Dubinsky T. Fetal skeletal dysplasia: An approach to diagnosis with illustrative cases. RadioGraphics. 2008;28(4):1061-77.
2. Inglis G, Jardine L, Davies M, Koorts P. Antenatal Consults, A Guide for Neonatologists and Pediatricians. Elsevier Publications; 2012.
3. Krakow D, Lachman RS, Rimoin DL. Guidelines for the prenatal diagnosis of fetal skeletal dysplasias. Genet Med. 2009;11(2):127-33.
4. Martin R, Fanaroff A, Walsh M. Musculoskeletal malformations of the neonate. Fanaroff and Martin Textbook of Neonatology, Volume 2. Amsterdam: Elsevier; 2019.
5. Paladini D, Volpe P. Skeletal dysplasias and muscular anomalies: A diagnostic algorithm. Ultrasound of Congenital Fetal Anomalies, Differential Diagnosis and Prognostic Indicators, 2nd edition. Boca Raton: CRC Press; 2014.

CHAPTER 11

Gastrointestinal Malformations

Naveen P Gupta, Chanchal Singh

INTRODUCTION

Congenital abnormalities affect 2–3% of the low-risk population. Gastrointestinal abnormalities encompass apparent abnormalities in the first trimester, such as anterior abdominal wall defects, to trachea-esophageal fistula (TEF) that may not manifest before the third trimester and are also suspected on indirect signs like polyhydramnios.

OBJECTIVES

- To understand the normal antenatal ultrasound findings of the fetal gastrointestinal tract
- How to suspect these disorders on antenatal ultrasound
- Antenatal follow-up, timing, and mode of delivery
- Immediate postnatal management
- Prognosis

FETAL GASTROINTESTINAL SONOGRAPHIC EXAMINATION

- Esophagus is collapsed in-utero and not visualized by imaging.
- A fluid-filled stomach is normally seen in the second and third trimesters since the fetus starts swallowing amniotic fluid between 11 and 14 weeks of gestation.
- Physiological midgut herniation can be seen between 9 and 11 weeks of gestation and its subsequent reduction by the 12th week. Any midgut hernia visible on ultrasound beyond 12 weeks is not normal. The bowel lumen is usually collapsed in the first trimester. Fluid is usually seen in the bowel by 20 weeks of gestation. Normal small bowel loops do not exceed 7 mm in diameter and 15 mm in length in the second and third trimesters. The diameter increases with advancing gestational age for the colon, achieving up to 23 mm filled with meconium at term. Peristalsis may be visible after 18 weeks of gestation. Dilated loops and vigorous peristalsis may suggest intestinal obstruction.
- Echogenic bowel is an ultrasound finding when bowel is visualized brighter (as bright as bone) in the second trimester. It may be a normal finding or marker of an abnormality, such as trisomy 21, congenital cytomegalovirus, parvovirus, cystic fibrosis, or severe intrauterine growth restriction.

ESOPHAGEAL ANOMALIES

Esophageal Atresia

Esophageal atresia (EA) refers to a congenital interruption of esophagus commonly associated with an abnormal connection with the trachea (tracheo-esophageal fistula). There are five types of tracheoesophageal anomalies:
1. *Type A*: EA without TEF (10%)
2. *Type B*: EA with a TEF to the proximal esophageal segment (<1%)
3. *Type C*: EA with a TEF to the distal esophageal segment (85%)
4. *Type D*: EA with TEF to both the proximal and distal esophageal segments (<1%)
5. *Type E*: TEF with no EA (4%)

Gross classification of EA; A, esophageal atresia without fistula; B, EA with proximal TEF; C, EA with distal TEF; D, EA with proximal and distal TEF; E, TEF (H-type).

When to Suspect Antenatally?

The following ultrasound findings are suggestive:
- Polyhydramnios
- Small or nonvisualized fetal stomach
- Pouch sign, which refers to visualization of a fluid-filled, blind-ending esophagus during fetal swallowing.

Type C variety is challenging to pick antenatally since the fistula allows fluid to flow into the stomach. Polyhydramnios accompanies one-third of cases of EA with distal fistula.

A systematic review noted that prenatal ultrasound detects only a third of cases of EA and there was a high rate of false-positive diagnosis. The sonographic signs suggestive of EA (polyhydramnios and small stomach) are neither sensitive nor specific. While 78% of fetuses with isolated EA are identified prenatally only 22% with an TEF was identified. It is essential to assess the fetus for associated anomalies that may be present in up to 50% of cases. The most common are cardiac malformations (25% of cases). It can be a part of the VACTERL association (vertebral, anal, cardiac, tracheoesophageal atresia, renal, limb malformation). Chromosomal abnormalities are noted in 6-10% of cases. Fetal MRI has a better diagnostic performance for the prenatal detection of EA. Additional tests include echocardiography and chromosomal microarray.

Postnatal Management

In the delivery room, a 10-12 French feeding tube should be passed through the esophagus to the stomach. Failure to pass the catheter beyond 11 or 12 centimeters is an important sign. Symptoms include excessive drooling, choking, and cyanosis especially if feeding is attempted. The neonate should be admitted to the neonatal intensive care unit (NICU). A continuous suction (Replogle catheter) should be applied in the upper pouch to prevent aspiration of secretions in the lung. Respiratory distress should be managed by intubation and ventilation. Continuous positive airway pressure (CPAP) should be avoided. Anteroposterior X-ray of the chest with abdomen demonstrates coiling of the catheter in the upper pouch. The presence of gas in the stomach suggests the presence of TEF associated with EA. Majority of infants with H-type TEF present in infancy or childhood with recurrent pneumonia. Because TEF/EA is part of a constellation of other abnormalities (CHARGE syndrome or VACTERL association), additional tests like echocardiography, renal ultrasound should be performed.

Surgical correction involves end to end anastomosis of the esophagus along with ligation of fistula. If the gap between the upper and lower end of the esophagus more than 3 cm or greater than the height of two vertebral bodies, then esophagostomy and gastrostomy are done, and primary repair is done later.

Prognosis

The outcome of EA with TEF has improved over the years. Reported survival rates have been 87-90%. The mortality rate is greater in infants with associated cardiac and chromosomal abnormalities.

ANOMALIES OF SMALL INTESTINE

Duodenal Atresia and Stenosis

The reported prevalence of duodenal atresia and stenosis is 1 in 5,000 births. It is the most common type of intestinal obstruction and presents as a "double bubble" sign in the ultrasound resulting from an enlarged stomach and duodenum on either side of the atresia. It is usually diagnosed in the late second trimester (>24 weeks) and polyhydramnios is seen in 50% of cases.

Associated anomalies include trisomy 21 (30% of cases), congenital heart disease (20-30% of cases), and renal and vertebral. Further investigations are microarray, echocardiography, and detailed ultrasound examination to look for renal and vertebral anomalies.

Jejunoileal Atresia and Stenosis

The reported prevalence of jejunal atresia is 1 in 5,000 births. It is usually diagnosed in the late second or third trimester when multiple fluid-filled bowel loops with dilatation of more than 7 mm are seen **(Fig. 1)**. Active peristalsis can be seen in the dilated bowel loops. If bowel perforation occurs, transient ascites, meconium peritonitis, and meconium pseudocysts may ensue.

Jejunal atresia/stenosis is not associated with an increased risk of chromosomal abnormalities and genetic syndromes. However, other bowel abnormalities may coexist, e.g., malrotation, gastroschisis, duplication, and meconium ileus. There is a 10% risk of cystic fibrosis, in which case up to 90% will have associated meconium peritonitis.

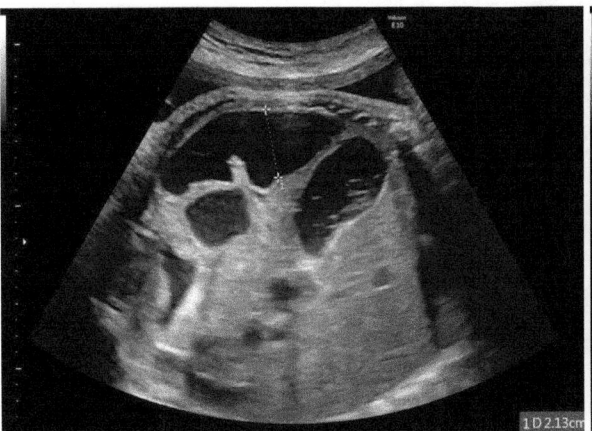
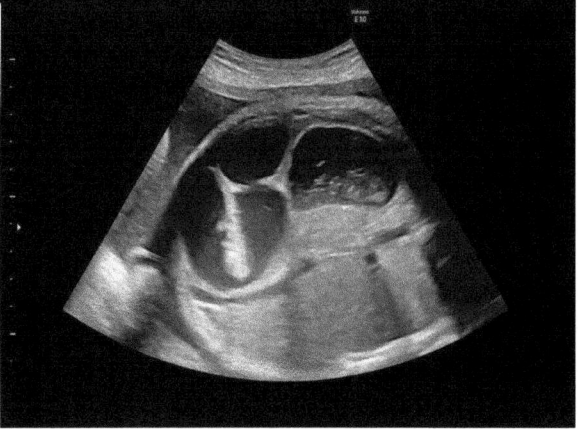

Fig. 1: 2D images showing dilated bowel loops in third trimester. Postnatally diagnosis of jejunal atresia was made.

Antenatal Management

After the initial diagnosis, periodic ultrasound examinations should be performed to look for any change in the appearance of the atresia or associated anomalies and to assess interval fetal growth and amniotic fluid volume. In severe polyhydramnios, therapeutic amnio-drainage should be considered. Delivery should be conducted in a tertiary care center. The aim is to deliver as close to 38 weeks as possible unless delivery is indicated earlier due to fetal growth restriction or progressive dilatation of intra-abdominal bowel defined as more than 20 mm in the transverse section.

Postnatal Management

Comprises initial stabilization followed by surgical correction. Feedings should be withheld and gut should be decompressed with an orogastric tube. Plain X-ray abdomen in erect posture and if needed, contrast upper gastrointestinal tract studies should be done. End to side or end to end duodenoduodenostomy should be done in duodenal atresia. For jejunal and ileal atresia end-to-end or end-to-back anastomosis is done.

Prognosis

In a large series, the long-term survival for duodenal, jejunoileal, and colonic atresia was 86%, 84%, and 100%, respectively. Major causes of mortality and morbidity are short bowel syndrome and associated prematurity, cardiac, chromosomal abnormalities.

DISORDERS OF THE LARGE INTESTINE

Obstruction in the colon may be due to Hirschsprung's disease, anorectal malformations of colonic atresia.

Hirschsprung's Disease

It is one of the most common causes of intestinal obstruction in the newborn. It is caused by the failure of ganglion cells to migrate cephalocaudally from the neural crest. It is characterized by severe constipation due to functional colonic obstruction with megacolon. The disease rarely manifests prenatally except the severe variety due to total colonic aganglionosis. Sonographic features include dilated loops of the small intestine occasionally with enterolithiasis. A quarter of patients may have associated anomalies. There is also a strong association with Down syndrome. Neonates present postnatally with a delay or failure to pass meconium during the first 24 hours of life and vomiting or abdominal distention.

Anorectal Malformations

The reported prevalence of anorectal malformation is 1 in 5,000 births. It is detected in the third trimester due to overdistention of the rectum and sigmoid colon (**Figs. 2A to C**). Amniotic fluid volume is usually normal. Sometimes

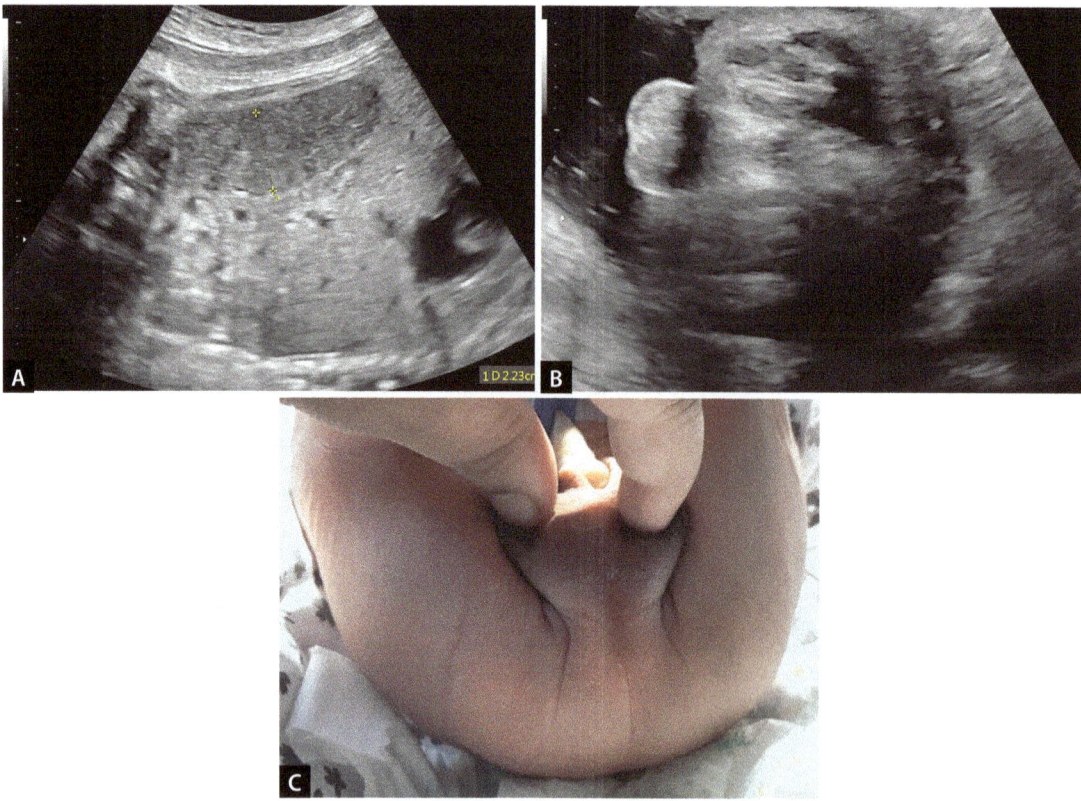

Figs. 2A to C: (A) 2D image showing dilated, meconium-filled dilated large bowel loop; (B) Absent target sign; (C) Postnatal image showing imperforate anus.

intraluminal calcifications due to meconium inspissation may be seen.

Anorectal malformations may be associated with chromosomal abnormalities in 3-4% of cases (mainly trisomy 21 and 18) and other defects such as urogenital malformations, vertebral anomalies and central nervous system abnormalities in up to 70% of cases. These may also be part of nongenetic syndromes, like VACTERL (sporadic; vertebral and ventricular septal defects, anal atresia, TEF, renal anomalies, radial dysplasia, and single umbilical artery), caudal regression syndrome (sporadic; sacral agenesis or hypoplasia, hypoplastic vertebral bodies, anal atresia), OEIS complex (sporadic; omphalocele, exstrophy of the cloaca, imperforate anus, and spinal defects). If the vesico rectal fistula is present, mixing of urine and meconium leads to calcification of meconium, forming enteroliths. Therefore, if intraluminal calcifications are identified, anal atresia with vesico rectal fistula should be suspected. MRI can help distinguish between cloaca and anorectal malformation.

Colonic Atresia

It is a rare cause of intestinal obstruction accounting for less than 15% of cases of bowel atresia. The majority occur proximal to splenic flexure with distal microcolon. Usually, it is missed prenatally because fluid is resorbed in the small intestine, and the lumen looks normal on ultrasound. It is also not commonly associated with polyhydramnios. Usually, it is isolated, rarely associated with anomalies like Hirschsprung's disease, gastroschisis, omphalocele, etc.

ANTERIOR ABDOMINAL WALL DEFECTS

Include exomphalos, gastroschisis, exstrophy of the bladder (Table 1).

Exomphalos or Omphalocele

Omphalocele (exomphalos) is a common congenital anterior abdominal wall defect. It is a midline defect at the umbilical ring containing midgut and other abdominal organs, such as the liver, spleen, and gonads. The contents are covered by three layers, amnion exteriorly, the Wharton's jelly in the middle, and peritoneal layer in the inside. The size of the omphalocele can range from 2 to 10 cm.

Ultrasound Diagnosis

It is diagnosed on ultrasound as a midline defect in the center through which a sac containing bowel and liver herniates into the amniotic cavity with the umbilical cord inserted at the apex of the sac. Omphaloceles in the epigastric region may have defects in the sternum or pericardial sac (pentalogy of Cantrell variant) and those in the hypogastrium have associated anomalies of the bladder, spine, or anus.

Associations and Further Investigations

Association with chromosomal and structural abnormalities is high in exomphalos. Almost 30–50% of exomphalos are associated with chromosomal abnormalities, mainly trisomy 18 and 13. It may be associated with genetic syndromes, especially Beckwith-Wiedemann syndrome, in 10% cases. About half are associated with anomalies in other organ systems such as the cardiac (most common), gastrointestinal, genitourinary, musculoskeletal, nervous system, and chromosomal defects.

Once an abnormality is diagnosed, a detailed ultrasound examination, including a fetal echocardiogram, should be done for associated structural abnormalities. Amniocentesis is offered for microarray and molecular testing for Beckwith-Wiedemann syndrome. Prognosis depends on the size of the defect and the associated anomalies.

Antenatal Management

The mother should receive standard antenatal care with a plan to deliver by 38 weeks. Frequent sonographic surveillance is done to monitor the fetal growth, amniotic fluid index and to look for signs of bowel ischemia. Formulae for estimating fetal weight (EFW) that incorporate abdominal

TABLE 1: Fetal anterior abdominal wall defects.

Abnormality	Gastroschisis	Omphalocele	Pentalogy of Cantrell	Bladder exstrophy	Cloacal exstrophy
Location of defect	Right paramedian	Midline	Midline supraumbilical	Midline infraumbilical	Midline infraumbilical
Relation to umbilical cord	The cord is normally inserted	Cord insertion at the top of herniated mass	Cord insertion at the top of herniated mass	Low insertion	Low insertion
Ultrasound features	Free-floating bowel loops	Midline sac with herniated abdominal organs covered by a membrane	Ectopia cordis, lower sternal defect, supraumbilical cardiac defect	Absent bladder with normal amniotic fluid	Absent bladder
Associated abnormalities	Uncommon	The majority have associated anomalies	Multisystem	Uncommon	Spinal, genitourinary

circumference (AC) are not applicable in these cases, and Sieme's formula can be considered as an alternate.

Delivery should be planned in a tertiary care center with intensive care and pediatric surgery facilities. Induction of labor can be done aiming for vaginal delivery. Cesarean should be reserved for giant exomphalos (sac containing more than 3/4th liver) to avoid sac rupture and hemorrhage.

Delivery Room Management

Avoid clamping the umbilical sac. The neonate or the omphalocele should be wrapped in a sterile plastic wrap to minimize insensible fluid loss. Insert an orogastric tube to decompress the stomach. Stabilize the airway and assess the need for ventilation. Establish peripheral intravenous access and start intravenous fluids. In case of signs of vascular compromise (hypotension, tachycardia, and dusky-bowel appearance), position the baby in lateral decubitus position. Place sterile gauze piece soaked in warm saline over the sac and cover it with plastic wrap.

Surgical Management

Small defects (2–3 cm) can be repaired in the first 2–3 days by primary closure. For large defects, apply silo in the first 24 hours, followed by delayed closure. Giant omphaloceles (greater than 5 cm defect, >75% liver out) require a combination of silo, skin graft, or formation of amniotic sac eschar by application of sclerosing solution (povidone-iodine) with the delayed repair. In the postoperative period, signs of raised intra-abdominal pressure should be monitored carefully.

Prognosis

Reported survival rates are more than 90% in isolated, small to moderate side effects. Large defects and one with associated anomalies carry poor outcomes.

Gastroschisis

Gastroschisis is seen in 1 in 3,000 live births. Substance abuse is associated with increased incidence. The defect will be seen as a paraumbilical abdominal wall defect, usually to the right side, along with a freely floating bowel in the amniotic fluid **(Figs. 3A and B)**. The umbilical cord is normally inserted in contrast with exomphalos.

Gastroschisis is not associated with an increased risk for chromosomal abnormalities or non-chromosomal genetic syndromes. However, with the availability of microarray, which has the advantage of picking up microdeletions and duplications not generally picked up on conventional karyotype, amniocentesis should be discussed with the parents.

Gastroschisis may lead to bowel atresia or obstruction secondary to volvulus, and ischemia at the hernial orifice in about 10–30% of cases. Fetal growth restriction may occur in 30–60% of cases. It may also be associated with spontaneous preterm birth in about 30% of cases. About 2–4% of pregnancies may result in intrauterine fetal demise.

Antenatal Management

A detailed anomaly scan including fetal echo should be done. Monthly ultrasound surveillance is recommended to monitor fetal growth, amniotic fluid volume, and fetal Doppler. Bowel dilatation and signs of bowel ischemia-like echogenic bowel, intra-abdominal calcifications should be looked for. In fetuses with abdominal wall defects, it is best to monitor growth through estimation of fetal weight by the Sieme formula, which uses biparietal diameter (BPD), occipitofrontal diameter (OFD), and femur length (FL).

Delivery should be conducted in a tertiary care hospital with NICU and pediatric surgery facilities. The aim is to deliver as close to 38 weeks as possible unless delivery is indicated earlier due to fetal growth restriction or progressive

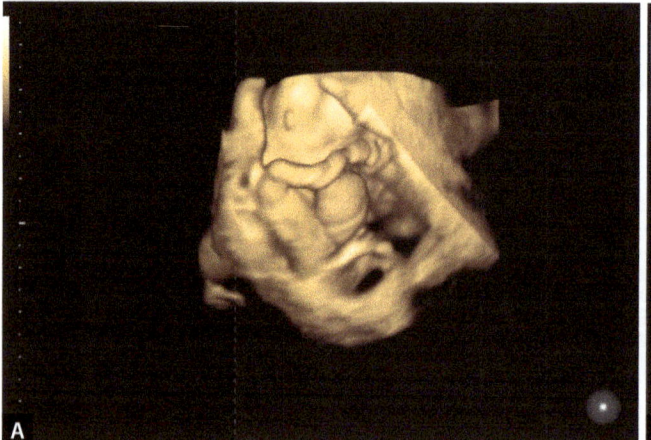
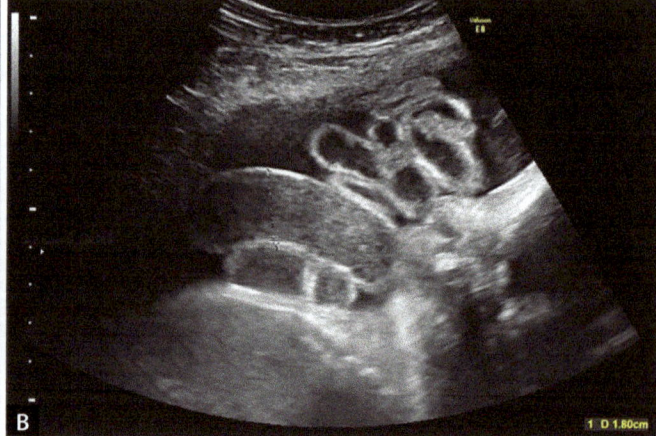

Figs. 3A and B: (A) 3D ultrasound image showing midline defect covered by membrane; (B) 2D image showing free-floating bowel loops in a case of gastroschisis.

dilatation of intra-abdominal bowel defined as more than 20 mm in the transverse section. Induction of labor and vaginal delivery should be aimed for and cesarean being reserved for obstetric indications.

Neonatal Management

The neonate should be received in a plastic bag covering its lower half to minimize fluid losses. An orogastric tube should be inserted to decompress the stomach. Peripheral intravenous access should be placed, and IV fluids (1.5–2 times maintenance) should be started. Primary closure should be done where ever it is feasible. When primary closure is not feasible because of edema, distended bowel loops, or small abdominal cavity, a silo is applied, followed by delayed closure.

Prognosis

Gastroschisis can be classified as simple or complex based on the absence or presence of intestinal atresia, stenosis, perforation, necrosis, malrotation, or volvulus. In simple cases, the prognosis is excellent. Complex gastroschisis is associated with a higher risk of in-hospital mortality, short bowel syndrome, necrotizing enterocolitis, and parenteral nutrition at discharge. There is a recurrence risk of about 3% in subsequent pregnancies, suggesting that genetic factors play a role in causation. First-trimester ultrasound should be advised in the next pregnancy.

OTHER GASTROINTESTINAL ANOMALIES

Fetal Intra-abdominal Cyst

Abdominal cystic masses are frequent findings at ultrasound examination. Renal tract anomalies or dilated bowel are the most common explanations, although cystic structures may arise from the biliary tree, ovaries, mesentery, or uterus. The correct diagnosis of these abnormalities may not be possible by ultrasound examination, but the most likely diagnosis is usually suggested by the position of the cyst, its relationship with other structures, and the normality of other organs.

Choledochal Cysts

Choledochal cysts represent cystic dilatation of the common biliary duct. Prenatally, the diagnosis may be made ultrasonographically by demonstrating a cyst in the upper right side of the fetal abdomen. There is communication between the bile duct and the cyst. The absence of polyhydramnios or peristalsis may help to differentiate the condition from bowel disorders. Postnatally, early diagnosis and removal of the cyst may avoid the development of biliary cirrhosis, portal hypertension, calculi formation, or adenocarcinoma. The operative mortality is about 10%.

Mesenteric or Omental Cysts

These cysts may represent obstructed lymphatic drainage. The fluid contents may be serous, chylous, or hemorrhagic. Antenatally, the diagnosis is suggested by finding a multiseptate or unilocular, usually mid-line, cystic lesion of variable size; a solid appearance may be secondary to hemorrhage. Antenatal aspiration may be considered in cases of massive cysts resulting in thoracic compression. Postnatal management is conservative, and surgery is reserved for bowel obstruction or acute abdominal pain symptoms following torsion or hemorrhage into a cyst. Complete excision of cysts may not be possible because of the proximity of major blood vessels, and in up to 20% of cases, there is recurrence after surgery. Although the malignant change in mesenteric cysts has been described, this is rare.

Hepatic Cysts

Hepatic cysts are typically located in the right lobe of the liver. They are quite rare and result from obstruction of the hepatic biliary system. They appear as unilocular, intrahepatic cysts, and they are usually asymptomatic, although they rarely may show complications, such as infections or hemorrhages. Hepatic cysts are found in 30% of the cases of adult polycystic kidney disease.

Hepatic Calcifications

Hepatic calcifications are uncommon, with a reported incidence of 1 in 2,000 at 20 weeks gestation. These are seen as solitary or multiple echogenic foci within the substance of the liver or in the capsule, where these appear as peripheral calcifications (**Figs. 4A and B**). The risk of chromosomal abnormalities is not increased with isolated hepatic calcifications. Parenchymal hepatic calcifications may be due to intrauterine infection. Once seen on ultrasound, a thorough ultrasound examination should be done to look for other signs of infection. Maternal TORCH IgM and IgG should be done. If it is suggestive of infection, amniocentesis for viral PCR should be offered.

The mother should receive standard antenatal care. Delivery should be planned at term with induction/cesarean to be reserved for usual obstetric indications. Prognosis is good for isolated cases.

Intestinal Duplication Cysts

These are quite rare and may be located along the entire gastrointestinal tract. They sonographically appear as tubular or cystic structures of variable size (**Fig. 5**). They may be isolated or associated with other gastrointestinal malformations. The thickness of the muscular wall of the cysts and the presence of peristalsis may facilitate the diagnosis. Postnatally, surgical removal is carried out.

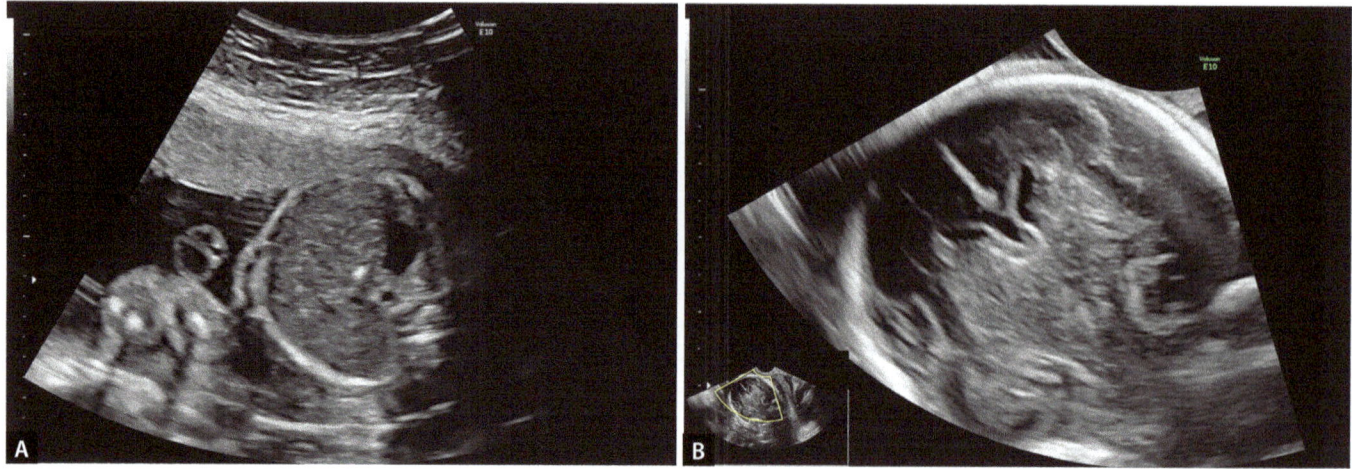

Figs. 4A and B: 2D USG images showing (A) transverse section of fetal abdomen with hepatic calcification; (B) Coronal view of fetal brain in same fetus showing periventricular calcification. CMV PCR was positive on amniotic fluid.

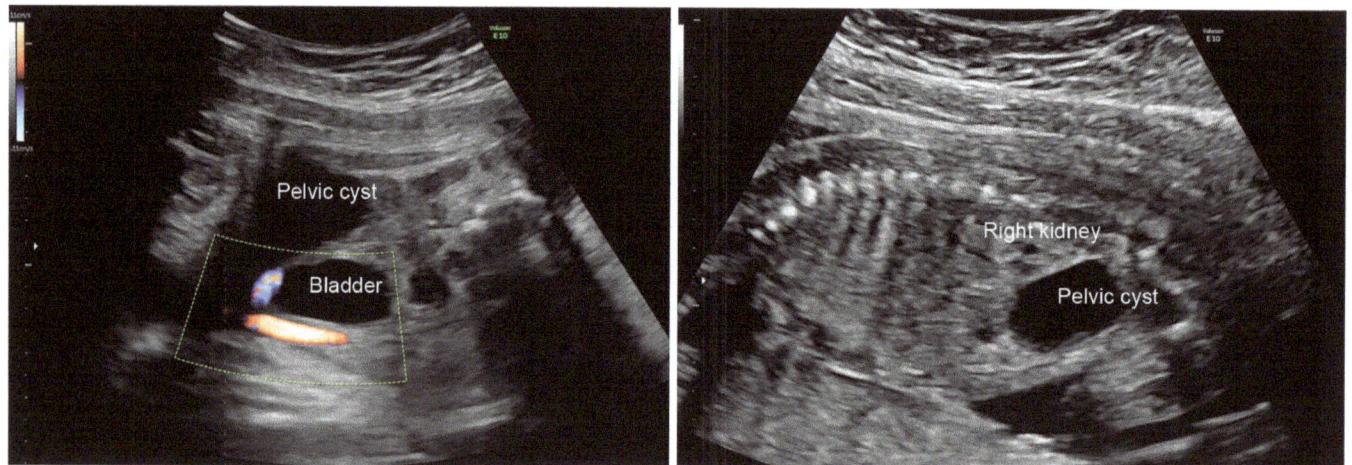

Fig. 5: Intestinal duplication cyst (found postnatally) appearing as cyst in pelvis in antenatal ultrasound.

Chapter at a Glance

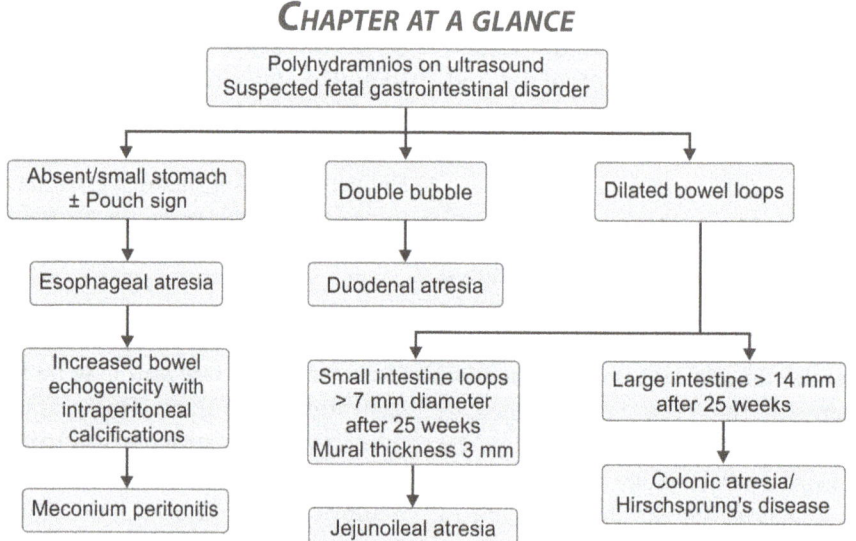

Antenatal diagnosis of fetal gastrointestinal disorders

KEY POINTS

- The absence of stomach bubble on antenatal ultrasound with associated polyhydramnios suggests EA.
- Dilated intestinal loops suggest intestinal atresia depending upon size and location.
- Many gastrointestinal malformations have associated anomalies. Fetal echocardiography, detailed ultrasound, and karyotyping/next-generation sequencing is required depending upon the disorder.
- Delivery should be done in a perinatal center with tertiary level NICU and pediatric surgery facilities.

SUGGESTED READING

1. Catania VD, Briganti V, Di Giacomo V, Miele V, Signore F, de Ware C, et al. Fetal intra-abdominal cysts: accuracy and predictive value of prenatal ultrasound. J Matern Fetal Neonatal Med. 2016;29(10):1691-9.
2. Furey EA, Bailey AA, Twickler DM. Fetal MR imaging of gastrointestinal abnormalities. Radiographics. 2016;36(3):904-17.
3. Laird A, Shekleton P, Nataraja RM, Kimber C, Pacelli M. Incidence of gastrointestinal anomalies and surgical outcome of fetuses diagnosed with echogenic bowel and bowel dilatation. Prenat Diagn. 2019;39(12):1115-9.
4. Lau PE, Cruz S, Cassady CI, Mehollin-Ray AR, Ruano R, Keswani S, et al. Prenatal diagnosis and outcome of fetal gastrointestinal obstruction. J Pediatr Surg. 2017;52(5):722-5.
5. Marrone L, Liberati M, Khalil A, Rizzo G, Leombroni M, Buca D, et al. Outcome of fetal gastrointestinal cysts: a systematic review and meta-analysis. Prenat Diagn. 2016;36(10):966-72.

CHAPTER 12

Fetal Growth Restriction

Pratima Anand, Sumitra Bachani

INTRODUCTION

World Health Organization (WHO) defines low birth weight (LBW) as neonatal weight <2.5 kg irrespective of gestational age as per the National Family Heath Survey (NFHS-4) about 18% of Indian children younger than 5 years are born with LBW in 2015–2016. To achieve the target of Sustainable Development Goal (SDG) in infant and under-5 mortality levels by 2030, an accelerated improvement is required in reducing the occurrence of LBW. It is therefore important to identify a fetus which fails to achieve its genetically determined growth potential in utero and a small for gestational age (SGA) fetus which is small, but its growth is not restricted. Fetal growth restriction (FGR) is an obstetrical condition with clinical variance in diagnosing, monitoring, and delivering a growth restricted fetus. There are multiple maternal and fetal variables and indices which must be assessed to determine the correct time and mode of delivering such a fetus. There is an added risk of prematurity associated with delivering at different gestational ages which adds to the neonatal morbidity.

OBJECTIVES

- To identify FGR versus constitutionally SGA, antenatally
- To discuss the evidence for management of FGR
- To discuss the time and mode of delivery of an FGR and SGA fetus
- To discuss postnatal management of neonates diagnosed as FGR antenatally

IDENTIFICATION OF "FETAL GROWTH RESTRICTION" VERSUS "(CONSTITUTIONAL)" SMALL FOR GESTATIONAL AGE

Antenatal screening can identify risk factors associated with FGR **(Table 1)**. Serial plotting of symphysio-fundal height against standard charts during antenatal examination can identify fetuses which are not growing appropriately. Clinical suspicion can be confirmed by ultrasonography biometry and Doppler examination of fetal vessels. Currently amongst available fetal growth charts Hadlock or INTERGROWTH 21st are commonly used. An SGA fetus lies between the 3rd

TABLE 1: Risk factors for fetal growth restriction

Maternal	*Fetal*	*Placental*	*Others*
Extremes of maternal age	Fetal genetic abnormalities	Ischemic placental disease	Teratogens
Short interpregnancy interval	Fetal infections	Gross cord and placental abnormalities	Alcoholism
Low pre-pregnancy weight, poor gestational weight gain, and poor nutritional status	Structural abnormalities	Placental mesenchymal dysplasia	Smoking
Maternal medical conditions, anemia, renal, cardiac, and autoimmune disorders	Multiple gestation		Drug abuse
Maternal obstetric conditions, preeclampsia, and uterine malformations			
Previous SGA baby, mother was SGA			
Abnormal maternal biomarkers, PAPPA, bhCG, AFP			

(AFP: alpha-fetoprotein; bhCG: beta-human chorionic gonadotropin; PAPPA: pregnancy-associated plasma protein A; SGA: small for gestational age)

and 10th centile as per the reference chart and has normal Doppler flow velocities in the vessels. A growth restricted fetus falls off the growth curve on the reference growth charts; however, an SGA fetus is small but continues to follow the growth curve.

Most guidelines [Royal College of Obstetricians and Gynaecologists (RCOG) and International Society of Ultrasound in Obstetrics and Gynaecology (ISUOG)] recommend that estimated fetal weight (EFW) and/or abdominal circumference (AC) is <10th centile and any one of the additional deranged Doppler parameters amongst the three namely uterine artery pulsatility index (UAPI) >95th centile, uterine artery pulsatility index (UtAPI) >95th centile, and cerebroplacental ratio (CPR) <5th centile to establish the diagnosis of FGR. A recently published DELPHI survey which incorporated opinions of 45 experts has reached a consensus for defining FGR and differentiating early and late-onset phenotype which most institutions utilize for diagnosing this condition **(Table 2)**.

Prediction and Prevention of FGR

Biomarkers such as pregnancy-associated plasma protein A (PAPPA), placental growth factor (PLGF), and uterine artery Doppler indices are combined with screening for aneuploidies in the first trimester. Accredited laboratories using specific software platforms such as Autodelfia and Rosche can predict the risk of preeclampsia (PE) and FGR which are closely linked along with the risk of aneuploidy in the fetus. Early assessment of risk for PE and FGR is beneficial because the prophylactic use of low-dose aspirin started in early pregnancy can potentially halve the incidence of PE but also that of SGA in the absence of PE. The World Health Assembly (WHA) Global Nutrition targets 2025 have listed interventions at country, region, community levels, and antenatal and postnatal period for prevention of low-birth-weight infants **(Table 3)**.

Indices for Fetal Assessment and Role in Management

These are ultrasonographically measured Doppler indices which are used for establishing the diagnosis of FGR (diagnostic indicators) and are relevant for the decision as to when delivery is indicated and possible neurodevelopmental outcomes (prognostic indicators).

Uterine Artery Doppler

High pulsatility index (PI) (>95th centile) is one of the factors included in the diagnosis of FGR **(Fig. 1)**.

Umbilical Artery Doppler

The umbilical artery (UA) Doppler **(Fig. 2)** is the only index that has both diagnostic and prognostic role in the management of FGR. Worsening of Doppler parameters to absent or reversal of end-diastolic flow have been reported to be present at least a week prior to acute deterioration. Reversed end-diastolic flow in the UA has a sensitivity and specificity of about 60% as a predictor of adverse perinatal outcome which is likely independent of prematurity. A 29% reduction in perinatal mortality on using UA Doppler in high-risk pregnancies has been reported. Once the pregnancy has crossed the period of viability (28 weeks in low-resource settings), the UA and ductus venosus (DV) Dopplers, fetal biometry, and biophysical profile including cardiotocograph are used for guiding the time of delivery in conjunction with the local neonatology support available.

Middle Cerebral Artery Doppler/ Cerebroplacental Ratio

A hypoxic fetus redistributes the blood flow to the most vital organ the brain. As more vasodilation marks the fall in resistance of middle cerebral artery (MCA), it is an indicator of redistribution of flow with brain sparing **(Fig. 3)**. It is a surrogate marker to determine the degree of fetal hypoxia. Abnormal MCA-PI (<5th centile) can be associated with adverse perinatal and neurological outcome; however, it is not established whether in preterm fetuses an early delivery before term will be of benefit. MCA Doppler has a

TABLE 2: DELPHI consensus for definition of intrauterine growth restriction/fetal growth restriction (FGR).

Early FGR (<32 weeks)	Late FGR (32 weeks or more)
• Solitary biometric • AC <3rd centile • EFW <3rd centile • *Solitary Doppler*: Absent end-diastolic flow in umbilical artery	• Solitary biometric • AC <3rd centile • EFW< 3rd centile
• Contributory biometric • AC <10th centile • EFW <10th centile	• Contributory biometric • AC <10th centile • EFW <10th centile • *Biometric relative*: AC or EFW crossing centiles more than two quartiles
• Contributory Doppler • UtrPI >95th centile • UAPI >95th centile	• Contributory Doppler • UAPI >95th centile • Abnormal CPR <5th centile
Algorithm: One solitary or two contributory one each of biometry and Doppler parameters	One solitary or two amongst three contributories including Doppler

Source: Gordijn SJ, Beune IM, Thilaganathan B, Papageorghiou A, Baschat AA, Baker PN, et al. Consensus definition of fetal growth restriction: a Delphi procedure. Ultrasound Obstet Gynecol. 2016;48(3):333-9.
(AC: abdominal circumference; CPR: cerebroplacental ratio; EFW: estimated fetal weight; UAPI: uterine artery pulsatility index)

TABLE 3: Interventions for prevention of low birth weight infant.

Country	Community	Antenatal	Postnatal	Selected cases
Support for women's empowerment and educational attainment	Adequate nutrition for adolescent girls	Protein energy supplementation	Early initiation of breast-feeding	Antiplatelet agents before 16 weeks for women at risk of preeclampsia
Improvement of clean and adequate water, sanitation, and hygiene	Community-based packages of care to improve linkage and referral for facility births	Fetal growth monitoring and neonatal size evaluation at all levels of care	Adequate spacing of births	Antenatal corticosteroids for preterm births
Support for national salt iodization programs to ensure that salt consumed by households is adequately iodized (for which there are new guidelines harmonizing iodine levels with reductions in salt consumption)	Intermittent iron and folic acid supplements for women of reproductive age and adolescent girls, in settings where the prevalence of anemia is 20% or higher	Decrease in nonmedically indicated caesarean delivery and induction		Cervical circle/progesterone for high risk of preterm birth
Improvement in facility-based perinatal care in regions with low coverage	Smoking cessation	Smoking cessation		Antibiotics for bacterial vaginosis
Universal simplified perinatal data-collection system with electronic feedback systems				

Source: WHA. Global Nutrition Targets 2025: Low Birth Weight Policy Brief. Evidence-based interventions to prevent low birth weight. [online] Available from: https://apps.who.int/nutrition/publications/globaltargets2025_policybrief_lbw/en/index.html. [Last accessed November, 2021].

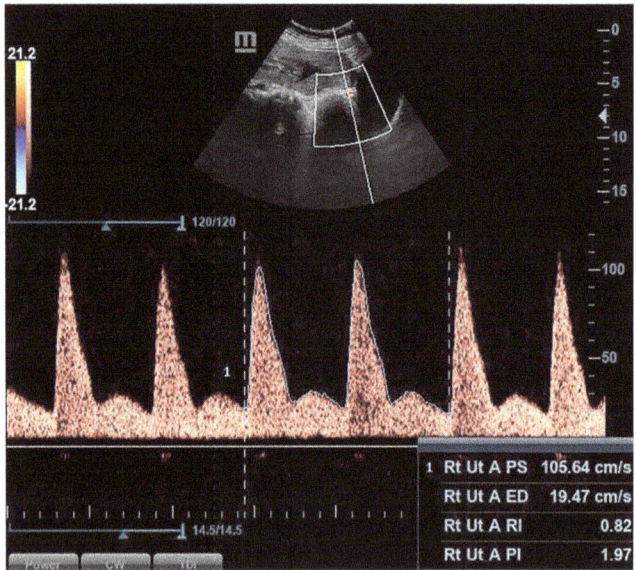

Fig. 1: Uterine artery Doppler.

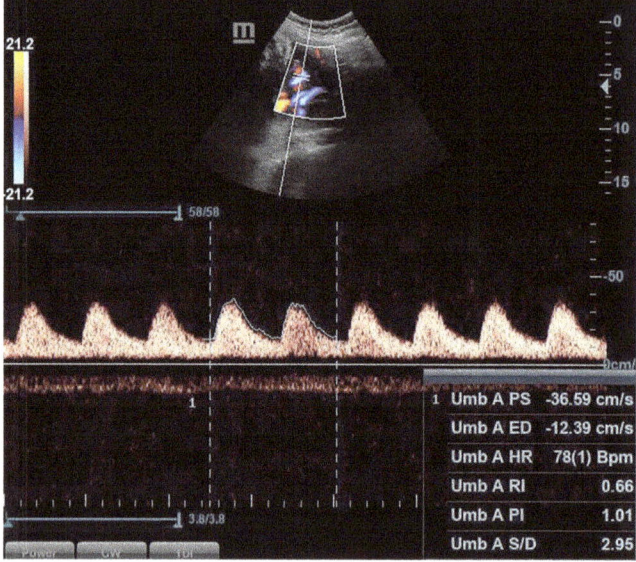

Fig. 2: Umbilical artery Doppler.

low sensitivity and acceptable specificity for the detection of FGR and it is improved using CPR. The ratio of MCA PI to UA PI improves upon the individual sensitivity of UA and MCA Doppler. The CPR can already decrease even when its individual components show mild changes but are still within normal ranges. Abnormal CPR (<5th centile) can be present before delivery in 20–25% of the cases of late-onset FGR and is associated with a higher risk of adverse perinatal outcome after labor induction.

Ductus Venosus Doppler

Ductus venosus flow waveforms **(Fig. 4)** become abnormal only in advanced stages of fetal compromise. Absent and reversed velocities (atrial contraction/a wave) are associated with perinatal mortality independent of the gestational age at delivery, with a risk ranging from 40 to 100% in early-onset FGR. Absent "atrial wave" in DV or reversal of "a" wave is an important indice to time the delivery in early-onset

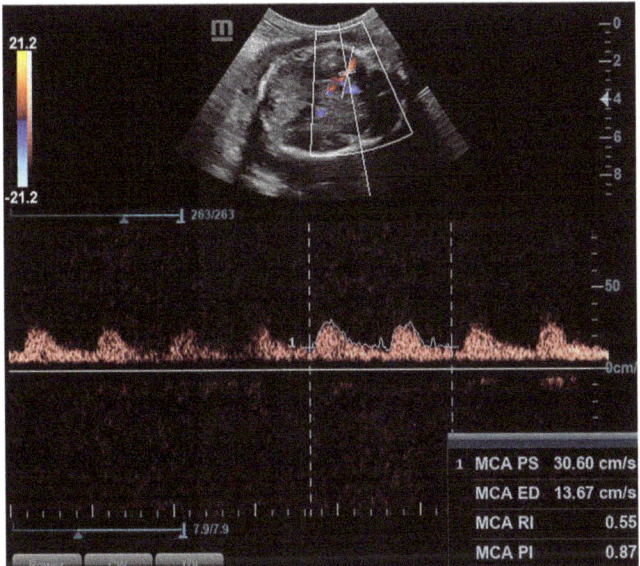

Fig. 3: Middle cerebral artery Doppler flow showing redistribution.

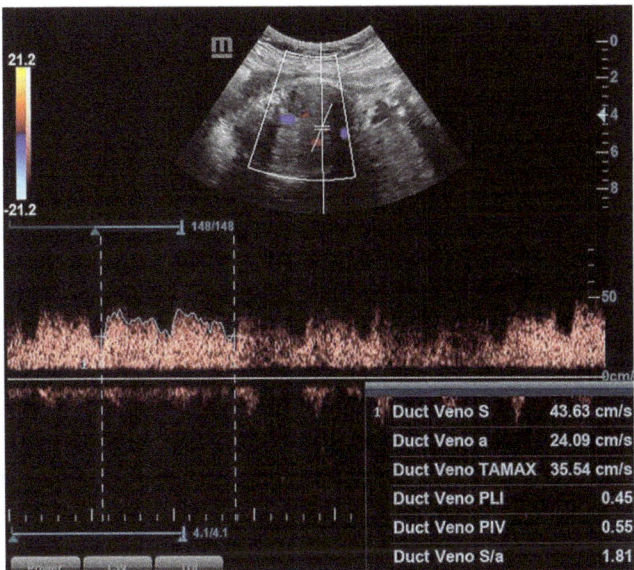

Fig. 4: Ductus venosus Doppler.

FGR in conjunction with all other parameters same as with abnormal UA Dopplers.

Aortic Isthmus Doppler

This area shows the balance between the impedance of the brain and systemic vascular system. Reverse aortic isthmus (AoI) flow is a sign of advanced deterioration, and it is follows in the sequence of abnormal Dopplers after UA and MCA Doppler. However, longitudinal studies show that the AoI Doppler abnormality precedes DV abnormalities by 1 week, and thus it is not as good as the latter to predict the short-term risk of stillbirth. In contrast, AoI seems to improve the prediction of neurodevelopmental outcome at 2–5 years of age. Among early-onset FGR with positive DV atrial velocities, a reversed AoI indicated an extremely high risk of late neonatal neurological complications including intraventricular hemorrhage and periventricular leukomalacia (57 vs. 9.7%).

TIMING OF DELIVERY IN FGR

There is currently no intervention to reverse the pathology leading to growth restriction. The main management strategy is to monitor the fetus for signs of deterioration and fine tune the time of delivery to balance prematurity and its consequences with perinatal morbidity, mortality including poor neurodevelopmental outcomes. At the same time, maternal comorbidity such as severe PE necessitating delivery is also to be considered.

Evidence for Timing Delivery in Early-onset FGR

Once an early-onset FGR is diagnosed, the pregnancy should be monitored and managed in tertiary-level fetal medicine and neonatal units according to a uniform management protocol. Multidisciplinary counseling by neonatologist and obstetricians or maternal–fetal medicine specialists is important. Evidence from a randomized trial [Trial of Randomized Umbilical and Fetal Flow in Europe (TRUFFLE)] reported that monitoring and delivery timing according to a specific protocol including DV Doppler and computerized cardiotocography (cCTG) improves outcomes. However, cCTG is not available in low-resource countries including India; hence, in addition to Doppler evaluation, assessment of conventional cardiotocography (CTG) and biophysical profile (BPP) scoring should be performed. The loss of fetal gross body movement in association with DV Doppler index alterations can predict fetal cord pH < 7.20, while loss of fetal tone is associated with pH < 7.00 or a base excess less than −12 mEq/L. The Growth Restriction Intervention Trial (GRIT) study was a multicenter randomized controlled trial including 548 pregnancies between 24 and 36 weeks with FGR, aimed to compare the effect of delivering early with delaying birth for as long as possible. The study observed that when obstetricians were uncertain about timing of delivery based on UA Doppler, the timing of delivery varied up to 4 days. However, the results of early delivery or delayed birth were almost similar terms of perinatal outcome.

Efficient recognition and management of severe PE may prolong some pregnancies with early FGR. The timely use of steroids, followed by magnesium sulfate, transfer to a tertiary care center, and consideration of the safest mode of delivery are the key concepts in early-FGR management.

Evidence for Timing Delivery in Late FGR

Regarding timing of delivery in late FGR, there is paucity of interventional management randomized trials based on Doppler indices, hence there is no international consensus regarding timing of delivery. The Disproportionate Intrauterine Growth Intervention Trial at Term (DIGITAT) study in which 650 women with suspected FGR > 36 weeks were randomized to induction or expectant management with Doppler surveillance carried out biweekly. There was no difference in the primary outcome of severe neonatal morbidity or in cesarean delivery. Women who were offered conservative/expectant management had a twofold increased risk of developing PE (7.9 vs. 3.7%, P < 0.05) and were more likely to have a baby with birthweight <3rd centile (30 vs. 13%, P < 0.001). The recommendation was that "it is rational to choose induction to prevent possible neonatal morbidity and stillbirth." There was no difference overall in neonatal morbidity between induction of labor and expectant management groups, but induction at <38 weeks was associated with increased admission in neonatal unit. It was recommended to continue pregnancy up to 38 weeks with close monitoring.

In pregnancies with late FGR and UAPI above the 95th percentile, expert opinion is that delivery should be considered when the gestation is beyond 36 + 0 weeks and not later than 37 + 6 weeks.

Timing of Delivery of SGA Fetus

The SGA fetus needs to be monitored closely; fortnightly assessment of fetal growth is recommended as some may cross over to FGR, especially the early-onset SGA fetuses. Even late-SGA fetuses with normal uterine artery PI can progress to brain sparing not identifiable by standard biophysical tools. ISUOG recommends universal induction of labor at term can be more beneficial than expectant management in terms of reduced perinatal mortality without increasing the rate of cesarean section or operative vaginal delivery. Hence, delivery should be considered between 38 + 0 and 39 + 0 weeks, to reduce the risk of adverse perinatal outcome in fetuses identified as SGA.

MODE OF DELIVERY IN FGR FETUS

There is a strong association with severe placental insufficiency and fetal hypoxemia hence planned cesarean section is conducted in most early-onset cases of FGR. Also, delivery is indicated based on maternal indications, mainly hypertensive disorders of pregnancy, that could adversely impact the perinatal and maternal outcome and mode of delivery is individualized as per the period of gestation, maternal co-morbid conditions such as previous cesarean section, eclampsia, pulmonary edema, and the local neonatal intensive care unit (NICU) set up. Depending on the clinical situation (parity, fetal weight, cervical findings), induction of labor may be undertaken, but this is not recommended in the context of critical UA Doppler findings [i.e., absent or reversed end-diastolic flow (AREDF)]. Continuous fetal heart rate monitoring during labor should be undertaken.

MANAGEMENT OF NEONATES DIAGNOSED AS FGR IN UTERO

Management at Birth

Fetal growth restriction is associated with risk of preterm delivery and hence preparation for resuscitation as for high-risk pregnancies is to be done. The growth restricted neonates are also reported to be associated with higher incidence of meconium aspiration, perinatal asphyxia, and hence resuscitation team should anticipate and prepare accordingly.

The standard practices (delayed cord clamping, skin-to-skin care after birth and early initiation of breastfeeds) should be followed in stable neonates, as defined in the Neonatal Resuscitation Guidelines. The neonates who need indications of admission to NICU are discussed in the next section of the chapter.

Placental Examination in the Delivery Room

The examination of placenta should be done as it provides vital clues to the underlying pathophysiology of FGR in each case.

The histological examination may reveal decidual vasculopathy, intervillous thrombosis, and infarction. Besides, placental may also reveal the changes due to intrauterine infections like cytomegalovirus (CMV), syphilis, and toxoplasmosis.

Postnatal Diagnosis of Neonates Born with FGR In Utero and Identification of at-risk Neonates

An experienced eye distinguishes healthy small for gestational age neonates from FGR (**Fig. 5**). While the FGR/intrauterine growth restriction (IUGR) is the terminology used in fetal life, a pediatrician/neonatology team would classify the product of conception after expulsion as appropriate-for-gestational-age (AGA), SGA, or large for gestational age (LGA). Since SGA is a statistical definition, i.e., <10th centile, all FGR (two major centiles downhill course in-utero) may not be born with the weight <10th centile at birth. However, many SGA neonates may not be FGR as they had slow but consistent fetal growth in utero, which remains <10th centile.

Growth Charts for Classification of Neonates at Birth, Further Clinical Assessment and Work Up

The Neonatal Cross-Sectional charts by Intergrowth 21st are the most recent growth standards to classify neonates as SGA, AGA, or LGA at birth.

Clinical assessment of neonates should include the following:

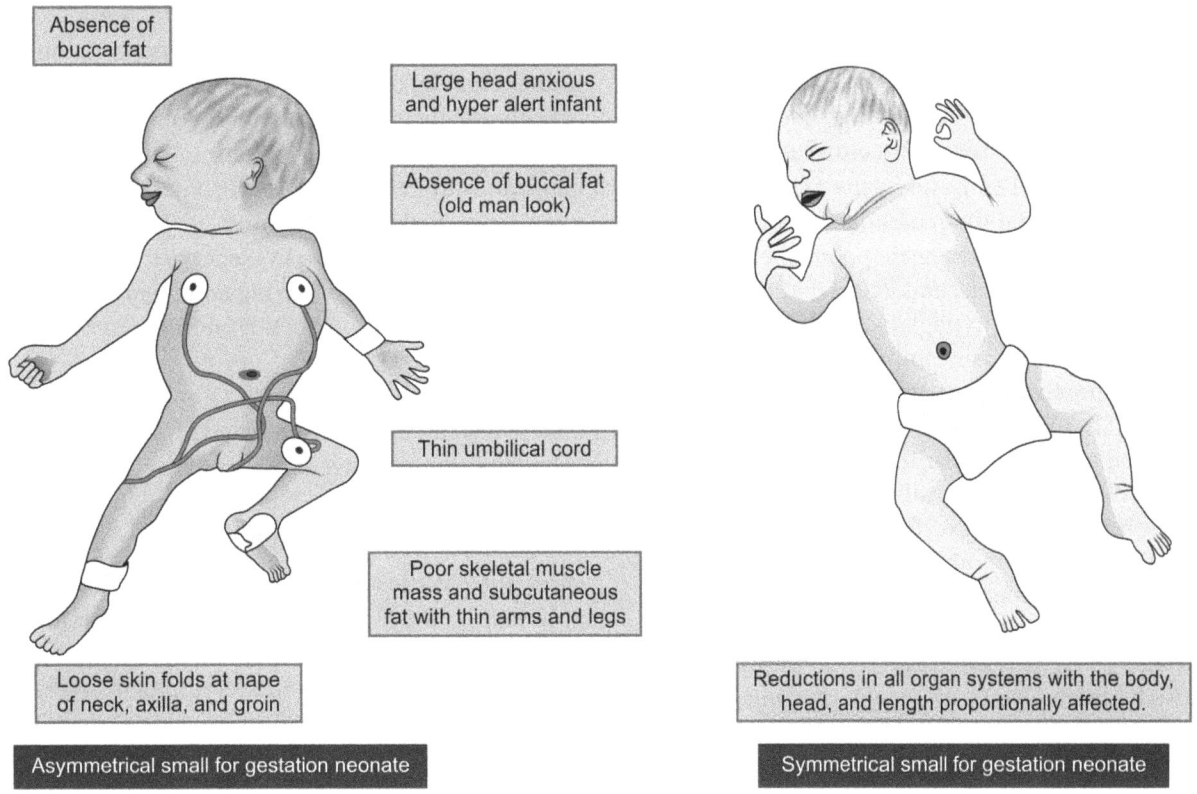

Fig. 5: Features of asymmetrical and symmetrical small-for-gestation neonates.

- Anthropometry at birth (weight, length, and head circumference) after stabilization
- Clinical features of growth restriction **(Fig. 5)**
- Calculation of indices (Ponderal Index, Cephalization Index, and CAN score)

Based on the Ponderal Index, neonates are classified as symmetrical or asymmetrical growth restricted:
- *Symmetric FGR (>2.0)*: The symmetrical FGR comprises 20–30% of cases, and it starts early in antenatal period and associated with reduction in overall cell number. As a result, there is reduction in all organ systems with the body, head, and length proportionally affected. Most of the underlying causes are intrinsic factors such as congenital infections or chromosomal abnormalities.
- *Asymmetric FGR (<2.0)*: The asymmetric FGR comprises 70–80% of FGR cases and has disproportionate growth restriction. In these cases, head circumference is preserved, length is affected to a smaller degree, and weight is reduced to a greater extent. As a result, the head appears relatively large compared to trunk and extremities. The cell number is normal in these cases, but cell size is reduced. Features of growth restriction are seen in the form of loose skin folds, loss of buccal fat, and the neonates have an old man look on examination.
- *Mixed FGR*: Decrease in both the number and cell size. Occurs mostly when FGR is affected further by placental causes in late pregnancy and has features of both symmetrical and asymmetrical FGR.

It should be noted that gestational assessment by Ballard scoring in neonates with FGR in utero may be fallacious due to the changes in physical parameters. For the corresponding gestation, compared to neonates with normal growth in utero. The growth restricted neonates have sole creases which are mature, the ear cartilage is thinner, and the female genitalia look underdeveloped due to reduced fat deposit in the labia majora.

Laboratory Investigations in Neonates with FGR In Utero

In majority of cases, the growth restriction is due to placental perfusion deficits, and no laboratory investigations are needed, except the detailed placental examination.

In situations where there is pointer toward a neonatal cause for FGR, like chromosomal anomalies, intrauterine infections such as TORCH group of infection and syphilis, multiple gestation (with/without twin-to-twin transfusion syndrome), inborn errors of metabolism, the neonate should be worked up accordingly, to decide the further management of the associated condition.

Monitoring During Hospital Stay

The growth restricted fetus who is found to be SGA in the postnatal period are at risk of immediate mortality and morbidities. Katz et al. in a pooled analysis of 20 cohorts (total population 2,015,019 live births) from Asia, Africa, and Latin America reported that in comparison with term

AGA infants, the RR for neonatal mortality was 1.83 [95% confidence interval (CI) 1.34-2.50] and postneonatal mortality RR was 1·90 (1.32-2.73) for SGA infants. The risk was maximum in babies who were both preterm and SGA in comparison to babies who were either SGA or preterm alone (15.42; 9.11-26.12). Besides, the SGA neonates are predisposed to impaired thermoregulation (less brown fat, poor thermoregulation mechanism, poor subcutaneous fat, deficiency of catecholamine, and associated complications such as hypoxia and hypoglycemia), hypoglycemia, polycythemia, hyperviscosity, impaired immune function, persistent pulmonary hypertension (PPHN), pulmonary hemorrhage, hypocalcemia, feed intolerance, renal problems such as renal tubular injury, bronchopulmonary dysplasia (BPD), and retinopathy of prematurity (ROP). Hypoglycemia (17%) and polycythemia (10%) were reported to be the most common morbidities by Deorari et al. on 144 SGA neonates. There was feed intolerance (22 vs. 12%, $p = 0.183$), necrotizing enterocolitis (NEC) (12 vs. 6%, $p = 0.295$), and mortality (8 vs. 2%, $p = 0.362$) in SGA group and these babies also had significantly more hypoglycemia ($p = 0.000$) and polycythemia ($p = 0.032$) and longer hospital stay ($p = 0.017$) as reported in yet another cohort.

Screening for hypoglycemia and polycythemia should be done as per standard unit protocols and managed accordingly. Work up for hypocalcemia is done in only symptomatic neonates.

Management of Sick Neonates and Feeding Protocols

Indications of Neonatal Intensive Care Unit Admission

Neonates born preterm (<34 weeks) and/or birth weight <1,800 g need continuous monitoring and hence need to be admitted in neonatal care units. The neonatal morbidities associated with prematurity are managed as per standard protocol.

Neonates with in-utero FGR, but gestation >35 weeks, can be roomed in with mother and provided with direct breastfeeds. There is no evidence that Doppler changes at gestation beyond 35 weeks have any impact on feeding of neonates, and hence direct breastfeeds can be initiated, on demand.

Growth-restricted fetus diagnosed as SGA postnatally, with Doppler changes in utero (reversal or absent Doppler flow), needs additional attention to their feeding and nutrition. The placental and adaptive hemodynamic changes in fetal circulation in utero in these neonates cause preferential distribution of blood flow to brain, heart, and adrenals at the expense of gastrointestinal tract, kidneys, lungs, and other organs. As a result, intestines and mesenteric circulation make it vulnerable to stasis and abnormal colonization and invasion by bacteria. It is also seen that the chances of NEC are twofold higher in neonates with AREDF when compared to infants with normal umbilical Doppler flow [odds ratio (OR) 2.13].

This concern leads to delay in enteral feeds and longer time to reach full enteral feeds and prolongation of duration of hospital, for neonates with gestation < 35 weeks **(Fig. 6)**.

Discharge and Follow-up

Discharge of these neonates should be as per the unit policy once the desired weight is gained, and all other discharge criteria are met as per respective unit protocol. A complete and elaborate neurodevelopment assessment and nutritional assessment should be done at each visit since growth restricted fetus, if diagnosed as SGA in the postnatal period, has a concern of long-term nutritional as well as neurodevelopmental lag.

Follow-up Visits

The schedule for follow-up should be planned keeping in mind the sickness of the neonate during hospital stay, the gestation, and other comorbidities, if any.

A broad guide for follow-up schedule is mentioned in **Table 4**.

Long-term Outcomes

The reported rates of cerebral palsy in term SGA neonates are almost double compared term AGA counterparts (2.4 vs. 1.2% at 18 months corrected age). This subgroup of neonates is also vulnerable to motor as well as developmental delay compared to AGA.

A higher proportion of infants in term SGA cohort have been documented to have undernutrition (weight for age z-score less than −2 SDs) and stunting (length for age z-scores less than −2 SDs) at 18 months of corrected age. The rates of neurodevelopmental delay and growth failure are higher in

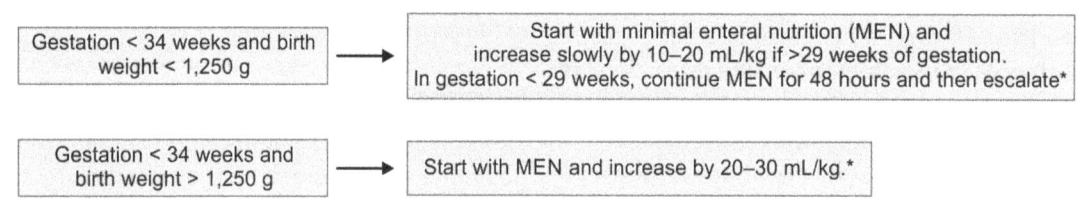

Fig. 6: Feeding protocol for neonates with antenatal Doppler changes and gestation <35 weeks.
*Fortification as per unit policy
(Based on findings of ADEPT trial and in Polin RA, Abman SH, Rowitch DH, Benitz WE, and Fox WW. (2017). Fetal and neonatal physiology)

TABLE 4: Guide for follow-up schedule of neonates.

	Neonates with gestation <32 weeks and/or birth weight <1,500 g	Neonates with gestation >32 weeks and/or birth weight >1,500 g
First visit	In the first 3–7 days	After 2 weeks
Subsequent visits	Every 2 weeks till the weight is 3 kg	Every 2 weeks till the weight is 3 kg
First 2 years visits	Combine with immunization visits as far as possible at 6, 10, and 14 weeks, followed by 6, 9, 12, 15, and 18 months of age	Combine with immunization visits as far as possible at 6, 10, and 14 weeks, followed by 6, 9,, 12, 15, and 18 months of age
2–5 years visits	Every 6 months/as needed	Every 6 months/as needed

preterm SGA compared to term SGA. Developmental origin of health and diseases (DoHaD) and Barker's hypothesis explain the fetal origin of adult disease and due to change in the metabolic milieu of FGR neonates, they are also predisposed to adult-onset diseases such as type 2 diabetes mellitus, metabolic syndrome, and hypertension. (Due to abnormal vascular development, postnatal excessive nutrition, and decreased beta cells of pancreas).

CHAPTER AT A GLANCE

Fetal growth restriction (FGR)

Definition: Fetus which has failed to achieve its biologically established growth potential
Early-onset FGR: Onset prior to 32 weeks of pregnancy
Late-onset FGR: At or after 32 weeks
Diagnosis: Based on DELPHI consensus considering EFW, AC, Doppler indices of uterine artery, umbilical artery, middle cerebral artery, ductus venosus in combinations. Solitary parameters are EFW/AC <3rd centile and/or absent end-diastolic flow in umbilical artery

Management: Stage-based approach (for early FGR)
Stage 1: FGR with UAPI/UtAPI >95th centile Weekly monitoring and delivery at 37 weeks. Consider induction of labor
Stage 2: UA AEDF: Biweekly monitoring. Deliver at or before 34 weeks. Offer cesarean section (CS)
Stage 3: UA REDF, DV PI >95th centile. Monitor daily and deliver at 30–32 weeks by CS
Stage 4: DV a wave reversal: Monitor 12 hourly till steroid cover is completed, deliver by CS
Late-onset FGR: Monitor weekly/biweekly. Consider delivery at 37–38 weeks. Offer induction of labor. In all cases deliver if maternal indication such as severe preeclampsia

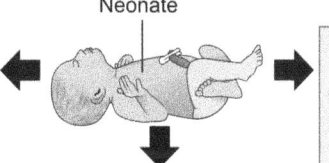

Neonate

Perinatal management in delivery room
• Watch for asphyxia, meconium aspiration
• Do placental examination

NICU management
• Detailed clinical examination
• Use anthropometric indices to classify as asymmetrical or symmetrical SGA
• Look for treatable neonatal causes of FGR
• Monitoring for short-term adverse outcomes during hospital stay (polycythemia, hypoglycemia, hypocalcemia, PPHN, and feed intolerance)
• Feeding as per protocol in neonates with Doppler changes and gestation < 35 weeks
• Discharge as per unit protocol

High-risk follow-up is needed
• At risk of neurodevelopmental delay compared to appropriate weight for gestation infants
• At risk of growth failure
• Neonates with FGR at risk of adult-onset diseases (DoHaD concept) such as metabolic syndrome, hypertension, and diabetes

(AC: abdominal circumference; CPR: cerebroplacental ratio; EFW: estimated fetal weight; UAPI: uterine artery pulsatility index; UtAPI: uterine artery pulsatility index; SGA: small for gestational age; PPHN: persistent pulmonary hypertensio; NICU: neonatal intensive care unit; DoHaD: developmental origin of health and diseases; REDF: reversal of umbilical artery end-diastolic flow)

KEY POINTS

- Fetal growth is a complex process controlled by many factors including genetic factors.
- FGR can be correctly diagnosed and differentiated from SGA based on the solitary and contributory parameters on biometry and Doppler indices.
- Certain Doppler indices have diagnostic while some indices predict the prognosis and neonatal outcomes and FGR or SGA fetus must be kept under close surveillance.
- Management of neonate includes postnatal classification as symmetrical and asymmetrical SGA, screening for immediate morbidities such as hypoglycemia and polycythemia. Feeding strategies to be followed for FGR with Doppler changes in gestation < 35 weeks.
- Neonates with FGR in utero are at risk of long-term neurodevelopmental delay and growth failure, so regular follow-up is mandatory, to ensure early intervention.

SUGGESTED READING

1. Gordijn SJ, Beune IM, Thilaganathan B, Papageorghiou A, Baschat AA, Baker PN, et al. Consensus definition of fetal growth restriction: a Delphi procedure. Ultrasound Obstet Gynecol. 2016;48(3):333-9.
2. GRIT Study Group. A randomized trial of timed delivery for the compromised preterm fetus: short term outcomes and Bayesian interpretation. BJOG. 2003;110(1):27-32.
3. ISUOG Practice Guidelines: diagnosis and management of small-for-gestational-age fetus and fetal growth restriction. Ultrasound Obstet Gynecol. 2020;56:298-312.
4. Jain S, Mukhopadhyay K, Jain V, Kumar P. Slow versus rapid enteral feed in preterm neonates with antenatal absent end diastolic flow. J Matern Fetal Neonatal Med. 2016;29(17):2828-33.
5. Leaf A, Dorling J, Kempley S, McCormick K, Mannix P, Linsell L, et al. Early or delayed enteral feeding for preterm growth-restricted infants: a randomized trial. Pediatrics. 2012;129(5):e1260-8.
6. Lees CC, Marlow N, van Wassenaer-Leemhuis A, Bilardo CM, Brezinka C, Calvert S, et al. 2 year Neurodevelopmental and intermediate perinatal outcomes in infants with very preterm fetal growth restriction (TRUFFLE): a randomized trial. Lancet. 2015;385(9983):2162-72.
7. Mari G. Fetal growth restriction: Evaluation and management. [online] Available from https://www.uptodate.com/contents/fetal-growth-restriction-evaluation-and-management. [Last accessed November, 2021].
8. van Wyk L, Boers KE, van der Post JA, van Pampus MG, van Wassenaer AG, van Baar AL, et al. Effects on(neuro)developmental and behavioural outcome at 2 years of age of induced labor compared with expectant management in intrauterine growth-restricted infants: long-term outcomes of the DIGITAT trial. Am J Obstet Gynecol. 2012;206(5): 406.e1-7.
9. WHA Global Nutrition Targets 2025: Low Birth Weight Policy Brief. Evidence-based interventions to prevent low birth weight. [online] Available from https://apps.who.int/nutrition/publications/globaltargets2025_policybrief_lbw/en/index.html. [Last accessed November, 2021].

Hydrops Fetalis

Raja Ashok Koganti, Anu Sachdeva

INTRODUCTION

Hydrops fetalis is defined as the accumulation of excessive fluid in two or more fetal serous cavities/sites **(Table 1)**. Hydrops fetalis is broadly classified into two categories based on its etiology: Immune hydrops fetalis (IHF) and nonimmune hydrops fetalis (NIHF). IHF is due to maternal alloimmunization, when mother develops antibodies against fetal antigen that is paternally inherited. Etiology of NIHF is diverse involving several primary diagnoses.

The above criteria represent the most commonly used definition of hydrops; some definitions include skin edema as a mandatory criterion while others do not include polyhydramnios.

OBJECTIVES

- To review the etiology of immune and nonimmune hydrops fetalis.
- To discuss the pathophysiology of immune and nonimmune hydrops fetalis.
- To discuss the antenatal monitoring and management of Rh isoimmunization and IHF.
- To discuss the prognostication and antenatal counseling aspects of hydrops fetalis.
- To discuss the delivery room and postnatal management of hydrops fetalis.
- To discuss the approach to diagnostic evaluation of nonimmune hydrops.

IMMUNE HYDROPS FETALIS

Etiology and Mechanism of Isoimmunization

Rh blood group antigens are the most clinically relevant antigens responsible for maternal isoimmunization. Out of >50 antigens described under Rh system D, C, c, E, and e are the most concerning ones. Atypical red blood cell antigens such as Duffy, Kidd, and Kell are rarely implicated. The inciting event to trigger maternal isoimmunization is most commonly some form of fetomaternal hemorrhage due to delivery and various obstetric events **(Table 2)**.

TABLE 1: Diagnostic criteria for antenatal hydrops fetalis.

Diagnostic criteria	Description
Abnormal fluid collections in two or more of the following sites:	
Ascites	Rim of fluid surrounding entire fetal abdomen on scan
Pleural effusions	Visualization of lung border unilaterally or bilaterally
Pericardial effusions	≥2 mm nonphysiological fluid
Skin edema	≥5 mm subcutaneous edema
Polyhydramnios	AFI ≥25 mm or single deepest pocket ≥ 8 mm
Placentomegaly	≥6 cm thickness

(AFI: amniotic fluid index)

TABLE 2: Obstetric events leading to fetomaternal hemorrhage.

Events leading to fetomaternal hemorrhage	
Abruptio placentae	Abdominal trauma
External cephalic version	Umbilical cord sampling
Amniocentesis	Manual removal of placenta
Chorionic villous biopsy	Internal podalic version
Spontaneous/Elective abortion	Placenta previa with bleeding
Ectopic pregnancy	Fetal death in utero

Even 0.25 mL of fetomaternal hemorrhage is sufficient to cause isoimmunization. As the primary maternal immune response is slow and involves immunoglobulin M (IgM) antibodies that do not cross the placenta, the initial event leading to sensitization does not normally lead to hemolysis. However, subsequent exposure to antigen leads to more rapid and strong IgG response that causes fetal hemolysis and anemia. Fetomaternal transfusion has been documented in 7, 16, 29, and 50% in first, second, third trimester, and peripartum period, respectively.

Pathophysiology of Immune Hydrops

Mechanism of hydrops in IHF involves a combination of fetal hypoxemia due to fetal anemia, high output cardiac failure, and hepatic dysfunction **(Flowchart 1)**. Pregnancies

Flowchart 1: Proposed pathophysiology of immune hydrops.

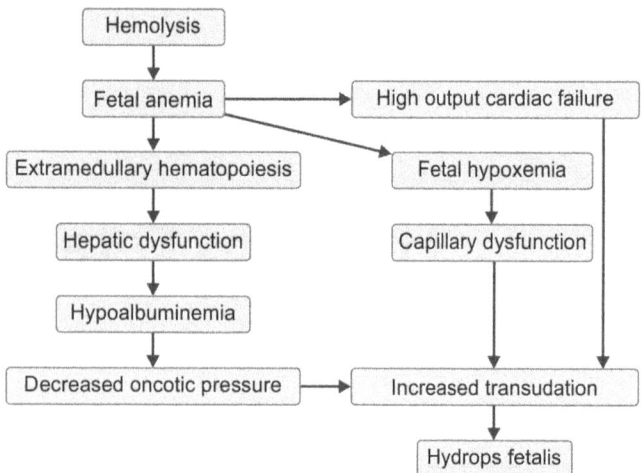

after the first alloimmunized pregnancy are characterized by increasingly severe fetal hemolytic disease due to the entry of fetal red cells into the maternal circulation at each delivery, which causes an anamnestic maternal antibody response. Maternal to fetal antibody transmission predominantly occurs after 22 weeks of gestation. Once these antibodies bind to fetal RhD antigens, it leads to hemolysis.

Most fetuses develop hydrops when the hemolysis is severe enough to cause the fetal hemoglobin (Hb) to fall below 5 g/dL or a hematocrit < 15%. As the mean Hb level varies with gestational age, an Hb value <0.5 times the median for gestation age is proposed as a more appropriate predictor for fetal hydrops.

Management of Immune Hydrops

Prevention

Anti-D immunoglobulin is passive IgG immunoglobulin against RhD antigen which is administered to the negative women to prevent isoummunization. It is given at a dose of 300 μg at 28 weeks of gestation and within 72 hours of delivery, if the baby has Rh-positive blood group. Anti-D immunoglobulin is also given following termination of pregnancy (medical or surgical), spontaneous abortion associated with repetitive episodes of bleeding, amniocentesis, chorionic villous sampling, or ectopic pregnancy. The recommended dose is 120–150 μg up to 12 weeks of gestation and 300 μg beyond 12 weeks of gestation. The risk of isoimmunization after antepartum and postpartum anti-D immunoglobulin prophylaxis is 0.1% against 16% without any prophylaxis. 300 μg of anti-D immunoglobulin can neutralize 30 mL of fetal blood or 15 mL of packed RhD-positive red blood cells (RBCs). There is no role of anti-D immunoglobulin in mothers who are already isoimmunized (i.e., positive indirect Coombs test—ICT), husband with RhD-negative blood group and antenatally diagnosed Rh-negative fetal blood group [either by cell-free fetal DNA (cffDNA) or amniocentesis or preimplantation diagnosis].

Antenatal Monitoring and Management

Preimplantation genetic diagnosis, paternal genotyping, cffDNA testing have been used in developed countries to clarify the fetal risk, facilitate counseling, and determining the need for intervention in RhD-negative women with RhD-positive husband. However, in Indian settings, these investigations are infrequently used. ICT is performed for anti-RhD antibodies in a setting of RhD-negative woman with RhD-positive husband. Testing for antibodies for all Rh antigens is reserved for situations with negative ICT against anti-RhD antibody and past history suggestive of isoimmunization.

Peak systolic velocity (PSV) of the middle cerebral artery (MCA) is used as proxy for detection of fetal anemia during antenatal monitoring of isoimmunized mothers. The sensitivity of this approach to predict moderate-to-severe anemia is 100% and false positive rate is around 12% making it a very useful tool for evaluation of at-risk fetus, its use has reduced the use of invasive procedures by 70%. Optimal threshold for mild, moderate, and severe anemia are 1.29, 1.5, and 1.55 multiples of median (MoM), respectively. However, this measurement does not have a good discriminative power after 35 weeks of gestation. Estimation of amniotic fluid bilirubin levels by delta OD 450 and its categorization into three zones with the help of Liley chart to estimate the severity of hemolysis is no longer practiced and is obsolete.

The antenatal management of RhD isoimmunization and immune hydrops (IH) is summarized in **Flowchart 2**.

Intrauterine transfusion (IUT) is commonly performed intravascularly. It is performed when the MCA PSV on Doppler is >1.5 MoMs and fetal hematocrit is <30%. A 20–22 G echogenic needle is used to enter the umbilical vein, with the preferred location being, cord insertion to the placenta. Type O, RhD-negative, irradiated, and leukodepleted packed red blood cells (PRBCs) crossmatched against maternal blood is used. The hematocrit is usually maintained >75% in the donor PRBC. The volume of blood to be transfused depends on the gestation, fetal hematocrit, and hematocrit of the donor PRBC.

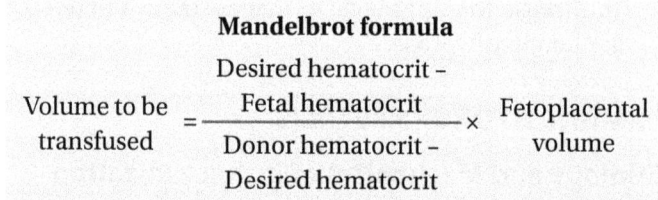

where fetoplacental volume (mL) = 0.14 × (estimated fetal weight in grams by ultrasound + 1.046)

It is estimated using nomogram's or with the help of Mandelbrot formula.

A post-transfusion hematocrit of approximately 40% is desirable. In case of lower gestations, a lower post-transfusion

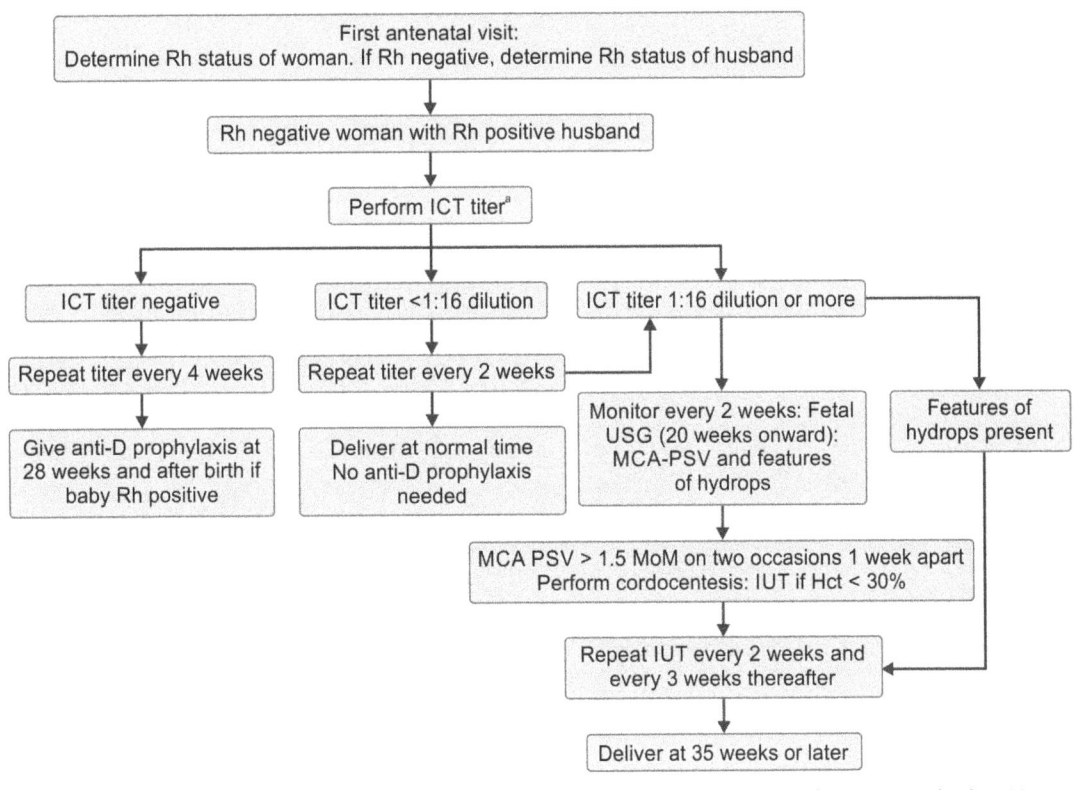

Flowchart 2: Antenatal management of Rh isoimmunization and hydrops fetalis.

[a]Typically laboratories set >1:16 titer as critical titer for isoimmunization, note the ICT titer mentioned is for anti-D antibodies. Management of isoimmunization due to other Rh antigens remains similar.
(Hct: hematocrit; ICT: indirect Coombs test; IUT: intrauterine transfusion; MCA: middle cerebral artery; MoM: multiples of median; PSV: peak systolic velocity; USG: ultrasonography)

hematocrit, i.e., not >25% increase in pretransfusion hematocrit is targeted to avoid cardiac decompensation. Typically, the fetal hematocrit falls by 1% per day and a repeat transfusion is usually necessary by 2 weeks and 3 weeks after the second IUT. A higher cutoff of 1.69 MoMs for MCA PSV is used for future IUTs. IUTs are not performed after 35 weeks of gestation, pregnancy is terminated in case IUT is required after 35 weeks.

Intraperitoneal transfusions are rarely performed only in exceptional circumstances when the umbilical vessel caliber does not permit placement of needle (usually <18 weeks) or when intrauterine transfusion is not possible due to abnormal fetal position or umbilical cord location.

Postnatal Management

The postnatal management of IH is summarized in **Flowchart 3**. Preparedness and immediate availability of blood products are crucial in the management of such neonates. Partial exchange is performed to rapidly restore the hematocrit to enhance oxygen-carrying capacity in hydropic neonates. A volume of 50 mL/kg of O negative PRBC crossmatched with baby's and mother's blood is used. Partial exchange transfusion is followed by double volume exchange transfusion (DVET). The details of DVET are summarized as next.

> **Double volume exchange transfusion**
>
> *Blood volume*: For example, for a term neonate weighing 3 kg
>
> 80 mL/kg (derived from Rawing's nomogram) × Weight (in kg) × 2 = 480 mL
>
> Add 50 mL additionally for priming the system = 530 mL to be ordered
>
> *Proportion of blood components*: 2/3 PRBC and 1/3 plasma
> *Choice of blood components*: O (or ABO as that of baby) Rh-negative PRBC suspended in AB plasma crossmatched against fetal and maternal blood

Hydropic neonates due to their altered physiological status require special considerations during ventilation, fluid balance, and shock management as summarized in **Flowchart 3**. There is insufficient evidence to recommend the use of intravenous immunoglobulin (IVIg) routinely in the management of Rh isoimmunization. Although a recent Cochrane review in 2018 did show a decrease in the need for exchange transfusion in neonates treated with IVIg, the quality of evidence was very low. Studies with low risk of bias included in the same review showed no benefit of IVIg in reducing need for exchange transfusions.

Flowchart 3: Algorithm for postnatal management of immune hydrops fetalis.

```
Fetus with immune hydrops due to deliver:
• Inform blood bank: Arrange for blood products
• Anticipate difficult resuscitation
• Delivery to be attended by atleast two neonatologists
• Be prepared for difficult airway, pleural and ascitic tap
• ECG leads preferable, as heart rate assessment may be obscured by pericardial effusion and skin edema
                                    ↓
Delivery room care:
• Resuscitate as per NRP
• Emergency pleural and ascitic tap may be required simultaneously to facilitate lung expansion
• PPV in setting of pulmonary hypoplasia and improper water seal during pleural tap may contribute to pneumothorax
• Collect cord blood for hematocrit, bilirubin, baby blood group and direct Coombs test (DCT)
• Shift to NICU
                        ↓                                                   ↓
NICU care:                                          • Respiratory: Poor chest wall compliance, pulmonary
• Ensure TABC (temperature, airway, breathing,        edema, surfactant deficiency, prone for air leak,
  circulation)                                        hemorrhage and PPHN. Requires high PEEP
• Partial exchange followed by double volume        • Restricted maintenance fluids, monitor Na, urine
  exchange transfusion                                output and daily weight
• Use dry weight for all calculations in severely   • Bedside ECHO: To guide fluid management by
  hydropic neonates                                   estimating intravascular volume and cardiac output
• Double surface intensive phototherapy             • Manage shock: Correct hypovolemia and impaired
• Monitor S. bilirubin, PCV, neurological monitoring  venous return
  for BIND
                                    ↓
Follow up care:
• Consider inspissated bile duct syndrome, if conjugated hyperbilirubinemia
• Hearing screening (AABR/BERA) at discharge
• ROP screening if gestation < 34 weeks
• High risk follow up clinic for development assessment, counsel mother regarding possible requirement
  of transfusions 4–8 weeks after discharge (hyporegenerative anemia)
```

(AABR: automated auditory brainstem response; BERA: brainstem evoked response audiometry; BIND: bilirubin-induced neurological dysfunction; ECG: electrocardiogram; NICU: neonatal intensive care unit; NRP: Neonatal Resuscitation Program; PEEP: positive end-expiratory pressure; PCV: packed cell volume; PPHN: persistent pulmonary hypertension of the newborn; PPV: positive predictive value; ECHO: echocardiography)

Short-term Outcomes

A retrospective review of fetuses treated for anemia due to Rh isoimmunization with IUTs showed a postnatal survival of 78% in hydropic fetuses. Early requirement of IUT, early appearance of hydrops, and antibodies against Kell antigen are associated with poorer outcomes. Neonates with hydrops may develop various other morbidities as illustrated in **Flowchart 4**.

Long-term Outcomes

The LOTUS trial evaluated the neurodevelopment outcomes of children with isoimmunization treated with IUT, cerebral palsy was detected in 2.1%, severe developmental delay in 3.1%, and bilateral deafness in 3.1%. Hydropic fetuses are at high risk of future neurodevelopment disability, hearing impairment, and require close follow-up after discharge as depicted in **Flowchart 3**.

NONIMMUNE HYDROPS FETALIS

Etiology

Etiology of NIHF is diverse and involves a wide range of conditions **(Table 3)**. Cardiovascular conditions (21% of all cases of NIHF) followed by idiopathic, chromosomal, hematological, and infections (in order of decreasing incidence) are the major contributors to NIHF.

Pathophysiology of Nonimmune Hydrops Fetalis

Increased central venous pressure, low plasma oncotic pressure, and reduced lymphatic flow are the main mechanisms contributing to the development of NIHF. The pathways for development are illustrated in **Flowchart 5**. Sometimes, NIHF is associated with generalized maternal edema. Since this "mirrors" the edema of the hydropic fetus and placenta, it is called mirror syndrome (also called Ballantyne syndrome). There is pulmonary involvement in mother in majority of the cases too. Although, this condition is usually associated with NIHF, it can also occur with immune-mediated hydrops. The pathogenesis has not been firmly established, but at least in some cases, the hydropic placenta increases production of soluble fms-like tyrosine kinase (sFlt1), which is an important mediator of maternal endothelial and vascular abnormalities in preeclampsia.

Flowchart 4: Postnatal morbidities and their mechanism in immune hydrops.

```
                                                    ┌─ Hyperglycemia, rebound hypoglycemia if CPD blood used
                                                    │
         ┌─ IUT's in antenatal period ─┐  ┌─ DVET in postnatal period ─┤
         │                             │  │                            ├─ Hypocalcemia if CPD blood used
         ▼                             ▼  ▼                            │
  Hemolysis due RhD      Suppression of erythropoiesis                 ├─ DVET using cold blood: Arrhythmia, arrest
    antibodies              Decreased EPO levels                       │
         │                             │                               ├─ Metabolic acidosis
         ▼                             ▼                               │
  Increased bilirubin     Hyporegenerative anemia                      └─ Thrombocytopenia
         │                 (between 2 and 6 weeks)
         ▼                             │
  Accumulates as Ca bilirubinate       ▼
   sludge in bile ducts         Requirement of
         │                   postnatal transfusions
         ▼
  Inspissated bile syndrome                      ( Decreased EPO and
         │                                         reticulocyte count
         ▼                                         Increased ferritin levels )
     BIND SNHL
```

(BIND: bilirubin-induced neurological dysfunction; CPD: citrate phosphate dextrose; DVET: double volume exchange transfusion; EPO: erythropoietin; IUT: intrauterine transfusion; SNHL: sensorineural hearing loss)

TABLE 3: Conditions associated with nonimmune hydrops fetalis.

Category	Specific conditions	Category	Specific conditions
Cardiovascular	• Structural • Hypoplasia, AV canal defect, single ventricle, transposition of the great vessels, TOF, Ebstein anomaly, septal defects, ductus arteriosus closure, truncus arteriosus, valvular stenosis • Arrhythmias • Atrial flutter/tachyarrhythmia, supraventricular tachycardia, Wolff–Parkinson–White syndrome, heart block, long QT syndrome • Cardiomyopathy	Syndromic/ malformation sequences/ chondrodysplasia	Noonan syndrome, arthrogryposis, multiple pterygium syndrome, myotonic dystrophy, Neu–Laxova syndrome, Pena–Shokeir syndrome, lymphedema distichiasis syndrome, Francois syndrome, type III homozygous achondroplasia, campomelic dysplasia, thanatophoric dysplasia, and achondrogenesis
Chromosomal	Trisomy of 13, 18, 21, Turner syndrome, monosomy (45X), duplications (18q+, 11p), and deletions (13q-, 17q-)	Metabolic	Gaucher disease, GM1 gangliosides, sialidosis, Hurler syndrome, mucopolysaccharide (MPS) IVa, mucolipidosis type I + II, galactosialidosis
Hematological	Alpha thalassemia, glucose-6-phsosphate deficiency, pyruvate kinase deficiency, and red blood cell aplasia	Gastrointestinal	Bowel obstruction with perforation/meconium peritonitis, small bowel volvulus/duplications, hepatic tumors/cysts, and fibrosis
Infection	Cytomegalovirus, parvovirus B19, syphilis, herpes simplex, rubella, coxsackie, toxoplasmosis, and leptospirosis	Urinary	Urethral stenosis or atresia, posterior urethral valves, prune belly syndrome, and congenital nephrotic syndrome
Thoracic mass/ lymphatic	Congenital cystic adenoid malformation, congenital diaphragmatic hernia, pulmonary sequestration, bronchogenic cyst, chylothorax, and pulmonary lymphangiectasia	Twin pregnancy	Twin-to-twin transfusion syndrome and acardiac twin

The list of conditions is nonexhaustive.
(AV: atrioventricular; TOF: tetralogy of Fallot)

SECTION 2 | Fetal Disorders

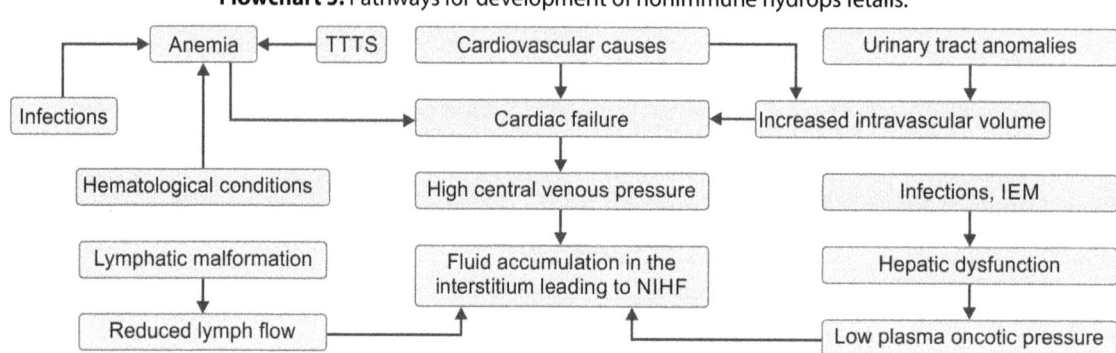

Flowchart 5: Pathways for development of nonimmune hydrops fetalis.

(IEM: inborn error of metabolism; NIHF: nonimmune hydrops fetalis; TTTS: twin-to-twin transfusion syndrome)

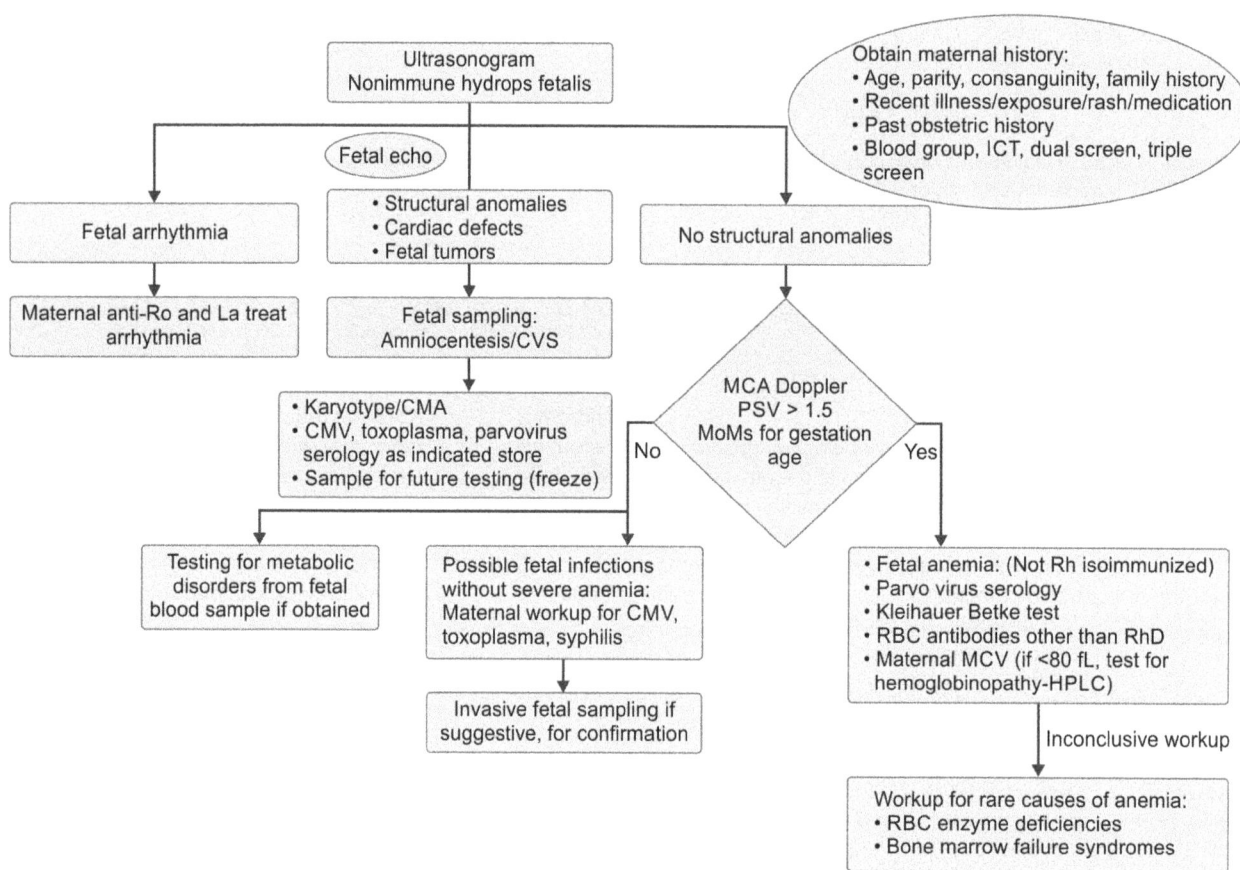

Flowchart 6: Antenatal diagnostic approach to nonimmune hydrops fetalis.

(CVS: chorionic villous sampling; CMA: chromosomal microarray; CMV: cytomegalovirus; HPLC: high performance liquid chromatography; ICT: indirect Coombs test; MCA: middle cerebral artery; MCV: mean corpuscular volume; MoM: multiples of median; PSV: peak systolic velocity; RBC: red blood cell)

Diagnostic Approach to Evaluation and Management of Nonimmune Hydrops Fetalis

Antenatal approach and investigations are summarized in **Flowchart 6**.

Table 4 summarizes the postnatal evaluations required for a newborn with nonimmune hydrops of unknown cause. The algorithmic approach to postnatal evaluation must be customized based on the clinical scenario after considering the examination findings of neonate and information gathered from antenatal evaluation.

Management

Antenatal management apart from diagnostics is conservative including fetal surveillance—nonstress test, biophysical profile, and serial ultrasonograms. When the etiology of hydrops is known, early consultations with

TABLE 4: Postnatal evaluation for a newborn with nonimmune hydrops fetalis.

System	Type of evaluation
Cardiovascular	Echocardiogram and ECG
Pulmonary	Chest radiograph and pleural fluid examination
Hematologic	Complete blood count, blood group, direct Coombs test, and peripheral blood smear
Gastrointestinal	Peritoneal fluid examination, abdominal ultrasound/X-ray, and liver function tests
Renal	Urinalysis, urea, and creatine
Genetic	Karyotype, infantogram, and dysmorphology analysis
Congenital infections	CMV PCR, serological testing, viral cultures, fundus evaluation, and cranial ultrasonogram
Pathologic	Placental examination and complete autopsy

(CMV: cytomegalovirus; ECG: electrocardiogram; PCR: polymerase chain reaction)

relevant subspecialty doctors (neonatologists, pediatric cardiologists, geneticists, and pediatric surgeons) is warranted. In-utero interventions such as shunt placements, fetal surgery is sometimes performed in conditions amenable to fetal therapy. Delivery is indicated in cases with progressive NIHF when gestation has crossed 34 weeks, although care must be individualized. In the absence of any maternal or fetal deterioration, or any reason for an earlier intervention, pregnancy may be continued up to 37 weeks, based on expert opinion. Maternal mirror syndrome or biophysical profile score persistently <6 is an indication for immediate termination. Cesarean delivery is indicated for obstetric reasons alone. Certain cardiac and thoracic malformations such as congenital high airway obstruction syndrome (CHAOS) benefit from ex utero intrapartum therapy (EXIT). In EXIT, procedures such as tracheostomy are performed, while the cord is still intact while fetus still receives uteroplacental blood flow. This procedure requires multidisciplinary collaboration and is performed in specialized centers.

Same principles apply in the management of these neonates in the delivery room and neonatal intensive care unit (NICU) as that of neonates with immune hydrops. Specific treatment varies based on the underlying cause of hydrops. The risk of recurrence is dependent on the underlying etiology, while hydrops due to viral infections have no risk of recurrence, the risk of recurrence can be high when the etiology is genetic. In cases where no etiology can be found, the chances of recurrence are low. It is reasonable to monitor by scanning in the mid trimester period for any features of hydrops.

Outcome

Prognosis in NIHF is largely dependent on the underlying condition causing this condition. Neonates with chylothorax, supraventricular tachycardia, parvovirus infection have highest survival rates, whereas hydrops from chromosomal cause has poor outcomes. Overall survival of a neonate with NIHF remains poor.

CHAPTER AT A GLANCE

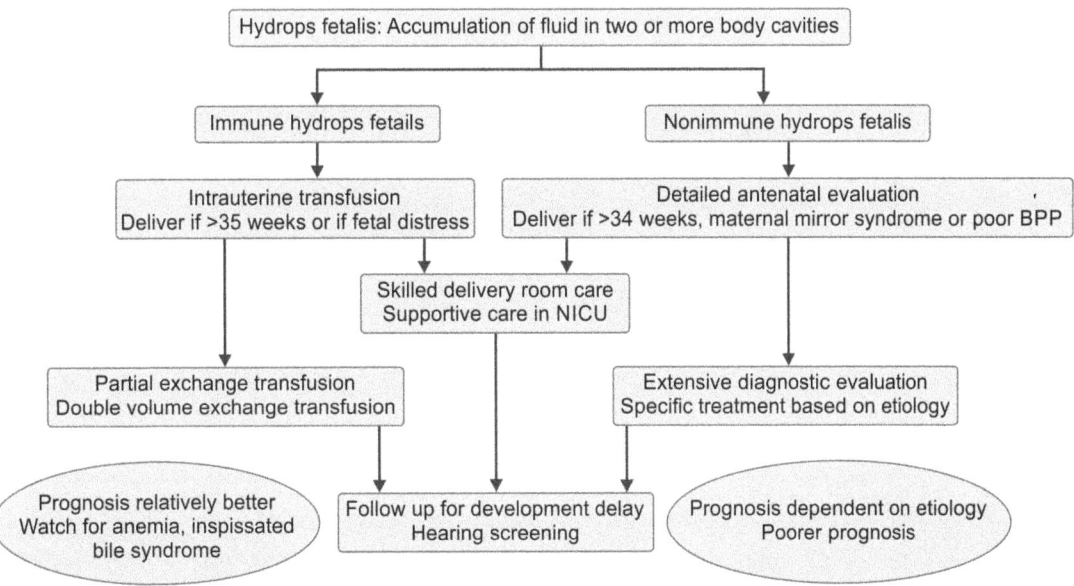

(BPP: biophysical profile; NICU: neonatal intensive care unit)

KEY POINTS

- Hydrops is defined as the accumulation of fluid in two or more body cavities.
- RhD antigen is the most common antigen responsible for immune hydrops.
- The etiology for NIHF is diverse with cardiovascular causes contributing to majority of the cases.
- High central venous pressure, low oncotic pressure, and reduced lymph flow are responsible for the development of hydrops.
- Skilled delivery room care and tertiary NICU with subspecialty support is necessary for management of hydropic neonates.
- Partial exchange and DVET soon after birth remain cornerstone of managing immune hydrops.
- The prognosis of nonimmune hydrops is dependent on the etiology.

SUGGESTED READING

1. Agarwal K, Rana A, Ravi AK. Treatment and Prevention of Rh Isoimmunization. J Fetal Med. 2014;1(2):81-8.
2. Lockwood CJ, Julien S. Non Immune Hydrops Fetalis. In UpToDate Post TW (Ed), Waltham, MA: UpToDate; 2021.
3. Martin RJ, Fanaroff AA, Walsh MC. Fanaroff and Martin's Neonatal-perinatal medicine: diseases of the fetus and infant. 11th edition, Volume 1. Amsterdam: Elsevier Limited; 2020. pp. 371-85.
4. Norton ME, Chauhan SP, Dashe JS. Society for Maternal-Fetal Medicine (SMFM) Clinical Guideline #7: nonimmune hydrops fetalis. Am J Obstet Gynecol. 2015;212(2):127-39.

CHAPTER 14

Antenatal Counseling for Fetomaternal Conditions

Umamaheswari Balakrishnan, Chitra Andrew

INTRODUCTION

Many conditions in pregnancy require detailed counseling to enable parents to make informed choices regarding the continuation of pregnancy, fetal therapy, timing and nature of the birth, and facility where delivery should occur and additionally understand the risk of recurrence. Antenatal counseling includes communicating to the parents the natural history of the disease, what to expect after birth, and plan for the neonatal care. A choice of termination of pregnancy versus continuation in an affected case depends on the severity of disorder, gestational age, and parental wishes. Antenatal diagnosis and counseling improve fetal and neonatal outcomes as care and delivery can be planned in advance.

OBJECTIVES

- Principles of counseling and approach
- Maternal medical conditions in pregnancy
  - Diabetes mellitus
  - Hypertensive disorders in pregnancy
  - Seizure disorder in pregnancy
- Special circumstances which influence fetal outcome
  - Isoimmunization
  - Teratogenicity
  - Fetal infections
- Fetal conditions which require counseling
  - Abnormal screening for aneuploidy in pregnancy
  - Structural anomalies
  - Direct testing
- Genetic disorders
  - Chromosomal, single gene, and mitochondrial disorders
  - Role of genetic testing
- Role of perinatal pathology

PRINCIPLES OF COUNSELING

Antenatal Counseling

The process of antenatal counseling aids the couple in making informed decisions about the pregnancy. Steps in counseling

BOX 1: Antenatal counseling and decision-making.
- Establishing trust
- Identify and explore individual and family values
- Avoid fixed counseling guidelines
- Facilitate collaborative decision-making
- Two-way communication process
- Reading nonverbal cues

BOX 2: Indications for antenatal counseling.
- Previous child with developmental delay of unknown etiology
- Suspected or confirmed genetic disorder in the family including inborn errors of metabolism and neuromuscular disorder
- Maternal medical disorders
- Exposure to teratogens
- Suspected or confirmed TORCH infections
- Fetal structural malformations
- Positive aneuploidy screening

(TORCH: toxoplasmosis, rubella cytomegalovirus, herpes simplex)

include gathering information, establishing the diagnosis, risk assessment, giving information, helping in decision making **(Box 1)**, and psychological and family support. Indications for antenatal counseling have been depicted in **Box 2**.

- *Gathering information*:
  - Detailed medical and family history
  - Three-generation pedigree charting
  - Detailed examination of the records
- *Establishing diagnosis*:
  - Examination of individuals—index child +/- Parents
  - Relevant and individualized investigations: Antenatal scan, genetic testing for the index child/fetus (karyotyping, chromosomal microarray, whole exome or whole genome sequencing), maternal investigation [e.g., glycated hemoglobin (HbA1C); TORCH (toxoplasmosis, rubella cytomegalovirus, herpes simplex, and HIV) screening, amniotic fluid viral polymerase chain reaction (PCR)]/parental testing.
- *Risk assessment*:
  - Depends on the type of condition—chromosomal/single-gene disorder/multifactorial/teratogenicity/environmental condition.

- This is an important step which helps in the current pregnancy as well as future pregnancies.
- *Giving information:* SPIKES (*S*etting up of scene; *P*erception checking; *I*nvitation to the context; *K*nowledge sharing-information in small boluses; *E*mpathy; *S*ummarizing and giving follow up plan) approach can be followed while breaking bad news.
- *Helping in decision-making:*
  - During the process of counseling, one respects the feelings of the couple and their autonomy.
  - All the ethical principles, namely autonomy, beneficence (best interest approach), nonmaleficence, justice, and equity, should be followed during the counseling process. On the majority of occasions, it should be nondirective.
  - Apart of ethical principles, values of parents including their personal beliefs and faith, family values, social, religious, financial concerns, and past experience should be considered while counseling.
  - Paternalistic imposition and fixed counseling guidelines should be avoided.
- *Psychological support:*
  - Approach should be empathetic with adequate time allotted for counseling in a nondisturbed environment.
  - Allowing additional family members to support them during counseling often helps. In an intense emotional state, their understanding might be hampered and they might feel overwhelmed and would often require more than one counseling session.

Role of Multidisciplinary Team

In complex situations, multidisciplinary team meetings discussing in detail about the maternal, fetal, and neonatal outcome would help. For example, in case of fetal malformation involving the upper airway, a team composed of a fetal medicine specialist, obstetrician, ENT specialist, anesthetist, neonatologist, and counselor have to plan the delivery and neonatal management and counsel the couple.

MATERNAL MEDICAL CONDITION IN PREGNANCY

Maternal Diabetes

Prevalence of gestational diabetes mellitus (GDM) varies widely between 1 and 14%. There is a 1.2- to 6-fold increase in the risk of congenital malformations, with lower risk observed in GDM and highest risk reported in preexisting diabetes with high HbA1C. Maternal glycemic control at the time of embryogenesis is crucial. The maternal, fetal, and neonatal complications are given in **Table 1**. Most common congenital malformations involve the cardiovascular system followed by central nervous system, spine, orofacial system, and renal, gastrointestinal, and skeletal systems. VACTERL (vertebral, anal atresia, cardiac, trachea-esophageal, renal/radial, limb abnormality) association occurs more frequency in maternal diabetes.

Counseling depends on whether the woman has GDM or preexisting diabetes. In preexisting diabetes, the factors which influence the decision-making include whether pregnancy is planned or unplanned, glycemic control at the time of conception, HbA1C levels (HbA1C of >10 is associated with poor prognosis), and time of diagnosis of preexisting diabetes (detected during or before pregnancy). In a woman with preexisting diabetes, preconceptional levels of HbA1C vary between different guidelines.

TABLE 1: Complications associated with maternal diabetes.

Maternal complications	Fetal/neonatal complications
• Severe hypoglycemia in first trimester • Preeclampsia • Complications including nephropathy, retinopathy, diabetic ketoacidosis, and thromboembolic disease • Increased risk of caesarean section • Risk of recurrence in future pregnancies • Risk of future type II diabetes	• Miscarriage, stillbirth, and neonatal death* • Macrosomia • Birth trauma and delivery complications • Congenital malformations* • Neonatal hypoglycemia, electrolyte imbalance, and hyperbilirubinemia • Long-term risks of insulin resistance, obesity, and type 2 diabetes

*Higher with high HbA1C.

HYPERTENSIVE DISORDERS IN PREGNANCY

Counseling depends on whether the woman has gestational hypertension (HT) or preexisting HT **(Table 2)**. Risk scoring in early pregnancy and initiation of low-dose aspirin for prevention of pulmonary embolism, fetal surveillance for fetal growth restriction (FGR), and well-being are important. Fetal surveillance is initiated at 26–28 weeks of gestation and done at regular intervals depending on the need **(Fig. 1)**. The timing of delivery depends on the maternal blood pressure control, severity of preeclampsia, and extent of Doppler abnormality in FGR fetus.

Maternal Seizure Disorder

Women with seizure disorders are at an increased risk of fetal malformations due to uncontrolled seizures or due to anticonvulsant therapy. As most of the anticonvulsants are teratogenic, a neurologist consultation should be obtained regarding the need for continuation of medication. If mandated, limiting the dose below a teratogenic threshold, monotherapy, or changing to an alternate drug with

TABLE 2: Summary of guidance on maternal medical conditions.

	Preconception	Early pregnancy	Fetal ultrasound	Factors influencing timing of delivery	Future risk
Maternal diabetes	Optimize HbA1C; folic acid supplementation	Glycemic control—avoid hypoglycemia and hyperglycemia	Detection of fetal malformation; monitor growth	• *Maternal*: Glucose control • *Fetal*: Growth—macrosomia	Yes; increased risk of GDM (30–60%) in future pregnancy
Maternal hypertensive disorder	Stop teratogenic medication	Preeclampsia risk scoring; initiate on aspirin if at-risk for preeclampsia	Detection of fetal malformation; monitor growth	• *Maternal*: Preeclampsia and eclampsia • *Fetal*: Fetal growth restriction and Doppler abnormality	Increased risk in future pregnancy (22%); need monitoring as increased risk of developing chronic HT and follow-up
Maternal seizure disorder	Stop highly teratogenic drugs; folic acid supplementation	Optimize seizure control	Detection of fetal malformation	Fetal growth	Risk of recurrence of teratogenicity if the same medication continued

(GDM: gestational diabetes mellitus; HT: hypertension)

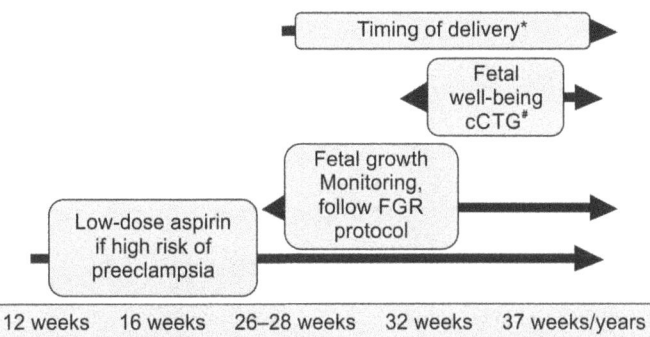

Fig. 1: Guidance in hypertensive disorder of pregnancy.
*Timing of delivery depends on the Doppler abnormality and maternal status.
#cCTG availability limited in an Indian setup.
(FGR: fetal growth restriction; cCTG: computerized cardiotocogram)

less teratogenicity should be done. Folic acid should be supplemented **(Table 2)**. Prevalence of birth defects is highest for sodium valproate (10.7%) followed by phenytoin (7.4%), phenobarbitone (4.9%), carbamazepine (4.6%), and lamotrigine (2.9%).

SPECIAL CIRCUMSTANCES WHICH INFLUENCE FETAL OUTCOME

Isoimmunized Pregnancy

Counseling a couple with isoimmunized pregnancy should include information on what is Rh incompatibility, need for serial indirect Coombs test (ICT) titers, and fetal testing by Doppler evaluation of the fetal middle cerebral artery (MCA) to identify fetal anemia. If the fetus is anemic, intrauterine transfusion (IUT) will be required. Delivery is usually planned between 37 and 38 weeks of gestation **(Flowchart 1)**. Delivery should be in a tertiary care center with neonatal intensive care unit (NICU) facilities. The neonatal cord blood testing of direct Coombs test (DCT), bilirubin, and hematocrit is done along with blood grouping and Rh typing. Management of the neonate includes intensive phototherapy, exchange transfusion if the rate of rise of bilirubin is >1 mg/dL/h despite intensive phototherapy, initiation of oral folic acid supplementation, and packed red cell transfusion if the infant develops anemia.

The couple must be aware there were no long-term consequences to the mother, however the infant can develop anemia needing packed red cell transfusion for which they should be under follow up with hematologist.

Teratogenicity

Teratogens interfere with normal development of the embryo usually early in pregnancy, but some can also damage the fetus later in pregnancy. Teratogen can be a chemical substance such as alcohol, an infection such as the rubella virus, or a physical agent such as X-rays. Exposure to teratogens is one of the important aspects in antenatal counseling in early pregnancy. However, a positive history from the mother and identification of congenital anomalies may give a clue to exposure to the specific teratogen late in pregnancy.

Various teratogenic agents and their effects on growing fetuses are enlisted in **Table 3**.

Prepregnancy counseling is ideal for maternal medical conditions such as preexisting diabetes, hypertension, and

Flowchart 1: Counseling in isoimmunized pregnancy.

```
All pregnant women—blood group and type at booking visit—Rh negative
           │                                    │
           ▼                                    ▼
      ICT negative                         ICT positive
      │        │                                │
      ▼        ▼                                ▼
Give routine   Additional anti-D          Do ICT titers
prophylaxis    if any sensitizing              │
with anti-D    events occur                    ▼
at 28 and 34                           Test ICT titer monthly till 28 weeks
weeks                                  Fortnightly from 28 weeks to delivery
      │                                         │
      ▼                                         ▼
Anti-D at birth if blood group is Rh +ve    Fetal MCA PSV 4 weekly
      │                                     if PSV MoM is <1.5
      ▼                ←── Deliver at term ──┘
Cord blood for DCT, Hb, bilirubin                │
                                                 ▼
Cord blood for DCT, Hb, bilirubin ← IUT and follow-up ← Fetal MCA PSV > 1.5
```

(DCT: direct Coombs test; ICT: indirect Coombs test; IUT: intrauterine transfusion; MCA: middle cerebral artery; MoM: multiples of median; PSV: peak systolic velocity)

TABLE 3: Teratogenic agents.

Maternal infections

• Rubella virus	• Congenital rubella syndrome
• Cytomegalovirus (CMV)	• Congenital CMV infection
• Toxoplasmosis	• Congenital toxoplasmosis
• Zika virus	• Congenital zika virus syndrome
• Varicella virus (chicken pox and herpes zoster)	• Congenital varicella syndrome

Maternal illnesses

• Diabetes mellitus	• Major malformations during early phase like holoprosencephaly, VACTERL association
• Maternal phenylketonuria	• Congenital heart defects and microcephaly

Radiation

• Excessive amounts of X-ray	Increased risk of miscarriage, malformation including microcephaly, IUGR, functional impairment, intellectual disability, childhood malignancy including leukemia
• Nuclear radiation (e.g., Chernobyl)	

Drugs

• ACE inhibitor	• Renal dysplasia
• Alcohol	• Cardiac defects, microcephaly, characteristic facies
• Chloroquine	• Chorioretinitis, deafness
• Diethylstilbestrol	• Uterine malformation, vaginal adenocarcinoma
• Lithium	• Ebstein anomaly
• Methotrexate	• Neural tube defects (NTD)
• Methimazole	• Aplasia cutis of scalp
• Penicillamine	• Connective tissue disorder, cutis laxa
• Phenytoin	• IUGR, dysmorphism, CNS anomalies, cleft lip and palate, distal limb defects, nail hypoplasia
• Retinoic acid	
• Streptomycin	• Ear and eye defects, hydrocephalus, heart defects
• Tetracycline	• Deafness
• Thalidomide	• Dental enamel hypoplasia
• Valproic acid	• Phocomelia, ear and cardiac anomaly
• Warfarin	• Spina bifida, atrial septal defect, cleft palate, hypospadias
	• Nasal hypoplasia, stippled epiphyses

Environmental pollutants

• Methyl mercury	Neurotoxicity and functional defects
• Lead	

(CNS: central nervous system; IUGR: intrauterine growth restriction; VACTERL: vertebral, anal atresia, cardiac, trachea-esophageal, renal/radial, limb abnormality) seizures. Preconceptional folic acid, avoiding unnecessary radiation exposure during reproductive age group, checking for rubella status, and vaccinating eligible women are some of the preventive care aspects. Health education is a key preventive measure. Prevention of birth defects can be summarized as PACT which stands for *P*lan ahead, *A*void harmful substances, *C*hoose healthy lifestyle, and *T*alk with healthcare providers.

Teratogenicity varies depending on the gestational age of exposure and earlier exposure during embryogenesis, causing maximal adverse effect. Careful evaluation of exposure history and clinical evaluation and counseling should be performed by specialists skilled in assessment of birth defects and capable of identifying characteristic patterns. Serology and ultrasound help in complete assessment. Four major manifestations of deviant development include fetal demise, malformation, growth retardation, and functional defect.

Teratogenic Drugs

Pregnancy is a crucial period where medication should be prescribed considering not only the maternal effects but also the fetal effects. Risk versus benefit should carefully be contemplated. There are certain medications such as isotretinoin where a wash-out period of 3 months is observed before pregnancy. The Food and Drug Administration (FDA) drug risk classification was widely used; however, as the pregnancy letter category system was overly simplistic, it is being replaced by pregnancy and lactation labeling rule (PLLR) where the relevant information is provided for individual medication which helps in critical decision-making.

Ionizing Radiation

In general, exposure occurs in women who get exposed without awareness of being pregnant. Radiation exposure is expressed in the units rad or millisievert (1 rad = 10 mSv). The dose of various radiological investigations varies widely, ranging from 0.01 rad for chest X-ray to 1 rad for CT of thorax **(Fig. 2)**. A thorough history of the type of exposure and the gestational age at exposure help in appropriate counseling. Radiation exposure of up to 5 rad is considered a threshold dose of safety. As majority of single-time exposure to radiation would be well below the threshold dose of safety, the couple could be counseled in the same to make informed choices **(Fig. 2)**. Fetal effects are summarized in **Table 3**.

Fetal Infections

The TORCH infections are a group of congenital infections that may have similar clinical presentations and affect the fetus. Other causes of intrauterine/perinatal infection include zika virus, enterovirus, varicella-zoster virus, and parvovirus B19. It is crucial for timely diagnosis as it has significant fetal and neonatal implications.

The scenarios where antenatal counseling is indicated include exposure to infection, overt maternal infection such as maternal varicella, fetal abnormalities suggestive of perinatal infection such as antenatal ventricular dilatation, hydrops fetalis, fetal anemia, microcephaly, and various CNS malformations. Majority of maternal infections which affect the fetus present with fever, rash, and mild maternal illness which often goes unnoticed, the exception being maternal varicella. Preconceptional consult of any woman should always include discussion on vaccination for rubella. The characteristics of maternal infection and guidance on counseling are summarized in **Table 4**.

FETAL CONDITIONS

Screening for Aneuploidy

All women should be offered aneuploidy screening irrespective of maternal age. The a priori risk is calculated

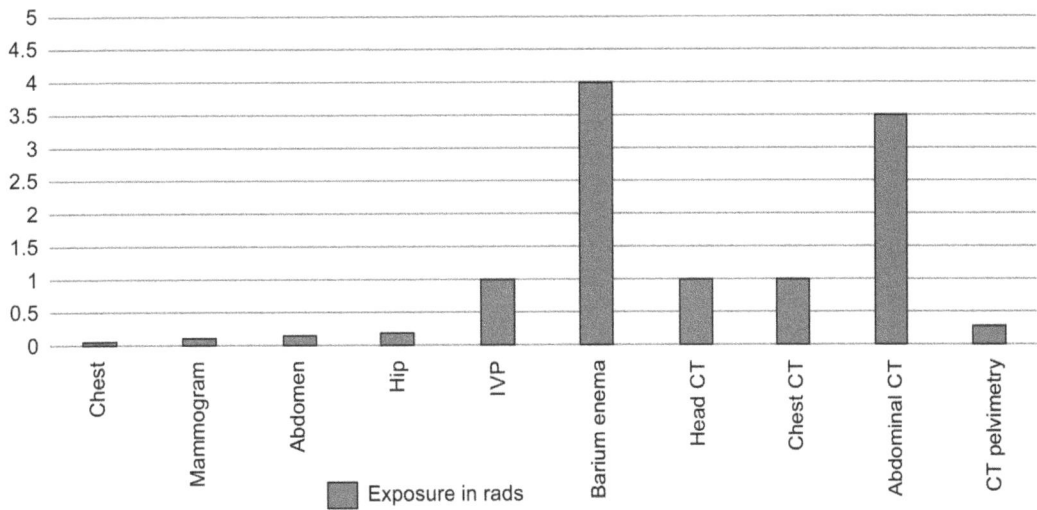

Fig. 2: Exposure of the conceptus from imaging studies.
(IVP: intravenous pyelogram)

SECTION 2 | Fetal Disorders

TABLE 4: Characteristics of maternal infection and guidance on counseling.

	Risk of transmission	Fetal features	Counseling guidance	Diagnosis	Prevention	Treatment-maternal
Toxoplasmosis	5–15% <13 weeks, 25% 13–28 weeks	• Intracranial calcifications • Hydrocephalus • Hydrops	Termination* offered in confirmed fetal infection	• *Serology*: IgG and IgM serology limited role • Positive amniotic fluid PCR	Hygiene measures,* early detection and adequate treatment during pregnancy	*<18 weeks*: Spiramycin gestation ≥18 weeks or affected fetus: Pyrimethamine, sulfadiazine, and folinic acid
Other—syphilis	>50% risk of transmission	Still birth, nonimmune hydrops, hepatosplenomegaly	Treatment options available	Serology, placental examination	Early detection and adequate treatment during pregnancy, healthy lifestyle*	Maternal antibiotics—penicillin adequate therapy
Rubella	75% < 8 weeks, 50% 9–12 weeks, 20% 13–20 weeks, 0–10% >20	Cardiac defects, cataracts, microphthalmia, growth restriction	Pregnancy termination may be an option when fetal infection is diagnosed within 16 weeks due to high risk of CRS; likely sequalae in neonate	Rubella-specific IgM or four-fold increase in IgG titers, cord blood rubella-specific IgM and PCR of amniotic fluid	Vaccination*	None
Cytomegalovirus	30–40% in primary infection; reinfection 1%	Placental enlargement, CNS malformations, periventricular calcification, ventricular dilatation	Available treatment for neonate and the likely sequalae	Anti-CMV IgM antibodies along with low avidity anti-IgG antibodies confirms primary infection, amniotic fluid PCR, fetal ultrasound	Hygiene measures,* ?CMV Hyperimmunoglobulin	Self-limiting illness in mother
Herpes	*Perinatal infection*: Primary infection >50% chance, recurrent infection <2% chance	Only <2% intrauterine infection, skin scarring, CNS-microphthalmia, retinal dysplasia, chorioretinitis, calcification, microcephaly	Need for caesarean section in active genital herpes	No fetal evaluation, neonatal evaluation	Caesarean section before rupture of membrane in active lesion	Acyclovir therapy
Varicella	*Congenital*: 0.4–2% within 20 weeks of gestation	Cicatricial skin lesion, cardiac defects, echogenic foci in liver, skeletal-limb abnormalities and CNS malformation	Low risk of infection, serial ultrasound though skin lesion cannot be picked up	Amniotic fluid PCR, fetal ultrasound	Vaccination*	Self-limiting illness; acyclovir therapy depending on the severity, usually self-limiting illness
	Perinatal: 5 days before and 2 days after delivery	Neonatal varicella	Need for IV Varicella IG to neonate	Clinical	Vaccination,* Varicella-specific immunoglobulin	IV varicella immunoglobulin, IV acyclovir once neonate develops infection
Parvovirus	10% and 35% risk of vertical transmission	Hydrops, cardiomyopathy, fetal anemia, If <20 weeks risk of still birth	Need for monitoring and intrauterine transfusion	Positive amniotic fluid PCR, IgG and IgM serology, Doppler MCA PSV	Hygiene measures*	Intrauterine transfusion

*Prevention of infection in the mother.
(PCR: polymerase chain reaction; CRS: congenital rubella syndrome; CNS: central nervous system; CMV: cytomegalovirus; MCA: middle cerebral artery; PSV: peak systolic velocity)

based on maternal age, previous birth of a baby with proven Down syndrome, and age of the donor and embryo freezing date in in vitro fertilization (IVF) conceptions. The couple should have pretest counseling to understand that screening tests have false-positive and false-negative rates and the need for further testing if the result is screen positive **(Flowchart 2)**.

Combined first-trimester screening has a detection rate of about 95% for a false-positive rate of 5%. The cutoff value for designating as high risk varies widely among different units (1 in 50 to 1 in 250). The algorithm for testing is depicted in **Flowchart 3**.

Noninvasive prenatal testing (NIPT) with maternal blood samples for cell-free fetal DNA (cf-DNA) has a detection rate of about 99% for a false-positive rate of 1% for trisomy 21. NIPT is an optional first-line investigation for those who are considered high risk. These include advanced maternal age, previous birth with Down syndrome, and maternal balanced translocation. NIPT can be also offered for those with intermediate risk between 1 in 250 and 1 in 1,000. NIPT is a screening test and not a definitive test, and amniocentesis to confirm the finding should be advised prior to any obstetric decision. NIPT is not advised when there is an increased nuchal translucency or a structural anomaly. Fetal fraction of >4% is required for an accurate cff-DNA report. This may be affected by sampling at early gestational age (<10 weeks) and maternal obesity.

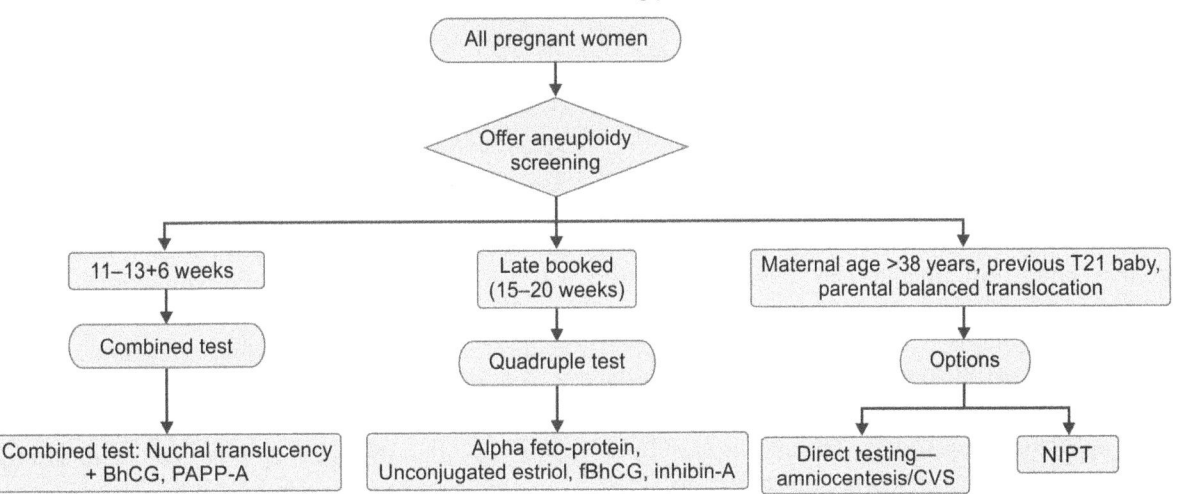

Flowchart 2: Screening protocol.

(CVS: chorion villus sampling; fBhCG: free beta human chorionic gonadotropin; PAPP-A: pregnancy-associated plasma protein A; NIPT: noninvasive prenatal testing)

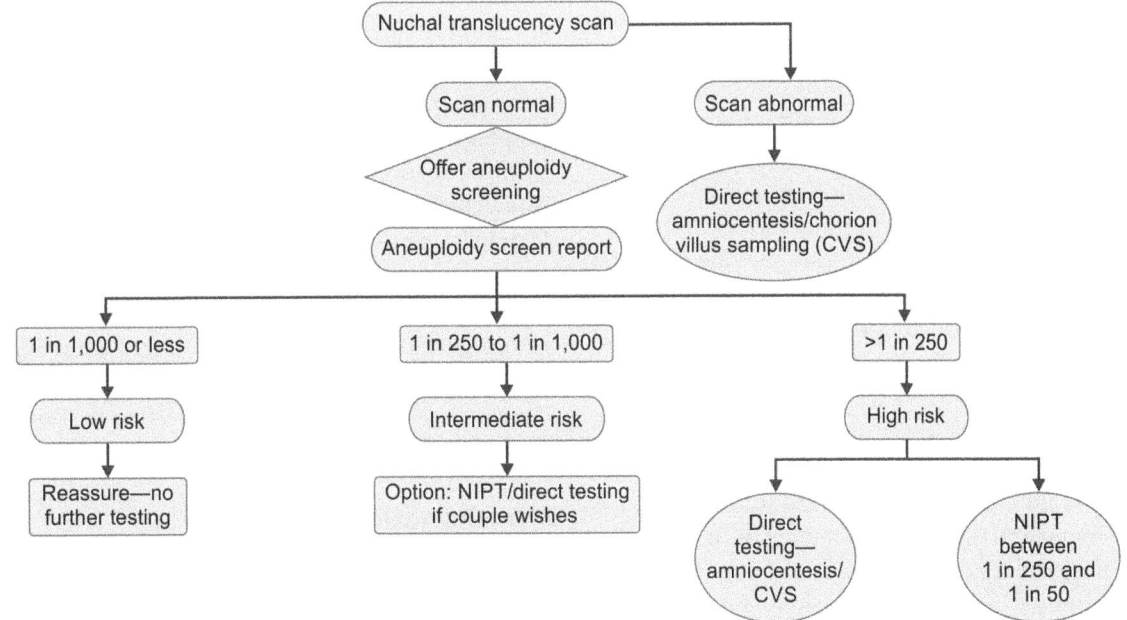

Flowchart 3: Follow-up of screening tests.

(NIPT: noninvasive prenatal testing)

Counseling is required in every step of screening. If the couple wishes to continue pregnancy in case of confirmed chromosomal abnormality, the family should know what extra care is needed for the baby once born.

Fetal Structural Anomalies

Fetal structural anomalies may be diagnosed in 11–13+6 weeks scan or targeted scan at 18–22 weeks. Counseling includes discussion of the lethality of the condition, the prognosis for the fetus, the availability and/or need for prenatal testing for genetic conditions, the need for treatment in utero if any, and the follow-up required for the neonate in various specialties **(Table 5)**.

Direct Testing

Direct testing or prenatal invasive testing includes chorion villus sampling (CVS), amniocentesis, and fetal blood sampling. Parents need to be counseled regarding the risks and benefits of direct testing. Testing is done to find a genetic cause for an anomaly, detect inherited disorder in the fetus, or if a screening test is positive or there are parental balanced chromosomal defects. Knowing the chromosomal or genetic abnormality helps decide regarding continuing the pregnancy and future pregnancies. The risks include loss of pregnancy (approximately 0.5–1%) and rare instances of infection or maternal bowel injury. Informed consent must be obtained and documented. Forms F and G of PCPNDT (preconceptional prenatal diagnostic test) should be obtained and stored for 5 years. The couple should be informed of the possibility of sample not being obtained or laboratory culture failure due to lack of cell growth or contamination.

Chorion villus sampling refers to sampling from the placental villi. This can be done transabdominally or transvaginally. CVS is done between 11 and 13+6 weeks. Sampling prior to this results in pregnancy loss and limb-reduction defects. Prior to genetic testing, the sample undergoes testing for maternal cell contamination (which may occur during sampling). Amniocentesis refers to transabdominal sampling of amniotic fluid using a 22-gauge needle after 16 weeks for diagnostic or therapeutic purposes. Amniocentesis before 15 weeks increases the rate of talipes. All Rh-negative women must be given anti-D prophylaxis after the procedure. Due to the legal implications of termination of pregnancy, the couple should be made aware of the time-bound nature of the test as termination may not be feasible after 24 weeks' gestation. Fetal blood sampling is useful for genetic testing and also for certain conditions where fetal hematological parameters are studied. It carries a loss rate of about 5%. Test results including the abnormality detected if positive result, implications of negative result, possible prognosis, and the recurrence risk should be discussed with the couple in a non-directional manner.

Due to the complex nature of the genetic testing and the additional information which might be obtained by perinatal pathology, storage of DNA is recommended in those who undergo direct testing for a suspected genetic disorder. A geneticist should be involved in counseling.

GENETIC DISORDERS

Chromosomal Disorders

Factors which influence the occurrence of chromosomal abnormality include advanced maternal age, high risk in screening tests, positive NIPT, major structural abnormality detected in the antenatal ultrasound, previous child with trisomy 21, and parents being carriers of balanced translocation. Counseling aspects of various genetic disorders and their risk of recurrence are depicted in **Table 6**. High-resolution karyotyping or chromosomal microarray [preferably single nucleotide polymorphism (SNP) array rather than comparative genomic hybridization (CGH) array] is the investigation of choice **(Table 7)**. While karyotyping typically provides information on the structure and number of chromosomes, microarrays provide additional information of copy number variation (CNV) and loss of heterozygosity. In families with a previous child having Down syndrome, karyotyping of the index child is a mandatory step to identify different etiologies of Down syndrome to decide on the approach **(Flowchart 4)**.

Detection of fetal cardiac anomaly, especially conotruncal anomalies, warrants ruling out DiGeorge syndrome (microdeletion disorder) by fluorescence in situ hybridization (FISH) technique or multiplex ligation-dependent probe amplification (MLPA) or prenatal BACs on beads (BOB) **(Table 7)**, and counseling should be done accordingly.

Single-gene Disorders

Situations where fetal single-gene disorders should be considered include parents with autosomal dominant (AD) disorder, previous child or family members with confirmed single-gene disorder, consanguineous couple with previous child with unknown disorder, and developmental delay **(Flowchart 5)**. Single-gene disorders typically follow the Mendelian inheritance pattern. Single-gene disorder can be autosomal recessive (AR), AD, X-linked recessive (XLR), or X-linked dominant disorder (XLD). Single-gene disorders with higher prevalence such as thalassemia and universal screening of all antenatal women could be carried out by Hb electrophoresis followed by testing in the partner and genetic analysis.

Mitochondrial Disorders

Mitochondrial disorders can be nuclear inheritance (single-gene disorder) or mitochondrial inheritance. Mitochondrial inheritance follows a non-Mendelian

TABLE 5: Congenital malformations.

Anomaly	Parameters	Prenatal care	Follow-up care
Congenital diaphragmatic hernia	• Side • Liver up/down • O/E LHR	Anomaly scan + ECHO *Good prognosis* Left sided Liver-down O/E LHR > 45 • Direct testing • Review scans for growth, polyhydramnios	• Delivery—tertiary care center • NICU • Surgery
Neural tube defects	Open NTD: • Guarded prognosis • Fetal surgery	Option of termination to be discussed with couple	• Folic acid 5 mg OD 3 months prior to conception • First-trimester scan in a fetal medicine unit for subsequent pregnancies
	Closed NTD	Association with chromosomal conditions is low	• Postnatal evaluation and surgery • Prognosis depends on level of lesion
Urinary tract dilation (UTD)	Renal pelvic dilation (UTD)	UTD A1: • 16–27 weeks renal pelvis 4–7 mm • 28 weeks renal pelvis 7–10 mm • No calyceal dilation	UTD A1: • Review at 32 weeks • If normal, no need follow-up • If dilation persists, follow 2–4 weekly depending on severity
		UTD A2/3: • 16–27 weeks renal pelvis >7 mm • 28 weeks renal pelvis >10 mm • Calyceal dilation • Parenchyma abnormal • Dilated ureter or bladder	UTD A2/3: • Review 4 weekly or oftener • Postnatal KUB scan 48 hours after birth, pediatric urologist opinion If single kidney with dilation or bilateral UTD postnatal scan immediately after birth and opinion
	Unilateral multicystic dysplastic kidney (MCDK)	• Follow-up scans 4–6 weekly • Look for UTD, liquor, and fetal growth	Postnatal KUB scan and follow-up
	Unilateral renal agenesis	• Scan to rule out other anomalies, VACTERL association • Direct testing not required	• Good prognosis if isolated • Postnatal KUB scan
	Bilateral renal agenesis or bilateral MCDK	Severe oligohydramnios—potter facies, pulmonary hypoplasia, limb abnormalities	Uniformly poor prognosis—termination may be discussed with couple
	Bladder outlet obstruction	Severe lower urinary tract dilation (LUTO) with anhydramnios	Poor prognosis
		Option of vesicoamniotic shunting	Not recommended at present
		Laser fulguration of posterior urethral valve by fetoscopy	• Available in some centers—may give a good outcome • Postnatal follow-up essential
Unilateral talipes, equinovarus	• Whether isolated • Family history	• Evaluate movement and limbs at 28–32 weeks • Counsel regarding favorable progress	• Pediatric orthopedic opinion • Ponsetti technique • Close follow-up • Favorable outcomes
Bilateral talipes equinovarus	• Whether isolated • Family history	• Direct testing—amniocentesis—microarray • Evaluate movement and limbs at 28–32 weeks • Counsel regarding favorable progress	• Pediatric orthopedic opinion • Ponsetti technique • Close follow up • Favorable-outcomes with proper follow-up and treatment
Cleft lip and palate	Complete scan to confirm it is an isolated finding	Amniocentesis for karyotype and microarray. Abnormal karyotype was found in 4.2% of isolated CL ± P compared to 11.1% in fetuses with complex CL ± P	Multidisciplinary approach with plastic surgery, orthodontist, speech therapist, and ENT teams is required

(KUB: kidneys, ureters, and urinary bladder; LHR: lung-to-head ratio; NICU: neonatal intensive care unit; NTD: neural tube defect; O/E: observed-to-expected; VACTERL: vertebral, anal atresia, cardiac, trachea-esophageal, renal/radial, limb abnormality)

TABLE 6: Counseling guidance on genetic disorders.

	Parental status	Risk of recurrence	Remarks
Chromosomal disorders:			
Chromosomal disorders, e.g., Down syndrome	If pure trisomy 21—no parental karyotype; if unbalanced translocation—parental karyotyping	• Pure trisomy 21 in index: 1% • *Balanced translocation in parents*: 2–10%	If normal variants such as satellite variants detected by karyotyping, parents are reassured
Microdeletion disorders, e.g., Di George syndrome	One of the parents may be affected	• 50% if one parent affected, • <1% if both parents normal	Some of the microdeletion disorders manifest late in pregnancy
*Single-gene/mitochondrial disorders:**			
Autosomal recessive	Parents are usually obligate carriers	25% if parents are carriers	Can be homozygous or compound heterozygous
Autosomal dominant	• One parent may be affected. • If both parents normal—de novo mutation	• 50% if one parent affected • <1% if both parents normal	Features like variable penetrance, skipped generation pose challenge in counseling
X-linked recessive	Mother may be the carrier	• 50% risk of being affected in male fetuses • 50% risk of carrier status in female fetuses	Counseling aspects should be handled sensitively
X-linked dominant	One parent may be affected	• *If father is affected*: Male fetuses not affected and all female fetuses affected • *If mother affected*: 50% risk of being affected in both male and female fetuses	Male-to-male transmission never occurs
Mitochondrial inherited disorders	Usually, the inheritance is from mother	Recurrence risk difficult to predict, both male and female fetuses can be affected	Prenatal diagnosis poses a challenge due to heteroplasmy

*Detected by Sanger sequencing.

TABLE 7: Genetic testing.

Disorder	Diagnostic testing	Indication	Turnaround time (TAT)	Resolution
Chromosomal	Cytogenetics (karyotyping/FISH/Qf PCR)	• High-risk prenatal screening (first-trimester combined/triple/quadruple screening) • NT > 3.5 mm • Structural anomaly suggestive of trisomy	• Karyotyping 14 days • FISH/Qf PCR 2–3 days	>5 Mb
Microdeletion syndrome (known)	• Fluorescent in situ hybridization (FISH)/multiplex ligation probe amplification (MLPA • Prenatal BOB	• Fetal cardiac anomaly (Di George syndrome) • Lissencephaly (Miller–Dieker syndrome) • Structural malformation specific to microdeletion syndromes	*FISH*: 2–5 days *MLPA*: 3–4 weeks	0.1–1 Mb
Copy number variation (CNV)	• Comparative genomic hybridization (CGH) array • Single nucleotide polymorphism (SNP) array	Fetal structural malformation	3 weeks	50–1 kb
Single-gene disorder—gene variant	• Molecular testing • PCR—first generation sequencing/exome sequencing—next-generation sequencing	• Previous sibling affected by single-gene disorder • Specific structural malformation specific to single-gene disorder (e.g., autosomal recessive polycystic kidney disease)	• *PCR*: 2–3 weeks • *Exome sequencing*: 4–6 weeks	0.5–1 kb

(BOB: BACs on beads; PCR: polymerase chain reaction)

Flowchart 4: *Counseling approach:* Index child with Down syndrome.

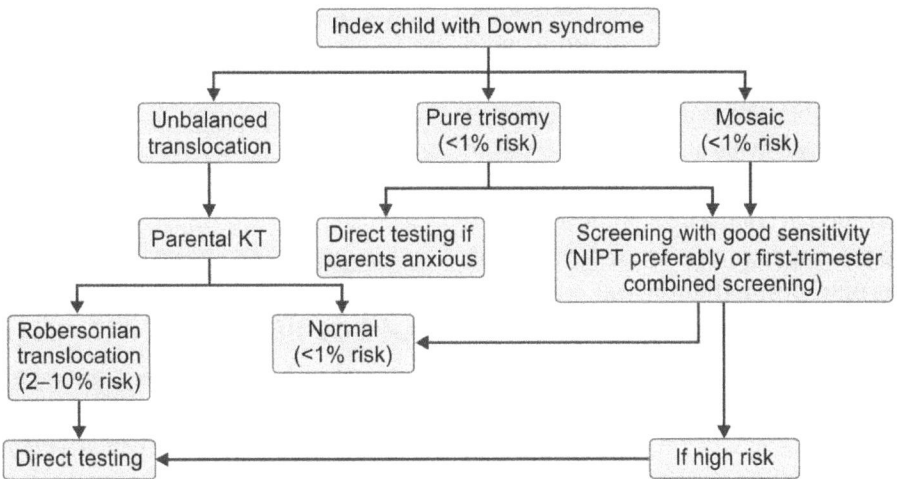

(KT: karyotype; NIPT: noninvasive prenatal testing)

Flowchart 5: Approach to suspected fetal single-gene disorders.

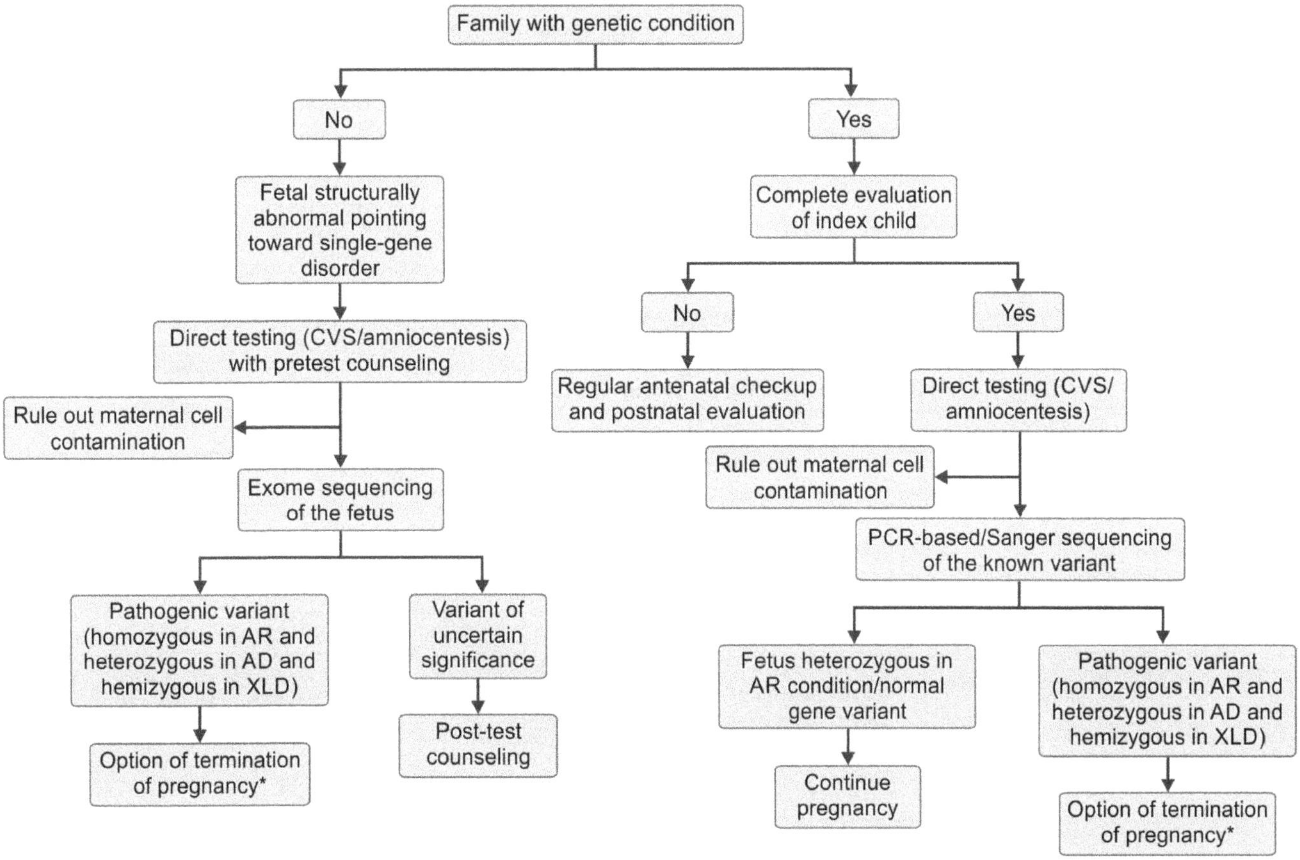

*Termination offered if gestational age ≤ 24 weeks.
(AD: autosomal dominant; AR: autosomal recessive; CVS: chorion villus sampling; XLD: X-linked dominant)

pattern and is inherited only from the mother as the ovum contains the mitochondrial DNA. Both males and females can be affected by the disease. It is difficult to predict accurate recurrence risks. In view of placental heteroplasmy and mosaicism, it is difficult to interpret CVS genetic report which thereby pose a challenge in prenatal diagnosis. IVF with donor oocytes can be given as an option during counseling.

Prenatal Genetic Testing

Prenatal genetic testing is unique in several aspects. In a clinical examination of an index child, clinical genetic testing is undertaken typically with a phenotypic abnormality to plan the management for that individual whereas in a prenatal setting, it is often done to gain information about the fetus with no known phenotype or incompletely defined phenotype due to limitation of prenatal imaging as the fetus may be at an increased risk of a chromosomal or other genetic condition. Another aspect of prenatal genetic testing is to enable the couple to take an informed decision regarding continuation or termination of pregnancy and to plan optimal antenatal, perinatal, and neonatal management. Treatment options during the prenatal period are very limited. Genetic testing results and the subsequent decision not only affect the well-being of the fetus but also that of the parents and extended family members.

Genetic testing in different genetic disorders is summarized in **Table 7**. Both CNV and gene variants are classified according to American College of Medical Genetics (ACMG) as benign, likely benign, variant of uncertain significance (VUS), pathogenic, and likely pathogenic variants. VUS particularly poses a challenge in interpretation and a pre- and post-test counseling is important. Index child evaluation is mandatory for prenatal testing. Prenatal testing should be avoided if the index evaluation shows VUS.

Preimplantation Genetic Testing

Preimplantation genetic diagnosis (PGD) is testing of preimplantation-stage embryos for genetic defects and offered to couples whose fetus is at risk of genetic disorder. PGD requires IVF, embryo biopsy, and either FISH or PCR testing at the single cell level. Parents should be adequately counseled about the limitations of PGD, the higher rate of false positivity and negativity, and the need for prenatal direct testing for confirmation.

ROLE OF PERINATAL PATHOLOGY

Perinatal pathology (autopsy) attempts to provide an answer to perinatal deaths, especially in unexplained still births, and it contributes significantly in >50% of the cases. The workflow of perinatal pathological examination includes fetogram (skeletal survey), clinical photographs, dysmorphology, and histopathological examination. This provides an insight into the mechanism of the events which led to the demise or anomaly which was noted in prenatal scan and gives a better understanding of the pathogenesis of the different conditions. It provides clues to the diagnosis of the condition and helps in deciding further genetic testing which in turn helps to predict the recurrence in the next pregnancy. Considering the limited phenotyping expression during fetal life, it provides information which is complementary to the prenatal scan.

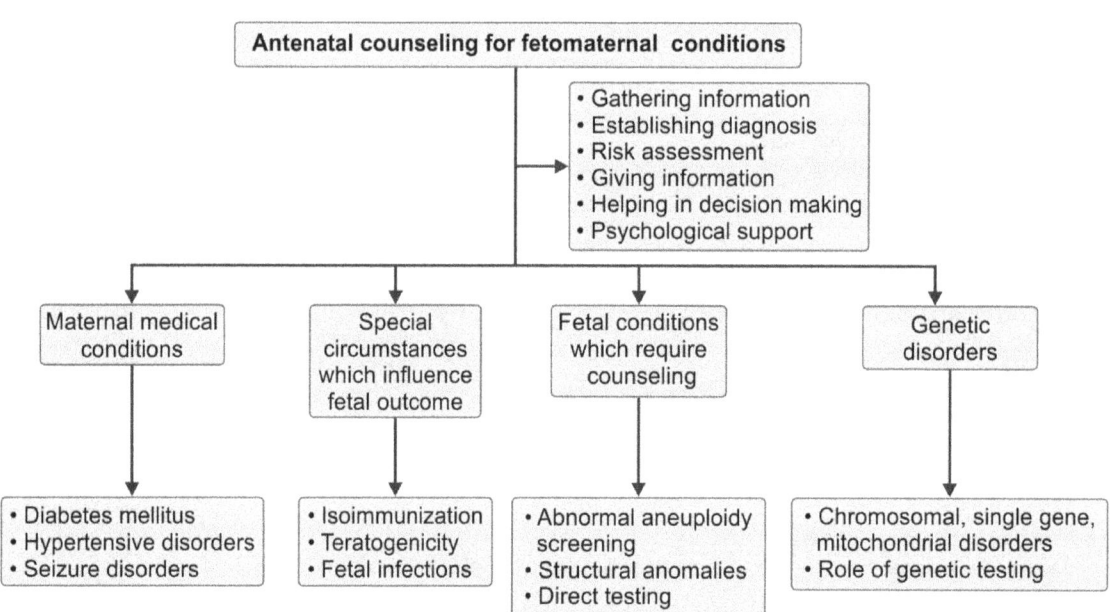

CHAPTER AT A GLANCE

KEY POINTS

- Antenatal diagnosis and counseling improve fetal and neonatal outcomes as care and delivery can be planned in advance.
- Aneuploidy screening should be offered to all women. Detection rates for first-trimester combined screening are up to 95% with false-positive rate of 5% and that for NIPT about 99% with false-positive rate of 1%.
- Antenatal scan showing a fetal anomaly should trigger to evaluate the underlying genetic etiology.
- Factors which influence the occurrence of chromosomal abnormality include advanced maternal age, high risk in screening tests, positive NIPT, major structural abnormality detected in the antenatal ultrasound, previous child with trisomy 21, and parents being carriers of balanced translocation.
- Index child evaluation is mandatory for prenatal testing of single-gene disorders. Genetic testing results and the subsequent decision not only affect the well-being of the fetus but also that of the parents and extended family.
- Perinatal pathology complements the genetic testing in the evaluation of fetal anomaly and unexplained still birth.

SUGGESTED READING

1. Alwan S, Chambers CD. Identifying human teratogens: An update. J Pediatr Genet. 2015;4(2):39–41.
2. American College of Obstetricians and Gynecologists. Preimplantation genetic testing. ACOG Committee Opinion No. 799. Obstet Gynecol. 2020;135:e133-7.
3. American College of Obstetricians and Gynecologists' Committee on Practice Bulletins—Obstetrics; Committee on Genetics; Society for Maternal-Fetal Medicine. Screening for Fetal Chromosomal Abnormalities: ACOG Practice Bulletin, Number 226. Obstet Gynecol. 2020;136(4):e48-e69.
4. Broughton C, Douek I. An overview of the management of diabetes from pre-conception, during pregnancy and in the postnatal period. Clin Med (Lond). 2019;19(5): 399-402.
5. NICE. (2019). Clinical guideline CG62. Antenatal care for uncomplicated pregnancies.
6. NICE. (2019). Hypertension in pregnancy: diagnosis and management. NICE guidelines [NG133]. [online] Available from https://www.nice.org.uk/guidance/ng133/resources/hypertension-in-pregnancy-diagnosis-and-management-pdf-66141717671365 [Last accessed November, 2021].
7. RCOG, Green-top Guideline No. 65. (2014). The management of women with red cell antibodies during pregnancy. [online] Available from https://www.rcog.org.uk/globalassets/documents/guidelines/rbc_gtg65.pdf [Last accessed November, 2021].
8. Rimoin DL, Pyeritz RE, Korf BR. Emery and Rimoin's Principles and Practice of Medical Genetics, 6th edition. Philadelphia: Elsevier; 2013.
9. Tian C, Ali SA, and Weitkamp JH. Congenital infections, Part I: Cytomegalovirus, toxoplasma, rubella, and herpes simplex. NeoReviews. 2010;11(8):e436-46.

SECTION 3
Maternal Medical Illness and Fetal Effects

Arjit Mohapatra, Princee Sahdev

- **Maternal Endocrine Disorders and Fetal Effects**
  K Sankaranarayanan, Lakshmi Shanmugasundaram
- **Anemia in Pregnancy**
  Rhishikesh Thakre
- **Thrombocytopenia in Pregnancy**
  Rhishikesh Thakre, Arjit Mohapatra
- **Autoimmune Disorders in Pregnancy**
  Laxman Basani, Prasanna Latha
- **Teratogenic Exposure**
  Brajagopal Ray, Pradip Goswami
- **Maternal Medications and Substance Abuse**
  Sanjay Wazir, Parul Chopra Buttan
- **Maternal Systemic Medical Illness and Fetal Effect**
  Santosh Kumar Panda, Mohini Sinha

CHAPTER 15

Maternal Endocrine Disorders and Fetal Effects

K Sankaranarayanan, Lakshmi Shanmugasundaram

INTRODUCTION

Several hormonal changes are critical for ovulation and for sustaining pregnancy and subsequently for maintaining lactation. Imbalances in the delicate balance between the various hormones involved in this physiologic state can affect the mother as well as the baby by various mechanisms. Early recognition and management of these conditions can lead to significant improvement in the outcomes.

OBJECTIVES

- To understand the potential effects of maternal endocrine disorders on perinatal outcome and understand their underlying mechanism.
- To understand methods of modifying the adverse impact so as to improve maternal and fetal outcomes.
- Further understanding about the benefits of early screening in preventing complications and improving the health of both the baby and the mother.
- To gain further understanding about the various interventions available to manage pregnancies complicated by endocrine disorders.

MECHANISMS BY WHICH MATERNAL ENDOCRINE ILLNESS CAUSE FETAL EFFECTS

- Endocrine function in the fetus is almost entirely dependent on the mother during the first trimester with the fetus becoming less reliant from the second trimester onward as fetal endocrine glands start production of hormones.
- Any one or combination of the following mechanisms causes the perinatal sequelae. So individualized care is essential:
  - Impact of the endocrine hormone imbalance via the transplacental transfer. For example, fetal hyperthyroidism as a consequence of Graves' disease is due to the autoantibodies transferred from the maternal circulation.
  - The maternal metabolic effects of the endocrine dysfunction. For example, the high blood glucose which is a metabolic effect of gestation diabetes can result in macrosomia and stillbirth and increase maternal infection risk. In diabetes insipidus (DI), electrolyte disturbance if unrecognized can even cause maternal death.
  - Role of associated comorbidities. For example, type 1 diabetes, complicated by nephropathy increases the risk for preterm, preeclampsia, and fetal growth restriction whereas large for gestational age occurs in diabetes without underlying vasculopathy or nephropathy.
  - Effect of medications used in treatment of endocrine dysfunction. For example, cabergoline and thyroxine in the treatment of hyperprolactinemias and hypothyroidism, respectively, are safe options. Hyperthyroidism management with carbimazole can cause embryopathy.

DIABETES IN PREGNANCY

The International Federation of Gynaecology and Obstetrics (FIGO) has recommended the use of the term "hyperglycemia in pregnancy" whether diabetes is known before pregnancy, during pregnancy, or because of the pregnancy **(Table 1)**. This is the new diagnosis of diabetes for the first time during pregnancy. Preexisting diabetes in pregnancy is less common compared to gestational diabetes mellitus (GDM) which affects approximately 7% of all pregnancies.

Gestational Diabetes

The Ministry of Health and Family Welfare, Government of India, recommends universal screening for GDM twice during pregnancy, once at first contact and once between 24 and 28 weeks **(Flowchart 1 and Table 2)**.

In GDM, the Hyperglycemia and Adverse Pregnancy Outcome (HAPO) study showed a clear relation between

TABLE 1: Incidence of hyperglycemia in pregnancy.

Type 1 diabetes	Type 2 diabetes	Gestational diabetes
7.5%	5%	85%

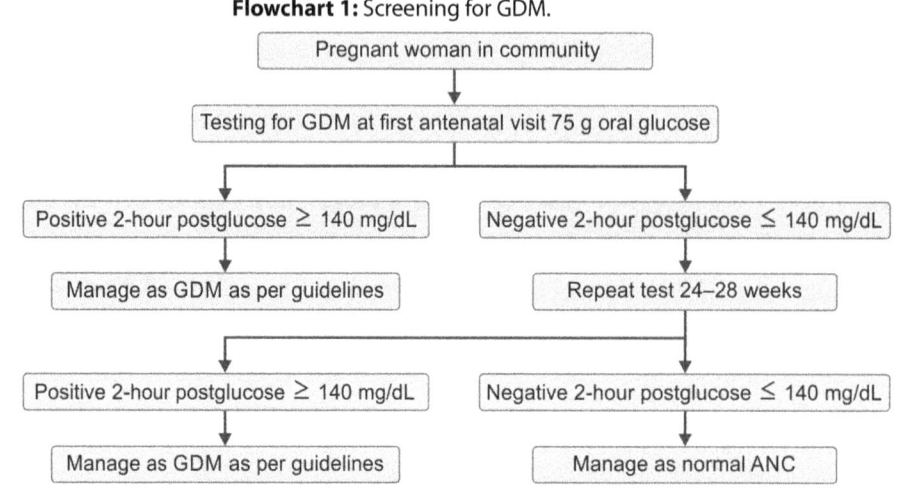

Flowchart 1: Screening for GDM.

(ANC: antenatal care in place of absolute neutrophil count; GDM: gestational diabetes mellitus)

TABLE 2: Complications of a diabetic pregnancy.

Maternal	Fetal	Neonatal
Infections	Congenital anomalies	Hypoglycemia
Preeclampsia	Prematurity	Hypothermia
Retinopathy (in type 1 and type 2 only)	Fetal growth disorders	Polycythemia
Vasculopathy (in type 1 and type 2 only)	Stillbirth	Hyperbilirubinemia,
Nephropathy (in type 1 and type 2 only)	Intrapartum birth trauma and hypoxia	Poor feeding

increasing increments of maternal blood glucose levels and all perinatal complications in GDM. Similar trend is observed in women with preexisting diabetes.

Jensen et al. in their study published in 2009 showed that the risk of congenital malformation was 16% when HbA1C was >10.4% and reduced to background population when the HbA1c levels were below 6.3%. In a large study of 1.2 million singletons published from Sweden, risk of congenital malformations increased with maternal overweight and increasing severity of maternal obesity.

PERINATAL MONITORING

Maternal

For good outcomes, control of diabetes prior to and during pregnancy/periconception is important. Women should be educated to check their blood glucose levels regularly and target fasting blood glucose < 95 mg/dL and 2-hour postprandial < 120 mg/dL. Regular evaluation of blood pressure, symptoms and signs of infections, and end-organ effects of diabetes must be undertaken serially.

Fetal

First-trimester anatomy scan at 12–13 weeks helps with early identification of anomalies, increased nuchal translucency measurement as screening for Down syndrome, congenital cardiac disease, and high resistance uterine artery Doppler for preeclampsia risk. The Federation of Obstetric and Gynaecological Societies of India (FOGSI) also recommends a fetal anatomy scan between 18 and 20 weeks' gestation. Fetal echo is required in women with poor glycemic control and obesity. The recommendations include serial fetal growth scans every 4 weeks from 28 to 30 weeks. Growth scans are necessary to exclude fetal growth disorders and polyhydramnios. Intrapartum continuous fetal heart rate monitoring is required in labor as there is a risk of hypoxia and still birth.

Management

The full description of the treatment of diabetes in pregnancy is beyond the scope of this chapter. We endorse the FOGSI recommendation that the management of the pregnant woman with diabetes should be done by a team comprising an endocrinologist, maternal-fetal medicine specialist, neonatologist, registered dietitian nutritionist, diabetes care, and education specialist nurse.

Prepregnancy

Women with preexisting diabetes ideally will need to have prepregnancy counseling. This allows for full evaluation for complications and gives opportunity to check their medications, optimize dose, and change medications that are not suitable for pregnancy use. This is ideal as it helps to discuss the effects of diabetes, its complications, motivate compliance, and start folic acid 5 mg daily orally. If needed, contraception can be advised if diabetes is poorly controlled until improvement is established for 3 months.

Oral Hypoglycemic Agents

Metformin and glyburide do not cause congenital anomalies in pregnancy despite transplacental transfer. Women on angiotensin converting enzyme (ACE) inhibitors and angiotensin receptor blockers (ARBs) for hypertension need to be switched to safer calcium channel blockers due to the teratogenic effects of ACE inhibitors. There is no clear evidence that maternal use of statins has deleterious effects on the fetus. Although previous studies had suggested a possible harmful effect, a more recent study published in 2014 has suggested no definite evidence of harm from the use of statins during pregnancy. Fibrates are not to be continued during pregnancy.

Medical Nutritional Therapy

For GDM, lifestyle modifications with diet and exercise—medical nutritional therapy (MNT)—is the mainstay in pregnancy. Women should be kept on metformin and/or insulin therapy if MNT fails during pregnancy and aim for optimal 2-hour target value of blood glucose is <120 mg%.

Women with preexisting diabetes usually require insulin but can be managed with metformin if stable levels of blood glucose are maintained.

Timing of Delivery

Elective delivery for preexisting diabetes at 37–38 weeks and uncomplicated GDM at 40 weeks is recommended. If fetal macrosomia exists, then elective cesarean delivery is required. Intrapartum avoidance of hyperglycemia is important to reduce neonatal hypoglycemia, early newborn feeding, and serial blood glucose monitoring is needed.

Postpartum Care

Mothers with GDM can stop treatment at delivery but need long-term surveillance for DM with regular blood glucose tests from 6 weeks postnatal. Babies of diabetic pregnancies are prone to diabetes and obesity.

Mechanism of Neonatal Problems

High maternal blood glucose in the mother has direct effects on the fetal organs. Chronic fetal hypoxia results in stimulation of fetal erythropoiesis resulting in polycythemia which can have several effects including neonatal hyperbilirubinemia. Elevated fetal glucose because of maternal hyperglycemia also leads to fetal hyperinsulinemia which stimulates lipogenesis from glucose. This leads to the fetus becoming macrosomic. Lipogenesis in turn leads to tissue hypoxia which stimulates release of catecholamines leading to hypertension and cardiac muscle hypertrophy.

Neonatal Problems

Neonates born to women with GDM are at increased risk of macrosomia, birth trauma, shoulder dystocia, neonatal respiratory distress syndrome (RDS), and neonatal hyperbilirubinemia. Further, pregnancies of women with GDM are also complicated by preeclampsia which further increase the risk of still birth, fetal hypoxia, and birth asphyxia. Perinatal asphyxia is a risk factor for neonatal hypocalcemia.

Monitoring of neonates born to diabetic mothers: Hence, monitoring of blood sugars, clinical examination for signs of birth trauma, respiratory distress and monitoring for development of complications related to hypocalcemia, polycythemia and being alert to the possibility of significant neonatal jaundice are important factors in the management of the babies born to infants of diabetic mothers.

THYROID DISORDERS (TABLE 3)

Thyroid dysfunction, i.e., hypothyroidism, is the second most common endocrine disorder. An intact hypothalamo-pituitary thyroid (HPT) axis produces about 100 µg of thyroid hormone predominantly as T4 to maintain normal body metabolism. Most of the thyroid hormone is in bound form with 0.04% of T4 and 0.5% of T3 being biologically active. Thyroid dysfunction is more common in those with diabetes.

Iodine is the main substrate for thyroid hormone production and in pregnancy there is an increased loss through kidneys. The WHO recommends daily iodine intake of 250–500 µg/day during pregnancy and breastfeeding. The main source of iodine is iodized salt. In India 70 million are estimated to be iodine deficient. Pregnant women must be advised to take only iodized salt during pregnancy and puerperium. Until 10–12 weeks, fetus depends on maternal thyroxine. Thereafter, fetal thyroid starts functioning and only iodine crosses the placental barrier.

Screening

Currently, risk factor-based screening with thyroid stimulating hormone (TSH), Ft4 is recommended based on living in an area of moderate-to-severe iodine deficiency, obesity, symptoms of hypothyroidism, history of diabetes infertility, recurrent miscarriage, history of goiter, neck radiation, and family history of thyroid disorder **(Tables 4 to 6)**.

Thyroid function test (TFT) analysis must be done following equilibrium dialysis and ultrafiltration to check for the free T4. Target TSH while on treatment is 0.5–2.5 mU/L.

TABLE 3: Incidence of thyroid disorders during pregnancy.

Subclinical hypothyroidism	Overt hypothyroidism	Subclinical hyperthyroidism	Overt hyperthyroidism
4.5%	6.4%	0.8%	0.9%

TABLE 4: Causes of thyroid dysfunction.

Hypothyroidism	Hyperthyroidism
Iodine deficiency	Graves' disease
• Autoimmune thyroid antibody activity (autoimmune thyroid disease) • Hashimoto thyroiditis	Drugs iodine, amiodarone, lithium
Iatrogenic—postradiation, antithyroid drugs, thyroidectomy	• Multinodular goiter • Solitary adenoma
Secondary to pituitary failure	Thyroiditis
Transient—postpartum thyroiditis	

TABLE 5: Normal levels of TSH and FT4.

Normal values	TSH (mU/L)	FT4 (ng/dL)
First trimester	0.1–2.5	0.8–1.2
Second trimester	0.2–3	0.6–1
Third trimester	0.3–3	0.5–0.8
Nonpregnant	0.3–4.3	0.8–1.7

(FT4: free thyroxine; TSH: thyroid-stimulating hormone)

TABLE 6: Effects of thyroid dysfunction on mother, fetus, and newborn.

Clinical manifestation	Maternal effect	Fetal effect	Newborn effect
Hypothyroidism	• Anemia • PIH • CS • Spontaneous abortion • Preterm birth • Abruption	• Fetal distress • IUGR • IUFD	• Congenital hypothyroidism (autoantibodies) • Neurodevelopmental delay • If severe can lead to cretinism
Hyperthyroidism	• Preterm labor • Thyroid storm	• Anomalies related to anti-thyroid drugs • IUGR	• Seizure disorder • ADHD

(ADHD: attention deficit hyperactivity disorder; CS: cesarean section; IUFD: intrauterine fetal death; IUGR: intrauterine growth restriction; PIH: pregnancy-induced hypertension)

Monitoring is needed 4–6 weeks after start of new treatment and check once in each trimester once stable. Antithyroid peroxidase antibodies are noted in 45–52% of hypothyroidism.

Hyperthyroid on medications require frequent monitoring every 4 weeks. In the initial phase of treatment, every 1–2 weeks, TFT should be performed as there is high risk of thyrotoxicosis.

Treatment

New clinical diagnosis in pregnancy of both hypo- and hyperthyroidism is difficult as symptoms overlap with normal pregnancy symptoms.

There is no clear conclusion from studies on benefit of treating subclinical hypothyroidism. But there is an association with miscarriage. Thyroxine sodium must be taken 30 minutes before breakfast, other medications, and caffeine-containing drinks. For those already on thyroid supplement, additional 25 µg may be needed in first trimester to meet the increased demand of pregnancy. Postdelivery dose can be changed back to the prepregnancy dose and TSH repeated at 6 weeks postdelivery.

In hyperthyroidism cases on treatment, stabilization to the lowest possible dose of prepregnancy is vital. Propylthiouracil (PTU) is preferred in pregnancy and restricted to first-trimester use due to hepatotoxicity and agranulocytosis risk. If treatment needed after 16 weeks, then switch to carbimazole. The lowest dose must be given to prevent fetal goiter and hypothyroidism. First-trimester use of methimazole/carbimazole (MMI/CM) causes embryopathy. PTU also has risks of urinary tract anomalies and facial and neck cysts but safer than CM. Hence, first- and second-trimester anomaly screening with ultrasound is essential along with joint care under an endocrinologist. Thiouracil is preferred for breast feeding in the lowest dose with regular maternal thyroid and neonatal developmental monitoring.

Disorders of Bone and Mineral Metabolism during Pregnancy

Changes during Pregnancy

During pregnancy, the pregnant woman' body undergoes several adaptations to meet the requirements of the rapidly growing fetus. 80% of the calcium and phosphorus present in the fetus is transferred during the last trimester.

During pregnancy, parathormone levels are decreased and calcitriol levels are high. PTH-related protein and estradiol are also elevated. Although total serum calcium levels are lower in pregnancy, albumin-corrected calcium and ionized calcium levels are normal.

Vitamin D deficiency: According to the FOGSI, low vitamin D levels are almost universal in pregnant women in India. Low vitamin D levels have several adverse outcomes both for the mother and for the fetus as shown in **Table 7**.

The FOGSI recommends Vitamin D supplementation during pregnancy at a dose of 4,000 IU/day to maintain 25(OH)D levels of at least 40 ng/mL in the mother.

Hyperparathyroidism

According to data from the US, 1% of all parathyroidectomies happen during pregnancy. Due to the expansion of the

TABLE 7: Maternal and fetal effects of vitamin D deficiency.

Stage of vitamin D deficiency	Serum 25 OHD	Maternal adverse events	Fetal adverse events
Severe deficiency	<10 ng/mL	Risk of preeclampsia, poor weight gain during pregnancy, myopathy	SGA, hypocalcemia, seizures, cardiac failure, rickets, enamel defects
Insufficiency	11–32 ng/mL	Bone loss	Neonatal hypocalcemia, infantile rickets
Adequate	32–100 ng/mL	None	None
Excess	>100 ng/mL	Hypercalcemia	Hypercalcemia

(SGA: small-for-gestational-age)

TABLE 8: Other disorders of bone and mineral metabolism and their effects of the fetus.

Disorder	Effects on mother	Effects on fetus
Familial hypocalciuric hypercalcemia	None	• Hypocalcemia and hypocalcemic seizures • If FHH is inherited, severe hypercalcemia
Dietary calcium excess >3 g	Hypercalcemia	Hypocalcemia
Magnesium sulfate	Hypotonia and muscle weakness	Hypotonia, respiratory depression

(FHH: familial hypocalciuric hypercalcemia)

intravascular volume, the diagnosis of hypercalcemia may be delayed. The effects of the hypercalcemia on the fetus include stillbirth, premature birth, miscarriage, and intrauterine growth retardation. The newborn baby is at a risk of hypocalcemia. Mothers must be closely monitored for hypercalcemia, especially during the third trimester. Primary hypoparathyroidism in pregnancy may be treated either medically or surgically. Neonates born to women with hyperparathyroidism should be monitored for neonatal hypocalcemia.

Hypoparathyroidism

According to available data, primary hypothyroidism may improve spontaneously or worsen during pregnancy. Hypoparathyroidism during pregnancy can significantly affect mineralization of the fetal skeleton with the possibility of fractures in utero, at delivery or after delivery. Serum calcium levels are to be monitored every 2–4 weeks. Pregnancy outcomes for the fetus are favorable if mothers have either normal or only slightly elevated serum calcium **(Table 8)**.

PITUITARY DISORDERS

Hyperprolactinemia

Hyperprolactinemia is usually associated with oligomenorrhea and subfertility and commonly drug induced or secondary to adenomas. Prepregnancy exclusion of macroadenoma is important when there is no other obvious cause evident.

Women planning pregnancy respond well to cabergoline and bromocriptine, both of which are safe in early pregnancy. Medications can be discontinued in microprolactinoma but continued for macroprolactinoma, especially if there is no prior surgical treatment/radiation.

Prolactin-producing adenomas are the most common pituitary tumor in pregnancy. There is a 31% risk of tumor growth for untreated macroadenoma in pregnancy compared to 2.6% for microprolactinomas and 1% for treated macroadenoma. Tumor growth is usually preceded by symptoms of headache and visual disturbance.

Intrapartum and postpartum care is the same as for general obstetric population. Course of the disease can improve in about 40% of the women after pregnancy. Prolactin levels should be reassessed only after cessation of breastfeeding. Breastfeeding should be encouraged and is not contraindicated.

Diabetes Insipidus

It is a rare condition. In pregnancy, new diagnosis can be difficult but pregnancy may unmask subclinical DI that preceded pregnancy. 50% of women with preexisting DI will deteriorate in pregnancy and improve following delivery.

Transient self-limiting DI may occur in the third trimester and resolve by 6 weeks postnatal without much clinical impact. Conditions like multiple pregnancy due to the larger placenta and causes of hepatic dysfunction, like PIH and HELLP (hemolysis, elevated liver enzymes, low platelets), can manifest as DI.

Diagnosis: Early detection with serum urea and electrolytes, calcium levels, thyroid function tests, plasma, and urine osmolality is required. If pituitary tumor is suspected, then imaging is necessary.

Complications are rare with three case reports of fetal death and polyhydramnios. Untreated DI may be life-threatening to the mother.

Acromegaly

Acromegaly is a rare condition and is primarily treated by surgery in the nonpregnant state. Prepregnancy planning is vital with cessation of octreotide/pegvisomant and screening for diabetes, hypertension, and cardiomyopathy. During pregnancy medical treatment, if required, dopamine agonist is preferred. There is a risk of fetal growth restriction. Pregnancy requires serial visual field assessment and fetal growth scans.

Pituitary Insufficiency

Diagnosis is based on low TSH, FT4, cortisol, and adrenocorticotropic hormone (ACTH). Magnetic resonance imaging (MRI) can be done if needed.

Causes:
- Postpartum pituitary necrosis
- Lymphocytic hypophysitis
- Tumor/surgery/radiation
- Rarely—pituitary bleed causing fatal apoplexy, as a complication of insulin-dependent diabetes mellitus (IDDM)

Management: L-thyroxine 100–200 µg daily to target mid-range FT4, hydrocortisone 15–25 mg/day. Serial endocrine follow-up. Urgent evaluation required if any acute intracranial signs manifest.

During labor, additional corticosteroids should be given due to the stress of delivery.

ADRENAL PATHOLOGIES IN PREGNANCY AND THEIR EFFECTS ON THE FETUS

Cushing's syndrome is extremely rare in pregnancy but is associated with high risk of maternal mortality. Fetal growth restriction, prematurity, fetal distress, fetal demise, neonatal respiratory distress, and neonatal sepsis are risk factors described following maternal Cushing's syndrome.

Adrenal insufficiency during pregnancy is associated with risk of delivering a premature baby as well as with the risk of delivering a baby who is small for gestational age.

PREGNANCY IN WOMEN WITH OBESITY AND POLYCYSTIC OVARIAN SYNDROME

The National Family Health Surveys in India indicated an increase in obesity from 10.6% in 1998–1999 to 14.8% in 2005–2006 and 20% in 2019–2020. Obesity can also be associated with several endocrine disorders and have further adverse effects on the fetus.

Obesity is associated with increased risk of hypertension, miscarriage, congenital malformations, prematurity, and still birth. Women with obesity are also more likely to have a cesarean delivery and their babies are also more likely to have macrosomia and have birth injuries.

There is also evidence that maternal obesity and nutrition during pregnancy can have long-term effects on the fetus **(Flowchart 2)**.

PREGNANCY IN TRANSGENDER INDIVIDUALS

While it is thought that between 0.3 and 0.5% of the population in the United States are likely to be transgender individuals, one estimate from India puts the number of transgender individuals at 490,000 in 2014. Very few health professionals are equipped to managing pregnancy of transgender individuals. Based on very small numbers, cesarean deliveries were more common in transgender individuals. Complications that were reported also include preterm labor, hypertension, and placental abruption. There are medical, social, and ethical issues to be addressed but limited published literature is available on this.

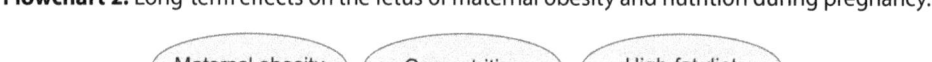
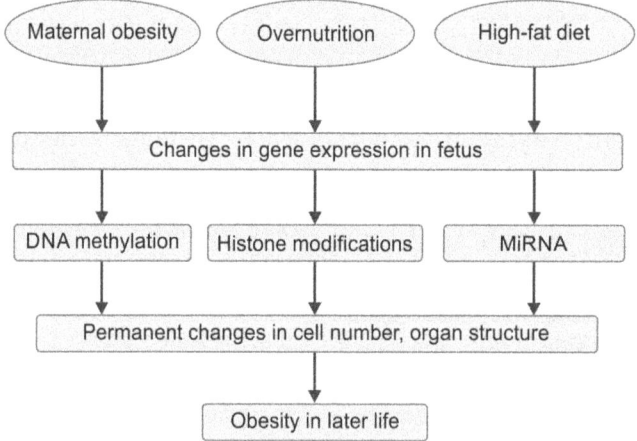

Flowchart 2: Long-term effects on the fetus of maternal obesity and nutrition during pregnancy.

CHAPTER 15 | Maternal Endocrine Disorders and Fetal Effects

Chapter at a Glance

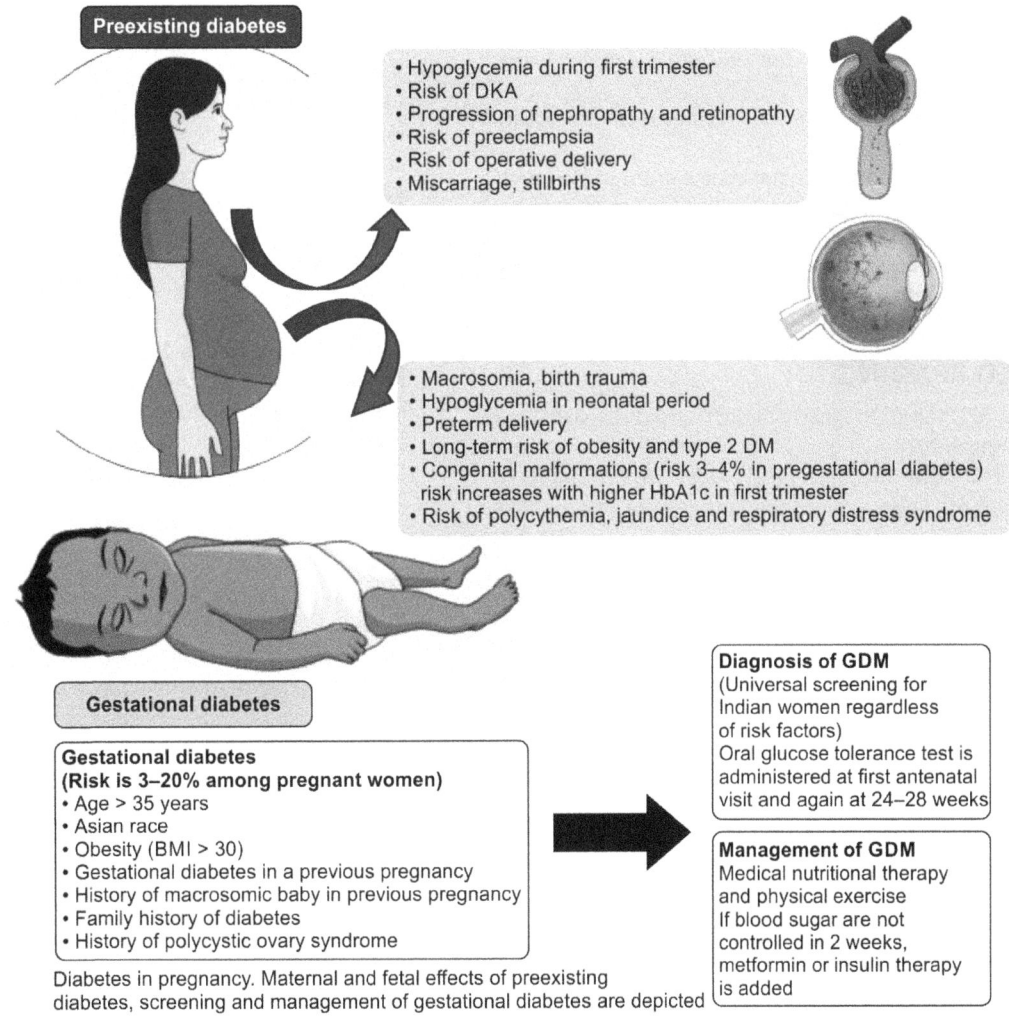

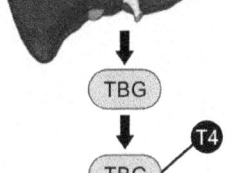

Diabetes in pregnancy. Maternal and fetal effects of preexisting diabetes, screening and management of gestational diabetes are depicted

Implications
- TSH reference levels in pregnancy are lower—use gestational specific cut-offs and not nonpregnant references
- Pregnant and lactating women should have a total daily iodine intake of 250 μg
- For overt hypothyroidism, initiate levothyroxine therapy (1.6–2.0 μg/kg/day)
- Maintain the target TSH levels ≤2.5 mIU/L
- Women with preexisting hypothyroidism may require higher dose of levothyroxine in pregnancy. If thyroid assessment cannot be done immediately increase dose by 30% as soon as pregnancy is diagnosed.

Source: Adapted from Thyroid physiology in pregnancy.
(BMI: body mass index; DKA: diabetic ketoacidosis; GDM: gestational diabetes mellitus; hCG: human chorionic gonadotropin; TBG: thyroxine-binding globulin; TSHR: thyroid-stimulating hormone receptor)

KEY POINTS

- Endocrine disorders in the mother affect the fetus by multiple mechanisms.
- Maternal diabetes and thyroid disorders are the commonest disorders affecting pregnancy.
- Early recognition of these disorders is necessary to avoid significant complications.
- Perinatal interventions to modify the course of these disorders can have significant benefits to the health of the mother baby dyad.
- Obesity is an increasing cause of multiple endocrine problems and can have long term consequences for the fetus.

SUGGESTED READING

1. Aggarwal S, Khan S. Pregnancy and Thyroid disease. New Delhi: Evangel; 2018.
2. Coustan DR, Lowe LP, Metzger BE, Dyer AR, International Association of Diabetes and Pregnancy Study Groups. The Hyperglycemia and Adverse Pregnancy Outcome (HAPO) study: paving the way for new diagnostic criteria for gestational diabetes mellitus. Am J Obstet Gynecol. 2010;202(6):654.e1-6.
3. FOGSI. [online] Available from https://www.fogsi.org/screening-for-gestational-diabetes/[Last accessed November, 2021].
4. Jensen DM, Korsholm L, Ovesen P, Beck-Nielsen H, Moelsted-Pedersen L, Westergaard JG, et al. Peri-conceptional A1C and risk of serious adverse pregnancy outcome in 933 women with type 1 diabetes. Diabetes Care. 2009;32(6):1046-8.
5. Kaur G, Anand T, Bhatnagar N, Kumar A, Jha D, Grover S. Past, present, and future of iodine deficiency disorders in India: need to look outside the blinkers. J Family Med Prim Care. 2017;6(2):182-90.
6. Kovacs CS, Deal C. Maternal-Fetal and Neonatal Endocrinology: Physiology, Pathophysiology, and Clinical Management. Cambridge: Academic Press; 2019.
7. Lakiang T, Daniel SA, Kurian CK, Horo M, Shumayla S, Mehra S. Generating evidence on screening, diagnosis and management of non-communicable diseases during pregnancy; a scoping review of current gap and practice in India with a comparison of Asian context. PLoS One. 2021;16(2):e0244136.
8. Persson M, Cnattingius S, Villamor E, Söderling J, Pasternak B, Stephansson O, et al. Risk of major congenital malformations in relation to maternal overweight and obesity severity: cohort study of 1.2 million singletons. BMJ. 2017;357:j2563.
9. Quigley J, Shelton C, Issa B, Sripada S. Diabetes insipidus in pregnancy. TOG. 2018;1.
10. Şanlı E, Kabaran S. Maternal obesity, maternal overnutrition and fetal programming: effects of epigenetic mechanisms on the development of metabolic disorders. Curr Genomics. 2019;20(6):419-27.

CHAPTER 16

Anemia in Pregnancy

Rhishikesh Thakre

INTRODUCTION

Anemia is a major public health problem in pregnancy. It is multifactorial in origin. Early detection, identification of cause of anemia, and its timely management is integral to optimizing the pregnancy and delivery outcomes. Active surveillance is required for early diagnosis in pregnancy.

OBJECTIVES

- Define anemia in pregnancy and identify the common causes.
- Know the consequences of anemia on maternal, fetal and neonatal health.
- Interpret red blood cell (RBC) indices to type and manage the anemia.
- Prevent and treat maternal iron deficiency.

MAGNITUDE OF THE PROBLEM

Globally, the most common cause for anemia in pregnancy is iron deficiency anemia (IDA). The prevalence of occult iron deficiency in the absence of anemia is estimated to be between 30 and 60% in pregnant women. Anemia is disproportionately concentrated in low socioeconomic group. India ranks at 170th in terms of anemia prevalence in women and accounts for 2.4% of total DALYs (disability adjusted life years) lost for females aged 15–44 years. Anemia contributes partly to 50% of all maternal deaths.

DEFINITION

The World Health Organization defines anemia as hemoglobin level of <11 g/dL antenatally and <10.5 g/dL postnatally **(Table 1)**. Indian Council of Medical Research (ICMR) classifies anemia as normal (11 g/dL or higher), mild (10–10.9 g/dL), moderate (7–10 g/dL), severe (<7 g/dL), and very severe (<4 g/dL).

TABLE 1: Hemoglobin cut off in pregnancy anemia (World Health Organization).

Pregnancy state	Normal range (g/dL)	Mild anemia (g/dL)	Moderate anemia (g/dL)	Severe anemia (g/dL)
1st trimester	≥11	10–10.9	7.9–9	<7
2nd trimester	≥10.5	–	–	–
3rd trimester	≥11	10–10.9	7.9–9	<7

CAUSES OF ANEMIA IN PREGNANCY

Physiologic Anemia

Plasma volume increases by 50% during pregnancy leading to dilution of hemoglobin and hematocrit values causing "pseudo" anemia. It peaks by the second trimester. There is also rise in RBC mass in pregnancy, although to a lesser degree. Anemia leads to decrease in the number of RBCs, and consequently their oxygen-carrying capacity to meet the body's requirement.

Nutritional Anemia

Iron Deficiency Anemia

Physiological iron requirements are three times higher in pregnancy. Age, nutritional status, dietary pattern, prior iron stores, and balance between iron absorption and losses influence the onset and degree of anemia. A recommended daily allowance in pregnancy is nearly 30 mg iron per day. Dietary iron is known to be inadequate to meet the iron requirement in pregnancy. Iron deficiency is the result of long-term negative iron balance **(Fig. 1)**. Majority of iron transfer to the fetus takes place during the second and the third trimester.

Vitamin B_{12} and Folate Deficiency Anemia

Folate deficiency usually results from imbalance between demand in pregnancy and supply from oral intake and leads

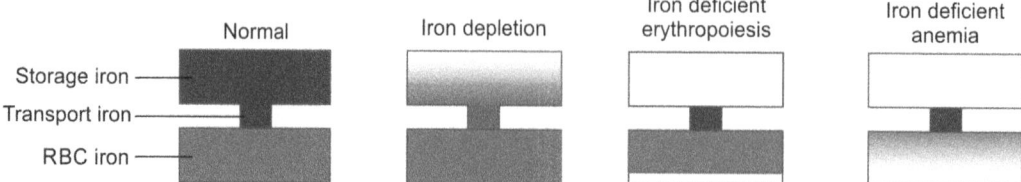

Fig. 1: Evolution of iron deficiency anemia.
(RBC: red blood cell)

to neural tube defects. True vitamin B_{12} deficiency is very rare due to body stores. Absence of meat, poultry, dairy products, and eggs in the diet, presence of gastrectomy, proton pump inhibitors, or malabsorption syndrome may predispose to vitamin B_{12} deficiency. Pernicious anemia is rare and disorder of old age. Growth retardation, hypotonia, and loss of neuromotor skills have been described in infants born to mothers with cobalamin deficiency.

Hemolytic Anemia

Thalassemia is a major hemoglobinopathy resulting in recurrent hemolytic anemia. It is caused due to decreased or negligible amount of globin chain in hemoglobin.

The sickle cell syndromes include sickle cell anemia (HbSS), sickle cell with hemoglobin C disease (HbSC), and hemoglobin S-beta-thalassemia (HbSβ0). There is increased risk of infection, vaso-occlusive painful crises, thrombosis, and maternal mortality as well as higher rates of preterm delivery, preeclampsia, and small for gestational age infants. RBC transfusion may improve maternal and fetal outcomes, but evidence for prophylactic indications is limited. Special attention to hydration is warranted.

Microangiopathic hemolytic anemia (MAHA) is characterized by intravascular mechanical fragmentation of RBCs leading to schistocytes on the peripheral blood film, thrombocytopenia, and organ dysfunction due to varied etiology. Hemolytic anemia, elevated liver enzymes, and low platelets (HELLP) is the most common cause of MAHA in pregnancy. It represents a severe manifestation of preeclampsia. HELLP predominantly is seen during the third trimester. Up to 30% of women may present within 48 hours of delivery.

Autoimmune hemolytic anemia is characterized by RBC destruction and may be secondary to warm [immunoglobulin G (IgG) autoantibodies], cold agglutinin disease, or a mix of warm and cold autoantibodies. Measurements of the fetal middle cerebral artery peak systolic velocity can provide reassurance of the absence of fetal anemia.

Other Causes

Malaria, HIV (human immunodeficiency virus), and tuberculosis are common infective causes of anemia. Advanced stage of HIV infection and antiretroviral use cause anemia. Chronic infection, inflammation and neoplastic disease, and chronic kidney disease contribute to anemia burden. Blood loss during and after delivery can also cause anemia.

> **BOX 1:** Consequences of iron deficiency anemia in pregnancy.
>
> *Antepartum complications:* Increased risk of preterm delivery, inadequate weight gain, premature rupture of membranes, preeclampsia, intrauterine death, intercurrent infection, antepartum hemorrhage, congestive cardiac failure, and maternal death.
>
> *Intrapartum complications:* Prolonged labor, increased rates of operative delivery and induced labor, fetal distress, and abruption.
>
> *Postpartum complications:* Postpartum hemorrhage, puerperal sepsis, lactation failure, pulmonary thromboembolism, and postpartum depression.
>
> *Consequences of iron deficiency anemia in fetus/neonate:* Low birth weight, prematurity, neonatal anemia, impaired cognitive development, autism, and schizophrenia

Consequences of Anemia

It is estimated that maternal anemia contributes to 18% of perinatal mortality and 20% of maternal mortality in South East Asia including India. Risk of maternal death is up to 20% in the peripartum period if the hemoglobin level is <5 g%. The effect of anemia differs based on timing of onset, duration, and severity **(Box 1)**.

CLINICAL FEATURES

Majority of the pregnant women are asymptomatic. Easy fatigability, tiredness, shortness of breath, and poor appetite are common manifestations. Pica may be present. Presence of icterus, splenomegaly, hepatomegaly, consanguinity, need for blood transfusion in the past, family history of blood disorders, petechiae, purpura, or bleeding from any site should alert to possibility of non-nutritional anemia. High blood pressure and pain in right upper abdominal quadrant or epigastric region with or without proteinuria in the third trimester should alert to MAHA. Nonresolution of MAHA postpartum by 3 days or appearance after 7 days of birth with renal or neurological dysfunction should alert to possibility of primary thrombotic microangiopathy (TMA).

TABLE 2: Blood indices to help differentiate microcytic hypochromic anemia.

	Iron deficiency anemia	B thalassemia	Sideroblastic anemia	Acute chronic inflammation
Hb	Decreased	Decreased	Decreased	Decreased
Ferritin	Decreased	Normal or increased		
S iron	Decreased	Normal or increased	Normal or increased	Normal or decreased
Total iron binding capacity	Increased	Normal	Normal	Slightly decreased
Mean corpuscular volume	Decreased	Decreased	Normal	Normal or decreased
Red cell distribution width	Increased	Normal to increased	Increased	Normal
Mentzer index	>13	<13	–	–

TABLE 3: Role of oral iron.

Indication	All pregnant women; postpartum period
Preparation	Ferrous gluconate (35 mg), ferrous sulfate (65 mg), ferrous fumarate (100 mg), and polysaccharide-iron complex (150 mg)
Timing	1 hour before meals on an empty stomach, with a glass of orange juice or other form of vitamin C
Response	Rise in Hb by 2 g% over 4 weeks in the absence of ongoing losses or increasing demand
Dose	See **Table 4**
Duration	• Starting after the first trimester, at 14–16 weeks of gestation • To be repeated for 100 days postpartum
Side effect	Nausea, gastric irritation, constipation, diarrhea, and metallic taste
Frequency	Weekly or daily is equally effective
Diet	Green leafy vegetables, whole pulses, jaggery, meat, poultry and fish, fruits and black gram, groundnuts, ragi, whole grains, milk, eggs, meat and nuts, etc.
Tip	• Ferric salts (III) have a superior GI tolerability • Ensure and emphasize compliance • Avoid enteric or sustained released preparation • Avoid with tea, coffee, legumes, nuts, and milk products • No superiority of one iron preparation over the other

(GI: gastrointestinal tract; Hb: hemoglobin)

TABLE 4: Ministry of Health and Family Welfare (MoHFW) recommendations.

	Prophylaxis	Treatment
During pregnancy	Daily 100 mg iron + 500 µg folic acid—for 100 days starting after the first trimester, at 14–16 weeks of gestation	*Mild anemia*: 2 IFA tablets/day—100 days *Moderate anemia*: IM iron therapy + oral folic acid
Postpartum	Daily 100 mg iron + 500 µg folic acid—6 months	

(IFA: iron and folic acid; IM: intramuscular)

INVESTIGATIONS

A complete blood count at 12 and 28 weeks' gestation is indicated in all pregnant women. Pregnant patients with nonresponsive IDA and of ethnic origins where thalassemia occurs, who have a microcytic hypochromic anemia, should be screened for hemoglobinopathy. Peripheral blood smear provides clue to type of anemia. Blood indices help differentiate microcytic hypochromic anemia **(Table 2)**. Up to 40% of pregnant women with true IDA have normocytic indices. Serum ferritin (<30 ng/mL) is the most sensitive and specific marker for iron deficiency than other iron indices. Serum folic acid concentrations <2 ng/mL are diagnostic of folic acid deficiency, whereas levels >4 ng/mL effectively rule out deficiency. Low cobalamin in pregnancy may not reflect true tissue deficiency.

After delivery, hemoglobin should be measured within 24–48 hours in persons with blood loss >500 mL and in those with uncorrected anemia detected during pregnancy.

DELIVERY OPTIONS

The mode of delivery, timing, and anesthesia is based on obstetric condition.

TABLE 5: Role of intravenous iron.

Indication	Absolute intolerance to oral iron, poor compliance to oral therapy, severe anemia in late pregnancy, iron deficiency in patients with inflammatory bowel disease, and patients on renal dialysis
Preparation	FCM, 50 mg elemental iron/mL
Test dose	Not required
Contraindication	First trimester or if there has been a severe or anaphylactic reaction to parenteral iron, iron overload condition
Dose	[2.4 × (target Hb-actual Hb) × pre-pregnancy weight (kg)] + 1,000 mg for replenishment of stores
Max dose	• Two doses of 750 mg, given 7 or more days apart (weight < 50 kg) • Two doses of 15 mg/kg (or 1,000 mg) given 7 or more days apart if weight >50 kg
Infusion time	15 minutes
Side effect	Itching, fever, lymphadenopathy, arthralgia, headache, malaise, and anaphylaxis
Prerequisite	Monitoring and resuscitation facility

(FCM: ferric carboxymaltose; Hb: hemoglobin)

BOX 2: Indication of packed cell transfusion.

Pregnancy <34 weeks:
- Hb < 5 g/dL with or without signs of cardiac failure or hypoxia
- Hb 5–7 g/dL – in presence of impending heart failure

Pregnancy >34 weeks:
- Hb < 7 g/dL even without signs of cardiac failure or hypoxia
- Severe anemia with decompensation

Acute hemorrhage:
- Always indicated if Hb < 6 g/dL
- Clinically unstable due to ongoing hemorrhage

Intrapartum period: Hb < 7 g/dL (in labor)

Postpartum period: Anemia with signs of shock/acute hemorrhage with signs of hemodynamic instability

Side effect: Circulatory overload, transfusion reactions, sensitization to antigens posing a risk of fetal hemolytic disease in a future pregnancy, and incompatible transfusions

(Hb: hemoglobin)

MANAGEMENT

A trial of oral iron in patients who are asymptomatic, with Hb concentration <11 g% in the first trimester and <10 g% in the second trimester is indicated (with a normocytic or microcytic anemia in the absence of a hemoglobinopathy). Oral iron is the first line of therapy **(Tables 3 and 4)** followed by parenteral iron **(Table 5)**. Blood transfusion is recommended in certain situations **(Box 2)**. Management is tailored according to the etiology, period of gestation, and severity of anemia **(Table 6)**.

PREVENTION

A healthy wholesome diet is essential in preventing anemia. Three servings a day of foods rich in iron, folic acid, and vitamin B_{12} is recommended in the diet. Foods that are high in vitamin C also help in the intake of iron from the gut. All healthy pregnant women are advised a prenatal multivitamin and mineral supplement containing 100 mg of elemental iron/day along with 500 μg of folic acid to achieve daily iron requirements. All mothers with sickle cell disease are started on 5 mg of folic acid daily.

TABLE 6: Definitive treatment of anemia in pregnancy.

Iron deficiency	Oral or parenteral iron, RBC transfusion, and diet
Folate deficiency	Folic acid supplementation
Vitamin B_{12} deficiency	Cobalamin supplementation
Sickle cell disease	Hydration, folic acid, RBC transfusion, and analgesia
Thalassemia	Folic acid, blood transfusion, and deferoxamine
Chronic renal failure	Erythropoietin
Autoimmune	Corticosteroids, IVIG, and RBC transfusion
Malaria	Antimalarial and blood transfusion

(IVIG: intravenous immunoglobulin; RBC: red blood cell)

Iron Supplementation

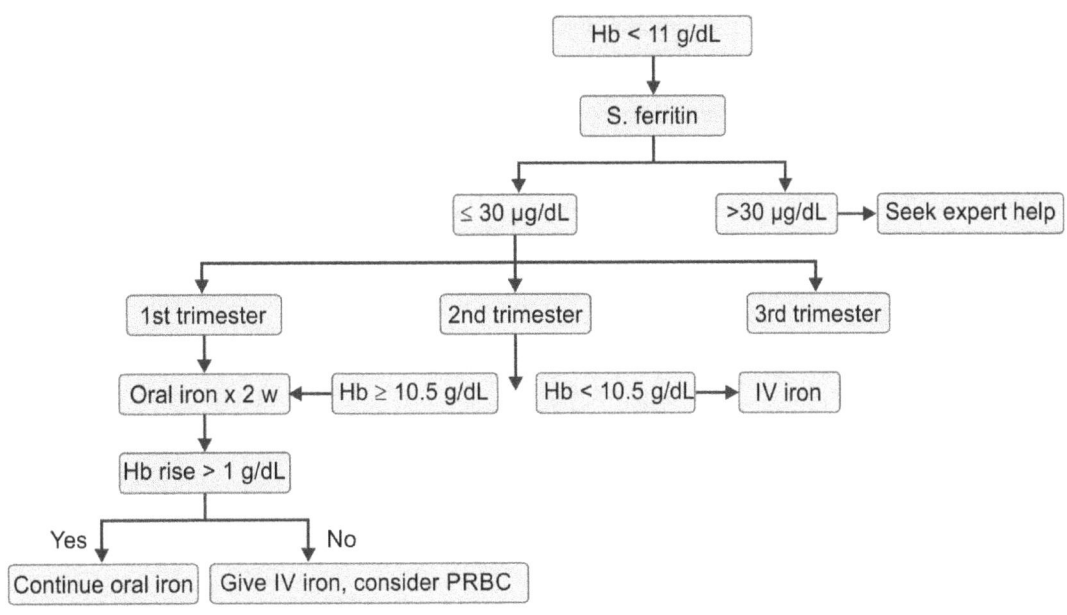

(Hb: hemoglobin; IV: intrvenous; PRBC: packed red blood cells)

CHAPTER AT A GLANCE

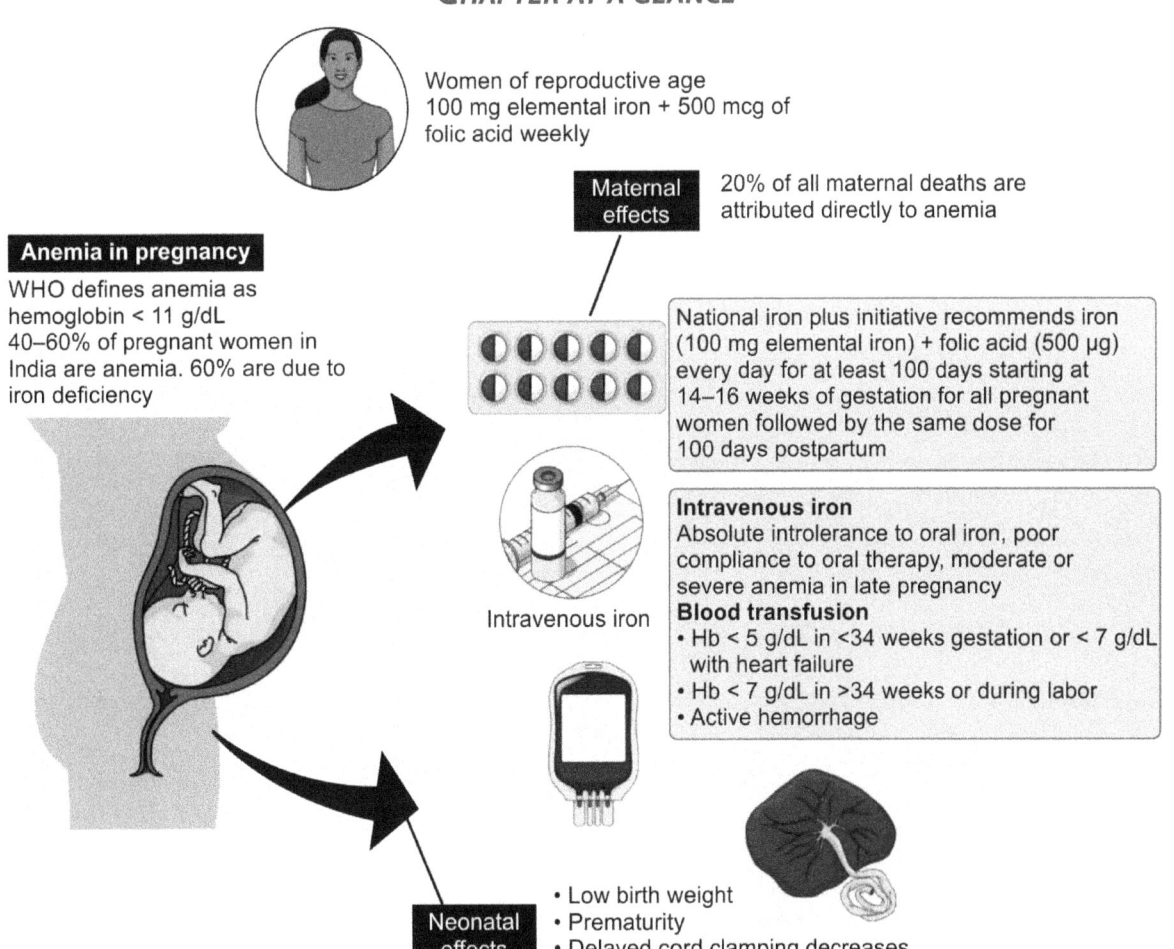

KEY POINTS

- Maternal anemia is common and is most commonly due to physiologic changes during pregnancy affecting the hematological parameters.
- Prompt detection and treatment of anemia is essential to prevent avoidable serious sequelae to mother and the fetus.
- Management is directed to the underlying cause. Oral iron is the preferred first-line therapy for most patients with iron deficiency anaemia.
- Prevention and control of anaemia is one of the key strategies to for reducing maternal, neonatal and childhood mortality and improving maternal, adolescent and childhood health status.

SUGGESTED READING

1. Achebe MM, Gafter-Gvili A. How I treat anemia in pregnancy: iron, cobalamin, and folate. Blood. 2017;129(8):940-9.
2. Sun D, McLeod A, Gandhi S, Malinowski AK, Shehata N. Anemia in Pregnancy: A Pragmatic Approach. Obstet Gynecol Surv. 2017;72(12):730-7.
3. Tandon R, Jain A, Malhotra P. Management of iron deficiency anemia in pregnancy in India. Indian J Hematol Blood Transfus. 2018;34(2):204-15.
4. Tran K, McCormack S. Screening and treatment of obstetric anemia: A review of clinical effectiveness, cost-effectiveness, and guidelines. Ottawa (ON): Canadian Agency for Drugs and Technologies in Health; 2019.

CHAPTER 17

Thrombocytopenia in Pregnancy

Rhishikesh Thakre, Arjit Mohapatra

INTRODUCTION

Thrombocytopenia is a common hematological disorder in pregnancy. It may be of varied etiology arising from pregnancy itself or secondary to a systemic disorder. The evaluation of thrombocytopenia helps to rule out any underlying systemic disorders which could adversely affect the outcome of the fetus. A thorough understanding of the pathophysiology, timing of onset, etiology, and severity is important in this regard.

OBJECTIVES

- Know the common causes of maternal thrombocytopenia
- Know the principles of treatment
- Know the impact on the fetus

DEFINITION

Thrombocytopenia is defined as a platelet count of $<150 \times 10^9/L$. It is classified as mild ($100-150 \times 10^9/L$), moderate ($500-100 \times 10^9/L$), and severe thrombocytopenia ($<500 \times 10^9/L$).

MAGNITUDE OF THE PROBLEM

Thrombocytopenia occurs in about 10% of all pregnancies. However severe thrombocytopenia occurs in <1% of pregnancies.

ETIOLOGY

Gestational thrombocytopenia is the most common cause of thrombocytopenia in pregnancy (75%), followed by preeclampsia (PEC) (20%), and immune thrombocytopenia (ITP) (up to 4%). The etiology varies with gestation **(Box 1)**.

PATHOPHYSIOLOGY (TABLES 1 AND 2)

Gestational thrombocytopenia is the most common cause of low platelets in the third trimester of pregnancy. It is thought to arise secondary to dilution from expanded plasma volume. It is self-limiting in nature and subsides 4–8 weeks

BOX 1: Causes of thrombocytopenia in pregnancy.

First trimester: ITP, hereditary thrombocytopenia (HT), and thrombotic microangiopathy (TMA)

Second trimester:
Platelet count $>100 \times 10/L$: Gestational thrombocytopenia, ITP, preeclampsia, HELLP, HT, and TMA
Platelet count $<100 \times 10/L$: ITP, HT, preeclampsia/HELLP, gestational thrombocytopenia, and TMA

Third trimester:
Platelet count $>100 \times 10/L$: Gestational thrombocytopenia, preeclampsia/HELLP, TMA, ITP, and HT
Platelet count $<50 \times 10/L$: Preeclampsia/HELLP, ITP, TMA, gestational thrombocytopenia, HT, and acute fatty liver

Other causes: Disseminated intravascular coagulation (DIC), bone marrow failure, antiphospholipid antibody syndrome, autoimmune conditions, type II Von Willebrand, infections (e.g., HIV, hepatitis C virus, *Cytomegaloviru*, *Helicobacter pylori*), drug-induced thrombocytopenia [e.g., heparins, thiazides, antimicrobials (ampicillin and rifampin), anticonvulsants (phenytoin and sodium valproate), digoxin, cimetidine, ranitidine, aspirin, indomethacin, etc.] and congenital thrombocytopenia

(HELLP: hemolysis, elevated liver enzymes, low platelet count; HIV: human immunodeficiency virus; ITP: immune thrombocytopenia)

postdelivery. It classically occurs in the third trimester, platelet counts rarely drop below $75 \times 10^9/L$, may recur in pregnancy, and remains a diagnosis of exclusion.

Preeclampsia with new-onset thrombocytopenia is associated with a state of platelet consumption and platelet activation. Thrombocytopenia resolves by urgent delivery and resolves by 2–6 days postpartum.

Immune thrombocytopenia is the most common cause of low platelets in the first trimester of pregnancy. It is predominantly an antibody-mediated disease but may also be secondary to malfunctioning T-cells or antigen-presenting cells. ITP may be primary with no cause and systemic findings or secondary where it may be associated with autoimmune disorders viz. systemic lupus erythematosus (SLE), rheumatoid arthritis (RA), scleroderma, antiphospholipid antibody syndrome (APLS), etc. It may be acute, persistent (duration of 3–12 months), and chronic (duration of 12 months or more). Maternal antibodies cross the placenta placing the fetus/newborn at risk for bleeding. Studies have identified several polymorphic, diallelic antigen systems that reside on platelet membrane glycoproteins to be responsible for fetal–neonatal alloimmune thrombocytopenia. The recurrence risk is related to paternal zygosity.

Thrombotic microangiopathy (TMA) is characterized by triad of microangiopathic hemolytic anemia (MAHA), thrombocytopenia, and organ injury. There is microscopic vascular damage with thrombosis. It may be associated with pregnancy-related condition viz. PEC, HELLP (hemolysis, elevated liver enzymes, low platelets) syndrome, and acute fatty liver of pregnancy (AFLP) or nonpregnancy-related conditions as thrombotic thrombocytopenic purpura (TTP), and atypical hemolytic-uremic syndrome (HUS). These are rare conditions. TTP is thought to be related to absence or inhibition of ADAMTS-13. Mutation in the function or expression of proteins controlling the alternative pathway C3 convertase leads to HUS.

Disseminated intravascular coagulation (DIC) is an imbalance between pro- and anticoagulant pathway and fibrinolytic system. It may be due to direct consequence of an obstetric complication [e.g., postpartum hemorrhage (PPH) and amniotic fluid embolism] or secondary to other pregnancy-related complications (PEC, HELLP, AFLP, etc.).

CLINICAL EVALUATION

The most common manifestations of thrombocytopenia are petechiae, ecchymosis, epistaxis, gingival bleeding, and abnormal uterine bleeding (either heavy or intermenstrual). Joint involvement is rare. It may be incidentally detected on blood count in an otherwise well patient. Clinically significant bleeding usually is rare and occurs in patients with very low platelet levels undergoing surgery. Presence of pallor, icterus, bleeding tendency, high blood pressure, chronic history, and organomegaly should alert to a systemic cause. There may be lag between appearance of thrombocytopenia and hypertension. Unexplained fetal or neonatal thrombocytopenia, hemorrhage, or ultrasonographic findings consistent with intracranial bleeding should raise suspicion of fetal neonatal alloimmune thrombocytopenia.

TABLE 1: Pathophysiolgy.

	Gestational thrombocytopenia	ITP
Onset	Mid late 2nd or 3rd trimester	Any time
Platelet count	$>80 \times 10^9$/L	$<100 \times 10^9$/L and progressive
Beyond pregnancy	Resolves	May be persistent
Neonatal affection	No	Possible

(ITP: immune thrombocytopenia)

TABLE 2: Pathophysiolgy.

	Preeclampsia	HELLP	AFLP	aHUS	TTP
Onset	Third trimester	Third trimester	Third trimester	Postpartum	Second to third trimester
Symptoms/signs					
Vomiting	+	+	++	+/−	+/−
Abdominal pain	+/−	++	++	+/−	+/−
Jaundice	+/−	+/−	++	+/−	+/−
CNS symptoms	+	+	+	+/−	++
High BP	+++	+++	+	++	+
Laboratories					
Proteinuria	+++	+++	+	++	+
Thrombocytopenia	+	+++	+	+++	+++
Hemolysis	+/−	+++	+	+++	+++
High bilirubin	+/−	+++	+++	+++	+++
High AST	+	+++	+++	+/−	+/−
High ammonia	+/−	+/−	+	+/−	+/−
Hypoglycemia	+/−	+/−	+++	+/−	+/−

[+/−: rare or absent (0–20% of cases); +: fairly common (20–50% of cases); ++: common (50–80% of cases); +++: very common (80–100% of cases); AFLP: acute fatty liver of pregnancy; aHUS: atypical hemolytic uremic syndrome; AST: aspartate aminotransferase; BP: blood pressure CNS: central nervous system; HELLP: hemolysis, elevated liver enzymes, low platelet count; TTP: thrombotic thrombocytopenic purpura]

IMPACT ON FETUS/NEWBORN

Gestational thrombocytopenia poses no risk of maternal or fetal hemorrhage or bleeding complications. Prematurity and fetal growth restriction is associated with an increased likelihood of neonatal thrombocytopenia (1.8%) independent of maternal platelet count in PEC. Studies show no relationship between maternal platelet count at delivery and infant platelet count at birth in cases of ITP. The nadir in platelet count for newborn takes place within 2 weeks after birth. Studies indicate medical therapies such as intravenous immunoglobulin (IVIG) and corticosteroids do not reliably prevent fetal thrombocytopenia or improve fetal outcome. There are no maternal test or clinical characteristics can reliably predict the severity of thrombocytopenia in infants born to mother with ITP. There has been no affection of TTP in infant born to mother with TTP. Delivery is necessary if there is no response to plasma therapy in TTP or for obstetric indications.

LABORATORY EVALUATION (BOX 2)

Complete blood count (CBC) helps rule out pancytopenia or bicytopenia. Peripheral smear confirms thrombocytopenia and rules out "clumping" suggestive of pseudothrombocytopenia. Bone marrow biopsy is rarely needed in pregnancy. Antiplatelet antibodies or platelet associated antibody assay are not routinely recommended. Repeat platelet count is done at each prenatal visit, 1-3 months postdelivery, and on clinical judgment. Human platelet antigen (HPA) type and zygosity of both parents, confirmation of maternal antiplatelet antibodies with specificity for paternal (or fetal-neonatal) platelets, and the incompatible antigen are indicated in suspected fetal neonatal alloimmune thrombocytopenia.

MODE OF DELIVERY

In gestational thrombocytopenia, the risk of bleeding to the mother and fetus is negligible. The decision is based on obstetric condition and not on platelet count. With thrombocytopenia associated with PEC/HELLP syndrome, delivery is recommended with severe features at or beyond 34 weeks of gestation, after maternal stabilization or with labor or rupture of membranes. The mode of delivery before 34 weeks is based on obstetric condition. For cesarean delivery, a platelet count of >50 × 10^9/L is desirable. The rate of intracranial hemorrhage is <1% in fetus born to mother with ITP. Use of fetal scalp electrodes or operative vacuum delivery should be avoided.

SPECIFIC TREATMENT

Thrombocytopenia associated with PEC or HELLP syndrome is treated by expediting delivery. Platelet transfusions are best reserved for patients with thrombocytopenia with active bleeding. Treatment with corticosteroids or uterine curettage has no effect on maternal morbidity or mortality.

Immune thrombocytopenia in pregnancy is best managed based on clinical status rather than platelet count. Treatment should be initiated when the patient has symptomatic bleeding, when platelet counts fall below 30 × 10^9/L, platelet count <50 × 10^9/L if cesarean section or count <70 × 10^9/L with epidural anesthesia. Prednisone (10-20 mg/day) is the standard initial treatment. It is individualized to a dose that raises the platelet count. Response is seen by 4-14 days and tapering is done after 21 days to lowermost dose that prevents major bleeding. IVIG (1 g/kg) is used for nonresponse to steroids, rapid fall in platelets or a more rapid rise in platelets is required. The response occurs in 1-3 days. Hematology consult guides further care.

Maternal treatment with IVIG with or without corticosteroids is indicated in fetal-neonatal alloimmune thrombocytopenia as it is associated with higher frequency of intracranial hemorrhage **(Box 3)**.

Thrombotic thrombocytopenic purpura/hemolytic-uremic syndrome management merits early plasma therapy (10-15 mL/kg) until the platelet count is >150 × 10^9/L for at least 3 days and serum lactate dehydrogenase (LDH) concentrations have returned to near normal levels. Serial fetal monitoring with uterine artery Dopplers is indicated. Prophylactic plasma exchange treatment is indicated if ADAMTS13 activity falls below <10% or the peripheral smear shows unequivocal red cell fragmentation.

BOX 2: Laboratory evaluation for maternal thrombocytopenia.

For all: Complete blood count, blood smear, retic count, liver function test, renal function test, B sugar, urine proteins, and direct antiglobulin test

First tier: HIV, HBV, HBC, antinuclear antibody, and antiphospholipid antibodies

Second tier: VWF activity (VWF:RCo) and antigen, ristocetin-induced platelet aggregation, and multimeric analysis of VWF

(HBV: hepatitis B virus; HBC: hepatitis C virus; HIV: human immunodeficiency virus; VWF: von Willebrand Factor)

BOX 3: Care of the newborn born to immune thrombocytopenia mother.

- Collect umbilical cord blood for platelet count. If normal, do not repeat, follow clinically
- If low platelet, repeat count daily. Expect drop in platelet by days 2–5
- If platelet <30 × 10^9/L or active bleeding, administer platelets and intravenous immunoglobulin (IVIG) (1 g/kg × 2 days)
- If platelet 30–50 × 10^9/L, administer IVIG only
- Avoid heel pricks as clotting may cause pseudothrombocytopenia
- Administer vitamin K once the platelet count is normal

CHAPTER AT A GLANCE

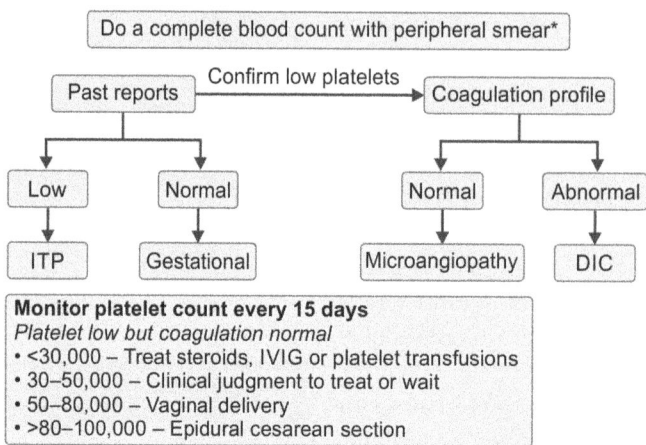

*If bicytopenia or pancytopenia or bleeding tendency seek expert help

(DIC: disseminated intravascular coagulation; IVIG: intravenous immunoglobulin; ITP: immune thrombocytopenia)

KEY POINTS

- Gestational thrombocytopenia is the most common cause of low platelets in third trimester and immune thrombocytopenia most common in first trimester of pregnancy.
- The decision making is based on clinical status and underlying cause rather than the platelet count in isolation.
- Treatment is directed towards the underlying cause.
- All infants born to mothers with immune thrombocytopenia should have cord blood platelet count done and if normal should be followed clinically. Anticipate drop in platelet count between 2 and 5 days but treat based on clinical status.

SUGGESTED READING

1. ACOG Practice Bulletin No. 207: Thrombocytopenia in Pregnancy. Obstet Gynecol. 2019;133(3):e181-93.
2. Fogerty AE. Thrombocytopenia in pregnancy: mechanisms and management. Transfus Med Rev. 2018;32(4):225-9.
3. Jodkowska A, Martynowicz H, Kaczmarek-Wdowiak B, Mazur G. Thrombocytopenia in pregnancy – pathogenesis and diagnostic approach. Postepy Hig Med Dosw. 2015;69:1215-21.
4. Stavrou E, McCrae KR. Immune thrombocytopenia in pregnancy. Hematol Oncol Clin North Am. 2009; 23(6):1299-316.

CHAPTER 18

Autoimmune Disorders in Pregnancy

Laxman Basani, Prasanna Latha

INTRODUCTION

Autoimmune disorders are characterized by tissue damage caused by antibodies and T cell-derived cytokines. Women are affected more often due to X chromosome characteristics, hormonal, and genetic factors.

During pregnancy Th2, Th17/Th2, and Treg cells from the decidua influence autoimmune diseases. Th1- and Th17-type autoimmune disorders improve in pregnancy [e.g., rheumatoid arthritis (RA), Graves' disease (GD) and multiple sclerosis] whereas Th2-type disorders worsen [e.g., systemic lupus erythematosus (SLE), Sjögren syndrome (SS)]. In the postpartum period, Th1- and Th17-type disorders might flare up, whereas Th2-type disorders could improve **(Fig. 1)**.

Fetal microchimerism is caused by fetal cells acquired by the mother during pregnancy. Maternal microchimerism acquired by the infant during pregnancy can cause type I diabetes.

OBJECTIVES

- To study pathophysiology of autoimmune disorders in pregnancy.
- Planned pregnancy and pre-pregnancy counseling prevents complications.
- To discuss the maternal management of the common autoimmune disorders in pregnancy.
- Multidisciplinary management ensures the best possible maternal and neonatal outcome.

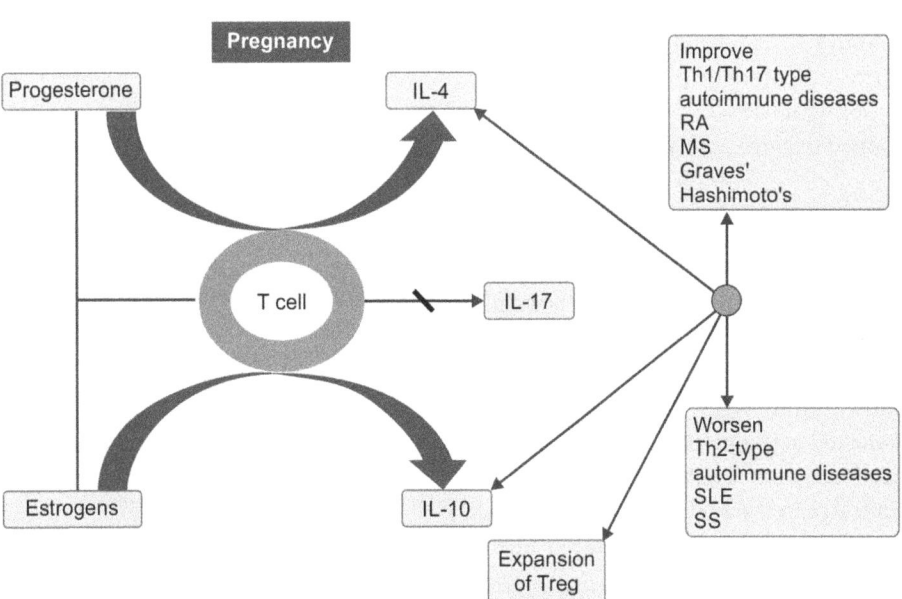

Fig. 1: Hormone-controlled T-cell responses influence the progression of autoimmune diseases.
Source: Adapted from Piccinni MP, Lombardelli L, Federica Logiodice F, Ornela Kullolli O, Paola Parronchi P, Sergio Romagnani S. How pregnancy can affect autoimmune diseases progression? Clin Mol Allergy. 2016;14:11.
(MS: multiple sclerosis; RA: rheumatoid arthritis; SLE: systemic lupus erythematosus; SS: Sjögren syndrome)

AUTOIMMUNE THYROID DISEASES

Thyroid autoimmunity affects 5-20% of women of childbearing age. Thyroiditis is associated with an increased risk of miscarriage, preterm delivery, perinatal death, intrauterine growth restriction (IUGR), respiratory distress syndrome (RDS), and impaired fetal neurodevelopment. Thyroid autoimmune disorders include Hashimoto thyroiditis (HT) and GD.

Graves' Disease

Graves' disease is the most common cause of hyperthyroidism in pregnancy caused by thyroid-stimulating antibodies that bind to thyroid-stimulating hormone (TSH) receptors causing excessive secretion of thyroid hormones. In 10% of women with GD, antibodies cross the placenta causing fetal and neonatal hyperthyroidism.

Antibody titers do not correlate with maternal thyroid status. Though the half-life of antibodies is 5-14 days, neonatal hyperthyroidism can persist for months to several years. Persistent fetal tachycardia and IUGR suggest fetal hyperthyroidism.

Management of GD in Pregnancy

The goal is to maintain clinical and biochemical euthyroid states.

Treatment options include:
- Thionamides—propylthiouracil (PTU), carbimazole, methimazole
- Beta blockers—propranolol
- Iodides
- Surgery (thyroidectomy)
- Radioiodine—contraindicated in pregnancy. Causes permanent fetal hypothyroidism
- Maternal 3'-triiodothyroacetic acid to mother to treat hypothyroid fetus

Complications of GD in Pregnancy

Graves' disease causes preterm birth and low birth weight (LBW), preeclampsia, and rarely thyroid storm. Thionamides can cause fetal hypothyroidism. Best opportunity is to treat with thionamides, radioiodine, or surgery prior to conception. PTU is preferred in pregnancy, but it crosses the placenta and can cause fetal goiter. The lowest possible PTU dose is used to maintain FT4 in the higher range of normal. In one third of patients, PTU can be discontinued in the second half of pregnancy.

Serial scans should be done to identify fetal goiter. Cord blood thyroid profile should be done. Neonatal thyrotoxicosis can occur in the first few days of life after clearance of maternal antithyroid drug and can last for several months.

Hashimoto's Thyroiditis

Hashimoto's thyroiditis is the most common autoimmune disorder in women of reproductive age with a prevalence of 2-17%. Antibodies in HT are antithyroid peroxidase antibodies (TPOAb) and antithyroglobulin antibodies (TgAb) which steadily decrease with increasing gestation and become undetectable in the third trimester.

TSH and free T4 levels are monitored every 4-6 weeks and dosage of thyroxine adjusted to keep free T4 and TSH within reference ranges. Untreated hypothyroidism causes maternal and fetal complications. Fetal hypothyroidism and fetal loss can occur in patients who are TPO antibody positive.

Pregnancy

- Drug of choice is levothyroxine
- Levothyroxine requirements decrease to prepregnancy levels 6-8 weeks postpartum.
- Serial ultrasound to identify fetal goiter
- Fetal cord blood sampling
- Intra-amniotic instillation of 250 µg thyroxine weekly or 600 µg fortnightly.

IMMUNE THROMBOCYTOPENIC PURPURA

Immune thrombocytopenic purpura (ITP) accounts for 3% of cases of thrombocytopenia in pregnancy. Antiplatelet antibodies cross the placenta and cause fetal and neonatal thrombocytopenia.

Diagnosis (Box 1)

Tests to detect platelet antibodies lack sensitivity, specificity, and do not predict thrombocytopenia. Careful history, physical examination, and laboratory tests help to exclude other causes of thrombocytopenia.

Management during Pregnancy (Table 1)

Maintain adequate platelet count to minimize risk of bleeding. Check platelet count monthly till second trimester,

---

BOX 1: Investigations in thrombocytopenia.

- CBC, peripheral smear, and reticulocyte count
- Liver function test
- Thyroid function test
- Viral studies (HIV, HCV, HBV)
- APLA, ANA
- *Helicobacter pylori* (breath test)
- PT, aPTT, fibrinogen, d-dimers
- VWD type IIB testing
- Direct Coombs test
- Quantitative immunoglobulin levels

(ANA: antinuclear antibody; APLA: antiphospholipid antibodies; aPTT: activated partial thromboplastin time; CBC: complete blood count; HBV: hepatitis B virus; HCV: hepatitis C virus; HIV: human immunodeficiency syndrome; PT: prothrombin time; VWD: von Willebrand's disease)

TABLE 1: Therapeutic options for immune thrombocytopenic purpura in pregnancy.

First line therapy	Second line	Other options		
		Relatively contraindicated	Not recommended	Contraindicated
• Steroids • IVIG	• Combination of steroids and IVIG • Splenectomy	• Anti-D immunoglobulin • Azathioprine	• Cyclosporine • Dapsone • Thrombopoietin receptor agonists • Campath-1 • Rituximab	• Mycophenolate • Cyclophosphamide • Vinca alkaloids • Danazol

(IVIG: intravenous immunoglobulin)

TABLE 2: Guidelines for intervention in immune thrombocytopenic purpura without bleeding.

Intervention	Platelet count (× 10^9/L)
Antenatal, no invasive procedures planned	>20
Vaginal delivery	>20
Operative or instrumental delivery	>50
Epidural anesthesia	>80

then fortnightly till 34 weeks, and weekly thereafter. Women without bleeding manifestations and platelet counts of ≥30 × 10^9/L do not require treatment. Prednisolone is started at lower dose (20 mg daily) and increased to 60 mg (if no response within a week). Intravenous immunoglobulin (IVIG) is given if platelet count is very low or if bleeding occurs. Anti-D is effective but causes hemolysis. Other options include platelet transfusions and splenectomy.

Management of Delivery (Table 2)

Mode of delivery is determined by obstetric indications. There is no safe platelet count, but at least 50 × 10^9/L is considered safe for delivery. If platelet count is <80 × 10^9/L, start prednisolone (10-20 mg/day) 10 days prior to anticipated delivery. Platelet transfusion and IVIG are considered if delivery is emergent or has bleeding manifestations.

Caesarean section does not reduce intracranial hemorrhage (ICH). Avoid head trauma (ventose, forceps) and fetal scalp electrodes. Fetal scalp and percutaneous umbilical blood sampling are not recommended. If cord blood platelet count is low, repeat counts on days 1 and 4. No further sampling if initial platelet count is normal.

Management of Neonate

Thrombocytopenia is seen in 14-37% of neonates. Approximately 5% of babies have counts <20 × 10^9/L and 10% have counts of 20-50 × 10^9/L. Maternal treatment (steroids or IVIG) has no effect on fetal platelet count. Give IM vitamin K after checking platelet count. Thrombocytopenia is more likely if sibling had thrombocytopenia.

If cord blood platelet count is <100 × 10^9/L, repeat platelet count daily until stable. If the platelet count is <50 × 10^9/L, perform cranial ultrasound. In case of ICH, give IVIG and steroids to maintain platelet count >100 × 10^9/L for 1 week and >50 × 10^9/L for next week.

SYSTEMIC LUPUS ERYTHEMATOSUS

Systemic lupus erythematosus is a chronic inflammatory disease that affects skin, joints, kidneys, liver, serosa, central nervous system (CNS), and other systems. Tissue damage is mediated by antibodies and complement system. It is 10 times more common in women and is familial. There is polyclonal B-cell activation, impaired T-cell regulation, and immune complex-mediated vasculitis.

The American College of Rheumatology criteria to diagnose SLE requires at least 4 out of 11 criteria.

Effect of Pregnancy on Systemic Lupus Erythematosus

Systemic lupus erythematosus flares occur in 15-60% of women who had active disease before conception. One third of patients with lupus nephritis experience SLE flare during pregnancy. Pregnancy should be avoided in patients with active lupus nephritis, pulmonary hypertension (HTN), heart failure, and chronic kidney disease (CKD) stages 4-5. Distinguishing lupus nephritis from preeclampsia is difficult **(Table 2)**, as both present with proteinuria, HTN, and multiorgan dysfunction. Elevated anti-dsDNA levels suggest active SLE. Normal or elevated C3 and C4 suggest preeclampsia.

Effect of Systemic Lupus Erythematosus on Pregnancy (Flowchart 1)

- HTN or preeclampsia in 20%
- Pregnancy loss (PL) in ~20%
- Antiphospholipid antibodies (APLAs) predict PL.
- Preterm birth due to preeclampsia, fetal distress, and PPROM (preterm prelabor rupture of the membranes),
- IUGR due to uteroplacental insufficiency, steroids, and HTN.

Neonatal lupus: Transient and presents with photosensitive rash, thrombocytopenia, hepatitis, and hemolytic anemia.

Flowchart 1: Recommendations and good clinical practice statements (GPS).

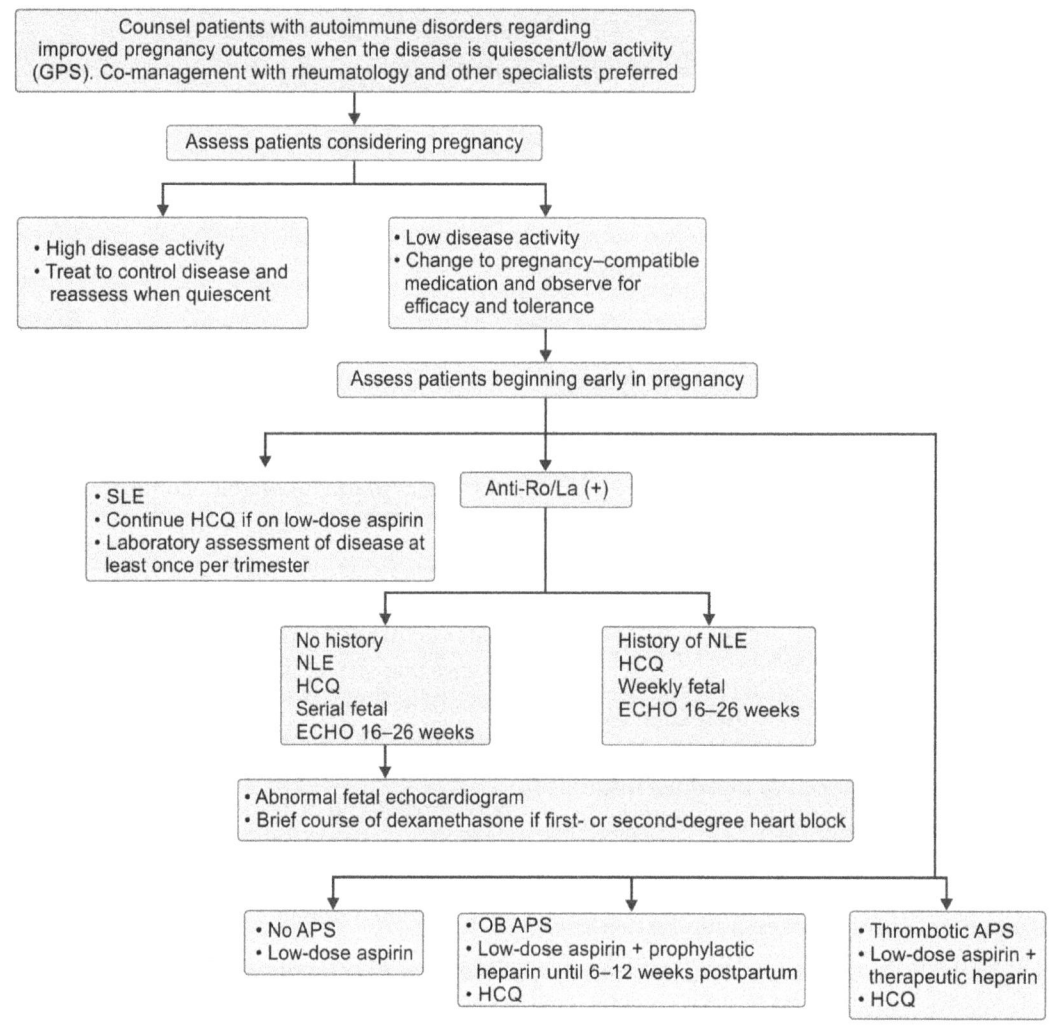

(APS: antiphospholipid syndrome; HCQ: hydroxychloroquine; NLE: neonatal lupus erythematosus; OB APS: obstetric APS; SLE: systemic lupus erythematosus)

Long-term Risk of Systemic Lupus Erythematosus

- Congenital heart block—seen in one third, usually permanent in presence of SSA or SSB antibodies.
- Risk of congenital heart block (CHB) is 1–3% with no history in family.
- Risk increases to 25–30% with one affected child.
- Dexamethasone is given but may not be effective. Hydroxychloroquine (HCQ) protects from CHB.
- Monitor fetal PR interval weekly from 17th week until delivery.
- Prolonged PR interval suggests first-degree heart block.
- Dexamethasone is recommended to prevent progression to CHB.
- Need permanent pacemaker in 47–64% in the first year.

Management of Systemic Lupus Erythematosus (Tables 3 and 4)

- Perinatal centers with multidisciplinary team
- Laboratory tests for anemia, thrombocytopenia, and APLAs
- Antenatal visit every fortnight till the second trimester and then weekly in the third trimester.
- In lupus nephritis, do a baseline 24-hour creatinine clearance and total protein.
- HCQ is effective and safe in pregnancy.
- Glucocorticoids (prednisolone, methylprednisolone) have adverse effects such as preeclampsia, placental insufficiency, IUGR, psychosis, infections, and diabetes.
- Nonsteroidal anti-inflammatory drugs (NSAIDs) cross placenta. Aspirin can cause intracranial bleed. Indomethacin given >32 weeks leads to premature closure of ductus arteriosus, oligohydramnios, and neonatal renal failure.
- Azathioprine and cyclophosphamide are used if steroids are ineffective. Methotrexate is contraindicated.
- *Postpartum period*: Look for SLE flare and start maintenance therapy.

CHAPTER 18: Autoimmune Disorders in Pregnancy

TABLE 3: Features differentiating preeclampsia and lupus nephritis.

Clinical and laboratory features	Preeclampsia	Lupus nephritis
Hypertension	>20 weeks of gestation	Any time during pregnancy
Complement	Normal-low	Low
Anti-ds-DNA	Absent or unchanged	Rising titers
Serum uric acid	Elevated (>5.5 mg/dL)	Normal
24-hour urine calcium	<195 mg/dL	>195 mg/dL
Urinary sediment	Inactive	Active
Other organs involved	Occasionally CNS or HELLP	Evidence of active nonrenal SLE
Response to steroids	No	Yes

(CNS: central nervous system; HELLP: hemolysis, elevated liver enzymes, low platelet count; SLE: systemic lupus erythematosus)

TABLE 4: Medicatiozns used in autoimmune disorders.

Medication	Preconception	During pregnancy	Breastfeeding
Hydroxychloroquine	++	++	++
Sulfasalazine	++	++	++
Colchicine	++	++	++
Azathioprine 6-Mercaptopurine	++	++	+ Low transfer
Prednisone	+ Taper to <20 mg/day by adding compatible immunosuppressants	+ Taper to <20 mg/day by adding compatible immunosuppressants	+ After a dose of >20 mg delay breastfeeding for 4 hours
Cyclosporine, tacrolimus	+ Monitor blood pressure	+ Monitor blood pressure	+ Low transfer
NSAIDs (COX 2 inhibitors not preferred)	+ Discontinue if women are having difficult conceiving	+ Continue in the first and second trimesters, discontinue in the third trimester	+ Ibuprofen preferred

(COX 2: cyclooxygenase 2; NSAIDs: nonsteroidal anti-inflammatory drugs)

Management of Systemic Lupus Erythematosus Flare

Mild or moderate flares are treated with prednisolone 10–30 mg/day.

For severe exacerbations, prednisolone 1–1.5 mg/kg/day in divided doses for 10 days and tapered.

For severe exacerbations (with CNS or renal involvement), IV methyl prednisolone 10–30 mg/kg for 5 days followed by 1–1.5 mg/kg/day in divided doses and tapered over 1 month.

Plasmapheresis and IVIG for cases refractory to steroids.

ANTIPHOSPHOLIPID ANTIBODY SYNDROME

Antiphospholipid antibody syndrome is characterized by thrombosis or fetal loss in the presence of lupus anticoagulant or anticardiolipin antibody.

Pathogenesis of Antiphospholipid Antibody Syndrome

The primary epitope for antiphospholipids is on $\beta2$-glycoprotein 1, which regulates coagulation and fibrinolysis. Placenta undergoes narrowing of spiral arterioles, intimal thickening, acute atherosis, and fibrinoid necrosis leading to fetal loss.

Diagnostic Criteria for Antiphospholipid Antibody Syndrome (Sapporo Revised Criteria)

- *Laboratory criteria*: At least one must be present
  - Lupus anticoagulant—positive
  - Anticardiolipin Ab-IgM and IgG medium/high positive
  - Beta-2 glycoprotein-1 ab-IgM and IgG > 99th percentile
- *Clinical criteria*:
  - Vascular thrombosis -arterial or venous, any size vessel
  - Unexplained fetal death ≥10 weeks
  - Unexplained fetal losses thrice <10 weeks (chromosomal abnormalities excluded)
  - Preterm delivery <34 weeks due to preeclampsia or IUGR

Diagnosis of APS requires ≥2 positive laboratory readings 12 weeks apart and one clinical criteria.

Effect of Pregnancy on Antiphospholipid Antibody Syndrome

- *Thrombotic complications*: Deep vein thrombosis (DVT), pulmonary embolism
- Transient ischemic attack (TIA), cerebrovascular accident (CVA), and venous thrombosis.

Effect of Antiphospholipid Antibody Syndrome on Pregnancy

- Gestational HTN/preeclampsia seen in 30%
- IUGR in 33%
- Preterm births in 30–60%
- Recurrent PL in 10–20%
- Catastrophic APS is rare and presents with skin lesions, acute respiratory distress syndrome (ARDS), disseminated intravascular coagulation (DIC), myocardial, and CNS microthrombosis with fatality of 50%. Diagnosis is confirmed by multiorgan involvement (>3) showing acute thrombosis and microangiopathy. Renal failure is common; ~80% require dialysis.
- Heparin and steroids along with IVIG or plasmapheresis are recommended. Acute thrombosis is treated with streptokinase or urokinase. Early delivery is planned in patients with catastrophic APS.

Management Strategies in Women with Antiphospholipid Antibody Syndrome

- Estimate prepregnancy levels of aPLs.
- Start anticoagulants as soon as cardiac activity is noted.
- Monitor every 2 weeks until 24 weeks and then weekly.
- Monitor for preeclampsia, thrombosis, and fetal well-being.
- Serial USG—every 3 weeks; nonstress test (NST) and amniotic fluid index (AFI) from 30 to 32 weeks.

Recurrent PL and APS should be treated with heparin and low-dose aspirin.

For thrombosis or preeclampsia, give thromboprophylaxis for 6 weeks with warfarin.

- Stop heparin at onset of labor and 24 hours prior to procedure.
- If activated partial thromboplastin time (aPTT) is prolonged, protamine sulfate should be given to reduce risk of bleeding.
- Stop anticoagulant 24 hours prior if on full anticoagulation.
- Anticoagulant is resumed 6 hours following vaginal delivery and 12 hours after cesarean section.

SJOGREN'S SYNDROME

- Lymphocytic infiltration of epithelial cells of various tissues leading to immune complexes of B-cell hyperactivity; female predominance.
- Primary SS immune complex deposition in salivary and lacrimal gland leads to oral/ocular dryness.
- Secondary SS—systemic or found with other autoimmune diseases like SLE.
- Can lead to B-cell hyperactivity, glomerulonephritis, neuropathy, and B-cell syndrome.

Maternal Morbidity

Usually uncomplicated but depends on primary or secondary SS.

Fetal/Neonatal Morbidity

Mainly secondary to presence of SSA and SSB antibodies:
- SSA in 60–80% of pts, SSB 30–40%
- SSA and SSB antibodies have affinity for fetal myocardial antigen epitope
- If SSA or SSB is positive, then monitor heart rhythm.

SCLERODERMA (SYSTEMIC SCLEROSIS)

- Uncommon disease with variable presentations affecting skin and internal organs.
- There is chronic inflammation with variable degree of collagen accumulation and obliterative vasculopathy of skin and viscera.
- Localized cutaneous form (morphea) on forearm and hands.
- Systemic sclerosis with Raynaud's phenomenon and organ involvement.
- CREST syndrome (Calcinosis, Raynaud's, esophageal, sclerodactyly, telangiectasia).
- Limited data since scleroderma usually develops after child-bearing age.
- Raynaud's disease tends to improve as a result of vasodilatation.
- *Renal crisis*:
  - Seen in 2–3% cases
  - Features similar to preeclampsia/HELLP (hemolysis, elevated liver enzymes, low platelet count)
  - Early delivery sometimes indicated due to renal failure
  - Increased risk of IUGR

Treatment: No specific therapy is available; low-dose aspirin.

RHEUMATOID ARTHRITIS (TABLE 5 AND FIG. 2)

It is a systemic autoimmune disease with chronic inflammation of joints and other structures. Extra-articular features include fatigue, vasculitis, subcutaneous (rheumatoid) nodules, and hematological abnormalities.

Female predominance: 3:1.

CHAPTER 18 | Autoimmune Disorders in Pregnancy

TABLE 5: The 2010 ACR/EULAR classification criteria for RA.

	Score
Target population who should be tested: • Have at least one joint with definite clinical synovitis (swelling) • With the synovitis not better explained by another disease	
Classification criteria for RA (score based algorithm: add score of categories A through D; a score of ≥6 out of 10 is needed for classification of a patient as having definite RA	
• Joint involvement:	
– One large joint	0
– Two to 10 large joints	1
– One to three small joints (with or without involvement of large joints)	2
– Four to 10 small joints (with or without involvement of large joints)	3
– >10 joints (at least one small joint)	5
• Serology (at least one test result is needed for classification)	
– Negative RF or negative ACPA	0
– Low positive RF or low positive ACPA	2
– High positive RF or high positive ACPA	3
• Acute phase reactants (at least one test result is needed for classification)	
– Normal CRP and normal ESR	0
– Abnormal CRP and normal ESR	1
• Duration of symptoms	
– < 6 weeks	0
– ≥ 6 weeks	1

(ACPA: anti-citrullinated protein antibody; CRP: C-reactive protein; ESR: erythrocyte sedimentation rate; RA: rheumatoid arthritis; ACR: american college of Rheumatology; EULAR: european league against rheumatism)

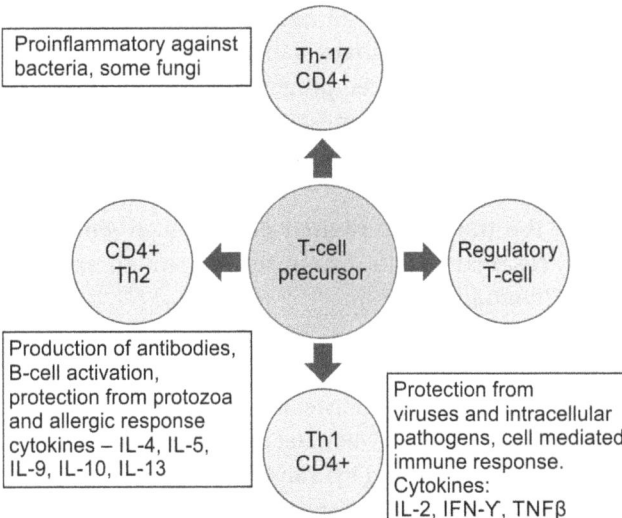

Fig. 2: The common lineage of CD4+ T-cells, a balance of these is required in pregnancy.

CD4 T cells produce cytokines and B cells produce rheumatoid factor (RF). There is association with HLA-DR4.

Effect of Pregnancy on Rheumatoid Arthritis

Antepartum: Arthritis symptoms improve in 50%, with complete remission in 20% of cases.

Symptoms may worsen if disease modifying anti-rheumatic drugs (DMARDs) are stopped.

Postpartum: Higher risk for flare; 90% in the first 4 months Glucocorticoids can be used for flares.

Effect of Rheumatoid Arthritis on Pregnancy

Increased risk for IUGR.

Management

- Stabilize woman's disease prior to conception, using medications that are safe in pregnancy.
- Drugs safe during pregnancy are NSAIDs, corticosteroids, and DMARDs, including sulfasalazine and hydroxychloroquine.
- Drugs contraindicated in pregnancy include methotrexate and leflunomide and anti-TNF agents such as rituximab and abatacept.

MYASTHENIA GRAVIS

Myasthenia gravis (MG) is an autoimmune disorder of neuromuscular junction (NMJ) with a prevalence of 150–250 per million. It is characterized by weakness of skeletal muscles due to antibody-mediated damage to acetylcholine receptors (AchRs) or other functionally related molecules on the postsynaptic membrane.

Myasthenia gravis affects women twice as often as men in reproductive age group. Severity ranges from pure ocular MG to generalized muscular weakness called generalized MG. Based on degree of weakness, MG is graded as mild, moderate, and severe. 10% of patients with MG have thymoma.

Other antibodies in MG are:
- Anti-MuSK (muscle-specific kinase) antibodies (40%)
- Antibody against lipoprotein receptor-related protein

Effect of Pregnancy on Myasthenia Gravis

Symptoms worsen in first trimester but improve in second and third trimesters. Symptoms again worsen 1 month after delivery.

Symptoms of MG worsen due to:
- Hypoventilation due to respiratory muscle weakness and elevation of diaphragm
- Puerperal infection
- Drugs
- Stress of labor and delivery

Effect of Myasthenia Gravis on Pregnancy

Duration of MG before pregnancy predicts maternal mortality. There is a risk of PPROM.

Management

- Optimal management by a multidisciplinary team
- Preconception counseling to all women with MG
- Thymectomy is the standard treatment in MG (with thymic hyperplasia or thymoma) and is done prior to conception.
- Antenatal check-ups every 2 weeks during the first two trimesters and weekly till delivery. They should avoid exertion, potassium-rich diet, and undue emotional stress. The list of drugs which can worsen MG should be given **(Box 2)**.

Pyridostigmine and neostigmine give symptomatic relief. Steroids are used in severe MG. Azathioprine/cyclosporine is used as alternate immunosuppressants. Severe exacerbations with crisis require plasmapheresis or IVIG with respiratory support.

BOX 2: Drugs which can worsen myasthenia gravis.

- Neuromuscular blocking drugs
- Aminoglycoside antibiotics like gentamycin, neomycin, amikacin, tobramycin
- Fluoroquinolones like levofloxacin, ofloxacin, ciprofloxacin, norfloxacin
- Vancomycin
- Beta-blocking drugs such as propranolol, labetalol, metaprolol
- Anti-arrhythmic drugs like procainamide, quinidine
- Magnesium
- Chloroquine and hydroxychloroquine
- Quinine
- Penicillamine
- Botulinum toxin
- Monoclonal antibodies such as nivolumab and pembrolizumab
- Inhalation and local anesthetic agents such as isoflurane, halothane, bupivacaine, lidocaine, and procaine
- Antibiotics like ritonavir, tetracyclines, macrolides, metronidazole, nitrofurantoin
- Antiepileptic drugs like carbamazepine, gabapentin, phenytoin, phenobarbitone, ethosuximide
- Glucocorticoids in high doses
- Antipsychotics like lithium, phenothiazines, butyrophenones
- Calcium channel blockers like verapamil
- Statins
- Cisplatin
- Riluzole
- Emetine
- Glatiramer
- Interferon alpha
- Iodinated contrast agents
- Topical ophthalmic solutions like timolol, tropicamide

Vaginal delivery is safe. Second stage may need assistance with forceps or vacuum. Cesarean section is reserved for obstetric indications. Nondepolarizing muscle relaxants, magnesium, sedatives, and opioids should be avoided. Epidural analgesia is preferred.

Neonatal effects: Maternal AchR antibodies cross the placenta and cause neonatal MG (10–20%) in the first 3 weeks. α-fetoprotein inhibits binding of anti-AchR antibodies to its receptors and protects the fetus.

Other rare complications are pulmonary hypoplasia, arthrogryposis multiplex congenita, and polyhydramnios due to impaired fetal swallowing.

PEMPHIGUS

Pemphigus is a rare autoimmune disease (incidence 0.68 cases per 100,000 persons per year) characterized by widespread bullae and erosions involving skin and mucosa membranes. Lesions are typically seen on scalp, face, axillae, groins, and pressure points. Antibodies directed against transmembrane glycoprotein desmoglein 3 hinder cell-to-cell adhesion causing blisters. Early diagnosis and treatment reduce risk to the mother and neonate.

It affects both sexes, especially elders, has genetic predisposition (*HLA-DR4* allele), and is frequently reported in Ashkenazi Jews and in patients with MG and SLE.

Diagnosis

Biopsy of the lesion shows acantholysis, supra basal cleft formation with deposits of IgG, and complement in the epidermis. Indirect immunofluorescence detects IgG antibodies against pemphigus antigen.

Effect on Pregnancy

Active pemphigus causes infertility (90% cases) and pregnancy is rare (only 26 cases reported). Pemphigus lesions may flare up, remain stable, or undergo remission during the pregnancy. Pemphigus vulgaris (PV) can cause miscarriage, IUGR, fetal demise, and preterm delivery.

Mode of Delivery

Though the trauma of vaginal delivery can worsen the lesions, cesarean section is not recommended except for obstetric contraindications.

Neonatal Pemphigus

There is no relationship between maternal disease severity and neonatal outcome. Neonatal pemphigus is a transitory blistering disease caused by transplacental transmission of PV IgG antibodies. Skin lesions are seen in 61% of cases and they improve in 2–3 weeks without scarring. No new vesicles or bullae appear after birth. Neonatal PV does not progress to adult disease.

Treatment

Steroids are effective and reduce mortality to 5–15%. Glucocorticoid (prednisolone) is the first-line agent. Azathioprine and cyclosporine are steroid-sparing agents. IVIG is used as an adjuvant to steroids. Plasmapheresis is tried if unresponsive to steroids and IVIG. Mycophenolate mofetil, cyclophosphamide, and methotrexate are contraindicated in pregnancy.

CHAPTER AT A GLANCE

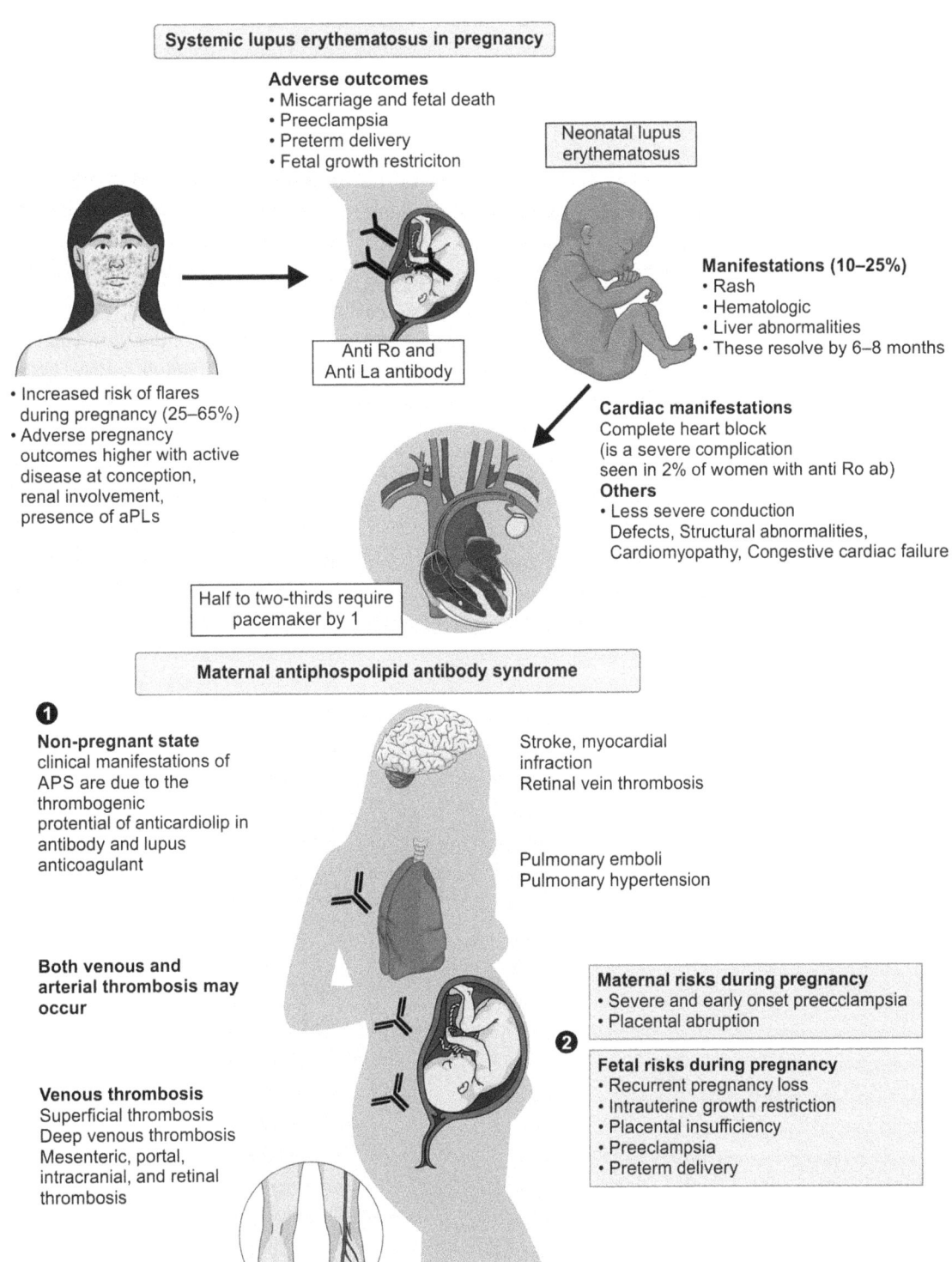

KEY POINTS

- Maternal autoimmune disorders can affect both health of the mother as well as growing fetus inter and during later life.
- Fetal effects can range from varying degree of malformation, risk of miscarriage, fatal growth restrictions and abnormalities, preterm delivery, perinatal death.
- Prompt detection and timely management can avoid deleterious effects in the baby.
- Safety and precautions of various maternal medications during preconceptional stage, pregnancy and lactation has to be kept in mind and monitored accordingly.

SUGGESTED READING

1. Ateka-Barrutia O, Nelson-Piercy C. Management of rheumatologic diseases in pregnancy. Int J Clin Rheumatol. 2012;7(5):541-58.
2. Gotestam Skorpen C, Hoeltzenbein M, Tincani A, Fischer-Betz R, Elefant E, Chambers C, et al. The EULAR points to consider for use of antirheumatic drugs before pregnancy, and during pregnancy and lactation. Ann Rheum Dis. 2016;75(5):795-810.
3. Izmirly P, Llanos C, Lee L, Askanase A, Kim M, Buyon J. Cutaneous manifestations of neonatal lupus and risk of subsequent congenital heart block. Arthritis Rheum. 2010;62(4):1153-7.
4. Miyakis S, Lockshin M, Atsumi T, Branch DW, Brey RL, Cervera R, et al. International consensus statement on an update of the classification criteria for definite antiphospholipid syndrome (APS). J Thromb Haemost. 2006;4(2):295-306.
5. Myers B. Thrombocytopenia in pregnancy. Obstet Gynaecol. 2009;11:177-83.
6. Nguyen CT, Sasso EB, Barton L, Mestman JH. Graves' hyperthyroidism in pregnancy: a clinical review. Clin Diabet Endocrinol. 2018;4:4.
7. Ostensen M, Cetin I. Autoimmune connective tissue diseases. Best Pract Res Clin Obstet Gynaecol. 2015;29(5):658-70.
8. Piccinni MP, Lombardelli L, Logiodice F, Kullolli O, Parronchi P, Romagnani S. How pregnancy can affect autoimmune diseases progression? Clin Mol Allergy. 2016;14:11.
9. Provan D, Stasi R, Newland AC, Blanchette VS, Bolton-Maggs P, Bussel JB, et al. International consensus report on the investigation and management of primary immune thrombocytopenia. Blood. 2010;115(2):168-86.
10. Smyth A, Oliveira G, Lahr B, Bailey K, Norby S, Garovic V. A systematic review and meta-analysis of pregnancy outcomes in patients with systemic lupus erythematosus and lupus nephritis. Clin J Am Soc Nephrol. 2010;5(11):2060-8.

19
Teratogenic Exposure

Brajagopal Ray, Pradip Goswami

INTRODUCTION

Teratogens are influences that interfere with normal in utero fetal growth, development, and functioning. The word teratogen originates from the Greek word of monster "teratos." Over the centuries, mankind has seen many abnormalities in the development of humans and animals, and they developed various theories about the causes for these abnormalities. They used to mostly relate these abnormalities to the persons associated with the devil or any other supernatural causes. The Greek philosopher Aristotle in the 4th century BC first described these abnormalities due to disturbances in the reproduction. At the beginning of the 19th century, the German scientist Joanne Frederick Meckel first asserted that the deviation from the normal development process leads to these malformations and he wrote his thesis in the journal dedicated to teratology in 1802. In the latter half of the 19th century, scientists started detecting teratogens and began several experimental studies. Throughout the 20th century, scientists identified several teratogens that may cause fetal abnormalities. However, it was only in the 1960s that the government in the US enacted regulations regarding the risk of exposure to human fetus, when several babies were born malformed following exposure to thalidomide.

OBJECTIVES

- To know what are teratogens
- Types of teratogens
- Mechanism of action of different teratogens
- Degree of impact on the developing fetus and newborn

PATHOPHYSIOLOGY

Teratogens affect morphogenesis, development, and differentiation of fetus, through cell death, failed cell separation, or alterations in the movement of the cells. There is an increasing recognition that stress, nutrition, and infections can alter the gene programming and expression during embryonic and fetal growth. The exact mechanism of how the organs can alter the normal development is not clear. Scientist postulated that certain biochemical mechanisms, for example, methylation, can alter the gene expression and subsequent gene regulation leading to abnormal development.

The effect of an environmental agent on the embryo or fetus depends upon the chemical or physical nature of the agent and several other factors, such as dose, route, and duration of exposure and more importantly the developmental stage at which the exposure occurs.

In 1977, James Wilson proposed six principles of the teratogenic exposure that were subsequently published in the handbook of teratology:

1. Susceptibility to teratogenesis depends upon the genotype of the conceptus and how it interacts with environmental factors.
2. Susceptibility to teratogenic agents varies with the developmental stage at the time of exposer.
3. Teratogenic agents act in specific ways on developing cells and tissue to initiate abnormal embryogenesis.
4. The final manifestations of abnormal development are death, malformation, growth retardation, and functional disorder.
5. The access of adverse environmental influences to developing issues depends on the nature of the agent.
6. Manifestations of deviant development increase in degree as the dosage increases from the no effect to that totally lethal effect.

CLASSIFICATION

Teratogens can be broadly classified into six categories:
1. Physical agents
2. Chemical agents
3. Infectious agents
4. Maternal conditions
5. Maternal substance abuse
6. Common prescription medicines

Physical Agents

Physical agents, such as ionizing radiation and elevated body temperature, can cause damage to the unborn fetus. Although there is no proof that human congenital malformation has been caused by diagnostic level of radiation, it is still advised to avoid exposure, especially during early gestation. The most critical period is between 8 and 15 weeks after fertilization.

- *Ionizing radiation*: Like X-rays, gamma rays that carry adequate energy to free an electron from the atom results in abnormalities at the cellular level. Because of the prolonged period of organogenesis, the central nervous system (CNS) remains the most vulnerable organ to the detrimental effects of radiation. Studies have also postulated that there might be an increased incidence of hematopoietic malignancies in later life.
- *Hyperthermia*: Agents that cause hyperthermia are also physical teratogens, like saunas, hot tubs, and infection that cause fever. Experiments on animals from the early 1970s to the early 1990s demonstrated that hyperthermia causes CNS malformations, microcephaly, abdominal wall defects, defects of the eye and palate, and limb reduction. One study by Smith et al. presented patients who had been exposed during pregnancy to hyperthermia caused by infections or by sauna bathing developed abnormalities in their fetus leading to mental deficiency, seizures, and midfacial anomalies. One study by Shiota et al. studied 100 embryos with CNS defects and found that 18% of mother with anencephalic infants had experienced hyperthermia during the critical embryonic period.

Chemical Agents

Exposure to various chemical substances is known to cause fetal anomalies.

- *Lead*: Prenatal exposure to a high level of heavy metals like lead is known to be associated with abnormalities like VACTERL association (vertebral, anal, cardiac, tracheoesophageal fistula, renal, and limb abnormalities). A small but significant increase in minor malformations, including hemangiomas, lymphangiomas, hydroceles, skin tags, skin papillae, and undescended testes, was seen in infants with high lead levels in the umbilical blood.
- *Mercury*: Mercury especially in an organic form, like methyl-mercury, can cause Minamata disease, seen in Japan. A similar incidence was reported in Iraq where contamination of wheat with methyl-mercury led to fetal cerebral abnormalities. Methyl-mercury poisoning produces atrophy of the granular layer of the cerebellum and spongiform softening in the visual cortex and other cortical areas of the brain.
- *Lithium*: Lithium, used in various psychiatric illness, can result in major cardiac defects in exposed fetus, e.g., Ebstein's anomaly, tricuspid atresia.
- *Toluene*: It is a chemical that can cause fetal embryopathy causing postnatal growth failure, microcephaly, developmental delay, cardiac, and limb defect similar to fetal alcohol syndrome.
- Various other chemicals, such as polychlorinated and polybrominated biphenyls (PCBs), can also cause skin discoloration, dark-colored nails, intrauterine growth restriction (IUGR), and exophthalmos in babies if mother is exposed.

Infectious Agents

The developmental effect of teratogenesis is the result of mitotic inhibition, direct cytotoxic effect, and a vascular disruptive event on the embryo or fetus. Some of these viruses do not result in congenital malformation but can cause fetal or neonatal death. These include coxsackievirus, poliovirus, echovirus, hepatitis, etc. The other group of viruses that mostly cause fetal malformations are rubella, cytomegalovirus, parvovirus B19, varicella zoster, etc.

- *Rubella*: The risk is highest in the first trimester. Affected infants suffer from cataracts, congenital heart disease, hearing impairment, and developmental delay. Infants often present with more than one of these signs but may also present with a single defect, most commonly hearing impairment.
- *Cytomegalovirus (CMV)*: CMV rarely causes problems in healthy people but if it infects pregnant women, it can cause various abnormalities in newborn babies. Babies develop hearing loss, intellectual disability, vision problems, and occasionally pneumonia.
- *Varicella*: It is caused by a herpes virus which gets transmitted from person to person by direct contact. This is contagious from 1 to 2 days before the appearance of the rash until the blisters have dried and become scabs. Affected infants present with scarred and malformed limb, small head size, blindness, seizures, and mental deficiency.
- *Mumps*: Although this is less harmful, mumps infection can still cause a condition called endocardial fibroelastosis in neonates.
- *Parvovirus B19*: They can cause a high incidence of stillbirth and also severe anemia leading to cardiac failure and hydrops.
- *Syphilis*: In untreated maternal syphilis in the primary or secondary stages, 50% are stillborn or die within 4 weeks after birth. Symptoms of congenital syphilis may present at birth or may be delayed as long as 5 years of age. Early presenters show signs of meningitis, fever, rash, and organomegaly and late presenters come with bony pain, teeth abnormality, saddle nose, and keratitis.
- *Toxoplasmosis*: This is one of the treatable conditions, where the affected fetus gets infection through placental transfer causing various CNS disorders like hydrocephalus, microcephalic, and cerebral calcification hepatitis.

Maternal Conditions

Maternal medical conditions are often ignored as potential teratogens. There are a number of maternal illnesses that can cause several birth defects, which can be minimized by repeated preconceptual counseling and intervention.

- *Diabetes mellitus*: It is well known that pregestational and early gestational glucose control greatly influence the rate of miscarriage and fetal anomalies. In a study performed by Hanson et al., hemoglobin A1c levels for those women seeking prenatal care were linearly correlated with the rate of miscarriage and anomalies. Hyperglycemia leads to inhibition of the myoinositol uptake that is essential for embryonic development. Infants of diabetic mothers are particularly prone to defects in the cardiovascular system, CNS, and skeletal system. The relative risk for cardiac anomalies is 4.3 times higher compared with normal glycemic controls. Transposition of the great vessels, ventricular septal defect (VSD), and dextrocardia occur with the greatest frequency. Anencephaly, spina bifida, and hydrocephaly are the major CNS malformations. Rare malformations include situs inversus and caudal dysplasia, vertebral and renal anomalies, imperforate anus, radius aplasia, and renal abnormalities including agenesis and dysplasia.
- *Thyroid disorder*: Thyroid disorders can cause a number of teratogenic problems on a developing fetus. Thyroid gland dysfunction like hypothyroidism, especially when induced by antithyroid drugs like propylthiouracil, carbimazole, radioactive iodine, etc., can affect fetal brain developments causing lower IQ. Hyperthyroidism or Graves' disease can also cause neonatal thyrotoxicosis with development of exophthalmos, tachycardia, hypothermia, cardiac failure, etc. Iodine deficiency in the mother, especially in the endemic regions, can lead to abnormal neonatal embryogenesis. Fetal iodine deficiency results in mental retardation, spastic diplegia, deafness, and strabismus.
- *Phenylketonuria*: Phenylketonuria in mother can also induce detrimental effect on growing fetus. If the level exceeds 20 mg/mL, it can cause mental retardation, microcephaly, IUGR, and cardiac malformation in the offspring.

Maternal Substance Abuse

- *Fetal alcohol syndrome (FAS)*: Alcohol is one of the most common teratogens that can affect the developing fetus. No amount of alcohol is safe while binge drinking has a poorer prognosis. FAS presents with postnatal growth retardation, typical facial anomalies, and CNS dysfunction. Acetaldehyde, an alcohol metabolite, is implicated to cause FAS by its inhibiting effect on DNA synthesis. However, there are some genetic predispositions where some fetuses are more vulnerable than others with the same amount of alcohol.
- *Marijuana*: The active ingredient of marijuana is 8,9 tetrahydrocannabinol, which is fat-soluble and can cross the placenta easily and may persist for as long as 30 days in the fetus. There have been reports of growth retardation and other malformation, especially if the fetus is exposed in the first trimester.
- *Tobacco smoking*: Nicotine is a vasoconstrictor that results in uterine vascular construction and can cause placental insufficiency. Infants are affected by IUGR and increased perinatal mortality and morbidity like abruptio placentae, spontaneous abortion, and premature delivery.
- *Cocaine*: Cocaine abuse is also dangerous during pregnancy. Cocaine blocks the presynaptic reuptake of neurotransmitters resulting in increased level of norepinephrine and dopamine. This causes reduced blood flow to the placenta and often results in abruptio placentae. It also produces cerebral hemorrhage, IUGR, limb effects, and necrotizing enterocolitis in newborns.

Common Prescription Medicines

Usually, prescription drugs are unlikely to cause teratogenic birth defects; however, there are a few medicines that can potentially cause damage to a developing fetus.

- *Antineoplastic agents*: Thalidomide: Although use of thalidomide during pregnancy has been prohibited for several decades, in the middle of the 20th century, women receiving thalidomide during pregnancy gave birth to children with multiple birth defect, also known as thalidomide embryopathy. These comprise limb reduction, hemangiomas, esophageal and duodenal atresia, cardiac defects, renal anomalies, and dental and ear anomalies. Mycophenolate mofetil is associated with external ear and facial defects; cleft lip and palate; heart, esophagus, kidney, and distal limb defects.
- *Folic acid deficiency/folic acid antagonist*: Folic acid deficiency can result in neural tube defect in developing fetus. Hence, this has been a routine practice to supplement women in childbearing age group with folic acid before they conceive. Women who have previously developed pregnancy with neural tube defect pose a higher risk of developing the same problem in subsequent pregnancies.
- *Ergotamine*: It has been frequently used for treatment of migraine; however, this can also cause constriction of fetal blood vessels and may develop IUGR and intestinal problems like jejunal atresia.
- *Retinoids*: Isotretinoin is often used as a treatment for acne. Although topical use is unlikely to cause any fetal damage, systemic use, especially during the first trimester, can cause severe damage to the developing fetus, including microcephaly, cerebellar dysgenesis,

TABLE 1: Classification of teratogenic agents.

Types	Subtypes	Potential effects on fetus
Physical	Ionizing radiation—increased risk beyond radiation exposure of 0.1 Gy (100 mGy, 10 rads)	• Miscarriage, malformations including CNS defects • Future hematological malignancies
	Hyperthermia	Microcephaly, abdominal wall defect, limb dysgenesis, seizures, mental deficiency
Chemical	Heavy metals—lead	VACTERL association
	Mercury	Minamata disease, cerebral cortical and cerebellar abnormalities
	Lithium	Cardiac anomalies
	Toluene	Similar to fetal alcohol syndrome
Infection	Rubella	Congenital rubella syndrome—cardiac defects, cataracts, microcephaly
	CMV	Congenital CMV infection—deafness, pneumonia, retinitis, hepatitis
	Varicella	Scars malformed limb, small head size, blindness seizures
	Parvovirus B19	Still birth, anemia leading to hydrops
	Mumps	Endocardial fibroelastosis
	Syphilis	Miscarriage, still born, congenital syphilis
	Toxoplasma	Brain malformation
Maternal medical condition	Diabetes mellitus	Miscarriage, preterm delivery, congenital heart defects, renal anomalies
	Thyroid disorders	Neonatal hypothyroidism, thyrotoxicosis, brain dysfunction
	Phenylketonuria	Mental retardation, micro carefully, IUGR, cardiac malformation
Maternal substance abuse	Alcohol	Fetal alcohol syndrome—typical facial features, CNS abnormalities
	Marijuana	Growth retardation
	Cocaine	Cerebral hemorrhage, IUGR, limb effects, and necrotizing enterocolitis
Common prescription medicine	Antineoplastic agents—thalidomide	Limb reduction, hemangioma, esophageal and duodenal atresia, cardiac defects, renal anomalies
	Antineoplastic agents—mycophenolate mofetil	External ear and facial defects, cardiac anomalies
	Folate antagonist/folic acid deficiency	Neural tube defect
	Ergotamine	IUGR and jejunal atresia
	Antiepileptic—phenytoin	Developmental delay, dysmorphic facial features, hypoplastic distal phalanges
	Antiepileptic—carbamazepine	Facial appearance, microcephaly, and limb defect
	Antiepileptic—valproic acid	Lumbosacral spina bifida with meningomyelocele or meningocele, often accompanied by midfacial hypoplasia, heart defects
	Mental health medication—lithium	Ebstein's anomaly
	Mental health medication—fluoxetine	Behavioral issue, PPHN
	Antihypertensive—ACE inhibitors, Captopril	Neonatal deaths, neonatal respiratory distress, PDA
	Antihypertensive—ARBs	Hypotension, renal dysplasia, anuria, fetal death
	Cholesterol-lowering agents—statin	Smith–Lemli–Opitz syndrome
	Anticoagulant—warfarin	Bony birth defects, like nasal hyperplasia, stippled calcification, CNS defects
	Antibiotic—tetracyclines	Dental staining
	Others—retinoic acid	Microcephaly, cerebellar dysgenesis, depressed nasal bridge, absent external ears, cardiac defects

(ACE: angiotensin-converting enzyme; ARB: angiotensin receptor blocker; CMV: cytomegalovirus; CNS: central nervous system; IUGR: intrauterine growth restriction; PDA: patent ductus arteriosus; PPHN: persistent pulmonary hypertension of the newborn; VACTERL: vertebral, anal, cardiac, tracheoesophageal fistula, renal, and limb abnormalities) depressed nasal bridge, absent external ears, cardiac defects including VSD, atrial septal defect (ASD), the tetralogy of Fallot, and hypoplastic adrenal cortex.

- *Sedatives*: Benzodiazepines group of medicines can produce IUGR, cleft palate, cleft lips, and other facial features similar to FAS and also congenital heart disease, specially with phenobarbital.
- *Antiepileptics*: Phenytoin: This medicine, often used in epilepsy, can rarely cause a combination of birth defects called fetal hydantoin syndrome. There is developmental delay, dysmorphic facial features, and hypoplastic distal phalanges. Chronic exposure over a long period of time increases the risk of developing a full-blown syndrome. Carbamazepine: It can also cause unique facial appearance, microcephaly, and limb defects, including complete or partial absence of a limb and overgrowth or underdevelopment of the fingers, toes, and nails. Valproic acid: It can produce lumbosacral spina bifida with meningomyelocele or meningocele, often accompanied by midfacial hypoplasia, deficient orbital ridge, prominent forehead, and congenital heart disease.
- *Mental health medication*: Lithium is associated with cardiac defects such as Ebstein's anomaly, selective serotonin reuptake inhibitor (SSRI), some SSRIs like fluoxetine can cause neonatal behavioral disturbances, and persistent pulmonary hypertension of the newborn (PPHN).
- *Antihypertensive medication*: Angiotensin converting enzyme (ACE) inhibitors: ACE inhibitors, specially captopril, can cross the placenta resulting in spontaneous abortion intrauterine and neonatal deaths, neonatal respiratory distress, patent ductus arteriosus (PDA), and renal tubular dysplasia. Angiotensin II receptor blockers (ARBs): These agents are potentially more dangerous and can cause hypotension, renal dysplasia, anuria or oliguria, oligohydramnios, IUGR, and even fetal death.
- *Statins*: Although no controlled studies have shown any teratogenic effects on human embryo, a number of syndromes associated with statin use during pregnancy have been documented. As cholesterol is an integral part of human brain development and its cell membrane, cholesterol-lowering agents have been implicated in causing disruption in fetal developments resulting in patterns like Smith–Lemli–Opitz syndrome and some skeletal dysplasia.
- *Anticoagulant*: Warfarin is commonly used as a long-term anticoagulant therapy. Warfarin metabolites interfere with calcium metabolism. As a result, the fetus exposed to warfarin during early pregnancy mainly shows the bony birth defects, like nasal hyperplasia, stippled calcification in proximal femur, tarsals, brachydactyly, and smaller nails. The fetus also develops microcephaly, optic atrophy, seizures, hypotonia, and mental deficiency.
- *Antibiotic*: Tetracyclines: Their use is associated with dental staining in later life **(Table 1)**.

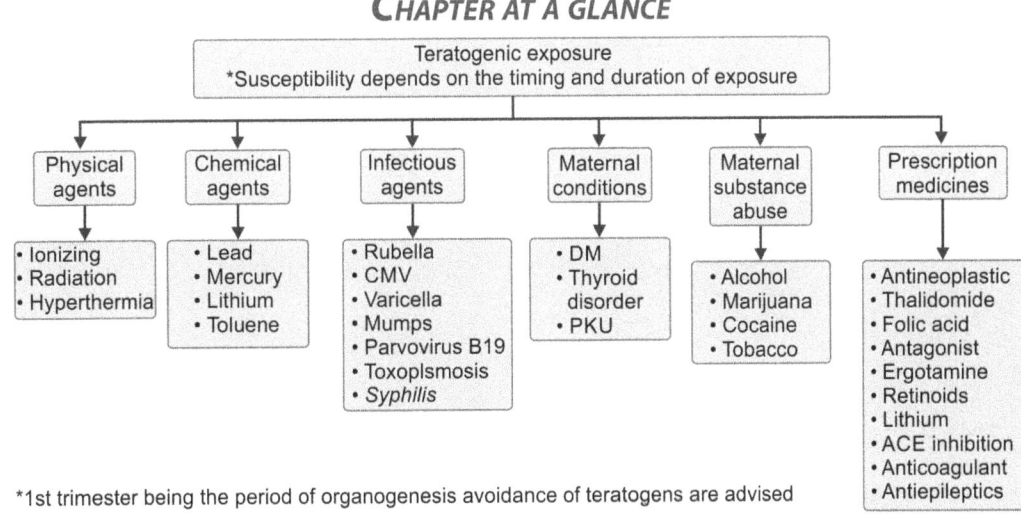

(ACE: angiotensin-converting enzyme; CMV: cytomegalovirus; DM: diabetes mellitus; PKU: phenylketonuria)

KEY POINTS

- Teratogens cause about 10% of all birth defects.
- Majority of the prescription medicines have not been adequately evaluated for the risk during pregnancy.
- Because of rapid organogenesis, first trimester carries the most vulnerable period of effect of teratogenic exposure.
- Brain and heart having long developmental stage takes the most brunt of teratogenic ill effects.

SUGGESTED READING

1. Beckman DA, Brent RL. Mechanism of teratogenesis. Annu Rev Pharmacol Toxicol. 1984;24:482-500.
2. Brent RL. The cause and prevention of human birth defects: what have we learned in the past 50 years? Congenit Anom (Kyoto). 2001;41:3-21.
3. Dauer LT, Miller DL, Schueler B, Silberzweig J, Balter S, Bartal G, et al. Society of Interventional Radiology Safety and Health

Committee; Cardiovascular and Interventional Radiological Society of Europe Standards of Practice Committee. Occupational radiation protection of pregnant or potentially pregnant workers in IR: a joint guideline of the Society of Interventional Radiology and the Cardiovascular and Interventional Radiological Society of Europe. J Vasc Interv Radiol. 2015;26(2):171-81.
4. Frias JL, Gilbert-Barness E. Human teratogens: current controversies. Adv Pediat. 2008;55:171-211.
5. Friedman JM. The principles of teratology: are they still true? Birth Defects Res Clin Mol Teratol. 2010;88(10):766-8.
6. Guidelines for diagnostic imaging during pregnancy and lactation. Committee Opinion No. 723. American College of Obstetricians and Gynecologists. Obstet Gynecol. 2017;130:e210-6.
7. Shiota K. Neural tube defects and maternal hyperthermia in early pregnancy: epidemiology in a human embryonic population. Am J Med Genet. 1982;12:281-8.

20
Maternal Medications and Substance Abuse

Sanjay Wazir, Parul Chopra Buttan

INTRODUCTION

Maternal substance abuse is a critical public health problem with consequences for both the mother and the child. The exposure to illicit drug abuse as well as prescription drugs has been rising. Substance abuse has grown among women, especially in metropolitan cities, because of lifestyle changes like increased work pressure and timings, economic stress, reduced community and family support system, and changing cultural values.

Drugs, both prescription and illicit, can directly affect fetal growth and maturation. Intrauterine asphyxia is perhaps the single most significant risk to the fetus. In addition, meconium-stained amniotic fluid is frequently encountered in pregnant addict and is a manifestation of fetal distress. Near the time of birth, maternal drugs can produce signs of acute toxicity in the newborn infant, cause persistent abnormal neurobehavior, or result in withdrawal signs. Other problems seen with increased frequency among such children include jaundice, aspiration pneumonia, meconium aspiration, persistent pulmonary hypertension of the newborn (PPHN) of the newborn, transient tachypnea, hyaline membrane disease, and infections.

OBJECTIVES

- To know the impact of maternal substance abuse in pregnancy and lactation on the neonate
- Strategies to reduce the substance abuse amongst pregnant mothers
- Management of infants born to mothers with substance abuse

SPECIFIC EXPOSURES

Antenatal Tobacco uses and Second-hand Smoke at Home

The percentage of women smokers in India is rising. The National Family Health Survey-3 (2005–2006) reported smoking in 9% of pregnant women, and 25% of women were exposed to second-hand smoke in India. The factors associated with smoking included lower education, lower socioeconomic status, and rural residence.

Both active maternal smoking and passive exposure to tobacco smoke are harmful to the fetus. The impact is mediated by reduced oxygenation of the fetus, reduced placental blood supply, and direct toxin effect on the developing brain and lungs of the fetus. In addition, active smoking is associated with reduced ovarian reserve, infertility, reduced in vitro fertilization success, and early onset of menopause. Fetal exposure to active maternal smoking is associated with placental dysfunction, spontaneous abortion, intrauterine growth restriction, preterm delivery, and congenital anomalies such as cleft lip and palate, cardiac defects, limb reduction defects. Maternal active smoking during pregnancy is associated with impaired cognitive functioning, auditory processing deficits, impulsivity, anxiety, depression, attention deficit hyperactivity disorder (ADHD), and conduct disorders in offspring. Active maternal smoking during pregnancy or exposure to second-hand smoke after birth is a significant risk factor for sudden infant death syndrome (SIDS).

Smoking cessation programs should focus on awareness, education and rehabilitation of preteens, adolescents, and women of childbearing age. In addition, because nicotine is a neurotoxin, nicotine replacement should be avoided to quit smoking during pregnancy. Nicotine from smoking or replacement therapy (e.g., patch) is transferred into breast milk along with its active metabolites. Therefore, breastfeeding women who have been unsuccessful in quitting smoking should be encouraged to use nicotine replacement therapy (lesser doses) to limit infant exposure to nicotine and addition because of other toxins in cigarettes.

Alcohol

Effects of alcohol on the fetus are extensive, devastating, and often permanent. Heavy alcohol consumption increases the risk of miscarriage and increases stillbirths. Fetal alcohol spectrum (FAS) disorder is an umbrella term that covers all diagnoses that pertain to children who were exposed to alcohol in utero. These include FAS as well as an alcohol-related neurodevelopmental disorder and alcohol-related birth defects. Fetal alcohol syndrome is defined by craniofacial abnormalities (including smooth philtrum, thin upper lip, and short palpebral fissures), growth deficiency (at or below the 10th percentile), and central nervous system (CNS) dysfunction (structural, neurologic, and functional).

The best advice is to abstain from alcohol exposure during pregnancy. Ethanol freely diffuses into breast milk and achieves levels equivalent to those in blood. Infrequent and moderate amounts of alcohol ingestion are not a contraindication to breastfeeding. For every drink consumed, the mother should avoid breastfeeding for at least 2 hours.

Opioid

Although less common than the developed countries, exposure to opioid has been rising in India. Opioids are not teratogenic. Common prenatal complications of opioid use include premature labor, premature rupture of membranes, antepartum hemorrhage, fetal demise, and low birth weight (LBW).

Neonatal abstinence syndrome (NAS) is the term that encompasses the constellation of clinical signs associated with opioid withdrawal. Because opioid receptors are concentrated in the CNS and the gastrointestinal (GI) tract, the predominant signs and symptoms of pure opioid withdrawal reflect CNS irritability, excessive autonomic activity, and GI tract dysfunction. The signs of CNS excitability are tremors, irritability, high-pitched crying, frequent yawning, exaggerated Moro's reflex, and seizures. In addition, neonates can present signs of GI dysfunction such as diarrhea, poor feeding, vomiting, dehydration, increased hunger, and poor weight gain. The onset of symptoms attributable to neonatal withdrawal from opioid usually presents at birth or begin within 24 hours of delivery, rarely beyond 7 days of life. Withdrawal signs in the newborn may mimic other conditions, such as infection, hypoglycemia, hypocalcemia, hyperthyroidism, intracranial hemorrhage, and hypoxic-ischemic encephalopathy. If none of these diagnoses is readily apparent, a diagnosis of NAS should be entertained.

Biologic testing is carried out using neonatal urine specimens in suspected cases, although it has a high false-negative rate. Other materials tested are meconium (highly sensitive and specific) and neonatal hair, but these are not readily available.

A plan to institute early supportive care is critical in infants who are at risk for withdrawal. Effective measures include minimizing environmental stimuli (both light and sound) by placing the infant in a dark, quiet environment; avoiding autostimulation by careful swaddling; responding early to an infant's distress signals; adopting appropriate infant positioning and comforting techniques; and providing frequent small volumes of hypercaloric formula or human milk to minimize hunger. The therapy goals are to ensure that the infant achieves adequate sleep and nutrition to establish a consistent pattern of weight gain and begins to integrate into a social environment.

For the infant who does not respond to the above non-pharmacologic management, drug therapy is appropriate to reduce the severity of signs of NAS to mild, tolerable levels and prevent complications such as fever, weight loss, and seizures. Many drug preparations have been used to treat NAS—an opioid (oral morphine or methadone) as the drug of choice. Clonidine and phenobarbital are second-line treatment modalities.

Heroin readily transfers into breast milk; a similar rationale is applied to the abuse of prescription narcotics (e.g., oxycodone, codeine), which are constituents of various over-the-counter products. Therefore, the use of such products should be minimized and carried out under the review of a registered medical practitioner.

Caffeine

It is found in coffee, tea, chocolate, cocoa, and numerous prescriptions and over-the-counter medications. It is a socially approved addictive substance, often perceived as harmless by expectant mothers. It readily crosses the placenta and is found in breast milk. Maternal caffeine consumption during gestation exerts an effect on birth weight through growth restriction in term newborns. Evidence indicates that caffeine is not a human teratogen and that caffeine appears to have no effect on preterm labor and delivery. There is a significant increase in the risk for spontaneous abortion and LBW infants in pregnant women consuming more than 150 mg caffeine per day. Caffeine ingested in large amounts [>4 cups (each cup of coffee = 8 Oz = 235 mL) of coffee per day or >300 g of caffeine per day] during pregnancy causes a dose-dependent decrease in birth weight. The current recommendation is to restrict coffee consumption to less than two mugs of brewed coffee.

Prescription Drugs

Over-the-counter availability of many prescription drugs, including antibiotics, leads to potential overuse and abuse by the general population. Access to the internet gives information that creates the illusion of power, often misleading young people into bypassing expert consultation for common health conditions. Several drugs harm the growing fetus in pregnancy and need caution when used in pregnancy. Some medications are known teratogens such as thalidomide (a sedative and hypnotic, causes phocomelia), retinoids (antiacne drug, causes severe eye, ear, brain defects), antiepileptic drugs such as phenytoin (cause fetal hydantoin syndrome—craniofacial anomalies, hypoplasia of distal phalanges, growth restriction, mental deficiency), and warfarin (anticoagulant causing fetal warfarin syndrome—microcephaly, hydrocephalus, growth restriction, nasal hypoplasia, stippling of the epiphysis, eye defects, postnatal developmental delay). Women with preexisting medical conditions should have preconception counseling by a multidisciplinary team to ensure medical optimization and switch over medications to pregnancy-safe ones where needed.

Substance abuse in pregnancy remains a significant public health problem, leading to several harmful maternal and neonatal outcomes. Women of childbearing age and their sexual partners should be screened for possible drug use and encouraged to discontinue those toxic substances before conception. Women who are pregnant should be counseled to seek prenatal care as soon as possible and abstain entirely from any illegal drugs. A multidisciplinary team approach is required in caring for these women and their families. The pediatrician also has an essential role in screening adolescent females for high-risk behaviors and providing information about the consequences of unhealthy lifestyle choices in a nonjudgmental manner. Pregnancy is a significant life event, and often, the motivation to prevent harm to her unborn baby makes the women receptive to interventions for deaddiction. From the drug user's perspective, addiction is not a problem. Instead, it is a solution to an underlying problem, albeit an unresourceful and harmful one. An informed, compassionate clinical team can facilitate healthier life choices impacting the present and future generations favorably.

CHAPTER AT A GLANCE

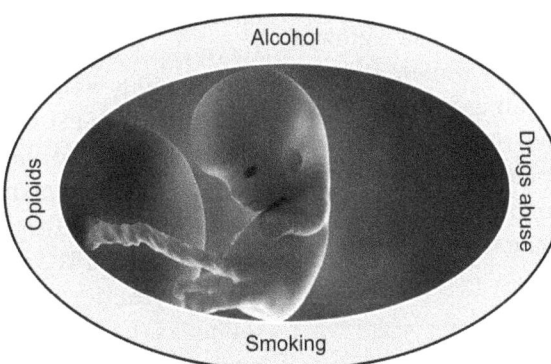

(ADHD: attention deficit hyperactivity disorder)
Comment: Although there is no exact dose dependent relationship between maternal alcohol consumption and effect on the fetus and hence there is no safe limit of intake of alcohol in pregnancy.

KEY POINTS

- Substance abuse is a growing problem amongst women in reproductive age group with significant implications for the fetus and the infant
- Screening both parents for the substance abuse should be part of pre-natal and antenatal counseling
- Counseling and multi-disciplinary approach is required for motivating the mothers to quit during pregnancy and lactation.

SUGGESTED READING

1. American Academy of Pediatrics Committee on Substance Abuse and Committee on Children with Disabilities: Fetal alcohol syndrome and alcohol-related neurodevelopmental disorders. Pediatrics. 2000;106:358-61.
2. Committee Opinion No. 711: Opioid use and opioid use disorder in pregnancy. Obstet Gynecol. 2017;130:e81.
3. Huybrechts KF, Bateman BT, Desai RJ, Hernandez-Diaz S, Rough K, Mogun H, et al. Risk of neonatal drug withdrawal after intrauterine co-exposure to opioids and psychotropic medications: cohort study. BMJ. 2017;358:j3326.
4. Jansson LM, Velez M. Neonatal abstinence syndrome. Curr Opin Pediatr. 2012;24:252.
5. Ostrea EM Jr, Knapp DK, Tannenbaum L, Ostrea AR, Romero A, Salari V, et al. Estimates of illicit drug use during pregnancy by maternal interview, hair analysis, and meconium analysis. J Pediatr. 2001;138:344.
6. Rogers JM: Tobacco and pregnancy: overview of exposure and effects. Birth Defects Res C Embryol Today. 2008;84:1-15.
7. Sachs HC, Committee On Drugs. The transfer of drugs and therapeutics into human breast milk: an update on selected topics. Pediatrics. 2013;132:e796.
8. Shankaran S, Lester BM, Das A, Bauer CR, Bada HS, Lagasse L, et al. Impact of maternal substance use during pregnancy on childhood outcome. Semin Fetal Neonatal Med. 2007;12:143-50.

CHAPTER 21

Maternal Systemic Medical Illness and Fetal Effect

Santosh Kumar Panda, Mohini Sinha

INTRODUCTION

A pregnancy should be considered high risk, if pregnant women are associated with a systemic medical illness. Evidenced-based disease-specific monitoring and intervention are considered to minimize maternal morbidities and fetal complications. Teratogenicity, growth impairment, and premature birth are common adverse fetal events in maternal systemic illness. Sometimes, early termination may reverse the deterioration of disease pathology in pregnancy. In this chapter, the fetal effects of maternal systemic diseases like cardiac, hepatic, specific neurologic disorders, mental illness, and renal disorders are described.

OBJECTIVES

- To discuss the adverse fetal complications in pregnant mother with various systemic illness, i.e., heart disease, liver disorder, epilepsy, neuromuscular disorder, psychiatric illness and renal disorder.
- To review about the safety of antiepileptic drug during pregnancy.

PREGNANCY WITH HEART DISEASE

Adverse fetal and maternal outcome are commonly found in pregnancy with heart disease (HD). Both structural, i.e., adult congenital heart disease (ACHD), and acquired heart diseases, i.e., cardiomyopathies, valvular heart disease (VHD), and pulmonary hypertension (PH), are complicated during pregnancy. VHD and ACHD are the most common types of cardiac problems during pregnancy reported worldwide. Maternal cardiomyopathy or pulmonary hypertension is usually associated with elderly mother, tobacco consumption, hypertension, and diabetes mellitus, which may have independent effect on neonatal outcome. There is an increased rate of intrauterine death, prematurity, and small for gestational age birth found in offspring of mothers with HD. The adverse fetal effects are more common in mothers with cardiomyopathy and PH, in comparison to VHD and ACHD. Pregnant mothers with ACHD have a risk of 3–5% congenital heart disease in their neonates. Some of the autosomal conditions, i.e., Marfan's syndrome, long QT, and hypertrophic cardiomyopathy, have 50% of inheritance risk to fetus from parents. The fetal survival risk is dependent on maternal desaturation, which is commonly associated with cyanotic heart disease or pregnancy with PH. Maternal SpO_2 < 85% implies high fetal demises, and fetal survival improved with maternal SpO_2 >90%. A high rate of miscarriage is found in mothers with cyanotic ACHD. The pharmacological therapy needs for management of HD during pregnancy, i.e., anticoagulant, antiarrhythmic, antihypertensive, and anticongestive therapies, have potential adverse effect on the fetus. In pregnant mothers with ACHD, presence of abnormal cardiac functions is associated with an abnormal uteroplacental Doppler abnormality. Hence, compromised uteroplacental Doppler may be the pathophysiology of small for gestational age and adverse fetal outcome. Majority of pregnancies with cardiomyopathy and PH are electively delivered by cesarean birth, and mothers with ACHD or VHD are usually supported with assisted vaginal delivery.

Echocardiography during the preconception period is recommended for risk stratification among women with HD. Preconception counseling, including genetic counseling by a cardiologist and an obstetrician, guides the women regarding the risk of hereditary cardiac defect and anticipated maternal complications. Pregnancy with HD, particularly ACHD, should be evaluated with maternal biochemical screening for chromosomal anomaly, nasal translucency scan at the first trimester, and total anomaly scanning along with fetal echocardiography at 18–20 weeks' gestational age. Maternal oxygen saturation and right ventricular function monitoring in pregnancy with HD are key to fetal survival. Presence of ventricular insufficiency in the first trimester is mandatory for therapeutic abortion. Pregnancy with HD is considered as high-risk pregnancy and should be taken care of by a multidisciplinary team involving a cardiologist, an obstetrician, and an anesthesiologist, and maternal cardiac status must be assessed between 28 and 32 weeks. From 32 weeks onward, weekly or biweekly nonstress test and biophysical profile should be done for fetal well-being. Delivery should be taken care of in a tertiary care hospital with support of the cardiac intensive care unit.

LIVER DISORDER IN PREGNANCY

Obstetric cholestasis, acute fatty liver of pregnancy, and HELLP syndrome (hemolytic anemia, elevated liver enzymes, low platelet) are pregnancy-specific liver disorders. Obstetric cholestasis (OC) is clinically manifested by pruritus in the second half of pregnancy with elevated serum bile acid. Increased adverse fetal or neonatal manifestation is associated with raised maternal serum bile acid > 40 µmol/L. Fetal distress, meconium aspiration, and respiratory distress are common fetal effects of OC. Surfactant depletion by bile acid is the hypothesis behind respiratory distress. Ursodeoxycholic acid used for management of OC relieves pruritus, improves liver function of mother, and decreases fetal bile acid level. The protocol of fetal monitoring of a high-risk mother should be followed to prevent stillbirth in OC. Early plan delivery is no more beneficial than spontaneous labor at term in management of OC to avoid stillbirth, which may be complicated with prematurity and respiratory distress.

Acute fatty liver of pregnancy (AFLP) is an uncommon hepatic condition in the third trimester of pregnancy. It is one of the causes of acute liver failure in pregnancy and clinically manifested by nausea, vomiting, abdominal pain, and jaundice. Around half of AFLP mothers have signs of preeclampsia. Presence of hypoglycemia and absence of thrombocytopenia in AFLP distinguish from HELLP syndrome. The pathogenesis of AFLP is recently linked to fetal genetics of fatty oxidation defect. AFLP is associated with high maternal and neonatal mortality. Fetal distress and prematurity are the major complications of AFLP. In a cohort of 55 mothers with AFLP with their 61 babies, 28 (45.4%) cases of fetal distress, 6 (9.4%) cases of fetal death, and 17 (26.4%) cases of neonatal asphyxia are noted.

PREGNANCY WITH NEUROLOGICAL DISORDER

Pregnancy with Epilepsy

Women suffering from epileptic disorder when become pregnant may have increased episodes of seizures in around one third of cases. There is alteration in serum concentration of antiepileptic drugs (AEDs) with physiological changes during pregnancy. Absorption of AED decreases, and its excretion increases during pregnancy. There is an apparent fall in the albumin level during pregnancy due to hemodilution, which exacerbates seizure due to a fall in total or free drug level of AED. A mother with well-controlled epilepsy prior to conception has less chance of seizure deterioration during pregnancy. Episodes of maternal seizure may cause fetal hypoxia and early termination of pregnancy.

TABLE 1: Effect of antiepileptic drugs on fetus.

Common antiepileptic drug	Fetal abnormalities
Phenobarbital	Orofacial clefts, cardiovascular anomaly, impaired cognitive functions, skeletal anomaly
Phenytoin	Fetal hydantoin syndrome, microcephaly, coagulopathies
Valproic acid	Limb defect, spina bifida, facial and cardiac anomalies, cognitive impairment

Exposure of AED during pregnancy may increase the risk of fetal congenital malformations. Use of multiple AEDs and higher serum concentration of AED may increase the teratogenicity. Congenital anomalies due to AED use are called fetal anticonvulsant syndromes (fetal valproate syndrome, fetal hydantoin syndrome), and the adverse effects of AED are listed in **Table 1**. Exposure of AED during pregnancy may cause fetal coagulopathy and manifested as early hemorrhagic disease of newborn (early HDN).

Maternal noncompliance with AED therapy may cause status epilepticus during pregnancy and need proper counseling during antenatal visit. Pregnant women with epilepsy need frequent monitoring of AED serum concentration and dose adjustment to avoid increased seizure frequency. Preferably low-dose monotherapy and AED should be used during pregnancy with epilepsy. Lamotrigine and Levetiracetam are the safest AEDs during pregnancy for the risk of congenital malformation. Valproate should be avoided in reproductive women considering its teratogenicity risk. Initiation of folic acid supplementation from the preconception period may prevent teratogenicity. Epilepsy-aggravating behavior should be avoided during pregnancy.

Total anomaly scan is to be done between 18 and 20 weeks of gestation for early detection of congenital malformation. Maternal vitamin K injection during the last month of pregnancy and neonatal vitamin K IM injection at birth prevent fetal coagulopathy and early HDN.

Pregnancy with Specific Neurometabolic and Neurological Disorders

An increased fetal phenylalanine level in uncontrolled maternal phenylketonuria results in microcephaly, miscarriage, and congenital cardiac malformation.

TABLE 2: Effects of antipsychotic drugs on fetus.	
Antipsychotic drugs	Effect on neonate
Selective serotonin reuptake inhibitor	Congenital heart defects, neonatal withdrawal syndrome, persistent pulmonary hypertension
Lithium	Teratogenic heart defects, Ebstein anomaly

Maternal hyperhomocysteinemia may be complicated with neural tube defect in fetus, and maternal supplementation of folate from the preconception period may prevent it. Some of the neuromuscular disorders in neonates are secondary to maternal diseases. The offspring of a mother with myotonic dystrophy may clinically manifest with neonatal myotonic dystrophy, congenital contractures, and respiratory insufficiency. Transient neonatal myasthenia results from transplacental passage of immunoglobulin to acetylcholine receptor from a mother with myasthenia gravis.

MATERNAL PSYCHIATRIC ILLNESS

Mental disorders in pregnancy have major consequences on maternal and fetal well-being. Mental illness is associated with around 10% pregnant women worldwide. Improper antenatal care and unhealthy lifestyles rather than mental illness of the mother influence the fetal outcome. In two meta-analyses, antenatal depression is associated with an increased risk for premature delivery; however, an increased risk of intrauterine growth restriction in antenatal depression is only noticed in low-middle-income countries. Schizophrenia has been associated with an increased risk of low birthweight, prematurity, stillbirth, and infant mortality. Maternal anorexia nervosa is associated with low birthweight neonates. There is a modest association between maternal anxiety disorder and prematurity. The effects of antipsychotic drugs on the fetus are given in **Table 2**.

The most commonly used antipsychotics in pregnancy, i.e., olanzapine, risperidone, and quetiapine, do not have teratogenicity effect. There is an association between gestational diabetes and antipsychotic in pregnancy. A fetus exposed to in-utero antipsychotic medication developed neonatal withdrawal symptoms and respiratory distress.

RENAL DISORDERS IN PREGNANCY

The physiological changes in the renal system during pregnancy make women prone to urinary tract infection (UTI). UTI including acute pyelonephritis, cystitis, and asymptomatic bacteriuria is the most common infection during pregnancy. Recurrent UTI may lead to preterm labor or preterm prelabor rupture of membrane. Maternal UTI increases the risk of intrauterine growth restriction (IUGR), preeclampsia, cesarean delivery, and preterm birth.

TABLE 3: Effect of immunosuppressive therapy on fetus.	
Immunosuppressive drug in pregnancy	Neonatal adverse effect
Cyclosporine	No teratopathy, usually well tolerated
Steroids	Prolonged use may lead to preterm birth, midfacial defect
Cyclophosphamide, chlorambucil, leflunomide	Should be avoided

Acute renal failure (ARF) during pregnancy is mostly due to secondary causes like preeclampsia, HELLP syndrome, AFLP, thrombotic microangiopathy, hemorrhage, or sepsis. Termination of pregnancy usually reverses the renal damage in some causes. Prematurity is the most common neonatal complication of maternal ARF.

Pregnancy with chronic kidney disease (CKD): Preconception renal function of pregnant women with CKD usually predicts pregnancy outcome. There is a risk of accelerated renal damage in CKD women during pregnancy. Pregnant women with CKD are complicated with anemia, chronic hypertension, vitamin D deficit, and secondary hyperparathyroidism and need renal replacement therapy. The adverse effect of maternal anemia on fetal health can be prevented by supplementation of erythropoietin. Pregnant women with CKD should be planned for termination of pregnancy between 34 and 36 weeks of gestation. Increased pregnancy loss, prematurity, and intrauterine growth restriction are common fetal complications in pregnancy with CKD.

Pregnancy in women with renal transplant: Women with renal transplant are planned for conception, usually 1 year after a successful renal transplant. Continuation of pregnancy beyond the first trimester increases the fetal survival around 95%. Fetal survival is prognosticated by the serum creatinine level of renal transplant mother during pregnancy. Antepartum exposure of immunosuppressive drug may lead to IUGR in the fetus. Chronic hypertension is usually associated with pregnant women with a chronic renal disorder. Monitoring of blood pressure during the antenatal period is most useful. Around half of renal transplant pregnancies are complicated with either preeclampsia, preterm labor, or fetal growth restriction. Immunosuppressive drugs used in renal transplant patients and their effect on newborn are listed in **Table 3**.

CHAPTER 21 | Maternal Systemic Medical Illness and Fetal Effect

CHAPTER AT A GLANCE

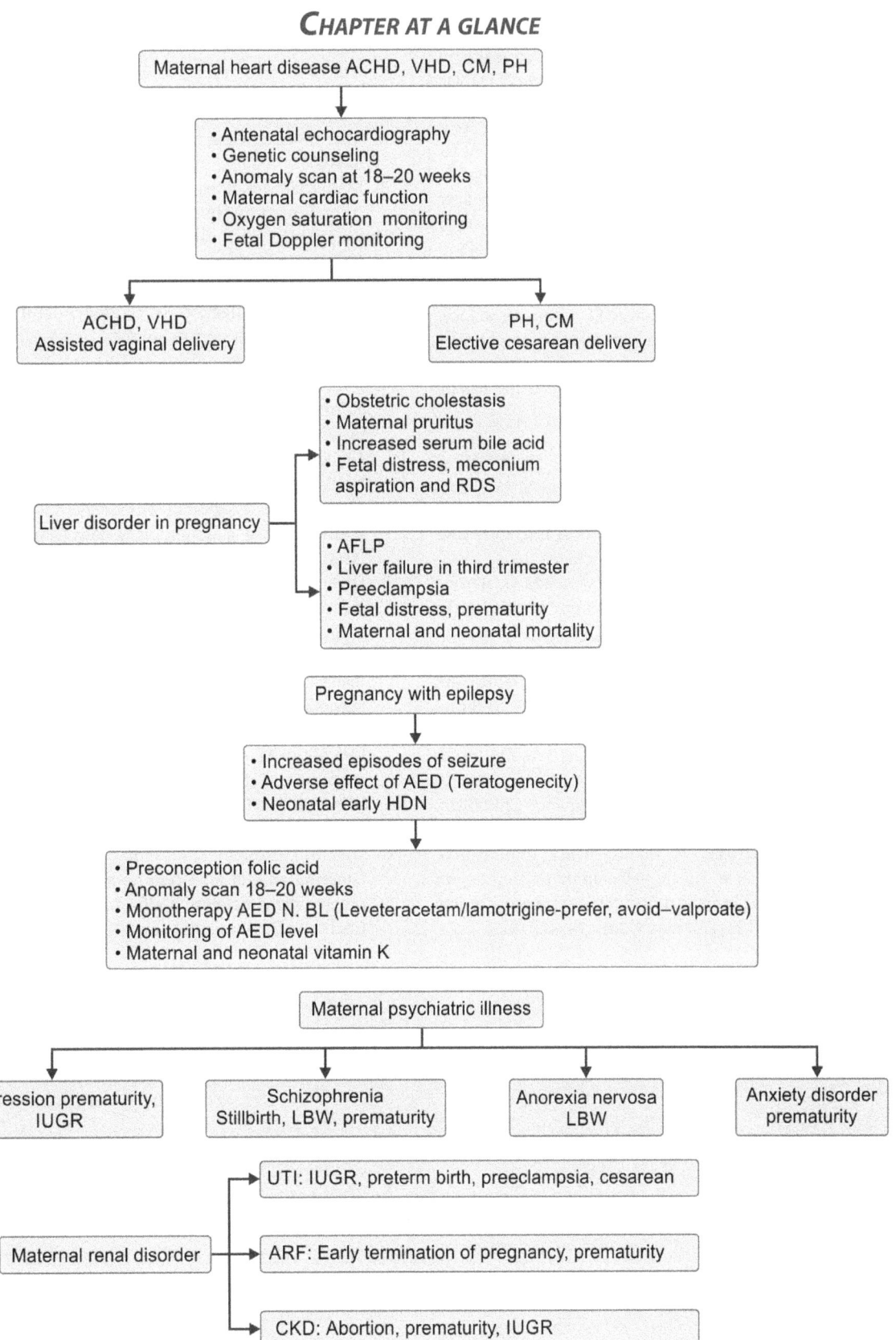

(ACHD: adult congenital heart disease; VHD: valvular heart disease; CM: cardiomyopathy; PH: pulmonary hypertension; AFLP: acute fatty liver of pregnancy; AED: antiepileptic drug; HDN: haemorrhagic disease of newborn; UTI: urinary tract infection; ARF: acute renal failure; CKD: chronic kidney disease ; IUGR: intrauterine growth restriction; LBW: lower birth weight; RDS: respiratory distress syndrome).

KEY POINTS

- Women with heart disease should have preconception echocardiography and frequent monitoring of maternal cardiac function and fetal wellbeing during pregnancy.
- Intrauterine death, prematurity and SGA are adverse fetal outcome among HD mothers.
- Fetal distress, meconium aspiration and respiratory distress are common fetal effect of Obstetric cholestasis. Acute fatty liver of pregnancy is associated with poor maternal and neonatal outcome.
- Seizure episodes increases during pregnancy in women with epilepsy. Some Antiepileptic drugs have teratogenic potential. Leveteracetam and Lamotrigine are safest AED during pregnancy.
- Prematurity and LBW are associated with maternal depression and schizophrenia.
- Urinary tract infection during pregnancy increases the risk of prematurity and IUGR.

SUGGESTED READING

1. Adab N. Therapeutic monitoring of antiepileptic drugs during pregnancy and in the postpartum period: is it useful? CNS Drugs. 2006;20(10):791-800.
2. Bianca I, Geraci G, Gulizia MM, Egidy Assenza G, Barone C, Campisi M, et al. Consensus document of the Italian Association of Hospital Cardiologists (ANMCO), Italian Society of Pediatric Cardiology (SICP), and Italian Society of Gynaecologists and Obstetrics (SIGO): pregnancy and congenital heart diseases. Eur Heart J Suppl. 2017;19(Suppl D):D256-D292.
3. Chang L, Wang M, Liu H, Meng Q, Yu H, Wu YM, et al. Pregnancy outcomes of patients with acute fatty liver of pregnancy: a case control study. BMC Pregnancy Childbirth. 2020;20(1):282.
4. Grigoriadis S, VonderPorten EH, Mamisashvili L, Tomlinson G, Dennis CL, Koren G, et al. The impact of maternal depression during pregnancy on perinatal outcomes: a systematic review and meta-analysis. J Clin Psychiatry. 2013;74:e321-41.2
5. Harden C, Lu C. Epilepsy in pregnancy. Neurol Clin. 2019;37(1):53-62.
6. Hladunewich MA. Chronic kidney disease and pregnancy. Semin Nephrol. 2017;37(4):337-46.
7. Joshi D, James A, Quaglia A, Westbrook RH, Heneghan MA. Liver disease in pregnancy. Lancet. 2010;375(9714):594-605.
8. Matuszkiewicz-Rowińska J, Małyszko J, Wieliczko M. Urinary tract infections in pregnancy: old and new unresolved diagnostic and therapeutic problems. Arch Med Sci. 2015;11(1):67-77.
9. Mazor-Dray E, Levy A, Schlaeffer F, Sheiner E. Maternal urinary tract infection: is it independently associated with adverse pregnancy outcome? J Matern Fetal Neonatal Med. 2009;22(2):124-8.
10. Montagnoli C, Zanconato G, Cinelli G, Tozzi AE, Bovo C, Bortolus R, et al. Maternal mental health and reproductive outcomes: a scoping review of the current literature. Arch Gynecol Obstet. 2020;302(4):801-19.
11. Nevis IF, Reitsma A, Dominic A, McDonald S, Thabane L, Akl EA, et al. Pregnancy outcomes in women with chronic kidney disease: a systematic review. Clin J Am Soc Nephrol. 2011;6(11):2587-98.
12. Owens A, Yang J, Nie L, Lima F, Avila C, Stergiopoulos K. Neonatal and maternal outcomes in pregnant women with cardiac disease. J Am Heart Assoc. 2018;7(21):e009395.
13. Parsonage WA, Zentner D, Lust K, Kane SC, Sullivan EA. Heart disease and pregnancy: the need for a twenty-first century approach to care. Heart Lung Circ. 2021;30(1):45-51.
14. Stein A, Pearson RM, Goodman SH, Rapa E, Rahman A, McCallum M, et al. Effects of perinatal mental disorders on the fetus and child. Lancet. 2014;384(9956):1800-19.
15. Westbrook RH, Dusheiko G, Williamson C. Pregnancy and liver disease. J Hepatol. 2016;64(4):933-45.
16. Weston J, Bromley R, Jackson CF, Adab N, Clayton-Smith J, Greenhalgh J, et al. Monotherapy treatment of epilepsy in pregnancy: congenital malformation outcomes in the child. Cochrane Database Syst Rev. 2016;11(11):CD010224.

SECTION 4
Obstetric Conditions and Fetal/Neonatal Effects

Archana Bilagi, Madhushree Vijayakumar

- **Preterm Labor and Preterm Prelabor Rupture of Membranes**
  Anita Nyamagoudar, Kirti M Hurakadli

- **Antenatal Steroids**
  Viraraghavan Vadakkencherry Ramaswamy, Vandana Hegde, Venkat Reddy Kallem

- **Prenatal Neuroprotective Strategies**
  Rema S Nagpal, Savita N Kamble

- **Antepartum Hemorrhage**
  Ashwini RC, Darshan Hosapatna Basavarajappa

- **Gestosis in Pregnancy**
  Pravin Singarayar, Saudamini Nesargi

- **Oligohydramnios and Polyhydramnios**
  Prathik BH, Ashok Kumar

- **Multiple Pregnancy**
  Anil Kallesh BR, Pruthvi Raj V

- **Bad Obstetric History**
  Kalyan Chakravarthy Balla, Bhagya Lakshmi

- **Chorioamnionitis**
  Deepti Thandaveshwar, KB Suma

Preterm Labor and Preterm Prelabor Rupture of Membranes

Anita Nyamagoudar, Kirti M Hurakadli

INTRODUCTION

Preterm birth is defined as the onset of regular uterine contractions associated with progressive cervical change from the period of viability up to 37 completed weeks of gestation. The incidence of preterm birth has relatively increased over the last two decades in both developed and developing countries. Prevention of preterm birth is the ideal yet elusive approach to prevent short- and long-term complications of prematurity. Pragmatically, identification of high-risk women and appropriate management are the key to better maternal and neonatal outcomes. Preterm prelabor rupture of membranes (PPROM) is defined as spontaneous rupture of the fetal membranes before 37 completed weeks of gestation and before onset of labor. PPROM and/or preterm labor have additional implications for prognostication and effective management of mother–infant dyad.

OBJECTIVES

- To discuss the etiology/pathways of preterm birth.
- To discuss the management of preterm labor and PPROM.
- To discuss the role of antenatal steroids, antimicrobials, tocolytics, and magnesium sulfate in preterm pregnancy.
- To discuss the most feasible preventive strategies for preterm birth.

PRETERM LABOR

Four Direct Causes of Preterm Birth

- Spontaneous unexplained preterm labor with intact membranes (40–50%)
- Idiopathic PPROM (20–30%)
- Maternal or fetal indications for preterm delivery (20–30%)
- Multifetal births

Though preterm birth resembles term birth in terms of cervical ripening/effacement and myometrial activation, preterm birth is not always an acceleration of normal process of labor. The various pathways of preterm labor are uterine distension, maternal–fetal stress, premature cervical changes, and infection. The most important risk factor for preterm delivery is prior history of preterm labor; hence, the timing of delivery cannot be reliably predicted in a primigravida.

Contributing Factors for Preterm Labor

- *Pregnancy factors*: Threatened abortion in early pregnancy, antepartum hemorrhage, fetal birth defects.
- *Lifestyle factors*: Extremes of maternal weight [low body mass index (BMI) <18 kg/m^2] and age (<17 years, >35 years), poverty, short stature, vitamin C deficiency, vitamin D deficiency, vitamin B$_{12}$ deficiency, maternal stress and cigarette smoking, manual labor > 8–10 hours/day.
- *Genetic factors*: Recurrent, familial, and racial nature of preterm birth.
- *Periodontal disease*: Showed significant association with preterm birth; treatment of the same does not prevent preterm births.
- *Interval between pregnancies*: Intervals of <18 and >59 months between pregnancies may be associated with preterm birth.
- *Prior preterm birth*: It increases risk of subsequent preterm birth by 3 times.
- *Infection*: Bacterial vaginosis: Increases the risk of preterm labor due to altered vaginal flora. However, treatment of the same does not reduce or prevent preterm birth. Asymptomatic bacteriuria, urinary tract infection (UTI), pyelonephritis, and malaria are also known risk factors.

Symptoms and Early Diagnosis of Preterm Labor

Uterine contractions associated with any of the other symptoms like pelvic pressure, menstrual-like cramps, watery vaginal discharge, and lower back pain suggest impending preterm birth.

Asymptomatic cervical dilation after midpregnancy may be associated with preterm birth. Though it could be a normal variant as well, the detection of cervical dilation does not improve pregnancy outcomes.

Fetal fibronectin: Though it indicates stromal remodeling of cervix, it has not been shown to improve perinatal outcomes when used as a screening tool for preterm labor.

Cervical length measurements: Shortening cervical canal with advancing gestation predisposes to preterm labor. This parameter is reliable in singleton pregnancies and is not applicable in multifetal gestation. Prior spontaneous preterm birth is one indication for monitoring cervical length measurements.

In clinical practice, identification of a woman with high risk for preterm labor is mainly based on obstetric history and management is predominantly related to treatment of bacterial vaginosis (if present) and two preventive interventions, namely cervical cerclage and vaginal progesterone.

Prevention of Preterm Birth

- *Cervical cerclage:* Instances when cervical cerclage is offered as an option are:
  - Women with mid-trimester pregnancy loss and diagnosed to have cervical incompetence.
  - Short cervix noted on sonological exam.

  "Rescue" cerclage is done when cervical incompetence is associated with impending preterm labor [contraindicated in antepartum hemorrhage (APH), chorioamnionitis, and active uterine contractions].

  The American College of Obstetricians and Gynecologists (ACOG) concludes that cervical cerclage may be considered in a woman with singleton pregnancy <24 weeks gestation with a prior spontaneous preterm birth at less than 34 weeks and has a cervical length <25 mm.

- *Progestogen compounds prophylaxis*: Progestogen compound has been found to reduce preterm labor by 30%. At present, progestogen compounds are recommended in women with singleton pregnancy who have a short cervix (<25 mm by transvaginal ultrasound between 16 and 24 weeks) with or without history of prior preterm birth.

  17-hydroxyprogesterone caproate is the first and the only drug approved by the Food and Drug Administration (FDA) for prevention of recurrent preterm labor in women with previous preterm delivery. This is the preferred therapy in women with history of preterm labor, with or without a short cervix. The dose is 250 mg IM weekly from 16 to 36 weeks' gestational age.

  In primigravidae women with short cervix, vaginal micronized progesterone 200 mg is recommended to be inserted daily at night until 36 weeks of gestation.

PPROM

Major Causes

Intrauterine infection, oxidative stress-induced DNA damage, and premature cellular senescence are the major predisposing factors. Lower socioeconomic status, lower BMI, nutritional deficits, and cigarette smoking are risk factors for PPROM. The risk of PPROM during the next pregnancy increases with history of PPROM in the present pregnancy. Chorioamnionitis and placental abruption pose additional risks. Neonatal problems associated with PPROM include prematurity, sepsis, cord prolapse, and pulmonary hypoplasia.

Diagnosis of PPROM

- History of per vaginal leak (either as a continuous stream or as a gush)
- Sterile speculum examination showing gross vaginal pooling of amniotic fluid or clear fluid from cervical canal or both.

Digital vaginal examination should be avoided when PPROM is suspected. If amniotic fluid is not visible on speculum examination, vaginal fluid may be tested for insulin-like growth factor binding protein-I (IGFBP-I) or placental alpha microglobulin I (PAMG-I).

The diagnosis of PPROM is accompanied by sonographic examination to assess amniotic fluid volume, identify presenting part, and to estimate gestational age.

The interval between PPROM to delivery is inversely proportional to the gestational age at which membranes rupture. The median time to delivery after PPROM is 7 days.

Intent for Delivery

Gestational age is an important determining factor of timing of delivery in case of PPROM. Expectant management is recommended in the absence of nonreassuring fetal status, clinical chorioamnionitis, or placental abruption. Expectant management can be offered until 37 completed weeks. However, timing of delivery should be individualized for each woman based on patient preference and ongoing clinical assessment.

Clinical Chorioamnionitis

Chorioamnionitis has many implications on maternal and newborn health like maternal sepsis, stillbirth, premature birth, neonatal sepsis, respiratory distress syndrome, chronic lung disease, and necrotizing enterocolitis.

The diagnosis of subclinical chorioamnionitis is challenging. Suggested risk factors are low parity, multiple digital vaginal examinations, use of internal fetal and uterine monitors, meconium-stained liquor, and presence of certain genital pathogens. Presence of chorioamnionitis is an indication for delivery.

A reliable indicator of clinical chorioamnionitis is maternal fever. Offensive vaginal discharge and fetal tachycardia are other indicators. Maternal leukocytosis is not a consistent finding in chorioamnionitis.

Overall, a combination of clinical assessment, maternal blood tests [leukocytosis and raised C-reactive protein (CRP)], and fetal tachycardia assessed by cardiotocography are used to diagnose chorioamnionitis in PPROM. Fetal tachycardia is usually a late indicator of infection. Abnormal biophysical profile (especially if absent breathing) and umbilical artery Doppler abnormalities are evaluated as tools of diagnosis of chorioamnionitis but have poor clinical correlation. High vaginal swabs (HVS) taken in suspected cases may be useful to guide antimicrobial therapy.

In 2015, the National Institute of Child Health and Human Development (NICHD) recommended to replace the term "chorioamnionitis" with "Triple I (*I*ntrauterine *I*nflammation, *I*nfection, or both)." The NICHD also recommended that antibiotics be given only for those meeting "Triple I" criteria. The ACOG guidelines (2017) stated that antibiotics should be considered in the setting of isolated maternal fever (maternal temperature between 38 and 38.9°C) unless a source other than intra-amniotic infection is identified and documented. However, there are ongoing studies that are evaluating the optimal utilization of antibiotics in this regard.

Women with PPROM, when cared for as outpatients, should be advised about symptoms of chorioamnionitis (fever, malaise, lower abdominal pain, abnormal vaginal discharge, and reduced fetal movements). They should be reviewed at least one to two times per week. They should be given an opportunity to discuss newborn care with the neonatologist.

Management of PPROM

Management of women with PPROM includes expectant management, steroids, magnesium, tocolysis, and antibiotics **(Table 1)**.

Antimicrobial Therapy

Antibiotics are recommended for women with PPROM and who are <$34^{0/7}$ weeks of gestation. They have been found to prolong pregnancy by >7 days and to reduce neonatal morbidities such as infection. However, there is no clear recommendation for the choice of antibiotics. Recommendations include erythromycin (WHO) and azithromycin/ampicillin combination.

Use of erythromycin is associated with improved outcomes like prolongation of pregnancy, reduced need for surfactant and oxygen, and fewer cerebral abnormalities on ultrasound (Oracle I RCT). Use of co-amoxiclav alone or in combination with erythromycin results in prolongation of pregnancy but is not associated with improved neonatal outcomes. Use of co-amoxiclav is associated with a higher rate of neonatal necrotizing enterocolitis. Hence, co-amoxiclav is not recommended in women with PPROM.

A HVS is recommended to be taken for culture which may potentially help to identify the causative organism. Periodic auditing of HVS reports may help in making policies regarding choice of antibiotics.

Antenatal Steroids

A single course of antenatal steroids is advised for women with PPROM from $24^{0/7}$ to $33^{6/7}$ weeks of gestation. Steroids could be considered as early as $23^{0/7}$ weeks of gestation with ruptured membranes if the delivery appears imminent in the

TABLE 1: Management of preterm prelabor rupture of membranes.

Gestation	Management
34 weeks or more	• Plan delivery, labor induction if no contraindication • Antenatal corticosteroid course may be considered up to $36^{6/7}$ weeks
32 weeks to 33 completed weeks	• Expectant management • Antenatal corticosteroid course • Antimicrobials to prolong latency
24 weeks to 31 completed weeks	• Expectant management • Antenatal corticosteroid course • *Tocolytics*: No consensus • Antimicrobials to prolong latency • MgSO$_4$ for neuroprotection recommended for $24^{0/6}$ to $29^{6/7}$ weeks* • Consider MgSO$_4$ for neuroprotection ($30^{0/6}$ to $31^{6/7}$ weeks)
<24 weeks	• Expectant management • Antenatal corticosteroid course (from $23^{0/7}$ weeks onward) • *Tocolytics*: No consensus • Antimicrobials to prolong latency

*MgSO$_4$ injection should be administered in case of established preterm labor or in a woman having a planned preterm birth within the next 24 hours.

TABLE 2: Antenatal corticosteroids.		
	Betamethasone	**Dexamethasone**
Dose	12 mg	6 mg
Route	IM	IM
Number	2 doses	4 doses
Timing	24 hours apart	Every 12 hours

(IM: intramuscular)

next 7 days. Controversies surround the use of steroids during late premature gestation. Steroids do not interfere with the diagnosis of chorioamnionitis when given in women with PPROM. Delivery occurring 24 hours and within 7 days after the last dose of steroid course will confer optimal benefit to the baby (**Table 2**).

Magnesium Sulfate

See Section "Magnesium Sulfate Therapy for Neuroprotection."

Tocolysis

Prophylactic tocolysis is not recommended in women with PPROM with no uterine activity.

Consider tocolysis in women with PPROM and uterine activity who need intrauterine transport or need time for antenatal steroids to act.

MANAGEMENT OF PRETERM LABOR WITH INTACT MEMBRANES

Differentiation of true and false labor may be difficult during preterm labor. However, association of regular uterine contractions with cervical changes helps diagnose preterm labor. Although amniocentesis can confirm the presence of intra-amniotic infection, utility of this test is limited considering the practical challenges.

Management of preterm labor involves:
- Establishing cause of premature onset of labor
- Ensuring delivery with appropriate care
- Evaluation of advantages and disadvantages of delaying delivery to increase gestational age
- Medications to optimize neonatal outcome (steroids, magnesium, tocolytics, antibiotics)

Corticosteroids for Fetal Lung Maturation

The ACOG recommends a single course of corticosteroids (betamethasone or dexamethasone) for women between $24^{0/7}$ and $33^{6/7}$ weeks of gestation who are at risk for delivery within the next 7 days. A single course of steroids may be considered for women starting from $23^{0/7}$ weeks of gestation with risk of delivery in the next 7 days.

The ACOG recommends considering the administration of betamethasone for women between $34^{0/7}$ and $36^{6/7}$ weeks (late preterm) at risk of preterm birth within the next 7 days and who have not previously received a course of antenatal steroids. However, there are short- and long-term implications on newborn health, especially in developing countries. It was found that antenatal steroids for late preterm deliveries increased the risk of neonatal hypoglycemia. In addition, although betamethasone was found to reduce the risk of transient tachypnea of newborn (TTNB), TTNB is a self-limiting condition. Hence, the use of antenatal steroids for late preterm deliveries has not been in uniform practice.

The Government of India guidelines recommend dexamethasone usage as it is available as an emergency drug even at primary health centers. Betamethasone acetate phosphate is not easily available in India. Betamethasone phosphate is available which is similar to dexamethasone with its short half-life and has no added advantage as compared to dexamethasone.

Rescue Therapy

Administration of an additional single dose of betamethasone may be considered when the delivery is imminent and more than 14 days have passed since the initial course of steroids and the gestation is still <34 weeks. It may also be considered in extreme preterm deliveries (<28 weeks' gestational age) if the initial course has been given more than 7 days ago. The effects of rescue therapy beyond 34 weeks are not known at present.

Repeated course of steroids is not advocated due to the risk of demyelination and cerebral palsy in the neonate.

Magnesium Sulfate Therapy for Neuroprotection

Magnesium sulfate therapy is given before early preterm delivery has been shown to reduce the incidence and severity of cerebral palsy.

Indication: Women with imminent preterm birth (<24 hours) due to PPROM or spontaneous onset preterm labor or obstetric/medical indication for delivery.

Gestational age: 24 weeks–32 completed weeks

Contraindications: Maternal myasthenia gravis, cardiac conduction defects, myocardial compromise, renal injury.

Dose: 4 g loading dose intravenously over 20 minutes followed by 1 g/h infusion for a maximum of 24 hours or until delivery, whichever comes earlier.

Antimicrobials

Antibiotics should not be routinely prescribed for women with spontaneous preterm labor with intact membranes and with no evidence of infection (ORACLE II trial). Antibiotics are recommended only if there is obvious evidence of infection or UTI.

TABLE 3: Tocolytic agents.

Tocolytic agent	Dose	Side-effects
Nifedipine	30 mg per oral followed by 20 mg followed by 10 mg 20 minutes apart with preloading fluids and 10–20 mg twice daily for 3 days	Headache, flushing, dizziness, nausea, transient hypotension
Magnesium sulfate	4 g IV bolus over 20 minutes followed by 2 g/h infusion	Flushing, headache, weakness, pulmonary edema, cardiac arrest. Neonatal: Lethargy, hypotonia, respiratory depression
Terbutaline	0.25 mg SC every 20 minutes for 3 hours	Arrhythmias
Indomethacin	50 mg oral followed by 25 mg twice daily for 48 hours	Nausea, severe neonatal side effects
Atosiban	6.75 mg IV bolus over 1 minute followed by infusion of 18 mg/h for 3 hours and then 6 mg/h for a maximum of 45 hours	Nausea, headache, vomiting

Studies have shown a higher incidence of cerebral palsy at 7 years of age in the group with fetal exposure to antimicrobials as compared to the group without fetal exposure.

Emergency or Rescue Cerclage

It is believed that cervical incompetence and preterm delivery are a part of continuum of events and hence, rescue cervical cerclage was evaluated as a preventive strategy. However, this practice needs to be done after appropriate counseling in women who have had poor pregnancy outcomes due to cervical incompetence in midgestation. This intervention can increase the risk of membrane rupture and intra-amniotic infection.

Tocolysis to Treat Preterm Labor

Tocolytic agents do not markedly prolong gestation but may delay delivery in some women for at least 48 hours. Tocolysis is mainly utilized in the context of transport of women to a center with better obstetric and neonatal care facilities and also to allow time for antenatal steroids to act. There is no evidence of any other major benefits with the use of tocolytics. Various agents have been tried as tocolytics for short-term effects. Maintenance tocolytic therapy after acute therapy has not shown any benefits and hence is not advised. Tocolytics are not recommended beyond 34 weeks of gestation as the pregnancy outcomes are generally good beyond late prematurity. Nifedipine and betamimetics should be avoided when magnesium sulfate is being given to avoid maternal side effects (**Table 3**).

DELIVERY

Delivery should be conducted in a tertiary care center with good neonatal care facilities; otherwise in-utero transfer to a tertiary care center is strongly recommended. Antenatal counseling by the NICU team is recommended before delivery. Continuous fetal heart monitoring is preferred in labor. Antibiotic prophylaxis should be considered if there is PPROM, evidence of chorioamnionitis, or UTI. Epidural analgesia may be offered for pain relief. One should not use fetal scalp electrode or do fetal blood sampling in preterm babies <34 weeks gestation. There is no role of routine episiotomy or forceps delivery. Vacuum should be avoided as it is associated with a high risk of intracranial bleed. Preferred mode of delivery is vaginal. Cesarean should be considered only for obstetric indications as studies have not shown an increased neonatal survival with cesarean as compared to vaginal delivery.

Limits of Viability

Most countries have their own guidelines for limits of viability. With advances in neonatology, the limits of viability have been lowered further. At present, considering the ACOG guidelines for antenatal steroids, the discussion of administration of steroids has been up to the gestational age of 24 weeks. However, at 23 weeks of gestation, discussion with parents regarding continuation of care, resuscitative efforts, and future implications of extreme prematurity should take place.

Whenever previability is complicated by PPROM or preterm labor, the first step is to confirm the gestational age. The best estimate of gestational age is a combination of last menstrual period (LMP) and the earliest available antenatal ultrasound scan. The risks of expectant management of PPROM at previability include chorioamnionitis, stillbirth, and umbilical cord compromise. The optimal method of delivery is based on patient factors such as gestational age, amnionitis, and prior caesarean. The pregnancy needs to be monitored for infection and abruption. Sonographic monitoring for persistent oligohydramnios and fetal growth should continue. Data on use of antimicrobials are not adequate.

SECTION 4 | Obstetric Conditions and Fetal/Neonatal Effects

CHAPTER AT A GLANCE

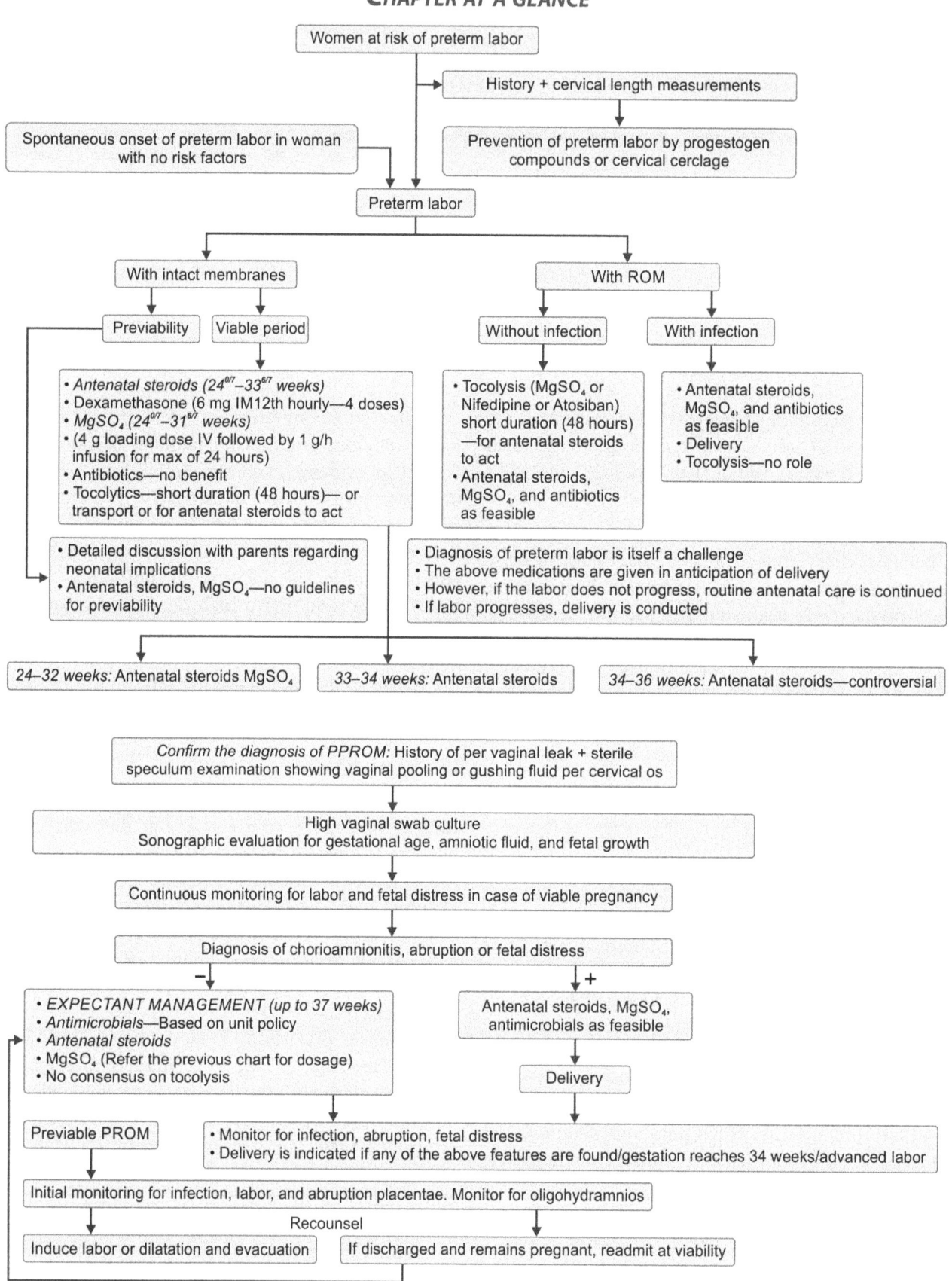

(PPROM: preterm prelabor rupture of membranes; IM: intramuscular)

KEY POINTS

- Preterm birth is multifactorial in causation. It carries a high risk of neonatal morbidity and mortality.
- The best possible prevention is to identify high-risk women. Treat bacterial vaginosis if present. Cervical cerclage and progestogens are used to prolong pregnancy.
- Established preterm labor needs careful management and decision-making to weigh the benefits over harm of prolonging the pregnancy. Delivery is indicated in case of amnionitis, abruption, and fetal compromise.
- Antenatal steroids, magnesium sulfate, and antimicrobials as indicated are beneficial in preterm labor and/or PPROM. There is no consensus on tocolysis.
- Antimicrobial therapy for PPROM with preterm labor has shown benefits. Antibiotics are not found to be useful in preterm labor with intact membranes.
- Women with PPROM beyond 24 weeks of gestation and who have no contraindications to continue pregnancy should be offered expectant management up to 37 weeks. Timing of birth should be individualized based on clinical scenario.

SUGGESTED READING

1. American College of Obstetricians and Gynaecologists Committee Opinion Number 713. Antenatal corticosteroid therapy for fetal maturation, August 2017. Obstet Gynecol. 2017;130:493-4.
2. American College of Obstetricians and Gynaecologists' Committee on practice bulletins – Obstetrics. Practice Bulletin No. 171: Management of preterm labour. Obstet Gynecol. 2016;128(4):e155-64.
3. Gibson KS, Brackney K. Periviable premature rupture of membranes. Obstet Gynecol Clin North Am. 2020;47(4):633-51.
4. Investigators of the Delhi Neonatal Infection Study Collaboration. Characterisation and antimicrobial resistance of sepsis pathogens in neonates born in tertiary care centres in Delhi, India: a cohort study. Lancet Glob Health. 2016;4:e752-60.
5. Magee LW, Silva DD, Diane Sawchuck RN, Synnes A, Dadelszen PV. Magnesium sulfate for fetal neuroprotection. SOGC Clin. Pract. Guideline. 2019;41(4):505-22.
6. Operational Guidelines for Use of Antenatal Corticosteroids in Preterm Labor (under specific conditions by ANM). Ministry of Health and Family Welfare. Government of India: 2014.

Antenatal Steroids

Viraraghavan Vadakkencherry Ramaswamy, Vandana Hegde, Venkat Reddy Kallem

INTRODUCTION

Antenatal corticosteroids (ACS) are one of the cornerstone strategies utilized in obstetric medicine in the management of anticipated preterm births. They act synergistically along with postnatal surfactant therapy in improving the outcomes of preterm neonates with respiratory distress syndrome (RDS) and have had a domino effect in ensuring morbidity-free survival of these infants since the past three decades. Despite decades of extensive research, there still exists a substantial knowledge gap related to ACS use and is often reflected in the differing recommendations put forth by the various national or international advisory bodies.

OBJECTIVES

- Historical perspective and evolution of practices related to ACS use
- Mechanism of action of ACS
- Dosing regimens and benefits of ACS in preterm births between $24^{0/7}$ and $33^{6/7}$ weeks
- Specific scenarios related to ACS in preterm births between $24^{0/7}$ and $33^{6/7}$ weeks
- Controversies and specific scenarios related to ACS in other preterm and term births
- Evidence on long-term risks of ACS
- Use of ACS in the Indian scenario
- Evidence gaps and future research avenues related to ACS

HISTORICAL PERSPECTIVE AND EVOLUTION OF PRACTICES RELATED TO ANTENATAL CORTICOSTEROIDS

Liggins and Howie in the follow-up to their animal research in premature lambs published their breakthrough work which was the first randomized controlled trial (RCT) of ACS in human subjects in 1969. It is an amusing fact that the dosing regimen of betamethasone phosphate/acetate used by them is still being continued in clinical practice. It took a mammoth two decades after their RCT that the medical fraternity came to a consensus accepting the beneficial effects of ACS for preterm births. Subsequently, the Royal College of Obstetricians and Gynaecologists (RCOG) in 1992 and the National Institute of Health (NIH) consensus conference in 1994 endorsed the use of ACS in anticipated preterm labor, basing their recommendation on meta-analyses of other RCTs published in the prior years. Thereafter, the RCOG in 2010 and American College of Obstetricians and Gynecologists (ACOG) in 2011 recommended the use of a rescue course of ACS in anticipated preterm births in mothers who had received a single course prior which was based on the best available evidence then. In sync with the rapidly expanding evidence on other areas of ACS use, the past decade has seen a flurry of new recommendations from many of these advisory bodies on different aspects of ACS use such as in periviable births, late preterm (LPT), and early term births. With many of the questions related to ACS still being contested and with many large multicentric RCTs on contentious topics ongoing, there might be many more changes in the existing recommendations.

MECHANISM OF ACTION OF ANTENATAL CORTICOSTEROIDS

Accelerating Lung Maturity

Antenatal corticosteroids have got several structural and biochemical effects on the developing fetal lung. The predominant effect is postulated to be due to its action on maturation of type II pneumocytes which appear during the saccular stage of lung development between 24 and 28 weeks of gestation and contain the precursors for surfactant. There are other presumed effects including decreased protein extravasation from the pulmonary vasculature into the alveoli, thinning of the mesenchyme of the alveolar-capillary structure promoting efficient gas exchange, and improving postnatal surfactant response by decreasing its clearance. ACS in LPT births act through a different mechanism where they increase the expression of sodium channels in the alveolar epithelium that are important in clearing the excessive fluid from the alveolar space into the interstitium.

Other Organ-specific Actions

The mechanism of action of ACS on other organ systems including the brain and the gut translating into better clinical outcomes of reduced risk of intraventricular hemorrhage (IVH) and necrotizing enterocolitis (NEC) is yet to be deciphered. In the rabbit models, ACS is postulated to decrease the vascular endothelial growth factor (VEGF) which is involved in angiogenesis (increases vascular fragility and risk of bleeding) in the germinal matrix area, thereby decreasing the risk of IVH. By accelerating the maturation of intestinal mucosal barrier, ACS is known to be effective in decreasing the risk of NEC. The mechanism of action of ACS on the various organ systems in the fetus is depicted in **Figure 1**.

DOSING REGIMENS AND BENEFITS OF ANTENATAL CORTICOSTEROIDS IN PRETERM BIRTHS BETWEEN $24^{0/7}$ AND $33^{6/7}$ WEEKS

Dosing Regimens of Antenatal Corticosteroids

- *Types of ACS, dosing regimens for single course*: The two commonly used ACS are dexamethasone sodium phosphate and betamethasone acetate/phosphate mixture. Both are fluorinated synthetic drugs with a high affinity toward the glucocorticoid receptors with minimal mineralocorticoid activity. While dexamethasone is administered intramuscularly at a dose of 6 mg at a 12-hourly interval for four doses, betamethasone mixture is given at 12 mg intramuscular dosage at a 24-hourly interval for two doses. There are not enough studies comparing different dosing regimens of either dexamethasone or betamethasone. The results of BETADOSE trial, a large multicentric RCT

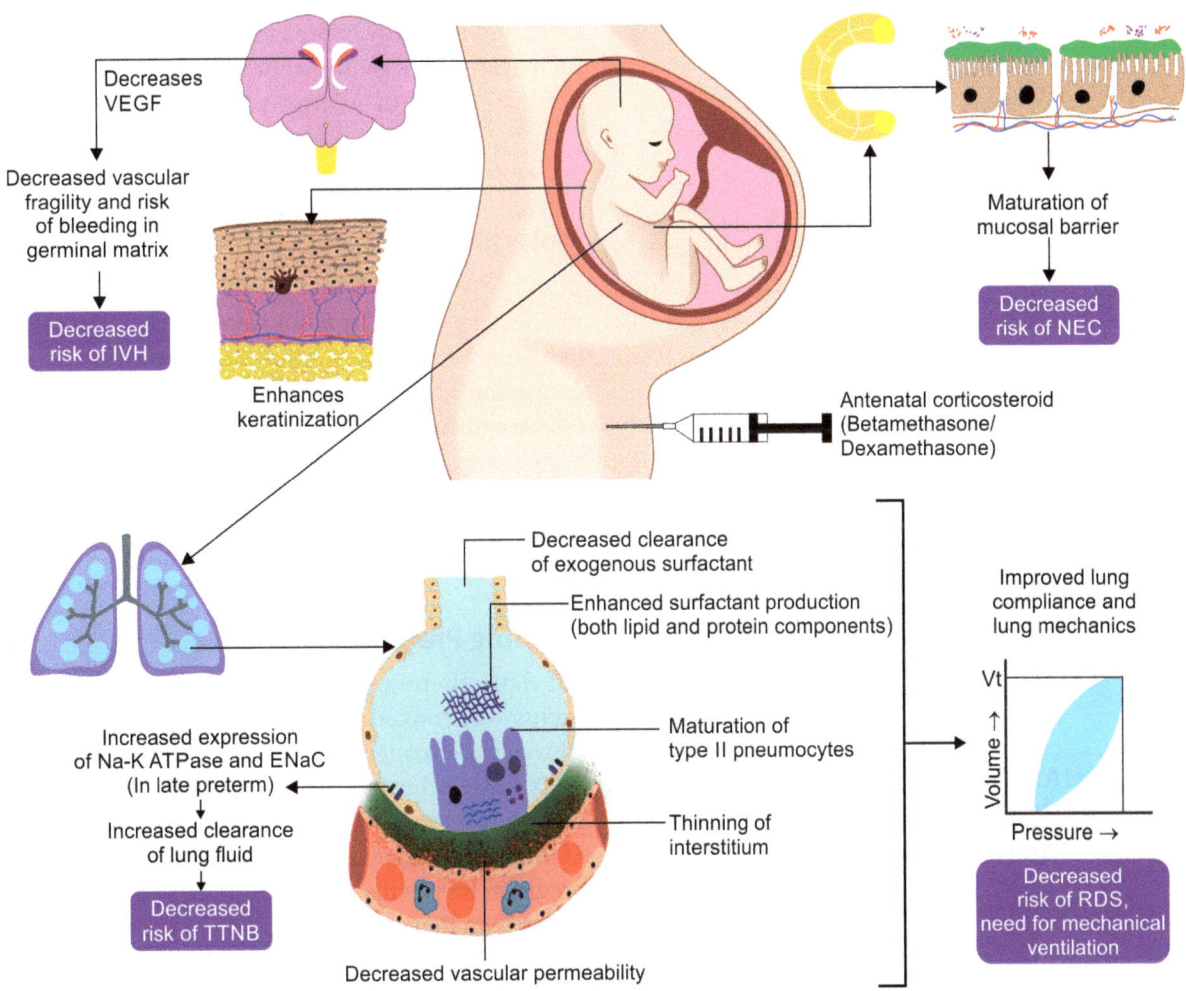

Fig. 1: Mechanism of action of antenatal corticosteroids on the fetus.
(IVH: intraventricular hemorrhage; NEC: necrotizing enterocolitis; RDS: respiratory distress syndrome; VEGF: vascular endothelial growth factor; TTNB: transient tachypnea of newborn)

evaluating a low dose of betamethasone compared to the currently used dosing regimen, is awaited. Though there have been studies questioning the safety profile of dexamethasone in relation to its association with chorioamnionitis and sepsis in mother, and IVH in preterm neonates when compared to the betamethasone mixture, none are conclusive. A large RCT is underway comparing these two drugs and the results of this study might add further insights into this subject. With the best available current evidence, both the drugs are considered to be equally efficacious with a similar safety profile.

- *Rescue course of ACS*: Evidence from meta-analysis of RCTs indicates that a single rescue course of ACS results in beneficial neonatal outcomes. These include decreased risk of RDS and composite serious neonatal outcomes. Hence, most of the advisory bodies recommend it in mothers who are at less than $34^{0/7}$ weeks, had received one course of ACS 7–14 days prior (WHO: 7 days, ACOG: 14 days), and are judged to be at risk of delivering in the next 7 days. The dose regimen is same as used for the first course.

Benefits of Antenatal Corticosteroids between $24^{0/7}$ and $33^{6/7}$ Weeks

The benefits of ACS use in pregnancies between $24^{0/7}$ and $33^{6/7}$ weeks of gestation are proven beyond doubt in this subgroup of preterm births and have become a staple component along with the other interventions used in preterm births. The best window of delivery is between 1 and 7 days following the last dose of the course.

Systematic reviews and meta-analyses have uniformly reported that ACS use results in decreased risk of RDS of varying severity, requirement of invasive mechanical ventilation, IVH, NEC, sepsis in the first 48 hours of life, and neonatal mortality. These studies have also shown no increased risk of maternal sepsis or chorioamnionitis with ACS. Published research has shown no long-term neurodevelopmental harm related to ACS exposure in the fetal period.

SPECIFIC SCENARIOS RELATED TO ANTENATAL CORTICOSTEROIDS IN PRETERM BIRTHS BETWEEN $24^{0/7}$ AND $33^{6/7}$ WEEKS

Scheduled or Serial Weekly Courses of Antenatal Corticosteroids

Scheduled or serial doses are different from rescue doses. Scheduled doses are given weekly even if the mother is not anticipated to deliver in the near future. Studies on scheduled doses have indicated that it increases the risk of maternal sepsis, suppresses the hypothalamic-pituitary-adrenal axis, decreases fetal birthweight, increases the risk of growth restriction, attention deficit hyperactivity disorder and cerebral palsy. Because of the possibility of harm, most guidelines uniformly advice against serial or scheduled weekly ACS doses.

Partial Courses of Antenatal Corticosteroids

Some studies have indicated beneficial effects of ACS even if the preterm birth happens within 24 hours of the first dose in the form of decreased neonatal mortality and morbidities. So, the first dose of ACS may be given even if it is anticipated that delivery might happen even before the completion of the course.

Prelabor Premature Rupture of Membranes

A single course of ACS is recommended as it has been shown to be associated with a decreased risk of RDS, IVH, NEC, and mortality in the neonates. Studies have shown no increased risk of maternal or neonatal infection. However, a rescue dose of ACS in preterm prelabor rupture of membranes (PPROM) is a subject of controversy and there is no international consensus.

Maternal Chorioamnionitis

In the setting of clinical chorioamnionitis, delivery should not be delayed for the administration of ACS. Meta-analysis of observational studies indicates that ACS use in clinical chorioamnionitis is not associated with any clear benefits for the neonate. Chorioamnionitis may alter the endogenous corticosteroid response in the fetus and hence may alter the effect of ACS. However, ACS has been shown to decrease neonatal mortality and morbidity in the setting of histological chorioamnionitis.

Multiple Pregnancy

Till date, there are no large multicentric RCT that has exclusively looked at ACS use in multiple pregnancies. However, retrospective studies and subgroup analysis of RCTs have indicated beneficial effects of ACS in multiple pregnancies as well. However, the advantageous effect of ACS in improving neonatal outcomes in multiple pregnancies seems to wane off after a period of 7 days (more than that observed in singleton pregnancies). So, it is more so important in multiple pregnancies than singleton pregnancies that delivery happens in the 1–7-day window after the first course of ACS.

With the best available evidence as of present, it is suggested that multiple pregnancies irrespective of the number of fetuses also receive ACS in the same dosing schedule as used for singletons. Single rescue course may be given as early as 7 days after the prior course instead of the usual 14-day time-gap suggested for singleton pregnancies. This is based on the aforementioned hypothesis that the therapeutic effect of ACS in twin pregnancies wanes off rapidly after 7 days of the first course.

Fetal Growth Restriction

Results of large cohort studies indicate that ACS use in the presence of fetal growth restriction (FGR) results in improved neonatal outcomes including decreased neonatal mortality, RDS, IVH as well as improved neurodevelopmental outcomes at 2 years. Hence, FGR is not a contraindication for ACS therapy.

Severe Preeclampsia/HELLP Syndrome

Antenatal corticosteroids has been studied well in HELLP (hemolysis, elevated liver enzymes, low platelet count) syndrome but not that extensively in severe preeclampsia and not at all in eclampsia. Studies have shown beneficial effects in neonates with no additional maternal harm when used in severe preeclampsia and HELLP syndrome. Hence, ACS could be used in severe preeclampsia and HELLP syndrome.

Gestational Diabetes Mellitus

Pregnancies complicated by gestational diabetes mellitus (GDM) have not been included in any of the large RCTs on ACS till date. Clinicians should be prepared to manage the increased blood glucose levels that usually happen 12 hours after starting ACS and can persist till 5 days after the completion of the course. Though there is no uniform protocol for management of ACS-induced derangement in glycemic profiles in GDM mothers, there is a uniform consensus that it should be managed with increased dosage of insulin. GDM pregnancies are also candidates for ACS with the dosage being similar to that used in other pregnancies.

CONTROVERSIES AND SPECIFIC SCENARIOS RELATED TO ANTENATAL CORTICOSTEROIDS IN OTHER PRETERM AND TERM BIRTHS

Use of Antenatal Corticosteroids in Preterm Births between $22^{0/7}$ and $23^{6/7}$ Weeks

With increasing survival of neonates born at threshold of viability, especially those born at $22^{0/7}$-$23^{6/7}$ weeks, the use of ACS in this subgroup has also been discussed extensively. A large cohort study from the National Institute of Child health and Development (NICHD) indicated that ACS exposure in $23^{0/7}$-$23^{6/7}$ weeks' births decreases the risk of death or neurodevelopmental impairment at 2 years' corrected age. However, such beneficial effects were not seen in $22^{0/7}$-$22^{6/7}$ weeks. Hence, ACS is advocated in preterm birth between $23^{0/7}$ and $23^{6/7}$ weeks, but after discussing with the family regarding the plans for postnatal resuscitation and type of care for such infants.

Use of Antenatal Corticosteroids in Late Preterm Births ($34^{0/7}$-$36^{6/7}$ Weeks)

Antenatal corticosteroids use in LPT births have been associated with a decreased risk of combined respiratory morbidity including RDS, transient tachypnea of newborn (TTNB), requirement of surfactant, and need for respiratory support. There is no international consensus on the use of ACS in LPT births. While ACOG, RCOG, and the Society for Maternal Fetal medicine recommend a single course of ACS in LPT births who are adjudged to deliver within the next 7 days, the WHO and New Zealand and Australian guidelines do not. The differing recommendations have their basis on the possible harm of increased risk of neonatal hypoglycemia as reported in the largest RCT [Antenatal Late Preterm Steroids (ALPS) trial] conducted till date. Neonatal hypoglycemia seen in LPT infants exposed to ACS in this trial were not associated with hypoglycemia-related adverse events. In line with the excluded population from this RCT, ACS may not be used in mothers with imminent LPT births as rescue course, who are complicated with GDM, multiple pregnancies, and chorioamnionitis. Also, tocolysis should not be started in these mothers to delay delivery for ACS administration. Finally, these neonates should be monitored for postnatal hypoglycemia as per the existing local protocols.

Use of Antenatal Corticosteroids in Early Term Births ($37^{0/7}$-$38^{6/7}$ Weeks) through Elective Cesarean Section

A Cochrane review which included the largest ACS RCT [antenatal steroids for term caesarean section (ASTECS)] in this population concluded that there was low certainty of evidence that indicated that ACS use in planned cesarean section in term births was associated with a decreased risk of RDS, TTNB, and neonatal intensive care unit (NICU) admissions. However, there are conflicting recommendations from different advisory bodies in relation to this. Though the RCOG stresses that an elective cesarean section should be delayed beyond at least 39 weeks, it does recommend ACS in scenarios where it is not possible. Most of the other academic bodies do not recommend for ACS in this subgroup of term births. The long-term neonatal outcomes reported by the RCT (ASTECS-2) did not indicate any major neurodevelopmental impairment in either of the two groups. However, a lower percentage of the children who were exposed to ACS were perceived to be represented in the top quartile of performance. Till further studies evaluating long-term outcomes are available, ACS may not be used in this subgroup of mothers.

LONG-TERM RISKS OF CORTICOSTEROIDS

Most of the studies on a single dose of ACS have not shown any long-term risks associated with fetal exposure of ACS. The 30-year follow-up data from the first RCT on ACS which had enrolled neonates of gestational age from 31 to 35 weeks did not show any adverse neurocognitive, pulmonary function, or cardiovascular outcomes. However, this cohort study concluded that ACS exposure might result in impaired glucose tolerance and insulin resistance in adult life. The NICHD Maternal-Fetal Medicine Units (MFMU) network trial on multiple serial weekly courses of ACS indicated that ACS exposure of four or more courses was associated with an increased risk of cerebral palsy. ACS in term cesarean deliveries might be possibly associated with an increased incidence of impaired school performance as indicated by the follow-up data from ASTECS-2 study. Also, another cohort study demonstrated that there might be an increased vulnerability to stress-related psychiatric disorders in children born at term gestation but exposed to ACS in fetal life for anticipated preterm birth. In conclusion, most of the studies evaluating long-term outcomes of a single course of ACS have been reassuring.

USE OF ANTENATAL CORTICOSTEROIDS IN THE INDIAN SCENARIO

The Ministry of Health and Family Welfare (MoHFW) guidance 2014 recommends dexamethasone as the preferred ACS over betamethasone. This is due to the fact that the betamethasone acetate/phosphate mixture (used in most of the RCTs) which is a combination of short- and long-acting salts is not presently available in India. Further, the available formulation of betamethasone which is the phosphate salt is short acting and its dosage has not been studied well. The other advantages of using dexamethasone include its easy supply chain as it is a part of the WHO essential medicines list, lesser cost, and good stability at higher temperature when compared to betamethasone. The MoHFW guidelines also recommends auxiliary nurse midwives (ANMs) to give the prereferral dose of dexamethasone for anticipated preterm births between $24^{0/7}$ and $33^{6/7}$ weeks in peripheral centers and then refer to a higher center if delivery is not imminent. In case of imminent delivery or refusal of referral, ANMs may continue the full course of dexamethasone and prepare for delivery. It should be noted that the large multicentric RCT (ACT trial) published after the MoHFW guidelines which came into force indicated that ACS use in community settings by trained health care workers (HCW) targeting pregnancies in which the fetus is presumed to less than 5th centile for birth weight (a proxy for preterm births) resulted in an increased overall neonatal mortality rate and maternal sepsis in the ACS group. This cautions against the overuse of ACS in peripheral settings at the community level without adequate assessment of gestational age and appropriate risk assessment for prediction of near-future occurrence of preterm birth.

Evidence Gaps and Future Research Avenues

- The overuse of ACS has been a subject of discussion. It is seen that only a fraction of those mothers who are given ACS for anticipated preterm labor in the next 7 days go on to deliver prematurely, thus exposing many of the fetuses to ACS who are then delivered at term. Future research needs to look at better ways of delineating mothers who are candidates for ACS and might deliver in the beneficial window period of 1–7 days.
- The dosing regimen that could yield the best possible neonatal outcomes for multiple pregnancy needs to be studied further.
- The use of ACS in LPT gestation in multiple pregnancy and those with diabetes mellitus needs further research as the infants born to these mothers in LPT gestation are at the highest risk of respiratory morbidity such as RDS.
- The use of rescue ACS course in PPROM is still controversial and needs to be explored further with adequately powered RCTs.

CHAPTER 23 | Antenatal Steroids

CHAPTER AT A GLANCE

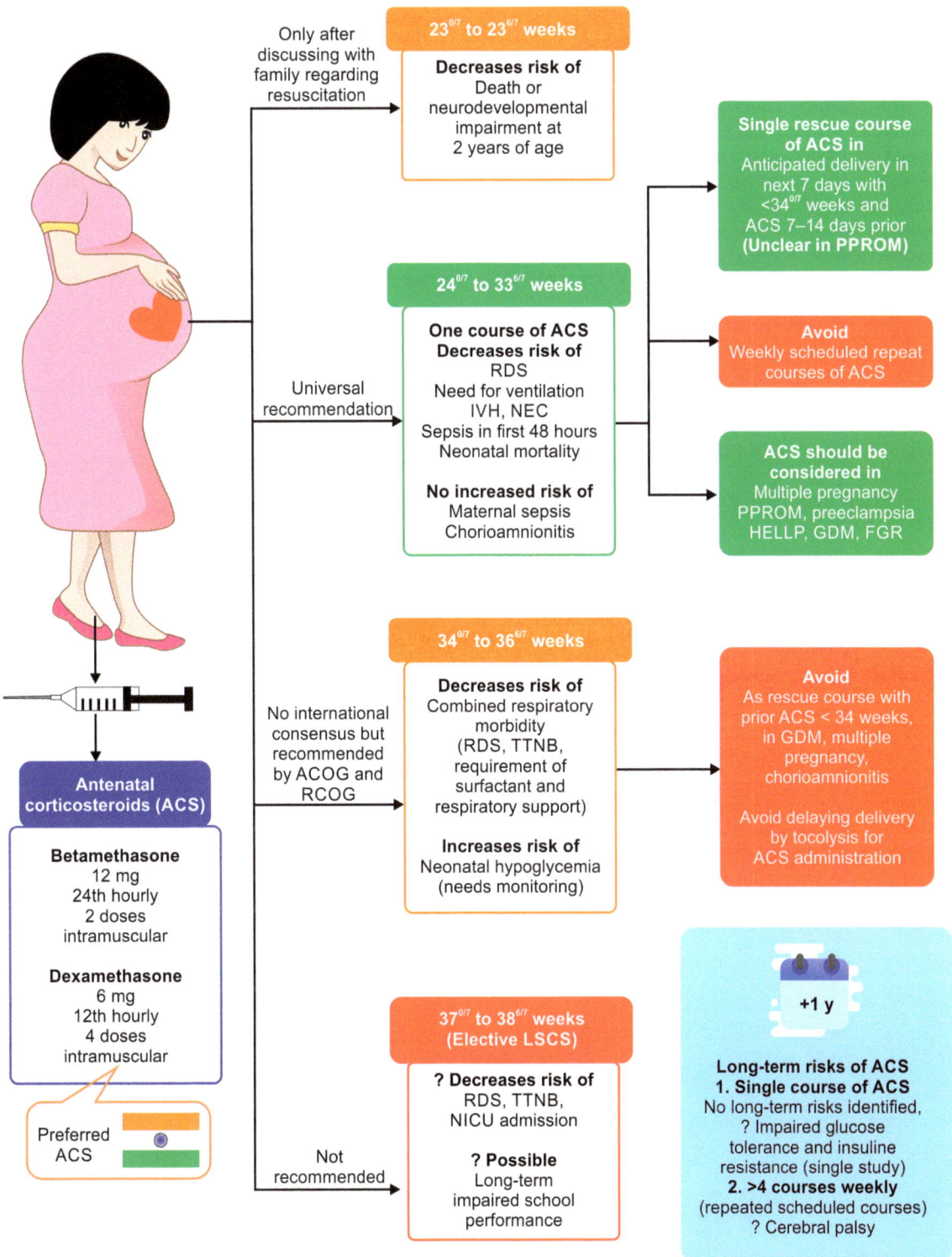

(ACOG: American College of Obstetricians and Gynecologists; ACS: antenatal corticosteroids; FGR: fetal growth restriction; GDM: gestational diabetes mellitus; HELLP: hemolysis, elevated liver enzymes, low platelet count; IVH: intraventricular hemorrhage; NEC: necrotizing enterocolitis; NICU: neonatal intensive care unit; PPROM: prelabor premature rupture of membranes; RDS: respiratory distress syndrome; RCOG: Royal College of Obstetricians and Gynaecologists; TTNB: transient tachypnea of newborn)

KEY POINTS

- ACS in preterm births between $24^{0/7}$ and $33^{6/7}$ weeks is a cost-effective strategy that could improve morbidity-free survival of preterm infants.
- Though both dexamethasone and betamethasone are equally efficacious with a similar safety profile, dexamethasone is preferred in Indian settings due to the unavailability of the betamethasone salt mixture which is proven to be of benefit in most of the trials.
- While a single rescue course of ACS could be given for mothers who had received a prior course of ACS 7–14 days back, are less than $34^{0/7}$ weeks, and are at risk of preterm delivery within the next 7 days, serial scheduled weekly multiple courses of ACS should not be given.
- ACS should be considered in preterm births $24^{0/7}$–$33^{6/7}$ weeks complicated by multiple pregnancy, preeclampsia, HELLP syndrome, diabetes mellitus, fetal growth restriction, and PPROM.
- ACS may be used in uncomplicated pregnant mothers of LPT gestation who are expected to deliver within the next 7 days. Tocolysis to prolong labor for ACS administration in these mothers should not be done.
- LPT neonates exposed to ACS need to be monitored for neonatal hypoglycemia.
- ACS is not advised in term neonates to be delivered through elective cesarean section and the primary aim should be to delay elective cesarean section beyond at least 39 weeks.

SUGGESTED READING

1. Deshmukh M, Patole S. Antenatal corticosteroids for impending late preterm (34-36+6 weeks) deliveries-a systematic review and meta-analysis of RCTs. PLoS One. 2021;16(3):e0248774.
2. Mwita S, Jande M, Katabalo D, Kamala B, Dewey D. Reducing neonatal mortality and respiratory distress syndrome associated with preterm birth: a scoping review on the impact of antenatal corticosteroids in low- and middle-income countries. World J Pediatr. 2021;17(2):131-40.
3. Rohwer AC, Oladapo OT, Hofmeyr GJ. Strategies for optimising antenatal corticosteroid administration for women with anticipated preterm birth. Cochrane Database Syst Rev. 2020;5(5):CD013633.
4. Shanks AL, Grasch JL, Quinney SK, Haas DM. Controversies in antenatal corticosteroids. Semin Fetal Neonatal Med. 2019;24(3):182-8.
5. WHO ACTION Trial. Antenatal dexamethasone for early preterm birth in low-resource countries. N Engl J Med. 2020;383(26):2514-25.

CHAPTER 24

Prenatal Neuroprotective Strategies

Rema S Nagpal, Savita N Kamble

INTRODUCTION

Significant improvement in neonatal care over the last few decades has led to an increasing survival of preterm neonates. The incidence of perinatal brain damage, however, remains high, leading to "neonatal encephalopathy," whose consequences range from cerebral palsy (CP), severe intellectual disability, sensorineural hearing loss, and blindness to more subtle behavioral and cognitive deficits. "Encephalopathy of prematurity" refers to nonhemorrhagic white and gray matter lesions, where the central pathology is periventricular white matter damage (PWMD) or periventricular leukomalacia (PVL). Other lesions that cause perinatal brain damage which often present in preterm neonates include germinal matrix-intraventricular hemorrhage (GM-IVH) and cerebellar disturbances. The area of prenatal or endogenous neuroprotection is a burgeoning area of research.

OBJECTIVES

- To review pathophysiology of perinatal brain damage
- To review the risk factors for perinatal brain damage
- To provide antenatal neuroprotective interventions

PATHOPHYSIOLOGY OF PERINATAL BRAIN DAMAGE

Cellular Architecture of Fetal Brain

The white matter of the brain is primarily made up of glial cells which include astrocytes, microglial cells, oligodendrocytes, and their progenitors. They play a major role in neuronal homeostasis, regulation of neurotransmitters, inflammation, immune responses, production of neuroprotective factors like antioxidants, and tissue remodeling/repair after injury. Oligodendrocytes, and its precursor preoligodendrocytes, are highly sensitive to oxidative stress injury between 24 and 32 weeks' gestation. The oligodendroglial progenitor cells are vulnerable to glutamate-mediated excitotoxicity resulting in cell death **(Fig. 1)**.

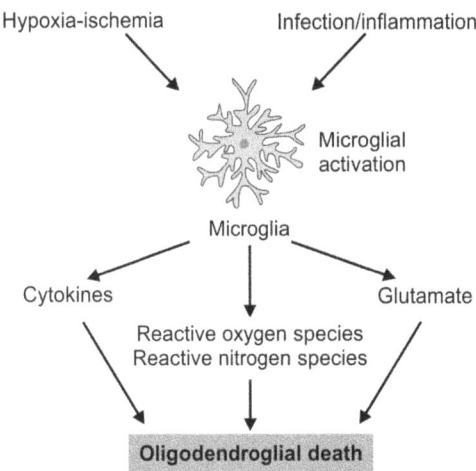

Fig. 1: Pathogenesis of oligodendroglial death.

Role of Hypoxia-ischemia and Infection/Inflammation in Periventricular White Matter Damage

Perinatal brain damage is multifactorial but principally involves two major molecular events: *hypoxia-ischemia (HI)* and *systemic inflammation*. HI leads to ion pump failure, glutamate release, calcium influx, and release of inflammatory mediators which leads to cell necrosis and apoptosis. Chorioamnionitis leads to a cascade of neurochemical processes called fetal inflammatory response syndrome (FIRS) causing PVL. The mechanisms of fetal brain injury include release of cytokines, free radical injury, glutamate release, and vascular injury associated with infection. The microscopic injury could be "white matter" and/or "neuronal injury," while extensive damage to the cerebral cortex, thalamus, and basal ganglia may also be seen. Damage to the three glial cell lines causes injury in two forms, i.e., focal necrosis deep in periventricular white matter manifesting as cystic changes **(Figs. 2A and B)** or a more diffuse non-necrotic white matter lesion characterized by astrogliosis, microgliosis, and loss of oligodendrocytes. With improved neonatal care, the diffuse white matter injury

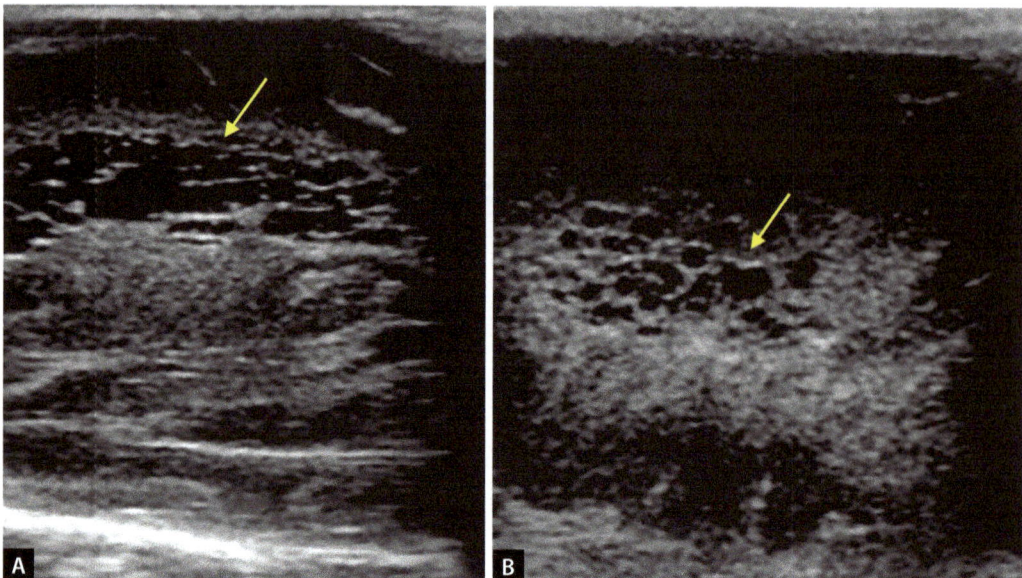

Figs. 2A and B: Cranial ultrasound images of periventricular leukomalacia (yellow arrow indicates the cystic lesions in the periventricular region).

is more common. This damage is called PWMD in preterm babies, which leads to PVL.

At birth, exposure to room air/oxygen leads to formation of the reactive oxygen species (ROS) molecules which including superoxide, hydroxyl, singlet oxygen, and H_2O_2. Superoxides are readily deactivated by the enzyme superoxide dismutase (SOD), which, if absent (as happens due to mitochondrial oxidative stress) or deficient as in preterm babies, leads to the accumulation of toxic-free superoxide radicals. The fetal oligodendrocyte progenitor and preoligodendrocytes are very vulnerable to this oxidative stress which leads to white matter injury and PVL.

RISK FACTORS FOR PERINATAL BRAIN DAMAGE

Antenatal Risk Factors

These include maternal infections, hypoxic-ischemic insult, malnutrition, anemia, stress, antenatal conditions like preeclampsia, diabetes, maternal thyroid dysfunction, placental abruption, maternal substance abuse, fetal chromosomal abnormalities, and growth restriction. These can cause either permanent damage to the developing brain or "sensitize" the brain, increasing susceptibility to damage following a future unfavorable event.

Perinatal Risk Factors

These include prematurity, hypoxic-ischemic insult, chorioamnionitis, prelabor rupture of membranes (PROM), and oxidative stress. Maternal infections and chorioamnionitis are all associated with an increased risk of CP. About 20–30% of all preterm labor is caused by chorioamnionitis. Preterm prelabor rupture of membranes (PPROM) is "associated" with intra-amniotic (IA) infections, while term PROM may be "followed" by IA infections. In preterm PROM, clinically evident IA infection occurs in 15–35% of cases. Fetuses exposed to clinical chorioamnionitis have a 140% increased risk of CP, while exposure to histological chorioamnionitis increases the risk by 80%.

Postnatal Factors

These include oxidative stress, inflammation, and genetic susceptibility.

ANTENATAL NEUROPROTECTIVE INTERVENTIONS FOR PREVENTION OF PERINATAL BRAIN INJURY

Prevention of Premature Birth and Role of Progesterone

Prevention of premature birth is the most decisive way to prevent PWMD. Identification of the woman at high risk for premature delivery with early treatment of premature labor is essential. Identification of modifiable risk factors (e.g., substance abuse, anemia, etc.) in early pregnancy, and appropriate interventions may help to prevent preterm labor.

Treatment with progestogens, such as 17-hydroxyprogesterone caproate (17P), reduces the risk of recurrent preterm birth **(Table 1)**. Progesterone, possibly, also has a neuroprotective role independently. In animal studies, progesterone and its derivative, allopregnanolone, have been shown to reduce inflammation and improve myelination. This could potentially be useful in neuronal and glial cell survival and repair.

TABLE 1: Progesterone in preterm labor—FOGSI (2017) and RCOG (2019).

Indication	Dose and route of administration
Prior spontaneous preterm birth	17-hydroxyprogesterone caproate depot 250 mg IM weekly start at 16–20 weeks, till 36 weeks' gestation
Cervical shortening <25 mm, at <24 weeks gestation	Progesterone suppository 200 mg or 90 mg gel vaginally each night from time of diagnosis till 36 weeks of gestation

(FOGSI: Federation of Obstetric and Gynecological Societies of India; RCOG: Royal College of Obstetricians and Gynaecologists; IM: intramuscular)

Dosage and Indications

Antenatal Magnesium Sulfate

Antenatal magnesium is a safe and feasible drug now recommended for fetal neuroprotection. It significantly decreases the incidence of moderate-severe CP and substantial gross motor dysfunction at 2 years of age in preterm babies less than 32 weeks of gestation. Number needed to treat (NNT) to prevent one CP is 63 [95% confidence interval (CI) 43-155]. There is no published evidence supporting the use of magnesium to prevent CP in term infants.

Mechanisms of the neuroprotective effect includes stabilization of cerebral circulation, antiexcitatory effect through impairment of neurotransmitter release and blocking NMDA receptors, antioxidant effect which protects against free radical injury, antiplatelet aggregation, and vasodilatation.

Evidence: The Cochrane meta-analysis (2009) of magnesium sulfate for fetal neuroprotection in women at risk for preterm birth included five seminal trials. These were the Australasian Collaborative Trial of Magnesium Sulphate (ACTOMgSO$_4$), the Beneficial Effects of Antenatal Magnesium Sulphate (BEAM) trial, and the PREMAG (PREterm brain protection by MAGnesium sulphate) trial. The fourth trial [Magnesium and Neurologic Endpoints Trial (MagNET)] looked at both, tocolysis and neuroprotection, and the MAGPIE (MAGnesium sulphate for Prevention of Eclampsia) trial looked at prevention of seizures in pre-eclamptic mothers. These trials, though heterogeneous in design, included 6,145 neonates (1,493 preterm babies). The major findings included:

- Significant reduction in "any" CP [relative risk (RR) 0.71, 95% CI 0.55-0.91] and moderate/severe CP (RR 0.64, 95% CI 0.44-0.92).
- Reduction in substantial gross motor dysfunction at 18 months to 2 years (RR 0.61, 95% CI 0.44-0.85).
- Death or CP was not reduced significantly overall but was reduced in the neuroprotection subgroups (RR 0.85, 95% CI 0.74-0.98).
- There was no reduction in risk of blindness, deafness, or developmental delay.
- There was no reduction in brain injuries due to IVH or cystic white matter injury.
- *Long-term outcomes at school ages*: While there is a reduced risk of CP at 2 years of age [odds ratio (OR) 0.63, 95% CI 0.42-0.95], similar long-term benefits at school ages have not been observed.
- There were no serious maternal side effects.

In a systematic review conducted by Shepherd et al. (2019), one randomized controlled trial (RCT) looked at a subgroup of babies born <32 week' gestation exposed to antenatal magnesium (n = 1,613); they had a 62% relative reduction in echo densities compared with unexposed babies (RR 0.38; 95% CI 0.19-0.79).

Administration and Dosage

Indications

- Gestational age <32 weeks (24^{+0}-31^{+6}) gestation at imminent risk (within 24 hours) of preterm birth (PPROM/preterm labor/obstetric indication). The Society of Obstetricians and Gynaecologists of Canada (SOGC) recommends to administer magnesium to women <33 + 6 weeks with imminent preterm birth.
- Delay administration of drug till cervical ripening is achieved. Do not delay emergency delivery of the baby for drug administration.
- If a mother is in active labor with ≥8 cm, cervical dilatation or the fetus has major anomalies and the administration may be deferred.

Contraindications

- Maternal myasthenia gravis (could precipitate a myasthenic crisis)
- Maternal myocardial compromise or conduction defects
- Mothers with impaired renal function

Dosage, Route, and Duration

The two regimens used for administration of magnesium sulfate are *Zuspan's regimen (IV magnesium)* and *Pritchard's regimen (IM magnesium)*, which were originally studied in mothers with severe preeclampsia and eclampsia. The recommendations by the Federation of Obstetric and Gynecological Societies of India (FOGSI), the American College of Obstetricians and Gynaecologists (ACOG), and SOGC all suggest that the intravenous regimen be used for magnesium administration in fetal neuroprotection. Intramuscular (IM) injections are painful and complicated by local abscess formation (0.5% cases). The IM regimen may possibly be a better option in peripheral hospitals, when infusion pumps are unavailable; however, there is no recommended dosage schedule for this.

Dose: Intravenous magnesium sulfate: 4 g loading dose over 20 minutes, followed by maintenance dose of 1 g/h, up to delivery or for 24 hours whichever is sooner. A repeat course is not currently advocated.

The SOGC in their recent practice guideline (2019) has recommended a dose of 4 g over 30 minutes with or without 1 g/h maintenance infusion for women with imminent preterm birth. For women with planned preterm birth (fetal/obstetric indication), the recommendation is to administer magnesium as a 4 g IV loading dose within 4 hours before birth.

Exposure to magnesium within 12 hours of delivery has reduced odds of CP compared to exposure more than 12 hours prior to delivery.

Monitoring:
- *Maternal*: Monitor for clinical signs of magnesium toxicity 4 hourly—pulse, BP, respiratory rate (should be at least 16/min), urine output (at least 100 mL in 4 hours), and deep tendon reflexes. Loss of patellar reflex is the initial sign of systemic hypermagnesemia. 1 g inj. calcium gluconate should be kept available as an antidote.
- *Neonate*: Hypermagnesemia can lead to hyporeflexia, poor suck, and rarely respiratory depression.

Antenatal Corticosteroids

Antenatal corticosteroids (ACS) administered to women at strong risk for preterm birth is associated with a decreased incidence/severity of neonatal respiratory distress syndrome (RDS) and mortality.

In a Cochrane systematic review (2020), the neuroprotective benefits of antenatal steroids included are:
- Probable reduction in IVH (1.9% vs. 3.3%, RR 0.58, 95% CI 0.45–0.75; 12 trials; 8,475 infants).
- Reduction in IVH (stage III/IV) or PVL at 23–24 weeks (this benefit was not seen in neonates born at 22 weeks).
- Probable reduction in developmental delay in childhood (RR 0.51, 95% CI 0.27–0.97; 600 children; three studies) without a clear improvement in intellectual impairment.

Administration of repeat courses of ACS showed no benefit on survival free of major neurosensory disability for children at 2–3 years (average RR 1.01, 95% CI 0.92–1.11) or major neurosensory disability at 2–3 years (RR 1.08, 95% CI 0.31, 3.76). Glucocorticoid receptors in the fetal brain are particularly vulnerable to steroids; when exposed to multiple courses of ACS, babies exhibited lower birth weight, length and head circumference, and a possible increased risk of CP.

The Antenatal Corticosteroids Trial (ACT) (2015), conducted in low- and middle-income countries (LMIC), reported the unexpected finding of increased neonatal mortality in steroid-exposed infants (RR 1.12, 95% CI 1.02–1.23). It is suspected that maternal and severe neonatal infections were higher in the ACS group leading to increased neonatal mortality. The recently published World Health Organization (WHO) ACTION-I trial (Antenatal Corticosteroids for Improving Outcomes in Preterm Newborns) (2020) has confirmed the benefits in LMIC, where the primary outcomes of stillbirth or neonatal death was also significantly lower in the dexamethasone group versus placebo (25.7% vs. 29.2%; RR 0.88; 95% CI 0.78–0.99). Possible maternal bacterial infection occurred in 4.8% in the dexamethasone group versus 6.3% in the placebo group.

In a population-based retrospective cohort study (2006–2017) from Finland, 14,868 children who were exposed to ACS had significantly higher cumulative incidence rates/hazards for any mental and behavioral disorder in a 11-year follow-up compared to nonexposed children [12.01% vs. 6.45%; absolute difference, 5.56% (95% CI, 5.04%–6.19%)]. The Finnish guidelines recommended ACS when birth was imminent before 34 + 6 days (34 + 0 in the pre-2009 guidelines), and yet 45.27% of the treatment-exposed children were eventually born at term. These findings seem to support an association between ACS and abnormal neurodevelopment, when administered in preterm mothers (but where babies were eventually born term). This suggests that we need to develop a better prediction model to diagnose those at imminent risk of preterm birth, so that unnecessary ACS is not administered.

Administration, Indications, and Dosage

- There is no specific or separate dosage for fetal neuroprotection as such. Dose and indications are the same as those used for fetal lung maturation. Betamethasone has been shown to have a clear reduction in IVH (RR 0.48, 95% CI 0.34–0.68). Dexamethasone has similar benefits, but confidence intervals are wide (RR 0.78, 95% CI 0.54–1.13).
- *Dose*: Inj. Betamethasone 2 doses of 12 mg IM 24 hours apart or inj. Dexamethasone 6 mg IM 12 hourly for 4 doses.
- The recommended combination of inj. Betamethasone acetate + phosphate is not available in India. Betamethasone phosphate is available but it is short acting, requires frequent doses, and is not beneficial over dexamethasone.
- Dexamethasone is cheaper and more stable at high temperatures and is recommended by the WHO and government of India (GOI).

Prelabor Rupture of Membranes and Role of Antibiotics

Clinical strategies to prevent maternal infections like chorioamnionitis could benefit in reduction of CP. Unfortunately, once diagnosed with chorioamnionitis, adequate antibiotic administration or immediate delivery does not appear to reduce the risk of CP. Other strategies which could be applied include treatment of maternal fever, induction of labor for patients at full term gestation with

TABLE 2: Management strategy for PROM.

Gestational age	Management strategy	Antibiotics
Term gestation	Induction of labor	Not required
Preterm < 34^{+0} weeks	• Expectant management, if no maternal or fetal contraindications • Antibiotics prolong latency (i.e., time between PROM and delivery)	• High incidence of penicillin resistance in Indian mothers • (FOGSI 2017) Erythromycin 250 mg four times/day for 10 days or till expected delivery • (ACOG 2018) IV Ampicillin + Erythromycin (followed by oral amoxicillin + erythromycin) for 7 days
Late preterm 34^{+0}–36^{+6} weeks	Expectant management or early delivery	Treat with antibiotics if mother has signs of infection. Latency antibiotics are not needed
Clinical chorioamnionitis	Delivery	Antibiotics (cephalosporins, metronidazole, aminoglycosides)

(ACOG: American College of Obstetricians and Gynaecologists; FOGSI: Federation of Obstetric and Gynecological Societies of India; PROM: prelabor rupture of membranes)

PROM, and avoidance of excessive vaginal examinations after rupture of membranes. The risk of chorioamnionitis is 10% if the fetus is delivered within 24 hours of PROM; this increases to 40% if delivered after 24 hours without antibiotic coverage **(Table 2)**.

Prevention of Hypoxemia-ischemia

The relation of cerebral WM injury to fetal metabolic acidosis indicates that optimal management during labor/delivery is required to prevent HI insults or development of cerebrovascular autoregulatory dysfunction that might lead to HI subsequently. This includes close fetal monitoring and appropriate resuscitation if required, by trained personnel.

Antioxidant Strategies

- *Reduction of reactive oxygen species:* To minimize ROS generation and hence oxidative stress, neonatal resuscitation protocols recommend resuscitation with room air in term neonates and FiO_2 0.21–0.30 for resuscitation in preterm neonates.
- *Free radical scavengers:*
  - *Melatonin* is an antioxidant, with anti-inflammatory and antiapoptotic properties, and possibly could protect the fetal brain against free radical-induced brain damage. Its use is under research.
  - *N-acetylcysteine (NAC):* NAC is a free radical scavenger. In experimental models of chorioamnionitis, prenatal administration of NAC has been shown to cross the blood–brain barrier, reduce oxidative stress, and reduce inflammation. In a recent trial (2020) by Buhimschi et al., administration of NAC to pregnant women at 23^{+0}–33^{+6} weeks' gestation with Triple I was found to be associated with reduced composite outcome of mortality and severe short-term neonatal morbidities including BPD and IVH, better Apgar scores, and lesser requirement for surfactant and resuscitation. Larger trials are required before recommendation for its use can be made.

- *Maternal vitamin D supplementation:* Vitamin D deficiency is implicated as a significant factor in preterm birth, preeclampsia, maternal diabetes control, and prolonged/obstructed labor. Vitamin D has a role in fetal brain development because of its antioxidant activity and its role in cell differentiation, cytokine regulation, and neurotransmitter synthesis. Studies have suggested a temporal association between maternal vitamin D levels and fetal morphological brain development.
  FOGSI recommends a daily intake of 600 IU of vitamin D during pregnancy and lactation.

Prevention of Inflammation

Research is ongoing with anti-inflammatory agents such as cytokine inhibitors like recombinant human (rh) IL-1Ra, IL-10, nuclear factor kappa B (NF-kβ) inhibitors like sulfasalazine and curcumin.

Prevention of Maternal Anemia

Systematic reviews suggest that maternal anemia in the first trimester increases the risk of premature birth [RR 1.65 (95% CI 1.31–2.08)]. However, this association is not significant in the second [RR 1.45 (95% CI 0.79–2.65)] and third [relative risk, 1.43 (95% CI 0.82–2.51)] trimesters. Prevention of maternal anemia is an important modifiable risk factor to prevent preterm birth.

Improved Antenatal Care and Resultant Neuroprotection

Good antenatal care with particular attention to prevention of maternal anemia, improved maternal nutrition, early diagnosis of Rhesus isoimmunization, and management to prevent bilirubin encephalopathy, screening to rule out maternal illnesses like diabetes and hypertension, early diagnosis of intrauterine infections in the fetus, etc., will have an indirect effect on prevention of brain damage in the neonate. Early recognition and management of fetal growth restriction are also important.

As per WHO recommendations, all women, from the time they try to conceive until 12 weeks' gestation, should take a folic acid supplement (400 µg) daily to prevent neural tube defects. To prevent recurrent neural tube defects, a dose of 4 g is recommended to be taken starting 3 months prior to conception until 3 months of pregnancy.

Uncontrolled maternal diabetes may possibly lead to language and motor impairments, attention deficit hyperactivity disorder, and problems in psychosocial development. While the causal relationship has not been proved, improved diabetes control could be a neuroprotective strategy.

Fetal exposure to preeclampsia is associated with an increased risk of CP (OR 2.5, 95% CI 2.0–3.2) if the baby is premature or small for gestational age. Preventive measures may benefit the baby in terms of neuroprotection.

There is some evidence of moderate quality that prophylactic antibiotic use in women with preterm labor with intact membranes results in an increase in CP in the children.

CHAPTER AT A GLANCE

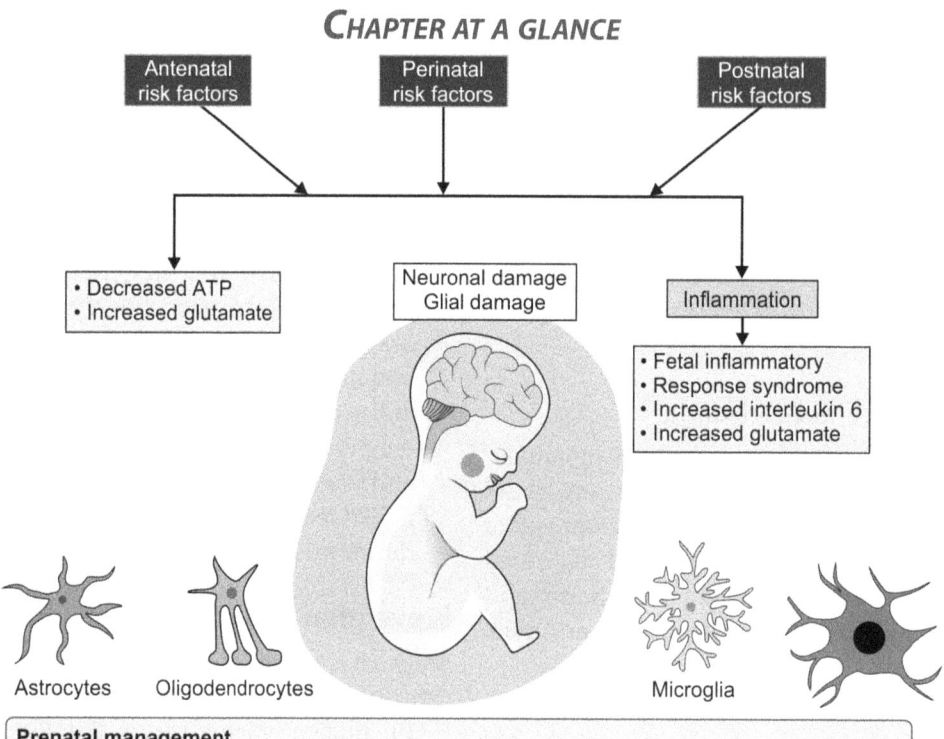

KEY POINTS

- Fetal brain cellular architecture, particularly glial cells, is very sensitive to two molecular events—hypoxia-ischemia and infection-inflammation.
- Preterm neonates are prone to PWMD, leading to PVL.
- Prevention of preterm birth is the most decisive way to prevent PWMD.
- Significant prenatal neuroprotective strategies include antenatal magnesium sulfate, antenatal corticosteroids, prevention of hypoxia and systemic inflammation, and antioxidant strategies.

SUGGESTED READING

1. Davis AS, Berger VK, Chock VY. Perinatal neuroprotection for extremely preterm infants. Am J Perinatol. 2016;33:290-6.
2. McGoldrick E, Stewart F, Parker R, Dalziel SR. Antenatal corticosteroids for accelerating fetal lung maturation for women at risk of preterm birth. Cochrane Database Syst Rev. 2020;12:CD004454.
3. Ranchhod SM, Gunn KC, Fowke TM, Davidson JO, Lear CA, Bai J, et al. Potential neuroprotective strategies for perinatal infection and inflammation. Int J Dev Neurosci. 2015;45:44-54.
4. Shatrov JG, Birch SCM, Lam LT, Quinlivan JA, McIntyre S, Mendz GL. Chorioamnionitis and cerebral palsy: a meta-analysis. Obstet Gynecol. 2010;116 (2 Pt 1):387-92.
5. Shepherd E, Salam RA, Middleton P, Makrides M, McIntyre S, Badawi N, et al. Antenatal and intrapartum interventions for preventing cerebral palsy: an overview of Cochrane systematic reviews. Cochrane Database Syst Rev. 2017;8:CD012077.
6. Wolf HT, Huusom LD, Henriksen TB, Hegaard HK, Brok J, Pinborg A. Magnesium sulphate for fetal neuroprotection at imminent risk for preterm delivery: a systematic review with meta-analysis and trial sequential analysis. BJOG. 2020;127(10):1180-8.

25. Antepartum Hemorrhage

Ashwini RC, Darshan Hosapatna Basavarajappa

INTRODUCTION

Antepartum hemorrhage (APH) is one of the catastrophic occurrences in obstetric practice that results in increased maternal and fetal morbidity and mortality. The initiated cascade of events is a consequence of maternal blood loss with multisystem damage resulting in acute kidney injury, stillbirth, perinatal asphyxia, or life-threatening consumptive coagulopathy. Hence, it is vital to understand the pathophysiology, follow an evidence-based protocol, and format a multidisciplinary care approach to prevent the perinatal adversities. APH, in particular abruption placenta, accounts for the highest stillbirths irrespective of gestational age and thus highlights the importance of effective perinatal management to reduce maternal and fetal/neonatal morbidity and mortality.

OBJECTIVES

- To discuss the prevalence, risk factors, pathophysiology and outcome of placenta previa, placental abruption, and placenta accreta spectrum.
- To discuss the overview of antenatal, natal, and postnatal management to improve neonatal outcomes.
- To manage APH using "Stepwise algorithm".

PREVALENCE OF ANTEPARTUM HEMORRHAGE

Antepartum hemorrhage is defined as bleeding from or into the genital tract of a pregnant female after 20 weeks of gestation until delivery of the fetus. It was a well-known clinical entity even in the 19th century where obstetricians of the era considered it a fatal event. But recent years have witnessed a significant rise in the prevalence from 1 in 1,000 births to 3–5% of all pregnancies at present as per the National Health Portal of India, 2019. A four-fold increase seems to be a direct consequence of increase in the risk factors contributing for this unusual clinical occurrence in an otherwise normal pregnancy.

RISK FACTORS AND PATHOPHYSIOLOGY OF ANTEPARTUM HEMORRHAGE

Bleeding could be from a placental or nonplacental source. Placental causes include placenta previa and abruption placenta which account for 80% of all the APH cases. The other causes could be of maternal or fetal origin as illustrated in **Flowchart 1**.

It has to be well understood that an abnormally located placenta or a prematurely separating placenta is an unnatural phenomenon and is always the result of an underlying pathogenic risk factor. Sometimes, the cause goes unnoticed and is clinically termed unidentified APH or indeterminate APH. For all practical purposes, this subgroup of cases should be clinically managed as mild revealed abruption.

There are obstetric and nonobstetric or general risk factors for the occurrence of APH. Nonplacental local causes are well characterized by their physical appearance and are diagnosed on clinical pelvic examination. Certain risk factors overlap for both placenta previa and abruption placenta while some are specific. **Table 1** illustrates the major risk factors and their relative importance.

The final common pathway of placenta previa and abruption is maternal bleeding, the clinical picture of which

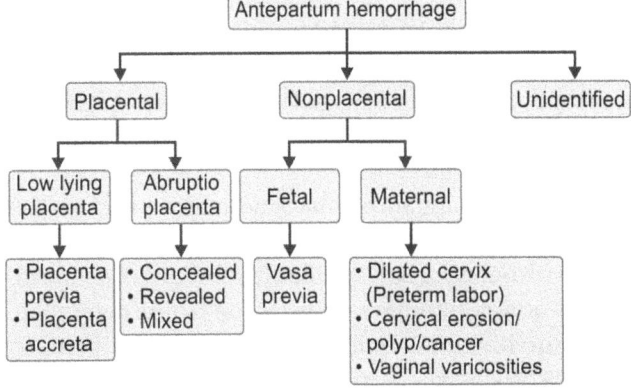

Flowchart 1: Major classification and different causes of antepartum hemorrhage.

TABLE 1: Major risk factors with their importance in placenta previa and abruption placenta.

Risk factor	Placenta previa	Abruptio placentae
Elderly mother (maternal age >35 years), IVF pregnancy	+++	+
Multiparity	+++	+
Maternal smoking	+	+++
Multifetal gestation	+	+++
Polyhydramnios	+	+++
Prior cesarean delivery, uterine curettage, endometrial ablation, manual removal of placenta	++++	+
Preeclampsia	Not applicable	+++
Maternal infections	Not applicable	+++
Preterm premature rupture of membranes	Not applicable	+++
Maternal trauma	Not applicable	++
Uterine leiomyoma	Not applicable	++
Prior antepartum hemorrhage	++	++++

(IVF: in vitro fertilization)

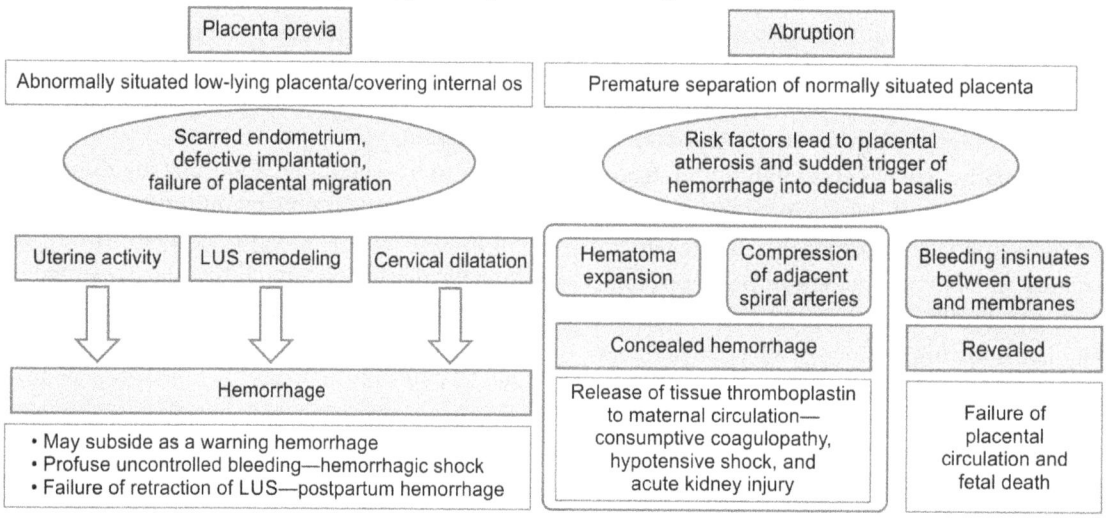

Flowchart 2: Pathophysiology of antepartum hemorrhage and multisystem involvement.

(LUS: lower uterine segment)

is quite complicated with the initiated cascade of events leading to severe maternal, fetal, and neonatal morbidity and mortality. **Flowchart 2** illustrates the pathophysiology of APH and multisystem involvement.

PERINATAL OUTCOMES OF ANTEPARTUM HEMORRHAGE AND THEIR PATHOPHYSIOLOGY

In placenta previa, the incidence of perinatal mortality has been reported to be higher and includes early term births, small for gestational age (SGA), fetal hemorrhage, low APGAR scores, and higher neonatal intensive care unit (NICU) admission rate.

In placental abruption, perinatal mortality varies from 4.4 to 67.3% depending on the neonatal care available. Placental abruption accounts for 20% of stillbirths and 15% of neonatal deaths. Severity of abruption and gestation at birth determine neonatal survival. Intrauterine growth restriction (IUGR) is seen in 80% of neonates born <36 weeks. Placental abruption accounts for 50-60% of preterm births, of which 50-80% are spontaneous. It is the fourth most common medical cause of premature birth. Other immediate neonatal outcomes include birth asphyxia, increased need for resuscitation, congenital malformations, especially involving central nervous system, and prematurity. Perinatal asphyxia has been found to be the leading cause of neonatal death. Among survivors, there is an increased risk of adverse long-term outcomes such as cerebral palsy and cystic periventricular leukomalacia (PVL). The pathophysiology of the perinatal outcome is illustrated in **Flowchart 3**.

PLACENTA ACCRETA SPECTRUM—"THE PRESSING PRIORITY"

Placenta accreta or morbidly adherent placenta is an entity where the abnormally located low-lying placenta fails to separate after the delivery of the fetus owing to the absence of Nitabuch's layer of separation. Incessant hemorrhage follows resulting in profound hemorrhage and shock necessitating hysterectomy as a lifesaving operation.

Flowchart 3: Pathophysiology of the perinatal outcomes.

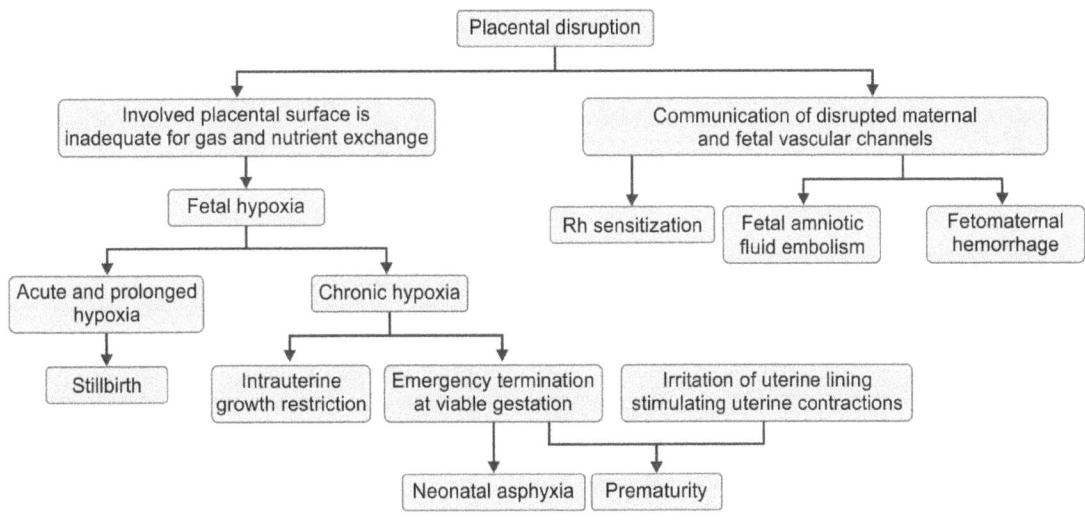

Placenta accreta is purely an iatrogenic complication which is a consequence of damage to the decidua basalis of the endometrium by either repeated cesarean section or overenthusiastic uterine curettages. The clear rise in the incidence of morbid adherent placenta by more than 15-fold from 1 in 4,000 in 1980s to 1 in 272 in a recent survey done in USA in 2016 (ACOG practice bulletin number 7, February 2021) speaks for the factors responsible subsequent to the increase in the incidence of cesarean section. Risk factors include advanced maternal age, multiparity, previous cesarean section, placenta previa, and previous uterine curettage.

Transvaginal and 3D abdominal ultrasonography are useful in diagnosis. Second-trimester biomarkers along with characteristic ultrasound features can be used to raise suspicion toward characterizing women as high risk for pathological placentation.

The perinatal importance of placenta accreta lies with the increase in adverse neonatal effects either as a direct hemorrhage-related complication or because of prematurity. Recent consensus and recommendations advocate scheduling an elective cesarean with an informed consent for hysterectomy should there be a life-threatening hemorrhage.

Involvement of a multidisciplinary team that includes urosurgeons, interventional radiologists for uterine artery embolization, and blood transfusion specialists is necessary for the delivery. Delivery should be scheduled to be performed at or after 34 completed weeks of pregnancy and before 36 weeks to avoid spontaneous onset of labor and hemorrhage due to uterine remodeling which could turn fatal. General anesthesia is generally favored.

In practice, the neonate of a mother with placenta accreta is a preterm either delivered electively or by emergency operation which results in a higher neonatal ICU admission rate and prematurity-related complications. Higher stillbirth rates have been reported in comparison to the gestation-matched controls at 32 weeks or earlier as per a population-based record linkage study from Australia in 2017.

STRATEGY TO IMPROVE NEONATAL OUTCOMES

To improve neonatal outcomes, the following considerations are suggested:
- Effective and timely communication between the obstetrician and the neonatologist regarding possibility of preterm birth.
- Antenatal counseling of expectant parents regarding risks and outcomes of preterm birth as per expected gestational age at delivery.
- Antenatal corticosteroids in view of anticipated preterm birth.
- Planned delivery in a hospital with a tertiary level NICU.

NEONATAL RESUSCITATION

- Anticipation and preparation for high-risk birth with possible need for advanced resuscitation by Neonatal Resuscitation Program (NRP) trained team.
- Team briefing regarding risks involved at birth and plan of management
- Resuscitation as per NRP guidelines
- *Special considerations:*
  - In the event of severe APH in mother, delayed cord clamping (DCC) is avoided.
  - Consider volume expansion with normal saline or O-negative blood cross-matched with maternal blood if severe blood loss is suspected or known or if the neonate does not respond to advanced resuscitation.

Golden hour management of preterm neonate with special focus on thermoregulation and optimal respiratory and cardiovascular support followed by ongoing care in the NICU by an experienced neonatal team would facilitate a good neonatal outcome with the goal of "intact" survival.

SECTION 4 | Obstetric Conditions and Fetal/Neonatal Effects

CHAPTER AT A GLANCE

Step-wise Algorithm for Management of Antepartum Hemorrhage

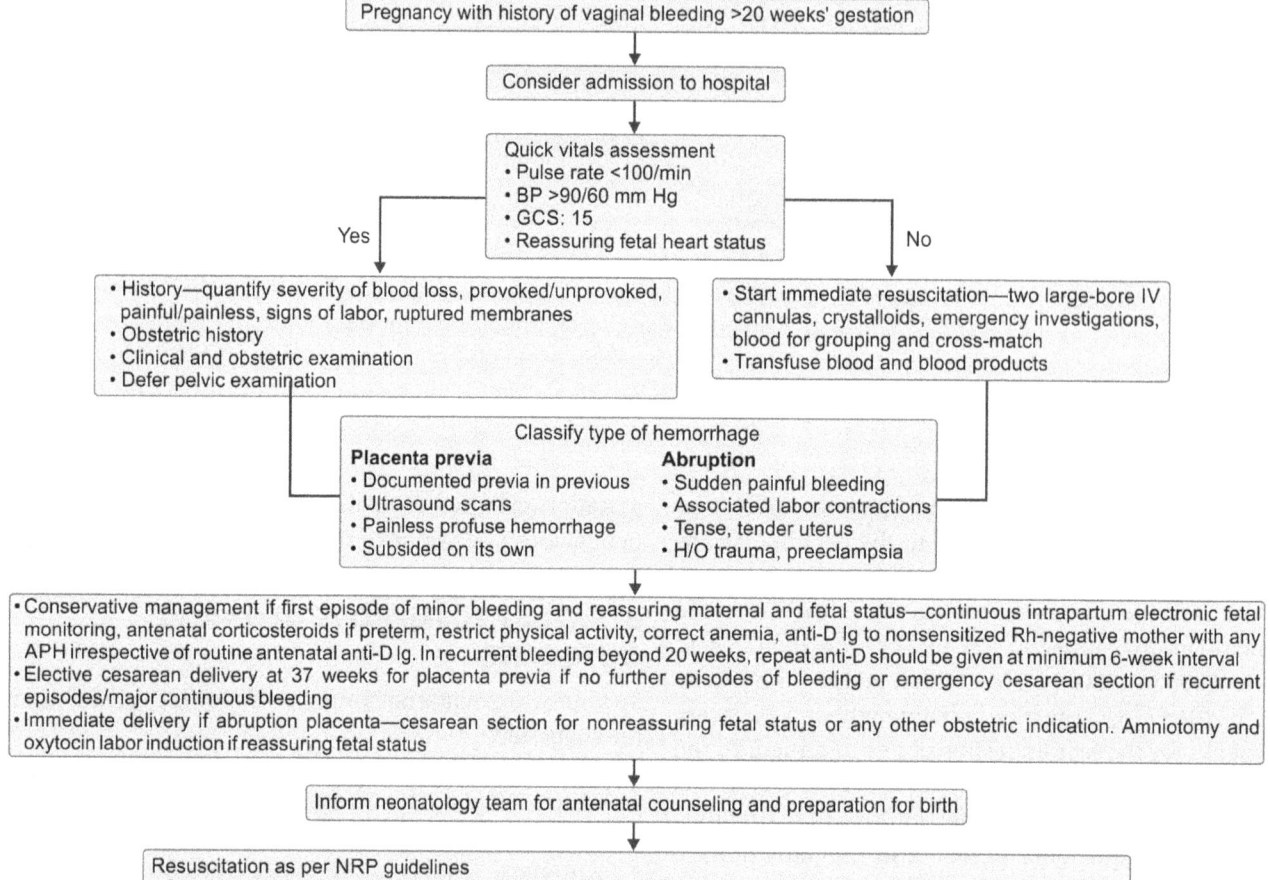

(APH: antepartum hemorrhage; BP: blood pressure; GCS: Glasgow Coma Scale; NRP: Neonatal Resuscitation Program)

KEY POINTS

- In mothers presenting with APH, classification of the type of bleeding and quantification of bleed with hospitalization and continuous electronic fetal monitoring are warranted.
- In minor bleeding, consider restriction of physical activity, counsel regarding preventive measures for deep vein thrombosis, administration of antenatal corticosteroids, correction of anemia, and anti-D Ig administration to nonsensitized Rh-negative mother.
- If maternal or fetal status is compromised and gestation is beyond the period of viability, consider emergency delivery.
- Deliver in a tertiary care hospital with level III NICU improves neonatal outcomes.
- Antenatal counseling of parents and resuscitation as per NRP guidelines to be done.
- Consider immediate cord clamping at birth and volume expanders if blood loss is suspected/known.

SUGGESTED READING

1. American College of Obstetricians and Gynecologists; Society for Maternal-Fetal Medicine. Obstetric Care Consensus No. 7: Placenta Accreta Spectrum. Obstet Gynecol. 2018;132(6):e259-75.
2. Aziz K, Lee HC, Escobedo MB, Hoover AV, Kamath-Rayne BD, Kapadia V, et al. Part 5. Neonatal resuscitation, 2020 American Heart Association Guidelines for cardiopulmonary resuscitation and emergency cardiovascular care. Circulation. 2020;142(suppl 2):S524-50.
3. Balayla J, Bondarenko H. Placenta accreta and the risk of adverse maternal and neonatal outcomes. J Perinatal Med. 2013;41(2):141-9.
4. Cunningham FG, Leveno KJ, Bloom SL, Spong CY, Dashe JS, Hoffman BL, et al. Obstetrical hemorrhage. William's Obstetrics, 25th edition. New York: McGraw-Hill Education; 2014.
5. Downes KL, Grantz KL, Shenassa ED. Maternal, labor, delivery and perinatal outcomes associated placental abruption: a systematic review. Am J Perinatol. 2017;34(10):935-57.
6. Rabe H, Gyte GM, Diaz-Rossello JL, Duley L. Effect of timing of umbilical cord clamping and other strategies to influence placental transfusion at preterm birth on maternal and infant outcomes. Cochrane Database Syst Rev. 2019;9:CD003248.
7. Redline RW. Placental pathology. In: Martin RJ, Fanaroff AA, Walsh MC, (Eds) Fanaroff and Martin's Neonatal-Perinatal Medicine: Diseases of the Fetus and Infant, 11th edition. Philadelphia, PA: Elsevier/Saunders; 2019. pp. 415-21.

CHAPTER 26

Gestosis in Pregnancy

Pravin Singarayar, Saudamini Nesargi

INTRODUCTION

Gestosis in pregnancy, also known as hypertensive disorders in pregnancy (HDP), is a spectrum of disorders ranging from chronic hypertension to preeclampsia and eclampsia. These are a major contributor to maternal mortality and fetal complications. The Indian Registry (2013) reported an incidence of preeclampsia at roughly 10%.

OBJECTIVES

- To understand the etiopathogenesis and theories of evolution of preeclampsia.
- To discuss the management of gestosis, from antenatal to postpartum care.
- To understand the prevention strategies which have been studied.
- To discuss some extreme forms of the disease such as HELLP (hemolysis, elevated liver enzymes, low platelet count) syndrome and eclampsia.
- To review the maternal and fetal complications of the disease.

CLASSIFICATION

Based on the onset of hypertension and its severity, gestosis can be classified as mentioned in **Table 1**.

HYPERTENSIVE DISORDERS IN PREGNANCY-GESTOSIS SCORING SYSTEM

A scoring system to calculate the risk of gestosis was developed depending on risk factors **(Table 2)**.

ETIOPATHOGENESIS AND ORGANS INVOLVED

Even though, the etiopathogenesis is not confirmed. It is proposed that it occurs in two stages. In the first stage, there is inadequate remodeling of the maternal spiral arteries by the invasive placental trophoblasts to result in reduced placental perfusion. In the second stage, there is increased maternal systemic vascular dysfunction, which leads to clinical features, including multiorgan involvement. The precise factor(s) linking stage I and stage II has been the focus of numerous studies.

The proposed factors are: Angiogenic factors which cause inactivation of vascular endothelial growth factor (VEGF) and placental growth factor reduce the vessel growth, immune mechanisms, endothelial dysfunction with vasoconstriction and activation of the coagulation cascade, and free oxygen radical injury.

Preeclampsia is a Multisystem Disease

Vascular and Cardiac Changes

Systemic vasospasm leading to hypertension, hemoconcentration, predisposition to fluid overload, exaggerated capillary permeability, and decreased plasma colloid osmotic pressure predisposing to pulmonary edema, left ventricular dysfunction resulting in a low output–high resistance state.

Kidneys

Glomerular endotheliosis leading to proteinuria, decrease in glomerular filtration rate (GFR) by almost 25% due to vasospasm of intrarenal vessels leading to oliguria, increased reabsorption of uric acid resulting in an increase in serum uric acid levels which serves as a marker for disease severity.

Liver

Intense vasospasms leading to ischemia, infarction, and hemorrhages in the liver results in swelling of the Glisson's capsule and the characteristic right upper quadrant/epigastric pain. Raised liver enzymes and serum lactate dehydrogenase (LDH) levels, and impaired coagulation may be seen in severe disease.

Hematology

Thrombocytopenia and hemolysis (LDH levels >600 IU/L). Platelets, a marker of disease severity, are decreased due to activation, aggregation, and consumption.

TABLE 1: Classification of gestosis.	
Preeclampsia	• BP ≥140 mm Hg systolic or ≥90 mm Hg diastolic on at least two occasions (4 hours apart) after 20 weeks of gestation in a woman with a previously normal BP, *OR* • BP ≥160 mm Hg systolic or ≥110 mm Hg diastolic; hypertension can be confirmed within a short interval (minutes) to facilitate timely antihypertensive therapy AND • Proteinuria ≥300 mg per 24-hour urine collection (or this amount extrapolated from a timed collection) *OR* protein/creatinine ratio of ≥0.3 *OR* dipstick reading of 1+ (used only if other quantitative methods not available) OR In the absence of proteinuria, new-onset hypertension with the new onset of any of the following: • Renal insufficiency with serum creatinine of >1.1 mg/dL or a doubling of the serum creatinine concentration in the absence of other renal disease • Impaired liver function with elevated blood concentration of liver enzymes to twice the normal concentration • Pulmonary edema • Persistent cerebral or visual symptoms • Platelets <100,000/μL
Severe features of preeclampsia (any)	• Systolic BP of ≥160 mm Hg or diastolic BP of ≥110 mm Hg on two occasions at least 4 hours apart while a patient is on bed rest (unless antihypertensive therapy is initiated before this time) • Thrombocytopenia (platelet count <100,000/μL) • Impaired liver function (elevated blood concentrations of liver enzymes to twice the normal concentration) • Severe persistent right upper quadrant or epigastric pain unresponsive to medication and not accounted for by alternative diagnoses • Progressive renal insufficiency (serum creatinine concentration of >1.1 mg/dL or a doubling of the serum creatinine concentration in the absence of other renal disease) • Pulmonary edema • Persistent cerebral or visual disturbances
Eclampsia	• Generalized seizures that occur in a preeclamptic woman that cannot be attributed to other causes
Superimposed preeclampsia (likely when any of these are present)	• A sudden increase in BP that was previously well-controlled or an escalation of antihypertensive therapy to control BP • New onset of proteinuria or sudden increase in proteinuria in a woman with known proteinuria before or early in pregnancy • Severe features (as in severe preeclampsia)
HELLP syndrome	Presence of *h*emolysis, *e*levated *l*iver enzymes, and *l*ow *p*latelets; may or may not occur in the presence of hypertension and is often considered a variant of preeclampsia
Gestational hypertension	• New onset of sustained elevated BP after 20 weeks' gestation in a previously normotensive woman (≥140 mm Hg systolic or ≥90 mm Hg diastolic on at least two occasions 6 hours apart) • No proteinuria

Source: Martin RJ, Fanaroff AA, Walsh MC. Fanaroff and Martin's Neonatal-Perinatal medicine, 11th edition. Amsterdam: Elsevier; 2020.
(BP: blood pressure)

Brain
- Hypertension and vasospasm leading to reduced cerebral perfusion, cytotoxic edema, ischemia, and infarction
- *Posterior reversible leukoencephalopathy syndrome (PRES)*: Acute onset of headache, seizures, vision problems, transient cortical blindness due to failure of autoregulatory mechanism of cerebral vasculature which results in vasogenic edema, hyperperfusion, and extravasation of erythrocytes and plasma.
- Intracranial hemorrhage

Placenta
Changes of acute atherosis, small placenta, and areas of ischemia and infarction.

SIGNS AND SYMPTOMS

Although screening using risk factor scoring may be prudent, most cases of preeclampsia occur in nulliparous women with no risk factors. Blood pressure (BP), weight check, and urinalysis for proteinuria are some of the commonly used basic screening tools which help to detect this often—asymptomatic problem.

Symptoms:
- Rapid weight gain (>1 kg/week)
- Swelling of feet/whole body
- Feeling unwell
- May be asymptomatic

Red alert symptoms:
- Symptoms of cerebral irritation (headache, blurring of vision/flashes of light)
- Epigastric pain
- Vomiting
- Reduced urine output
- Altered consciousness
- Difficulty in breathing

Signs:
- Hypertension
- Pedal edema

Red alert signs:
- Brisk tendon reflexes/clonus
- Anasarca
- Features of pulmonary edema
- Features of placental abruption

TABLE 2: Gestosis scoring system.

Risk factor	Score
• Age older than 35 years • Age younger than 19 years • Maternal anemia • Obesity (BMI > 30) • Primigravida • Short duration of sperm exposure (cohabitation) • Woman born as small for gestational age • Polycystic ovary syndrome • Family history of cardiovascular disease • Interpregnancy interval >7 years • Conceived with assisted reproductive (IVF/ICSI) treatment • MAP > 85 mm Hg • Chronic vascular disease (dyslipidemia) • Excessive weight gain during pregnancy	1
• Maternal hypothyroidism • Family history of preeclampsia • Obesity (BMI > 35 kg/m²) • Gestational diabetes mellitus • Multifetal pregnancy • Hypertensive disease during previous pregnancy	2
• Pregestational diabetes mellitus • Chronic hypertension • Mental disorders • Inherited/acquired thrombophilia • Maternal chronic kidney disease • Autoimmune disease (SLE/APLAS/RA) • Assisted reproductive (OD or surrogacy) treatment	3

When total score is ≥3; pregnant woman should be considered as—at risk for preeclampsia

Source: Martin RJ, Fanaroff AA, Walsh MC. Fanaroff and Martin's Neonatal-Perinatal medicine, 11th edition. Amsterdam: Elsevier; 2020.

(APLAS: antiphospholipid antibody syndrome; BMI: body mass index; ICSI: intracytoplasmic sperm injection; IVF: in vitro fertilization; MAP: mean arterial pressure; RA: rheumatoid arthritis; SLE: systemic lupus erythematosus)

LABORATORY INVESTIGATIONS

Following tests are done to assess the severity of the disease:
- Urine for proteinuria:
  - *Urine dipstick (≥2+; since 1+ has a high false positive rate of 71%)*: Quick results
  - *Ideal*: Spot urine protein:creatinine ratio (>0.3 is diagnostic)
  - *Gold standard*: 24-hour urine-protein quantification (>300 mg/dL proteinuria)
  - Do not use the first morning void to quantify proteinuria
  - Once significant proteinuria has been established, there is no need to repeat measurements.
  - Not mandatory for diagnosis if other severe features of preeclampsia are present
- Hematological tests:
  - *Complete blood count*: Raised hematocrit and hemoglobin (hemoconcentration)
  - Anemia (microangiopathic hemolytic anemia)
  - *Thrombocytopenia*: Both absolute number and trend of fall are important
  - *Peripheral smear*: Evidence of hemolysis-schistocytes and Burr cells
  - *Coagulation profile and fibrinogen*: Done if platelet count is <1.5 lakh/µL, significant hepatic dysfunction, or placental abruption
- Renal function tests:
  - *Serum creatinine*: Renal insufficiency is diagnosed when the serum creatinine concentration is >1.1 mg/dL or a doubling of the baseline value in the absence of other renal disease.
  - Blood urea nitrogen (BUN)
  - *Serum uric acid*: Increased. May prognosticate fetal outcomes. Raised values should not be used as an indication for delivery.
- *Serum electrolytes*: In severe disease
- Liver function tests:
  - *Serum bilirubin*: >1.2 mg/dL in case of hemolysis. Values >5 mg/dL are seldom seen in preeclampsia.
  - *Aspartate aminotransferase (AST) and alanine aminotransferase (ALT)*: >70 IU/L or twice the upper limit of normal suggests hepatic periportal necrosis. AST is raised more than ALT initially—this may point in favor of the diagnosis of preeclampsia. In other parenchymal liver diseases, ALT is raised more than AST.
  - *Serum LDH*: >600 U/L may suggest hepatic necrosis or hemolysis.

MANAGEMENT

Outpatient and Inpatient

It is advisable to admit all patients with preeclampsia to complete a full maternal and fetal assessment, stabilize BP, and finalize a plan of care prior to considering outpatient follow-up and management. Home monitoring may be considered in patients with gestational hypertension and preeclampsia without severe features. They must have easy access to health care in times of emergency.

Outpatient Monitoring

- *Daily monitoring*: BP, fetal kick count, and worsening of symptoms. Home BP measurement gives a better idea about the hypertension than a single office reading.
- *Twice weekly*: Nonstress test (NST)/biophysical profile (BPP)
- *Weekly*: Clinic visits, ultrasonography (USG) for amniotic fluid index (AFI), laboratory parameters to look for worsening/HELLP features, and urinalysis for proteinuria.
- *Every 2–3 weeks*: USG for fetal growth surveillance

Inpatient Monitoring

- To be done in all patients with preeclampsia/gestational hypertension at diagnosis, severe hypertension, abnormal laboratory parameters, signs of fetal complications, signs and symptoms of worsening of disease, and in those unable to follow-up/monitor at home.
- Allows frequent BP monitoring, fetal monitoring and early detection of severity.
- *Disadvantages*: Increased risk of thromboembolism (due to longer bed rest periods), disruption of regular and family life, cost, boredom, monotony of hospital food and routine, and depression.

Assessment of Fetal Well-being

As the severity of preeclampsia worsens, the perinatal morbidity also increases. Fetal assessment is crucial to decide timing of delivery. Although expectant management has no maternal benefits, there are tremendous benefits to the fetus.

- *Fetal growth scans*: Every 3–4 weeks
- AFI to know how the fetus has been coping in the preceding 2 weeks. Done at diagnosis and then every week
- *BPP/NST*: Done at diagnosis and then twice weekly or as frequently as the clinical picture indicates
- *Obstetric Doppler*: Done at diagnosis and weekly or biweekly as the clinical picture indicates. Reversal of ductus venosus flow beyond 26 weeks, reversed end-diastolic flow (REDF) beyond 30 weeks, or absent end-diastolic flow (AEDF) beyond 34 weeks warrant delivery. Severe fetal growth restriction (FGR) with no Doppler abnormalities may be induced at 37 weeks of gestation. In preeclampsia, the worsening of Doppler parameters may be more rapid and may not follow a predicted pattern.
- Daily fetal movement count

Pharmacological Management of Hypertension

While the definitive treatment is delivery, antihypertensive treatment will protect the mother from dangerous complications such as cerebral hemorrhage but will not alter the course of preeclampsia or prevent eclampsia. There is inadequate evidence that treatment of nonsevere hypertension improves maternal and fetal outcomes. Treatment exposes the woman and fetus to potential harm without clear evidence of benefit.

- BP must be obtained at least twice >4 hours apart. In case of severe hypertension (>160/110 mm Hg), repeat readings within a shorter interval and institute treatment within minutes (ideally within 1 hour).
- It is reasonable to treat hypertension if systolic blood pressure (SBP) > 150 and/or diastolic blood pressure (DBP) > 100 mm Hg.
- During labor, antihypertensives may be given parenterally.
- Magnesium causes only a transient fall in BP and should not be used as antihypertensive (**Table 3 and 4**).

TABLE 3: Blood pressure (BP) values for instituting treatment.

BP cutoffs	ACOG (2019)		RCOG (2019)	
	Antepartum	Postpartum	Antepartum	Postpartum
SBP	160	150	140	150
DBP	110	100	90	100

(ACOG: American College of Obstetricians and Gynecologists; DBP: diastolic blood pressure; SBP: systolic blood pressure)

TABLE 4: Oral maintenance treatment of antihypertensives.

	Drug	Pregnancy category	Dose	Side effects	Remarks
First line	Labetalol	C	200–2,400 mg/day 8–12 hourly (start with 100 mg BD, titrate up to 800 mg TID)	• Bradycardia • Nausea • Fatigue • Insomnia • Headache	• Contraindicated in: • Asthma • Congestive cardiac failure • Heart block
Second line	Nifedipine (slow release)	C	20–120 mg/day OD	• Flushing • Headache • Hypotension • Tachycardia • Inhibition of labor • Constipation • Edema	Do not use sublingually
Third line	Methyldopa	B	500–3,000 mg/day (divided 6–12 hourly)	• Hypotension • Depression • Sedation • Blurred vision • Dryness of mouth • Hemolytic anemia • Elevated liver enzymes	Do not use in postpartum period

Management of Hypertensive Emergencies (Flowchart 1)

- Persistent severe hypertension needs to be confirmed after at least 5-15 minutes of rest.
- Reasonable first-line agents for acute lowering of BP in hospital: Labetalol intravenously (IV) and hydralazine
- *When intravenous (IV) access is not available*: Oral immediate release nifedipine
- *When both oral nifedipine and IV access not available*: Tablet labetalol 200 mg; repeat after 30 minutes if required.
- Perform fundoscopy to look for papilledema and hemorrhages
- Monitor fetal heart rate (FHR)
- *Goal*: To achieve a range of 140-150/90-100 mm Hg
- Do not lower >25% of mean arterial pressure (MAP) within minutes to hours
- Initiate oral therapy once severe hypertension has been treated
- Monitor BP every 10 minutes for 1 hour, then every 15 minutes for the next hour, then every 30 minutes for another hour, then every hour for 4 hours.

Management of Gestational Hypertension/ Preeclampsia without Severe Features (Flowchart 2)

Women with both these conditions may be managed similarly. About 50% of women with gestational hypertension progress to preeclampsia, more likely if detected preterm.

Antenatal Steroids

Even a single dose of corticosteroid 1 hour prior to delivery has benefits compared to no steroids. Delivery should not be delayed for the sake of steroids in the late preterm period. Steroids may be considered in case of elective cesarean section (CS) up to $38^{6/7}$ weeks.

Management of Gestational Hypertension/ Preeclampsia with Severe Features (Flowchart 3)

Expectant management is intended to provide neonatal benefit at the expense of maternal risk. The notion that gestational hypertension is less concerning than preeclampsia is fallacious.

Intrapartum Care

Parturients with preeclampsia/gestational hypertension have a higher risk of placental insufficiency and subsequent fetal hypoxic stress during labor. In some women, severe features may develop during labor. It is important to note that induction of labor/CS does not control hypertension. Maternal stabilization is a must before delivery even in urgent circumstances.

Maternal Monitoring

- Urine for proteinuria
- BP measurement hourly in labor
- Continue antihypertensive drugs
- Monitor intake/output
- Limit IV fluids to 80 mL/hour
- In case of severe hypertension, parenteral drugs are preferred due to delayed gastric emptying.
- Monitor for severe symptoms
- Consider epidural catheter for labor analgesia
- Preanesthetic check-up

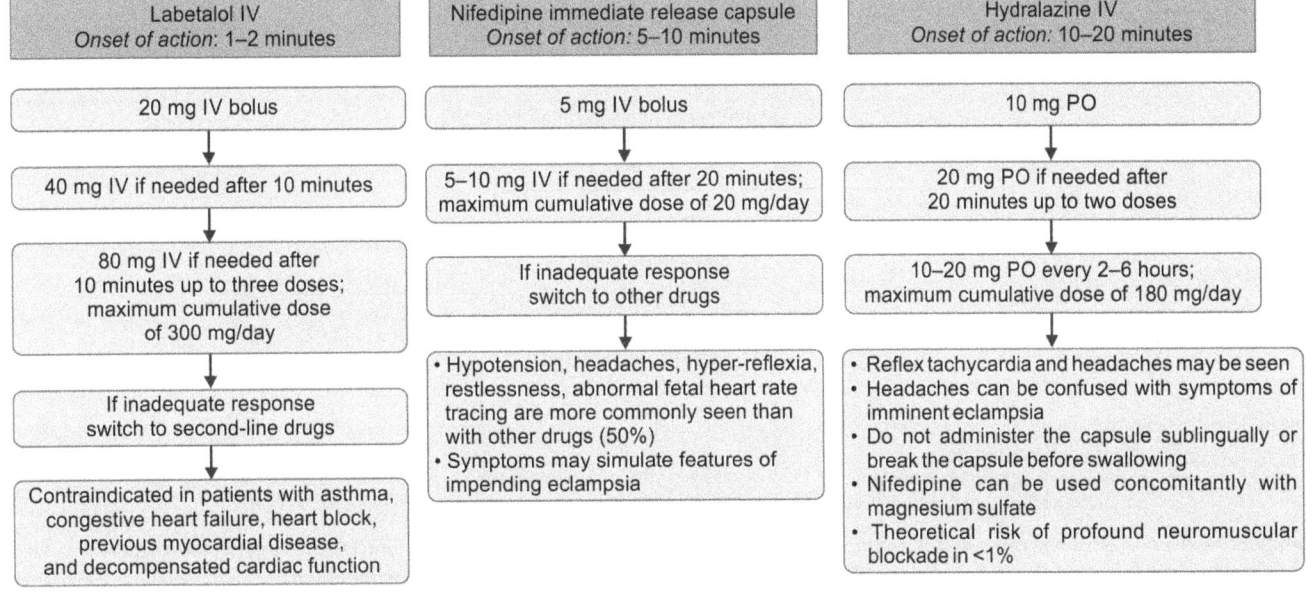

Flowchart 1: Management of hypertensive emergency.

Flowchart 2: Management of gestational hypertension/preeclampsia without severe features.

```
                    Gestational hypertension/preeclampsia without severe features
                                                │
                        ┌───────────────────────┴───────────────────────┐
                  <37 weeks of gestation                         ≥37^(0/7) weeks of gestation
                           │                                              │
                           ▼                                          Deliver
        • Start antihypertension if BP >150/100 mm Hg
        • Check CBC, RFT, and LFT
        • USG to look for FGR/OB Doppler/oligohydramnios
        • Give steroids for fetal lung maturity*
        • Watch for severe symptoms
                           │
                           ▼
            Stable for >48 hours and no signs of severity
                           │
             ┌─────────────┴─────────────┐
            Yes                          No
    Consider outpatient          • Continuous assessment
    management with              • Maternal: BP 4th hourly, daily weight check
    regular follow-up            • CBC, LFT, RFT twice weekly
                                 • Fetal: DFMC, NST twice weekly
                                 • Doppler and AFI weekly
                                 • Growth scan 3-4 weekly
                                            │
                                            ▼
                                      Stability:
                                Yes: continue expectant
                                management and deliver at 37^(0/7) weeks
                                No: Early delivery
```

*Delivery should not be delayed for the sake of steroids in the late preterm period

(AFI: amniotic fluid index; BP: blood pressure; BPP: biophysical profile; CBC: complete blood count; DFMC: daily fetal movement count; FHR: fetal heart rate; LDH: lactate dehydrogenase; LFT: liver function test; NST: nonstress test; RFT: renal function test)

Flowchart 3: Management of gestational hypertension/preeclampsia with severe features.

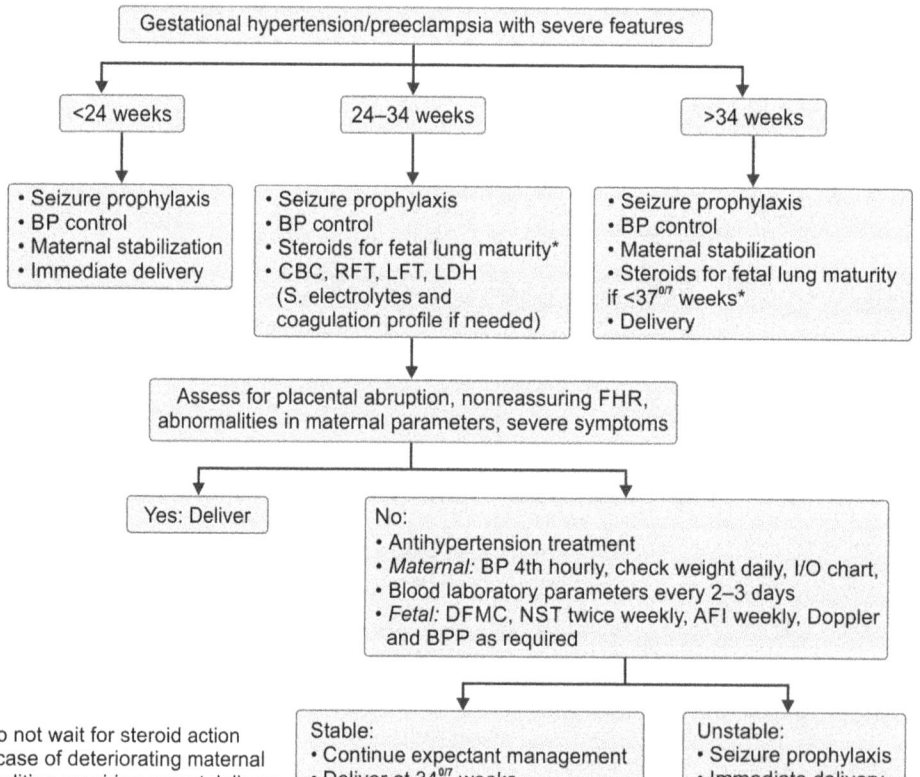

*Do not wait for steroid action in case of deteriorating maternal condition requiring urgent delivery

(AFI: amniotic fluid index; BP: blood pressure; CBC: complete blood count; DFMC: daily fetal movement count; FGR: fetal growth restriction; LDH: lactate dehydrogenase; LFT: liver function test; NST: nonstress test; RFT: renal function test; USG: ultrasonography)

- Arrange blood and blood products
- Watch for signs and symptoms of placental abruption
- Eclampsia prophylaxis in case of severe hypertension or if symptoms of imminent exlampsia.
- Instrumental delivery to cut short second stage of labor may be considered in cases of uncontrolled hypertension or if neurological symptoms are present.
- Use of methylergometrine for postpartum hemorrhage (PPH) is contraindicated in women with preeclampsia/gestational hypertension even if the BP is normal at the time of delivery.

Fetal Monitoring
- Electronic fetal monitoring is recommended so as to diagnose early fetal distress, hyperstimulation, and placental abruption.
- Neonatologist/trained pediatrician to be present for neonatal resuscitation.

Thrombophilia and Preeclampsia
Antiphospholipid antibody syndrome (APS) is the most common acquired thrombophilia in pregnancy. Gestational hypertension/preeclampsia occurs in about 30% of APS pregnancies. Preeclampsia is usually more severe and occurs at an earlier gestational age in APS. Women with APS with preeclampsia should receive low-dose aspirin and low molecular weight heparin during pregnancy, along with frequent monitoring for complications and fetal well-being.

Prevention
- Pregnant women with risk factors for preeclampsia should be offered first trimester uterine artery Doppler screening between $11^{0/7}$ and $13^{6/7}$ weeks. High pulsatility index (PI) (>90th centile) is associated with 50% risk of preterm preeclampsia. These women should be closely monitored and offered aspirin 150 mg at bedtime till 36 weeks.
- *Aspirin*: This antiplatelet drug causes selective inhibition of platelet thromboxane production. There is compelling evidence that there is a small-to-moderate benefit in reducing the incidence of preeclampsia, SGA, preterm birth, intrauterine fetal demise (IUFD), and neonatal death. The risk reduction is more in women at high risk for preeclampsia [numbers needed to treat (NNT) for women at high risk: 39].
Advise women with 1 high risk factor or ≥2 moderate risk factors to start aspirin **(Table 5)**.
Recommended dose: 150 mg once a day at bedtime until 36 weeks. Optimal time to start therapy is before 16 weeks. Contraindicated in women with bleeding disorders and peptic ulcer disease.
- *High-dose calcium supplementation*: To be given to women with low dietary calcium intake, especially those at high risk for preeclampsia (Dose: 1.5–2 g/day).

TABLE 5: Risk factors for aspirin prophylaxis.

High-risk factors	Moderate-risk factors
• Hypertensive disease in previous pregnancy • Chronic kidney disease • Autoimmune disease (SLE and APLA) • Type 1 or type 2 diabetes • Chronic hypertension • Multi-fetal pregnancy	• First pregnancy • Age ≥ 35 years • Pregnancy interval >10 years • BMI ≥ 30 kg/m² at first visit • Family history of preeclampsia

(APLA: antiphospholipid antibody; SLE: systemic lupus erythematosus)

The following interventions are NOT recommended in the prevention of preeclampsia: Salt restriction, bed rest, garlic, fish oil, vitamin D, vitamin C, vitamin E, magnesium, folic acid, progesterone, statins, heparin, metformin, sildenafil, and nitic oxide donors.

ECLAMPSIA
Pathophysiology
Eclampsia, a form of hypertensive encephalopathy, describes the extreme end of the preeclampsia spectrum. Although not all cases of preeclampsia progress toward eclampsia, it remains one of the most dreaded complications of the disease process. Theories suggest that it could be due to a result of loss of cerebral autoregulation due to malignant hypertension combined with endothelial damage resulting in vasogenic edema [threshold MAP: 140 mmHg (180–190/120–130)]. The effects are seen predominantly in the occipital and parietal regions.

In about 15% of cases, there may not be hypertension or proteinuria. Hypertension, although not the primary cause, can certainly potentiate the problem.

Management and Prevention
Seizure in pregnant women without a history of seizure disorder should be diagnosed with eclampsia unless proven otherwise. It is often accompanied by elevated BP and proteinuria.

Most women have preceding imminent symptoms of cerebral irritation such as headache, blurring of vision, scotoma, epigastric pain, and vomiting.

Goals of management include: Protection of airway, control of seizures, control of hypertension, and expedite delivery.

General Principles
- Maintain airway, breathing, and circulation
- Keep in left lateral decubitus position/recovery position (to avoid aspiration)

- Measures to avoid trauma to the tongue
- Elevate bed rails
- O₂ at 8–10 L/min
- Suction secretions/vomitus

Magnesium Sulfate Therapy

This is the drug of choice for the treatment of eclampsia and prophylaxis in case of severe hypertension or if symptoms of imminent eclampsia are present (NNT for asymptomatic cases: 129, for symptomatic cases: 36). In patients with impaired renal function, the loading dose can be given irrespective of the renal function but the maintenance dose has to be titrated based on serum magnesium levels. In case the patient is being shifted to another hospital, give the loading IV + intramuscular (IM) dose before shifting (VIMS regime).

Dose

- *Preferred*: IV—loading 4 g over 20 minutes; maintenance: 1 g/hour
- *IM*: Loading 10 g (5 g in each buttock deep IM using 20 G needle)
- *Maintenance*: 5 g in alternate Buttock q 4 hours

Duration

Until 24 hours after the seizure or 24 hours after delivery, whichever is later.

For Recurrent Seizures within 20 Minutes of Loading Dose

Continue with regular maintenance dose and administer additional 2 g IV over 5 minutes. Further recurrence: administer injection phenobarbitone 300 mg slow IV. Any further seizures: Intubation is warranted.

Contraindications

Myasthenia gravis, hypocalcemia, moderate-to-severe renal failure, cardiac ischemia, heart block, and myocarditis. Use lorazepam or phenytoin instead.

Clinical Monitoring During Magnesium Therapy

Deep tendon reflexes, urine output (at least 30 mL/hour), respiratory rate (at least 14/min), and SpO₂: >96%.

Serum Magnesium Levels (Table 6)

Routine monitoring is not required in all patients. Should be monitored only in patients with impaired renal function (reduced urine output, creatinine >1.0 mg/dL), somnolence, or slurred speech.

TABLE 6: Serum magnesium level and toxicity.

Serum magnesium levels (mEq/L)		
Normal level: 1.5–2	Loss of patellar reflex: >7	Cardiac arrest >25
Therapeutic level: 4–7	Prolonged PQ interval and wide QRS: 5–10	Respiratory paralysis >10

Magnesium Toxicity

- Loss of deep tendon reflex (DTR) is the first sign of magnesium toxicity
- *Absent patellar reflex*: Discontinue drug until reflex reappears
- *Urine output <20 mL/hour*: Discontinue drug and measure serum magnesium levels
- *Respiratory depression*: IV 10% calcium gluconate 10 mL over 10 minutes; consider intubation and mechanical ventilation; IV furosemide 40 mg to enhance urinary excretion of magnesium. Using diuretics in patients with impaired renal function does not excrete magnesium although the urine output increases.

Normal therapeutic levels of magnesium can cause loss of FHR variability. FHR accelerations with contractions or on scalp stimulation are interpreted as normal.

Expedite Delivery

Plan delivery only after maternal stabilization. Eclampsia itself is not an indication for CS. Magnesium within therapeutic levels does not increase the chances of CS, PPH, or prolonged labor.

Cesarean is performed if any of the following are present: Obstetric indication, abruption, unfavorable Bishop score, status eclampticus, and nonreassuring fetal status.

Complications of Eclampsia

- *Maternal*: Abruption, disseminated intravascular coagulation (DIC), cerebral hemorrhage, pulmonary edema, aspiration pneumonia, and death.
- *Fetal*: Hypoxia and stillbirth

Role of Imaging

Imaging is neither essential for diagnosis nor management of eclampsia. Some situations warranting imaging studies include:

- Atypical eclampsia (occurring later than 48 hours postpartum, before 20 weeks of gestation, or without hypertension and other features of preeclampsia).
- Focal neurological deficits
- Prolonged coma
- Unilateral pupil dilatation

Hyperthermia following seizure is an ominous sign as it may suggest a cerebral hemorrhage.

HELL P SYNDROME

The syndrome of hemolysis, elevated liver enzymes, and low platelet counts is a more severe form of preeclampsia. In about 15% cases, there is no hypertension or proteinuria and in 30%, it may progress or present postdelivery. It should be considered in any women in the third trimester or immediate postpartum with new-onset epigastric/upper abdominal pain, even in the absence of hypertension.
- *Clinical features*: Malaise and right upper quadrant pain (90%), nausea, and vomiting (50%)
- *Diagnosis*:
  - *Hemolysis*: Evidence of hemolysis on peripheral blood smear (schistocytes and Burr cells), serum bilirubin ≥1.2 g/dL, and LDH ≥600 IU/L.
  - Low-serum haptoglobin
  - *Elevated liver enzymes*: AST and ALT >70 IU/L or twice the upper limit of normal
  - *Thrombocytopenia*: Platelet count <1 lakh/μL
- *Monitoring*: Laboratory parameters every 12 hours. Platelet counts drop by 40% a day. AST >2,000 IU/L and LDH >3,000 IU/L suggest an increased mortality risk. Peak intensity of the disease: First 2 days postpartum. Watch for pulmonary edema, acute respiratory distress syndrome (ARDS), and renal failure.
- *Delivery*: It is the mainstay of treatment. Delivery can be postponed up to 24–48 hours for benefit of corticosteroids for fetal lung maturity under careful monitoring. Deliver in case of worsening. Arrange adequate blood and blood products.
- *Maternal complications include*: Eclampsia, abruption and DIC, acute renal failure, ARDS, pulmonary edema, hepatic rupture, and death. *Fetal*: Stillbirth, hypoxia and acidosis, growth restriction, and prematurity

Postpartum care: Recovery may have rebound hypercoagulability causing fatal thrombosis. Use of thromboprophylaxis is advised. Monitor laboratory parameters. Platelet counts and liver function tests (LFTs) normalize by 7th postpartum day.

CHRONIC HYPERTENSION IN PREGNANCY

The pregnancy-induced reduction in systemic vascular resistance causes a fall in BP, which has a nadir at 16–18 weeks of gestation and returns to prepregnant levels by the third trimester. First antenatal visit late in pregnancy may cause misdiagnosis of chronic hypertension as hypertensive disease of pregnancy. The incidence of chronic hypertension in parturients is increasing due to late pregnancies and the obesity epidemic.

Preconception Care

Preconception care includes evaluating for cause of hypertension and for evidence of end-organ damage. Management includes optimizing body mass index (BMI), replacement of antihypertensive medications with labetalol, nifedipine, or methyldopa if SBP > 150 mm Hg or DBP >100 mm Hg.

Antenatal Care

Advise on weight management, salt restriction, and exercise. Plan weekly visits if hypertension is poorly controlled and every 2–4 weeks if well-controlled. Advise obese women not to lose weight during pregnancy. Advise restricted nonstrenuous work with extra 1–2 hours of rest during the day. Offer aspirin. BP should be monitored at home and urine checked for proteinuria periodically. Fetal growth should be assessed with scans from 28 weeks inward.

Complications

Incidence of preeclampsia in women with congenital hypothyroidism (CHT) is 20–50%. The risk of preeclampsia is higher in chronic hypertensive women with obesity, smokers, hypertension >4 years, baseline DBP > 100 mm Hg, and previous history of preeclampsia.

Timing of Delivery

- $38^{0/7}$ weeks for women with CHT not on medication and between $37^{0/7}$ and $39^{0/7}$ weeks for those with CHT well-controlled on medications
- *CHT with superimposed preeclampsia with severe features*: Can manage expectantly up to 34 0/7 weeks
- *CHT with superimposed preeclampsia and no severe features, stable maternal and fetal condition*: Expectant management up to $37^{0/7}$ weeks
- *At any general anesthesia (GA) if*: Uncontrollable severe hypertension, eclampsia, pulmonary edema, DIC, new or increasing renal insufficiency, abruption or abnormal fetal testing.

Intrapartum Care

Continue antihypertensives. Monitor for acute elevations in BP during labor, proteinuria, urine output, and FHR. Epidural analgesia can reduce BP by 15%. The duration of first stage of labor may be prolonged.

Postpartum Care

Monitor BP daily for the first 2 days and at least once between days 3 and 5. Maintain BP < 150/100 mm Hg. Angiotensin-converting enzyme (ACE) inhibitors, angiotensin receptor blockers (ARBs), and diuretics can be used safely during lactation. Avoid atenolol and metoprolol in the postpartum period. Avoid methyldopa due to possibility of postural hypotension and depression. Blood loss should be ruled out if there is an acute drop in BP.

OBSTETRIC ANALGESIA AND ANESTHESIA

General Principles

- Gross intravascular volume contraction in parturients with preeclampsia may pose challenges.
- No clear evidence on optimal fluid or fluid rate (do not give >80 mL/hour)
- Overhydration contributes to maternal mortality from pulmonary edema and ARDS. Caution in oliguria, renal impairment, or pulmonary edema.
- Aspiration prophylaxis to be given
- Maintain left uterine displacement
- Do not discontinue magnesium drip during delivery or cesarean section
- Avoid opioids since they lower the seizure threshold
- Effective postoperative analgesia is required since it facilitates BP control, promotes early ambulation, and reduces the risk of thromboembolism.

Regional Anesthesia

- Preferred over GA
- *Concerns*: Hypotension, fluid overload, and aortocaval compression
- Contraindicated in patients with thrombocytopenia <50,000/µL and in coagulopathy. It can be safely given in patients with platelet count >75,000/µL.
- The platelet count at removal of the catheter is as important as during insertion.
- Epidural analgesia is suitable for providing pain relief for labor and delivery. With pain relief, the serum concentration of catecholamines decreases resulting in an increase in uteroplacental and intervillous blood flow.
- Regional anesthesia need not be delayed in patients on low-dose aspirin or on prophylactic doses of low-molecular weight heparin.

General Anesthesia

- Used only when regional anesthesia is contraindicated (coagulopathy), when there is inadequate time to perform a block (fetal distress), has failed, refusal of regional anesthesia, maternal hemodynamic instability, or altered consciousness.
- *Challenges with GA include*: Gross upper airway edema causing difficulty during intubation, drug interaction between magnesium and muscle relaxants, and exaggerated hypertensive response to endotracheal intubation.

POSTPARTUM CARE

It is important to remain vigilant in the postpartum period for complications such as eclampsia, PPH, HELLP, pulmonary edema, cardiovascular, cerebrovascular events, and thromboembolism. In about 5% of patients, gestosis may appear de novo in the postpartum period (up to 6 weeks postpartum), even without hypertension or proteinuria during pregnancy.

Monitoring

Blood pressure decreases within 48 hours following delivery but increases again 3-6 days postpartum. BP should be monitored for at least 72 hours postpartum and again 7-10 days after delivery.

Management of Hypertension

- BP > 150/110 mm Hg over 4 hours should be treated with antihypertensives
- BP > 160/110 mm Hg should be treated within 1 hour; eclampsia prophylaxis is to be considered
- Reduce antihypertensive treatment if BP < 130/80 mm Hg.
- If BP remains normal for > 48 hours, antihypertension treatment can be stopped.
- All antihypertensives (ACE inhibitors, ARBs, and diuretics) can be used safely during lactation.
- Avoid methyldopa (depression and fatigue) and atenolol (secreted in higher concentrations in breast milk).
- Nonsteroidal anti-inflammatory drugs (NSAIDs) can be used for pain relief
- Home BP monitoring

FETAL EFFECTS

Fetal effects are the result of poor perfusion from the placenta. Short-term effects are: Intrauterine growth restriction (IUGR), prematurity (often iatrogenic) with increased risk of morbidity and mortality. Babies with IUGR and prematurity are at increased risk for metabolic syndrome.

LONG-TERM PROGNOSIS

Women with gestosis have an increased risk of recurrent preeclampsia, cardiovascular disease [stroke and ischemic heart disease (IHD)], and renal disease.

CHAPTER AT A GLANCE

```
Gestosis in pregnancy
├── Organs involved: Heart, liver, kidneys and brain
├── Gestosis score > 3: High risk
├── Aspirin if risk factors present
├── Fetal effects: Growth restriction, prematurity, low birth weight
│
├── Gestational hypertension
├── Preeclampsia
│     ├── Features: Edema, hypertension, proteinuria
│     └── "Red alert" symptoms: Headache, epigastric pain, blurring of vision
├── Preeclampsia with severe features
│     └── Features include: Severe hypertension, thrombocytopenia, abnormal liver or renal function tests, cerebral or visual disturbances, epigastric pain, pulmonary edema
├── Chronic hypertension superimposed with preeclampsia
├── Eclampsia
│     ├── Seizures
│     └── Emergency
└── HELLP syndrome
      └── Hemolysis, elevated liver enzymes and low platelet counts
```

Investigations	Management	Management	Delivery	Postnatal care
• Urine examination for proteinuria • CBC for thrombocytopenia • Renal function • Liver function test	Indications for hospital admission: • At the time of first diagnosis • Severe hypertension, abnormal lab parameters • Signs of fetal complications • Worsening of disease • Unable to follow-up/monitor at home	• Antenatal steroids if GA < 34 weeks • Magnesium sulfate if GA < 31^{+6} weeks • Labetalol: Drug of choice for hypetension • Magnesium sulfate if seizures or severe features of preeclampsia • Delivery only after maternal stabilization	• If GA > 37 weeks • If < 37 weeks, delivery if: – Unstable or worsening hypertension – Abnormal fetal well-being tests – Worsening lab parameters	• Continue BP monitoring for at least 72 hours • Stop antihypertensive drugs if BP normal for > 48 hours • If severe hypertension, prophylaxis with magnesium

KEY POINTS

- Gestosis in pregnancy affects ~10% of all pregnancies.
- Appropriate diagnosis and management are crucial.
- Preeclampsia arises from a systemic inflammatory response that causes endothelial dysfunction: This response is common to all pregnancies, and preeclampsia is simply the extreme end of the spectrum.
- Preeclampsia affects various organs and can progress to life-threatening eclampsia.
- Hypertension is one of the problems of this varied systemic disease.
- Principles of management include antihypertensive drugs, magnesium sulfate for seizure prophylaxis, corticosteroids for fetal lung maturity, and appropriate timing of delivery.
- If delivery is imminent, use of corticosteroids decreases both mortality and morbidity in the fetus.
- Prevention may be by using low-dose aspirin in high-risk pregnancies
- To date, no single test predicts preeclampsia and no single preventive measure is definitive.

SUGGESTED READING

1. American Heart Association. Recommendations for blood pressure measurement in humans and experimental animals. Hypertension. 2005;45:142-61.
2. Gestational Hypertension and Preeclampsia: ACOG Practice Bulletin, Number 222. Obstet Gynecol. 2020;135(6): e237-60.
3. Gupte S, Wagh G. Preeclampsia-eclampsia. J Obstet Gynaecol India. 2014;64(1):4-13.
4. Martin RJ, Fanaroff AA, Walsh MC. NICE guidelines 133 Hypertension in pregnancy: Diagnosis and Management. Fanaroff and Martin's Neonatal-Perinatal medicine, 11th edition. Amsterdam: Elsevier; 2020.

Oligohydramnios and Polyhydramnios

Prathik BH, Ashok Kumar

INTRODUCTION

Amniotic fluid acts a cushion around the fetus which protects from trauma, compression of umbilical cord, and infection. It has a role in fetal lung and musculoskeletal development also. Any changes in amniotic fluid volume can have serious consequences in maternal and fetal health.

OBJECTIVES

- To review the amniotic fluid regulation in fetus
- To review the methods of amniotic fluid estimation
- To review the conditions associated with oligohydramnios and management
- To review the conditions associated with polyhydramnios and management

AMNIOTIC FLUID REGULATION IN FETUS

Major part of amniotic fluid is water (98–99%) with changes in its solute concentration occurring throughout the gestation. The volume of amniotic fluid mainly depends on the fetal organ functions and it is tightly regulated to maintain the fluid status of the developing fetus. Hence, it should be considered as a part of fetal body fluid compartment. In the earlier part of gestation, amniotic fluid is isotonic to maternal plasma indicating that majority is contributed by transudation from fetal skin or placenta. As the skin barrier of fetus matures in second half of pregnancy, the major contribution of amniotic fluid is from fetal kidneys (urine) and a minor proportion by fetal lungs (fetal lung fluid). About 800–1,200 mL of urine is produced per day during this time. The osmolarity also decreases from 290 mOsm/kg in the first trimester to 255 mOsm/kg near term due to increased production of hypotonic fetal urine. Fetal lungs secrete about 300–400 mL of fluid per day of which half is egressed from the trachea and swallowed by the fetus and the other half enters the amniotic cavity. Amniotic fluid in this half of gestation is removed mainly by fetal swallowing and absorption from the fetal surface of the placenta. Swallowing by fetus removes about 500–700 mL of fluid and about 400 mL is removed by absorption from fetal membranes (intramembranous pathway). Amniotic fluid is also regulated by maternal circulation via placenta (transmembranous pathway), but this pathway has a miniscule role in amniotic fluid dynamics. The pathways of production and absorption of amniotic fluid are depicted in **Figure 1**.

Amniotic Fluid in Fetal Nutrition

Amniotic fluid contains many nutrients which aid in fetal development. In the latter part of pregnancy, nearly 10–15% of the nutritional requirement of the fetus is met by amniotic fluid. This is supported by many animal studies where ligation of esophagus resulted in growth restriction in the fetus and it was reversible by intragastric feeding. In addition, the neonates who had proximal intestinal obstruction had more severe growth restriction as compared to those with distal obstruction. Amino acids in amniotic fluid such as glutamine and arginine also aid in fetal intestinal growth. Glycoproteins such as transferrin and lactoferrin deliver iron to intestinal epithelium. The dead fetal cells in amniotic fluid after degradation may supply lipid to the growing fetus in the third trimester. Growth factors such as insulin-like growth factor (IGF) present in amniotic fluid aid in fetal growth. The functions and role of amniotic fluid are depicted in **Figure 2**.

AMNIOTIC FLUID MEASUREMENT

There are many methods of amniotic fluid measurement. It can be measured at the time of delivery by direct measurement, dye dilution technique, magnetic resonance imaging (MRI), or ultrasound. Direct measurement even though accurate can be done only once at the time of delivery and hence not useful. Dye dilution technique is invasive and hence not recommended. MRI, even though accurate in volume estimation, is not practical for estimating the amniotic fluid volume. Ultrasound is the preferred method as it is noninvasive, accurate, user-friendly, noncumbersome, and can be repeated for serial monitoring.

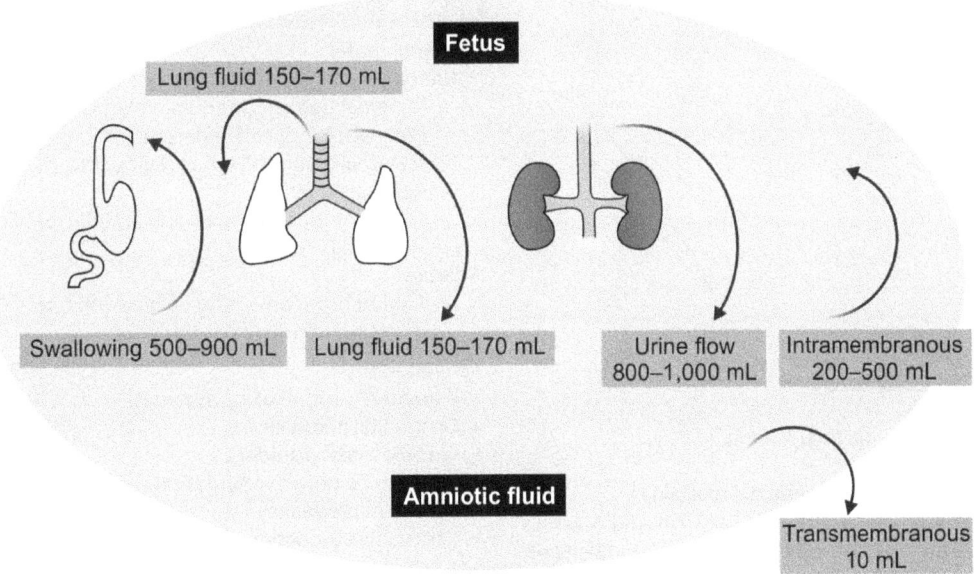

Fig. 1: Pathways of amniotic fluid production and removal.

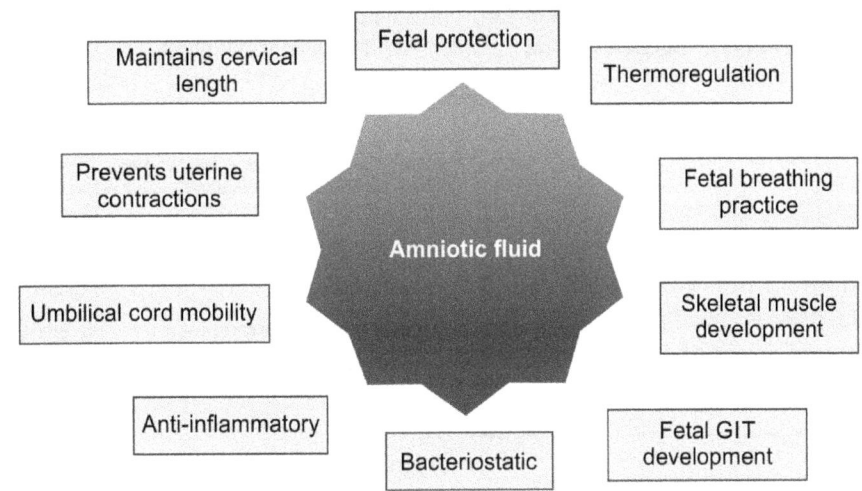

Fig. 2: Role and functions of amniotic fluid.
(GIT: gastrointestinal tract)

The main methods of amniotic fluid estimation using ultrasound are: (1) Amniotic fluid index (AFI), (2) two diameter pocket, (3) deepest vertical pocket (DVP) or single deepest pocket (SDP) or maximal vertical pocket (MVP), and (4) subjective assessment.

Subjective assessment is based on the overall visual impression by the experienced sonologist and is categorized as normal, increased, or decreased. Two diameter pocket, which is a value obtained by multiplication of horizontal and vertical measurement of maximum vertical pocket, is no longer used.

Currently two common methods used for amniotic fluid estimation are AFI and DVP. In AFI, the abdomen is divided into four halves using umbilicus and linea nigra as landmarks. The maximum vertical pocket of fluid (in centimeters) is measured in each quadrant and added to get the AFI (in cm). DVP is obtained after measuring the single largest vertical pocket in any one of the quadrants after global assessment in all the four quadrants. The width of such pocket should be at least 1 cm when such measurement is taken. AFI is approximately three times the DVP.

Although both AFI and DVP are commonly used methods by clinicians for amniotic fluid estimation, most of the studies have shown that AFI overestimates oligohydramnios and might result in unnecessary interventions without any change in the perinatal outcome. Hence, DVP should be considered for making clinical decisions, especially in high-risk pregnancies.

ABNORMALITIES OF AMNIOTIC FLUID VOLUME

Any deviation in the amniotic fluid volume will have an impact on perinatal outcome depending on the severity as shown in **Figure 3**.

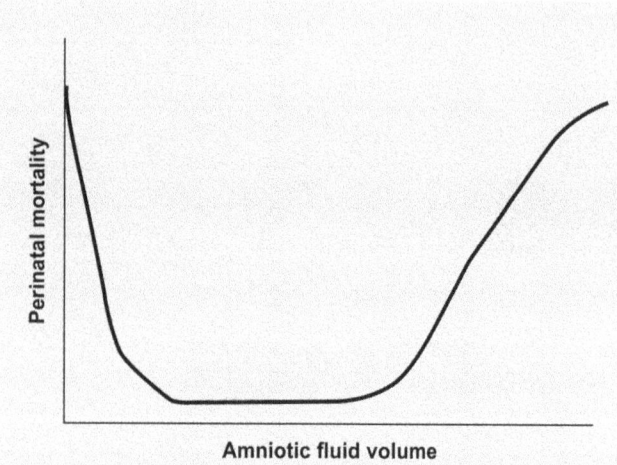

Fig. 3: Amniotic fluid and perinatal mortality.
(*Source:* Martin RJ, Fanaroff AA, Walsh MC. Fanaroff and Martin's Neonatal-Perinatal Medicine, 11th edition. Amsterdam: Elsevier; 2019)

TABLE 1: Amniotic fluid abnormalities.

Amniotic fluid volume	Amniotic fluid Index	Deepest vertical pocket
Normal	8–25 cm	2–8 cm
Oligohydramnios	<8 cm	<2 cm
Polyhydramnios	>25 cm	>8 cm

BOX 1: Etiology of oligohydramnios.

Maternal causes:
- Uteroplacental insufficiency:
  - Maternal dehydration/hypovolemia
  - Pregnancy-induced hypertension
  - Maternal diabetes with vasculopathy
  - Renal disease
  - Autoimmune conditions and antiphospholipid antibody syndrome
- Drugs:
  - Angiotensin-converting enzyme inhibitors
  - Prostaglandin synthase inhibitors

Fetal causes:
- Premature rupture of membranes
- Congenital anomalies
- Chromosomal disorders
- Intrauterine growth retardation
- Post-term pregnancy
- Obstructive uropathy

Placental causes:
- Twin-to-twin transfusion syndrome
- Placental infarction
- Multiple gestation (placental insufficiency)
- Abruption (long-standing)

Idiopathic

TABLE 2: Classification of oligohydramnios.

Amniotic fluid volume	Amniotic fluid index	Deepest vertical pocket
Oligohydramnios	<8 cm	<2 cm
Moderate oligohydramnios	5–8 cm	1–2 cm
Severe oligohydramnios	<5 cm	<1 cm

A decrease in amniotic fluid volume is called oligohydramnios and an increase is called polyhydramnios. The common abnormalities of amniotic fluid volume are depicted in **Table 1**.

OLIGOHYDRAMNIOS

Oligohydramnios is defined sonographically as an AFI < 8 cm or DVP < 2 cm. The incidence varies from 1 to 3%. There are three main reasons for decreased amniotic fluid volume—decreased production, loss, and idiopathic cause. The important causes of oligohydramnios are depicted in **Box 1**.

Among the causes mentioned in **Box 1**, the most common causes are prelabour rupture of membranes (PROM), intrauterine growth restriction (IUGR), and congenital anomalies. When oligohydramnios is diagnosed in the early second trimester, it usually indicates a fetal renal problem or a placental abnormality that affects perfusion. However, ruptured membranes must also be excluded. Oligohydramnios in the latter part of second trimester or in third trimester is usually due to uteroplacental insufficiency. The severity of oligohydramnios based on AFI and DVP is depicted in **Table 2**.

Complications and Pregnancy Outcomes

There is increase in incidence of stillbirth rate, growth restriction, nonreassuring fetal heart rate, meconium aspiration syndrome, preterm birth, and perinatal asphyxia as compared to normal pregnancies. Perinatal mortality is increased by nearly 47 times when oligohydramnios is associated with growth restriction in the fetus.

Approach to Oligohydramnios

When the diagnosis of oligohydramnios is made, a complete history along with physical examination and a detailed ultrasound should be performed to identify the cause. A history of leakage of clear or blood-stained fluid should be asked. If in doubt, a sterile speculum examination should be performed. The presence of fluid in the posterior part of vagina indicates rupture of membranes as the possible cause. There are other tests such as microscopy, pH estimation of the fluid, and a few commercial tests. However, these tests are seldom used in clinical practice.

The next step is to do a detailed ultrasound examination to evaluate the amniotic fluid volume, assess the fetal anatomy, and look for growth parameters in the fetus. If the growth of the fetus is appropriate for gestational age with overall normal anatomy including kidneys and a well-visualized bladder, then the chances of PROM are very likely. Nonvisualization of kidneys and bladder points to congenital renal anomalies and has a poor prognosis. Sometimes, it is difficult to visualize the kidneys in cases of renal agenesis or enlarged adrenal glands can be mistaken as kidneys, especially when there is anhydramnios. In such situations, Doppler of the renal arteries should be done to rule out renal agenesis.

Another important aspect is to evaluate the growth of the fetus. Apart from PROM and congenital malformations, IUGR due to uteroplacental insufficiency is an important cause of oligohydramnios. Hence, a detailed ultrasound examination including Doppler should be done to assess fetal growth.

Pulmonary status should be assessed in all the cases of oligohydramnios. The risk of pulmonary hypoplasia is increased if oligohydramnios is prolonged or if it occurs between 16 and 26 weeks during the canalicular phase of lung development. Even though ultrasound does not accurately rule out pulmonary hypoplasia, there are many sonographic parameters which can predict pulmonary hypoplasia such as lung length and chest circumference, thoracic to abdominal circumference, and lung area ratio. MRI has emerged as a promising mode to detect pulmonary hypoplasia and can be useful in cases where findings of lung ultrasound are equivocal. Whatever technique used, it is important to rule out pulmonary hypoplasia in pregnancies complicated by oligohydramnios, especially when it is long-standing.

Management

The management of oligohydramnios depends on the etiology, gestation, and severity. Pregnancy can be induced if oligohydramnios is detected at term. In preterm pregnancies, if the oligohydramnios is due to PROM and there is evidence of infection, the fetus should be delivered. If there is no evidence of infection, then the patient should be hospitalized and should be observed till 34 weeks of gestation. Antibiotics should be administered and steroids should be given for lung maturity.

When oligohydramnios is accompanied by Doppler abnormalities, fetal heart rate abnormalities, or abnormal biophysical profile, immediate delivery should be considered.

Maternal hydration and left lateral positioning have been shown to transiently increase the amniotic fluid volume. These studies have shown that increase in the amniotic fluid volume was documented when oligohydramnios was diagnosed by AFI and not by DVP criteria. The increase was mild in nature, not sustained, and there was no much change in the perinatal outcome; hence hydration is not used in routine clinical practice.

Tissue sealants for PROM and amnioinfusion are no longer recommended for management of oligohydramnios.

POLYHYDRAMNIOS

Polyhydramnios is defined as amniotic fluid volume >2,000 mL. It is defined sonographically as AFI > 25 or MVP > 8 cm or amniotic fluid volume >95th centile for gestational age. There are three main mechanisms for development of polyhydramnios: Increased production, decreased absorption, and idiopathic cause.

The overall incidence of polyhydramnios is 1–2%. The perinatal mortality and morbidity is directly related to the time of occurrence, with earlier presentation and larger volume resulting in poor outcome. Most of the cases are idiopathic in nature. Among the other common causes are fetal anomalies and diabetes, both of which account for nearly 15% of the cases. Polyhydramnios can also be a component of hydrops fetalis and the conditions leading to it should be excluded. Multiple gestation per se can cause polyhydramnios in about 16–18% of cases; it can also be a part of twin-to-twin transfusion syndrome. The common causes of polyhydramnios are depicted in **Box 2**.

Polyhydramnios increases the risk of preterm delivery and preeclampsia by 2.7-fold, intrauterine fetal death and neonatal death by 7.7-fold, postpartum hemorrhage by sixfold, and caesarean section by fourfold. It also increases the risk of malpresentation due to excess fetal mobility and of abruptio placenta.

Some authors have classified polyhydramnios based on MVP into three subcategories based on both AFI and MVP (**Table 3**). The chances of identifying a specific cause is more with moderate-to-severe polyhydramnios.

Approach and Management

Polyhydramnios should be kept in the list of differential diagnosis when a pregnant woman presents with a rapidly enlarging uterus on clinical examination especially in mid-trimester. A detailed ultrasound examination must be performed to assess complete fetal anatomy. Attention should be given to rule out gastrointestinal and central nervous system anomalies. Stomach bubble should be looked for and its absence suggests esophageal atresia or external compression of esophagus by mass. Presence of "multiple bubble" or multiple cystic structures point toward intestinal atresia. Fetal swallowing must also be assessed during the scan; decreased swallowing may point toward trisomies, neuromuscular disorders, and skeletal dysplasia. Fetal cardiac anatomy should be evaluated when there is associated hydrops fetalis. Placenta should be evaluated to rule out chorioangiomas. Polyhydramnios in association with fetal growth restriction is a dangerous association and, in such circumstances, chromosomal abnormalities and other malformations must be ruled out.

Maternal diabetes must be ruled out when poly-hydramnios is found in an otherwise normal scan. New

BOX 2: Etiology of polyhydramnios.

Maternal: Diabetes mellitus and gestational diabetes mellitus

Fetal:
- *Gastrointestinal anomalies:* Esophageal atresia/trachea-esophageal fistula, duodenal atresia, gastroschisis, omphalocele, and diaphragmatic hernia
- *Central nervous system anomalies:* Anencephaly, holoprosencephaly, and hydranencephaly
- *Pulmonary:* Congenital pulmonary airway malformation, chylothorax, congenital diaphragmatic hernia, and pulmonary sequestration
- *Cardiac:* Congenital heart disease and arrhythmias
- *Craniofacial:* Cleft lip/palate and micrognathia
- Congenital high airway obstruction
- Hydrops fetalis
- Fetal anemia (severe)
- Neuromuscular disorders
- Tumors (hemangioma, teratoma, and mesoblastic nephroma)
- Skeletal dysplasia
- Bartter syndrome

Placental:
- Chorioangioma
- Twin-to-twin transfusion

TABLE 3: Severity of polyhydramnios.

Amniotic fluid volume	Amniotic fluid index	Deepest vertical pocket	Patients affected
Mild polyhydramnios	25–29.9 cm	8–11 cm	65–70%
Moderate polyhydramnios	30–34.9 cm	12–15 cm	20%
Severe polyhydramnios	>35 cm	>16 cm	15%

appearance of polyhydramnios in the third trimester is usually mild and not associated with any structural defect.

Complications

A patient who develops polyhydramnios gradually may tolerate it very well in contrast to acute overdistension which may need intervention. It may induce preterm labor with or without rupture of membranes. These patients may present with symptoms due to effects of overdistension of uterus on other organs. Pressure on diaphragm can lead to dyspnea and orthopnea which reduce only in upright position. Edema of lower limbs, vulva, and abdominal wall may develop due to compression of venous system by the enlarged uterus. These patients are at increased risk of complications during labor such as placental abruption (especially after rapid decompression), uterine atony, and postpartum hemorrhage. There is also an increased rate of cesarean section, macrosomia, and increased perinatal mortality in these pregnancies.

Treatment

In patients with mild idiopathic polyhydramnios with an otherwise normal fetal anatomy, the outcome will be similar to a patient with normal amniotic fluid volume. In patients with polyhydramnios, uterine overdistension may induce rupture of membrane and preterm labor with associated risk of cord prolapse. Hence, these patients should be counseled for signs and symptoms of preterm labor.

Delivery in women with severe polyhydramnios should be considered in a tertiary care center as the risk of fetal anomalies is higher in these pregnancies. In cases of mild idiopathic polyhydramnios, delivery should occur spontaneously and induction should not be considered at <39 weeks of gestation in the absence of other indications. The mode of delivery should be based on routine obstetric indication.

In patients with severe polyhydramnios (AFI > 40), amnioreduction, and prostaglandin inhibitors are considered in the presence of maternal complications such as dyspnea or severe discomfort. Amnioreduction may result in complications such as preterm labor and abruption. There are also chances of reaccumulation of fluid and repeated procedures may be needed. Prostaglandin inhibitors such as indomethacin decrease amniotic fluid volume by reducing the urine output and has been used in pregnancies <32 weeks but it is associated with many neonatal complications such as decreased urine output, increased creatinine, periventricular leukomalacia, and intraventricular hemorrhage. Hence, indomethacin should not be used for the sole purpose of decreasing amniotic fluid in polyhydramnios.

CHAPTER 27 | Oligohydramnios and Polyhydramnios

CHAPTER AT A GLANCE

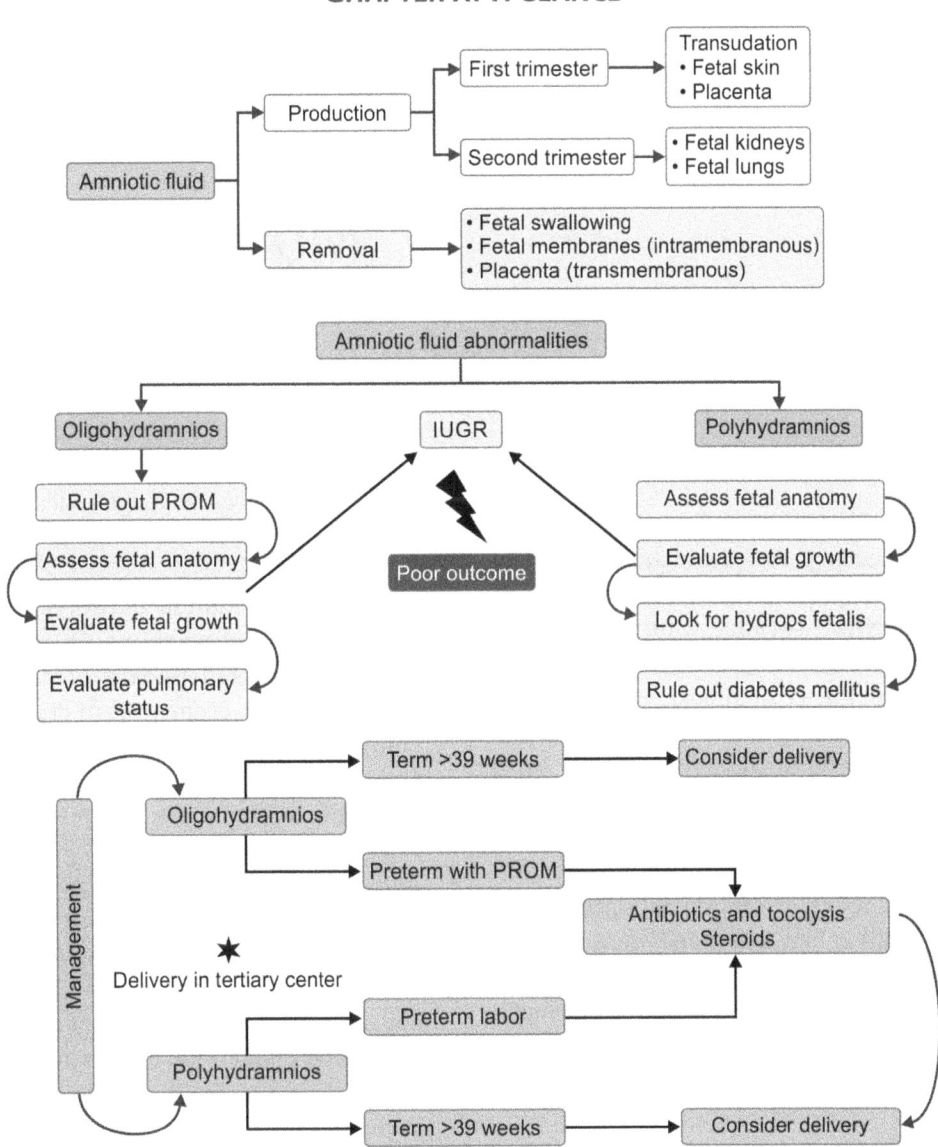

KEY POINTS

- Amniotic fluid is a dynamic in nature and is closely regulated by the fetus, placenta, and mother.
- Amniotic fluid has an important role in the growth and development of fetus.
- MVP/DVP is a better indicator than AFI in the diagnosis of oligohydramnios.
- Oligohydramnios associated with fetal growth restriction is associated with significant perinatal morbidity and mortality.
- Polyhydramnios in early pregnancy is associated with malformations, aneuploidy, and poor perinatal outcome.

SUGGESTED READING

1. Dashe JS, Pressman EK, Hibbard JU. SMFM Consult Series #46: Evaluation and management of polyhydramnios. Am J Obstet Gynecol. 2018;219(4):B2-8.
2. Figueroa L, McClure EM, Swanson J, Nathan R, Garces AL, Moore JL, et al. Oligohydramnios: a prospective study of fetal, neonatal and maternal outcomes in low-middle income countries. Reprod Health. 2020;17(1):19.
3. Sagi-Dain L, Sagi S. Chromosomal aberrations in idiopathic polyhydramnios: A systematic review and meta-analysis. Eur J Med Genet. 2015;58(8):409-15.
4. Underwood MA, Sherman MP. Nutritional characteristics of amniotic fluid. Neoreviews. 2006;7(6):e310-e316.
5. Yeast JD. Polyhydramnios: Etiology, diagnosis, and treatment. Neoreviews. 2006;7(6):e300-4.

28

Multiple Pregnancy

Anil Kallesh BR, Pruthvi Raj V

INTRODUCTION

The occurrence of twin and triplet births has been increasing due to rise in use of assisted reproductive techniques (ARTs) and an increasing number of women delivering at advanced age. Multiple pregnancy is associated with an increased risk to both mother and fetus. Except for postmaturity and macrosomia, a higher incidence of almost every potential complication of a singleton pregnancy is encountered in multiple pregnancy. Preterm birth (PTB) and low birth weight are the most commonly encountered complications leading to increased perinatal, neonatal, and long-term morbidity and mortality. Determining zygosity and chorionicity is of utmost importance, owing to the presence of shared placental circulation between monochorionic twin fetuses, predisposing them for unique complications. After birth, breastfeeding of twins and triplets poses a challenging situation to both the mother and the healthcare provider.

OBJECTIVES

- To review global incidence of multiple births and risk factors for its occurrence.
- To discuss the antenatal care of pregnant mother and monitoring the complications of multiple gestation.
- To discuss the perinatal management of multiple births.
- To discuss the hurdles in breastfeeding the multiples and techniques to overcome the challenge.

EPIDEMIOLOGY, PREVALENCE, AND RISK FACTORS

Prevalence

The occurrence of multiple pregnancies is heterogeneous across the globe varying between countries and populations. This variation is primarily due to the change in frequencies of dizygotic twins. Various overview studies (since the early 1970s) reported that twin birth rates are less than 8 twin births per 1,000 births in south-east Asia, whereas in Europe, USA and India, it is 9–16 per 1,000 live births; it is 17 and more per 1,000 births in African countries. Monozygotic twin births have been relatively constant (3.5–4 per 1,000 births) with little variation across geographical region and race.

Risk Factors

- *ARTs*: Over one-third of all twin births can be attributed to iatrogenic interventions. Due to multiple embryo transfer increased release of oocytes by ovulation induction drugs, occurrence of dizygotic twins are more common following ARTs in comparison to naturally conceived pregnancies (95% vs. 70%). The increasing risk of monozygotic twins appears to be due to embryo cleavage.
- *Advanced maternal age*: With advanced age at conception, there will be an increase in follicle-stimulating hormone concentration and also increased use of fertility-enhancing treatments. Maternal age does not appear to affect the outcomes of twin gestation.
- *Race/geographic area*: Spontaneous twinning is more common in the Black population than in the White population. Naturally conceived dizygotic twins accounted for 1.3 per 1,000 births in Japan, 8 per 1,000 births in the United States and Europe, and 50 per 1,000 births in Nigeria.
- *Parity*: Multiparous women are at an increased risk for dizygotic twin birth in comparison to primiparous women even after adjustment for maternal age.
- *Family history*: Gene-mapping studies have found that specific genetic variants expressed by oocytes and family history of dizygotic twinning in the maternal side were partly responsible for twin gestation.
- *Maternal weight and height*: Obese and tall women [body mass index (BMI) ≥30 kg/m^2 and height >164 cm] are at a greater risk for dizygotic twin birth.

TERMINOLOGIES IN TWIN PREGNANCY AND DIAGNOSIS

Zygosity and Chorionicity

Zygosity: It reflects the type of conception and determines the shared risk for genetic abnormalities among fetuses.

Fertilization of one ovum by one sperm creates a single zygote, which splits into two genetically identical twins resulting in monozygotic twins, which are always of the same sex. Fertilization of two separate ova by two separate sperms creates two different zygotes, which result in dizygotic twins (fraternal twins). They may be of the same or different sex.

Chronicity (placentation): Dizygotic twins will always develop as dichorionic-diamniotic (DCDA) pregnancy resulting in two separate placentas and two separate amniotic sacs. In monozygotic pregnancy, splitting of zygote occurs following fertilization. The developmental stage of zygote splitting determines the chorionicity and the emerging complexity and outcomes of the pregnancy **(Fig. 1)**. Monozygotic splitting may give rise to dichorionic diamniotic (DADC), dichorionic monoamniotic (DCMA), or monochorionic monoamniotic (MAMC). Overall, 80% of monozygotic twins are DC and 20% are monochorionic.

Diagnosis of Multiple Gestations

Twin pregnancy is usually diagnosed during routine first-trimester antenatal ultrasonography (USG). As early as 5 weeks of gestation, USG can show single gestational sac containing multiple yolk sacs or two separate gestational sacs, each containing a separate yolk sac. At 6 weeks, one gestational sac with multiple fetal poles and cardiac activity or separate gestational sacs, each containing a fetal pole with cardiac activity, confirms multiple pregnancy. Accuracy of first-trimester USG to determine the chorionicity and amnionicity is higher (sensitivity > 98%) which dips to (sensitivity ≥ 90%) in the early second trimester. Sonographic identification of fetal membranes is less accurate in the third trimester owing to the presence of oligohydramnios in one or both gestational sacs.

Estimation of Gestational Age

It is essential to accurately time various screening and diagnostic tests, determine fetal growth, and time the delivery. Ultrasound assessment before 22 weeks of gestation provides an accurate estimation of gestational age. If there is a discrepancy between the twins in biometric measurements used for estimating gestational age, if, the consensus is that the gestational age and expected delivery date (EDD) should be based on the measurements for the larger twin.

Determining Zygosity and Chorionicity

Determining zygosity and chorionicity is of utmost importance, due to the presence of shared placental circulation between monochorionic twin fetuses, which predispose them for unique complications discussed later.

- In early sonography, the presence of two discrete placentas is highly suggestive of dichorionic twins. At later gestations, placentas often appear fused precluding accurate identification of chorionicity. Rarely, separate placentas can become fused early in pregnancy. So single

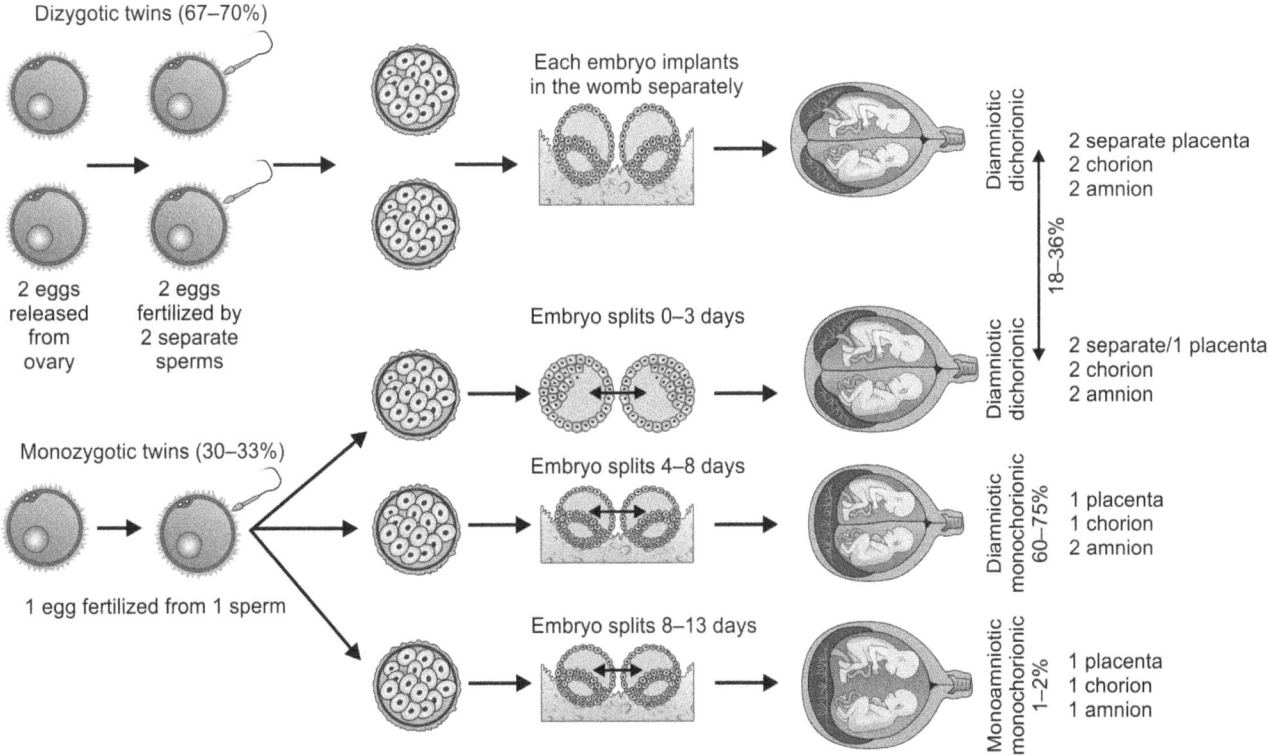

Fig. 1: Zygosity and chorionicity. Formation of monozygotic and dizygotic twins.
Source: Modified from Twin pregnancy in raisingchildren.net.au; the Australian parenting website.

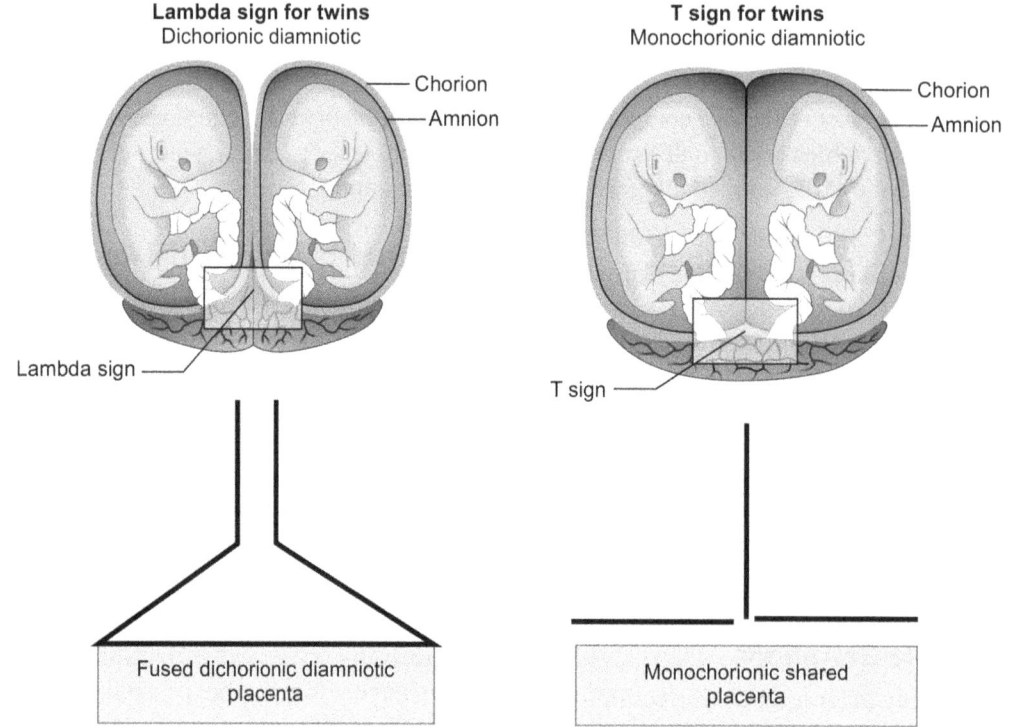

Fig. 2: Lambda sign and "T" sign used in diagnosis of dichorionic diamniotic and diamniotic monochorionic twins.
Source: Modified from Fahad AlQabba's blog on FHYR.

visible placental mass is not diagnostic of a monochorionic pregnancy as occasionally, a monochorionic placenta may be bilobed or has a succenturiate lobe mimicking as two discrete placentas.
- Sonographic presence/absence of the intertwin membrane (lambda sign and T sign).

DADC twins: "Twin peak" or "lambda (λ)" sign in sonography occurs due to the triangular extension of tissue between layers of the intertwin membrane from a fused dichorionic placenta **(Fig. 2)**. The presence of this sign indicates dichorionic twins. It is best appreciated between 10 and 14 weeks, becomes less prominent after 20 weeks of gestation, or may even disappear.

Monochorionic/diamniotic (MCDA) twins: "T" sign on USG appears due to a membrane comprising two amnions as they take off from a monochorionic placenta at a 90° angle **(Fig. 2)**. The presence of "T" sign suggests a MCDA placenta.

Monochorionic monoamniotic: Nonvisualization of intertwin membrane and presence of intertwined umbilical cords (M-mode with two different heart rates in adjacent loops of cord) are diagnostic of monoamniotic twins.

FETAL SURVEILLANCE AND COMPLICATIONS
Antenatal Monitoring of Multiple Pregnancy

Serial ultrasonographic surveillance to identify growth discordance, amniotic fluid levels, cervical length, and other specific complications of monochorionic twins is warranted in twin pregnancy. Serial monitoring should begin from 18 weeks of gestation for uncomplicated dichorionic twins and from 16 weeks for monochorionic twins. The frequency of monitoring is once in every 3–4 weeks. Growth of the twins is usually concordant till 30 weeks of gestation, after which it becomes discordant due to unequal sharing of placenta. Growth charts of singleton pregnancy can be used to label growth abnormality in fetus; discordance in growth is expressed as a percentage. Extent of growth discordance among twins is directly proportional to fetal and perinatal mortality. More than 20% discordance or selective intrauterine growth restriction (IUGR) warrants more frequent fetal surveillance twice weekly with a nonstress test (NST), biophysical profile (BPP), and umbilical artery Doppler flow velocimetry. Routine cervical length measurement between 16 and 24 weeks can help to identify women at risk of preterm delivery. Due to absence of robust evidence, the American College of Obstetricians and Gynecologists (ACOG) does not recommend routine use of cervical cerclage placement or progesterone supplementation for women with twin gestation and a short cervix to prolong pregnancy in these women. For those in preterm onset of labor, tocolytics can be used to facilitate action of antenatal steroids or transfer of pregnant women to a tertiary care center. Antenatal corticosteroids should be administered to women between 24 and 34 weeks if delivery is imminent within the next 7 days and a repeat dose of steroids can be considered for women who remained without delivery after at least 14 days have passed from the administration of the first course of steroids and expected to deliver in the next 7 days and remained at less than 34 gestational weeks of gestation. Magnesium sulfate injection for neuroprotection of the fetus should be used in women at less than 32 weeks and have documented evidence of imminent preterm labor.

Maternal Complications

- Increased risk of physiological anemia and pulmonary edema
- Increased incidence of gestational hypertension, preeclampsia (13% in twins vs. 5–6% in singletons), and HELLP (Hemolysis, Elevated Liver enzymes and Low Platelets) syndrome.
- Increased risk of gestational diabetes mellitus (GDM). Screening, diagnosis, and management of GDM are similar to those in a singleton pregnancy.
- *Others*: Increased incidence of intrahepatic cholestasis of pregnancy, acute fatty liver of pregnancy, hyperemesis gravidarum, abruption, and thromboembolism; pruritic urticarial papules and plaques of pregnancy (PUPPP) is seen.

FETAL COMPLICATIONS

Prematurity

More than 50% of twin and a higher percentage of triplet pregnancies culminate in PTB. The mean gestation age at birth is 36, 33, and 29 weeks, respectively, for twins, triplets, and quadruplets. There is an 8- and 33-times increased likelihood of very low birth weight (VLBW) birth (<1,500 g) in twins and triplets, respectively.

Twin-to-twin Transfusion Syndrome

Twin-to-twin transfusion syndrome (TTTS) is a unique and most serious complication occurring in approximately 8–10% of monochorionic pregnancies. Pathophysiology is attributed to the presence of arteriovenous anastomoses between the two fetuses on the placental surface, allowing transfusion of blood between the donor and the recipient fetus. Diagnosis is made during surveillance USG twin pregnancy. In early stages, a recipient twin amniotic pocket is found to have polyhydramnios showing maximal vertical pocket (MVP) of fluid of >8 cm, and the donor twin has oligohydramnios/anhydramnios and restriction of growth with an MVP of fluid of <2 cm, giving a "stuck-twin" appearance on ultrasound. Fetal echocardiography may depict fluid overload signs like biventricular hypertrophy and progressive cardiac failure. Among many different staging systems proposed, the Quintero staging system is most widely followed to monitor progression in TTTS **(Table 1)**. If TTTS remains untreated or in cases diagnosed at < 20 weeks' gestation, mortality for both twins approaches 80–100%. Management of TTTS is fast evolving and depends on gestational age at diagnosis and stage and includes expectant management and delivery, amnioreduction, termination of pregnancy, selective fetal reduction, and fetoscopic laser (FLS) surgery **(Table 1)**. In the Eurofetus trial that included 142 women, FLS improved perinatal survival (76% vs. 56%), decreased cystic periventricular leukomalacia (PVL; 6% vs. 14%), and caused fewer neurological complications at 6 months of age, compared to serial amnioreduction.

Neonatal management includes and may need packed red blood cells (PRBC) transfusion in donor twin to treat anemia and partial exchange transfusion in recipient twin.

Twin Anemia-polycythemia Sequence

It is characterized by discordance in hematocrit between MC twins in the absence of amniotic fluid abnormality. Twin anemia-polycythemia sequence (TAPS) is seen in

TABLE 1: Quintero staging, management of TTTS, and outcome.

Stage	Findings on ultrasonography	Management	Outcomes
I	Oligohydramnios with the deepest vertical pocket (DVP < 2 cm) in donor sac and polyhydramnios (DVP > 8 cm) in recipient sac	Conservative management (75% regress or remain stable). Weekly monitoring of fetal bladder, UA Doppler, and for hydrops	86% perinatal survival
II	As in I plus bladder of the donor twin not visible	• Referral to tertiary center, for laser photocoagulation • If between 16 and 26 weeks—laser	10% risk of cotwin death 10–30% risk of neurological complications in both twins
III	As in I plus, Doppler studies are critically abnormal, AEDF/REDF in donor abnormal ductus venous flow, a pulsatile umbilical vein in the recipient	• If between 16 and 26 weeks—laser • If no expertise available, serial amnioreduction is tried	
IV	Stage III plus hydrops in one twin	Management same as stages II and III	
V	Death of one or both twin	Conservative management	

(AEDF: absent end diastolic flow; DVP: deepest vertical pocket; REDF: reversal of end diastolic flow; TTTS: twin-to-twin transfusion syndrome; UA: umbilical arteries)

10-13% of cases following fetoscopic laser ablation for TTTS but may occur spontaneously in 3-5% of MC twins. Due to the presence of tiny (<1 mm) arteriovenous anastomoses, chronic and slow transfer of blood occurs between the donor and the recipient, thus delaying the presentation until after 26 gestational weeks or 1-5 weeks after laser therapy for TTTS. Diagnosis is made prenatally by middle cerebral artery peak systolic velocity (MCA-PSV) Doppler discordance or postnatally by hematocrit and reticulocyte count discordance between the twins. Optimal management strategy is still not established.

Twin Reversed Arterial Perfusion Sequence

It is a unique complication of monochorionic twin pregnancy, wherein a morphologically normal cotwin (called "pump twin") exists alongside an acardiac twin (lacks a complete cardiac structure) and supplies both circulations. Incidence of twin reversed arterial perfusion (TRAP) sequence is 1 every 9,500-11,000 pregnancies, and approximately 2.6% of monozygotic twins. The term "reversed arterial perfusion" is used to denote the opposite blood flow direction in the acardiac twin in comparison to normal blood supply of the fetus. In TRAP sequence, oxygenated blood enters towards abnormal twin through the umbilical artery, which usually carries blood away from the fetus towards placenta. The blood then exits through the umbilical vein, which normally carries blood from the placenta to the fetus. The acardiac twin being nonviable, poses significant threat to the pumping twin by increasing workload on its heart. Larger the size of acardiac twin, higher is the risk to the pumping twin. This may eventually lead to (1) polyhydramnios and congestive heart failure and of the pump twin, (2) overdistension of uterus resulting in preterm prelabour rupture of membranes (PPROM) and preterm delivery (3) IUGR of the pump twin due to hypoxia caused by the deoxygenated blood that comes back to the pump twin through vascular anastomosis. Management of TRAP involves interrupting the vascular supply to the acardiac twin. Ultrasound guided laser coagulation or radiofrequency ablation of intrafetal vessels are the preferred approaches. Timing of intervention is still a controversy. The ongoing TRAP Intervention Study (TRAPIST), comparing treatment at 13-15 weeks versus 16 weeks, is expected to define the optimal timing of treatment.

Intrauterine Fetal Demise

Death of one of the twins significantly influences the prognosis and survival of the surviving twin. In monochorionic twins, due to shared placental circulation, death of one fetus causes significant hypotension in the other fetus, leading to death or severe neurologic morbidity in the surviving twin in 26% of cases. Neurologic injury may not be preventable by immediate delivery of the surviving fetus. Due to high risk of stillbirth for the surviving twin, delivery at 34-36 weeks of gestation is reasonable.

In dizygotic twins, since there is no shared placental circulation, death of one dizygotic twin has minimal effect on the surviving cotwin. If the death occurs early in the first trimester, the cotwin may be completely resorbed "vanishing twin" or compressed between the amniotic sac and the uterine wall (fetus papyraceus). The demised twin genetic material can affect the results of cell-free DNA testing when used to screen for the common fetal aneuploidies.

Higher Order Multiple-gestation Triplets and Quadruplets

Triplets, quadruplets, and higher order multiple gestations carry a proportionately increasing risk of gestational hypertension, GDM, antepartum, premature rupture of membranes, antepartum and postpartum hemorrhage, and PTB. Since robust data to support vaginal delivery of triplets or quadruplets are lacking, delivery by cesarean section is the preferred mode. Due to the above-mentioned increased risks to both the mother and the fetus, reducing multifetal pregnancy to twin or singleton has been shown to improve perinatal outcomes.

Conjoined Twins

Splitting of a monozygotic embryo after 14 days of fertilization results in conjoined twins, present within a monochorionic and monoamniotic gestational sac. Conjoined twins are classified based on the anatomical site of union (e.g., head, chest) and adding a suffix "pagus" [meaning fixed (e.g., craniopagus)]. USG shows monoamnionicity, shared organs at the site of fusion, and contiguous skin. Fetal anomaly scan and echocardiography, along with additional magnetic resonance imaging (MRI), are essential to counsel the parents about prognosis and survival and plan for possible postnatal surgical management. Cesarean section is the mode of delivery of all viable conjoined twins.

MODE OF DELIVERY, MORBIDITY, AND MORTALITY

Delivery Plan

Because of the increased risk of stillbirth in twin pregnancy with increasing gestation age, delivery is typically considered at 37-38 weeks. Ultrasonographic examination should be done to confirm the presentation of both twins to plan the mode of delivery. Induction of labor can be done by prostaglandins, intracervical Foley balloon, and oxytocin infusion. In 40-45% of cases both twins will be in the vertex position and, in such cases vaginal delivery can be attempted. If the first twin is nonvertex or both the twins are in a nonvertex position and in all monochorionic monoamniotic twins, cesarean section is the preferred mode of delivery.

Continuous cardiotocography (CTG) of both twins throughout labor should be attempted in women going for vaginal delivery. The first twin is better monitored by fetal scalp electrode, unless it is contraindicated. Twin two should be monitored by an abdominal external transducer. Delivery should take place in an operation theater setting where backup for cesarean section with an anesthetist and a neonatologist is alerted. The delivery of the second twin should not be rushed if there is no visible cord prolapse or bleeding and if the fetal heart rate remains normal on a cardiotocograph. The delivery interval between first and second twins should generally be less than 30 minutes but may be prolonged if the fetal heart rate tracing is normal. One may attempt stabilization of lie, internal podalic version, breech extraction, or immediate cesarean section based on the skilled expertise available. Active management of the third stage of labor is advised.

Neonatal Morbidity and Mortality and Long-term Morbidities

Prematurity and IUGR are associated with an increased risk of necrotizing enterocolitis, bronchopulmonary dysplasia, retinopathy of prematurity, and intraventricular hemorrhage among the neonates. The risk of cerebral palsy (CP) in twins is 7.4% in comparison to singleton (1%). Twins account for 5–10% of all cases of cerebral palsy. Twins have a higher risk of learning disability, even after controlling for CP and low birth weight.

Feeding in Multiple Pregnancy

Rates of breastfeeding are lower in women with multiple births (twins, triplets, or more) compared to a singleton pregnancy. Both antenatal and postnatal education of pregnant women and family members and good lactational support have been found to increase any/exclusive breastfeeding rate and duration. PTB and need for neonatal intensive care unit (NICU) admission of one or both twins can lead to delayed starting or early stoppage of breastfeeding. Current recommendations for energy supplementation during breastfeeding are 2,100–2,500 kJ (500–600 kcal) per baby per day. The infants do not necessarily have the same sucking ability, and the new situation is often quite overwhelming for the parents. It is preferable to alternate breasts when breastfeeding twins. This ensures that each breast receives balanced stimulation from the different babies and that the milk yield for each baby will be the same.

Commonly used positions for simultaneous breastfeeding:
- Double football
- Double cradle
- Combination of the cradle with football

CHAPTER AT A GLANCE

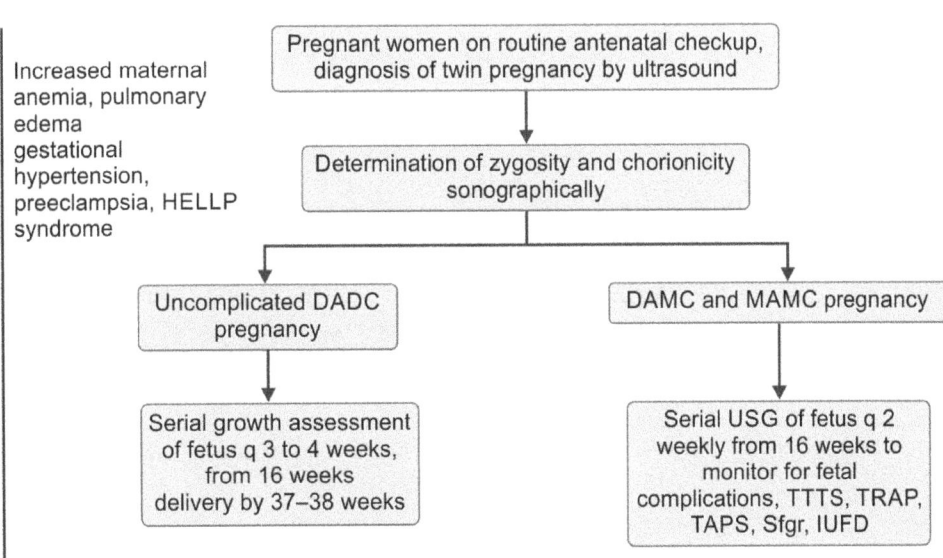

(DADC: diamniotic dichorionic; DAMC: diamniotic monochorionic; HELLP: Hemolysis, Elevated Liver enzymes and Low Platelets; IUFD: intrauterine fetal demise; MAMC: monochorionic monoamniotic; TAPS: twin anemia-polycythemia sequence; TTTS: twin-to-twin transfusion syndrome; USG: ultrasonography; TRAP: twin reversed arterial perfusion)

KEY POINTS

- Incidence of multiple pregnancy is rising due to use of ARTs and are associated with increased maternal and fetal complications.
- Determination of zygosity and chorionicity is of utmost importance to monitor growth of twins and identify complications of monochorionicity.
- Both antenatal and postnatal education of pregnant women and family members and good lactational support have been found to increase any/exclusive breastfeeding rate and duration.

SUGGESTED READING

1. American College of Obstetricians and Gynecologists' Committee on Practice Bulletins—Obstetrics, Society for Maternal-Fetal Medicine. Multifetal gestations: twin, triplet, and higher-order multifetal pregnancies: ACOG practice bulletin, Number 231. Obstet Gynecol. 2021;137:e145.
2. Chauhan SP, Scardo JA, Hayes E, Abuhamad AZ, Berghella V. Twins: prevalence, problems, and preterm births. Am J Obstet Gynecol. 2010;203:305-15.
3. D'Alton M, Breslin N. Management of multiple gestations. Int J Gynecol Obstet. 2020;150:3-9.
4. Khalek N, Johnson MP, Bebbington MW. Fetoscopic laser therapy for twin-to-twin transfusion syndrome. Semin Pediatr Surg. 2013;22:18-23.
5. Senat MV, Deprest J, Boulvain M, Paupe A, Winer N, Ville Y. Endoscopic laser surgery versus serial amnioreduction for severe twin-to-twin transfusion syndrome. N Engl J Med. 2004;351(2):136-44.

29: Bad Obstetric History

Kalyan Chakravarthy Balla, Bhagya Lakshmi

INTRODUCTION
Pregnancy loss is a challenging problem for both couples and clinicians. The scenario gets complicated if there are multiple such events with the same couple. The subsequent pregnancies are labeled high risk and tend to have statistically higher chance of poorer outcomes than otherwise. These could be abortions, stillbirths, or premature deliveries. The emotional burden on the family also becomes an important factor to be considered by the treating physician. In this chapter, we try to understand the causes and evaluation of common scenarios labeled together as "Bad Obstetric History" (BOH).

OBJECTIVES
- To define the heterogeneous group of conditions labeled together as BOH.
- To identify risk factors for recurrent abortions, previous stillbirths, preterm deliveries, and early neonatal deaths (END).
- To evaluate and manage pregnancy in women with BOH.

DEFINITIONS
The optimal natural outcome of a conception is a full-term delivery. However, recurrent unfavorable fetal outcomes are not uncommon. The term "Bad Obstetric History" is loosely used to indicate that the outcome of current pregnancy is likely to be affected adversely by the nature of the outcome of the previous pregnancy. These "adverse" outcomes could include miscarriages which happen in first or second trimester, stillbirth, or preterm delivery.

The various definitions used in clinical practice are as follows:
- *BOH*: Two or more adverse outcomes with pregnancies (Consensus definition).
- *Recurrent pregnancy loss (RPL) or miscarriage*: Two or more pregnancy losses before 24 weeks of gestational age.
- *Stillbirth*: Pregnancy loss after 24 weeks of gestational age.
- *Preterm delivery*: Delivery of a live newborn after 23 weeks of gestational age and before 37 weeks of gestational age.
- *END*: Death of a newborn in the first 7 days of life.

RECURRENT PREGNANCY LOSS OR MISCARRIAGE

Incidence
The true incidence is uncertain. The reported incidence is 15% of all pregnancies. It affects about 1% of couples. With an increase in the number of abortions, the subsequent risks of miscarriages are higher **(Table 1)**.

Risk Factors
- *Epidemiological factors (Fig. 1)*:
  - Maternal age and previous miscarriages are two independent risk factors. Advancing maternal age is associated with a higher risk of RPL. The incidence of miscarriage at 12–19 years is 13% as compared to 25% at 35–39 years of age. The incidence further increases to 93% for women over 45 years of age.
  - Advanced paternal age is also identified as a risk factor. The risk of miscarriage is the highest among couples where the woman is >35 years and the man is >40 years of age.
  - *Previous reproductive history*: The risk increases with each subsequent pregnancy loss with the risk being over 40% after three previous pregnancy losses. A previous live birth does not preclude a woman developing miscarriage.

TABLE 1: Risk for recurrence after previous miscarriage.

With no history of previous miscarriage	15%
After 1 abortion	19%
After 2 abortions	35%
After 3 abortions	47%

Source: Adapted from RCOG guidelines on recurrent pregnancy loss (updated in 2017).

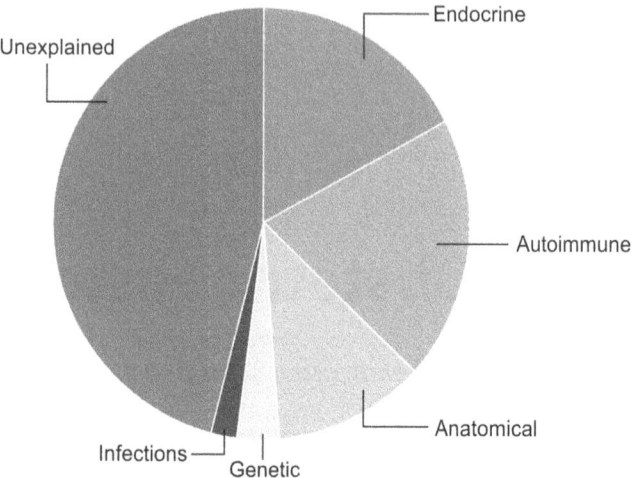

Fig. 1: Etiology of recurrent pregnancy loss.

- Environmental factors are usually risk factors for sporadic rather than recurrent miscarriage. Maternal smoking, caffeine consumption, and heavy alcohol consumption are associated with increased risk. Obesity is shown to increase the chance of both sporadic and recurrent miscarriage in retrospective studies.
- *Antiphospholipid antibody (APLA) syndrome or antiphospholipid syndrome (APS)*: This is the most important treatable cause of recurrent miscarriage. This syndrome refers to association between antibodies and adverse pregnancy outcome or vascular thrombosis.
  Adverse pregnancy outcomes include:
  - Three or more consecutive miscarriages before 10 weeks
  - One or more morphologically normal fetal losses after 10 weeks of gestation
  - One or more preterm birth before 34 weeks of gestation due to placental disease

  The mechanism of morbidity in APS is inhibition of trophoblastic function and differentiation in early pregnancy, and thrombosis of uteroplacental vasculature in the later period of gestation.

  The APLA syndrome has been observed among 15% of all women presenting with recurrent miscarriages and 2% of low obstetric risk women. In women with APLA syndrome with recurrent miscarriages, less than 10% deliver a live birth baby with no pharmacological intervention.
- *Genetic factors*:
  - *Parental chromosomal rearrangements*: About 2–5% of couples. Balanced structural chromosomal anomaly is the most common finding.
  - *Embryonic chromosomal abnormalities*: The risk increases with advancing maternal age. In couples with recurrent miscarriage, embryonic chromosomal abnormalities account for 30–57% of further miscarriages.
- *Anatomical factors*:
  - *Congenital uterine malformations*: The prevalence is varied across various studies (1.8–37.6%). The prevalence of uterine malformations appears to be higher in women with second-trimester miscarriages. Arcuate uteri tend to miscarry more in the second trimester, while septate uteri are more likely to miscarry in the first trimester. A retrospective study showed that women with uterine anomalies tend to have higher miscarriage rates or preterm deliveries. Term delivery occurs in only about 50%.
  - *Cervical weakness*: This results in spontaneous recurrent second-trimester abortions or spontaneous rupture of membranes.
- *Endocrine factors*: Systemic maternal endocrine disorders such as diabetes mellitus and thyroid disease are associated with miscarriage. Polycystic ovary syndrome has been linked to an increased risk of miscarriage.
- *Infective agents*: Any severe bacterial or viral infection can result in sporadic miscarriage. Bacterial vaginosis is associated with second-trimester miscarriage and preterm delivery. A randomized controlled trial (RCT) showed that treatment of vaginosis early in the second trimester significantly reduces the incidence of miscarriage or preterm delivery.

  It is important to note that TORCH [Toxoplasmosis, Other (syphilis, varicella-zoster, parvovirus B19), Rubella, Cytomegalovirus (CMV), and Herpes infections] infections do not result in RPL.
- *Inherited thrombophilic defects*: Both inherited and acquired thrombophilias are possibly associated with RPL. Activated protein C resistance, deficiency of protein C/S, antithrombin III, hyperhomocysteinemia, and prothrombin gene mutation are established causes of systemic thrombosis.

Evaluation of Couples with Recurrent Pregnancy Loss (Table 2)

- *Antiphospholipid antibodies*: Screen for antiphospholipid antibodies in:
  - All women with recurrent first-trimester miscarriage
  - All women with one or more second-trimester miscarriage

  The updated International Consensus (Sydney) Classification (ICS) criteria for definite APS require the presence of:
  - A lupus anticoagulant (LA) and/or
  - IgG or IgM anticardiolipin antibodies (aCL) present in medium or high titer (i.e., >40 GPL or MPL or >99th percentile) and/or anti-β_2 glycoprotein-1 (aβ_2GPI) (IgG and/or IgM) >99th percentile.

  These should be persistent, defined as being present on two or more consecutive occasions at least 12 weeks apart.

TABLE 2: Evaluation of recurrent pregnancy loss.

Etiology	Recommended evaluation
Genetic	Karyotype of both parents
Anatomic	Hysterosalpingography, hysteroscopy 2D or 3D ultrasound, saline-infusion sonohysterography
Endocrine	• TSH • Possible testing for insulin resistance, serum prolactin level, ovarian reserve testing, antithyroid antibodies
Infections	No evaluation recommended unless patient has chronic endometritis/cervicitis or is immunocompromised
Autoimmune	• Anticardiolipin antibody levels (IgG and IgM) • Lupus anticoagulant
Non-APS thrombophilia	Homocysteine, factor V Leiden, prothrombin promoter mutation, activated protein C resistance

Source: Adapted from Ford HB, Schust D. Recurrent pregnancy loss: etiology, diagnosis and therapy. Rev Obstet Gynecol. 2009;2(2):76-83.
(APS: antiphospholipid syndrome; TSH: thyroid stimulating hormone)

TABLE 3: Therapeutic intervention for recurrent pregnancy losses—etiology based.

• Genetic • Balanced translocations	• Genetic counseling • IVF with preimplantation genetic diagnosis • Donor gametes
• Anatomic • Mullerian anomalies • Asherman syndrome	• Hysteroscopic resection of septa, adhesions, and submucosal fibroids • Myomectomy for intramural and subserosal fibroids >5 cm
Endocrine—PCOS/hypothyroidism/diabetes, luteal phase defects	• Appropriate control • Progesterone supplementation
Infections	Antibiotics
Autoimmune—APS	Low-dose aspirin plus prophylactic LMWH in women without a history of a systemic autoimmune disease such as SLE or a history of thrombosis
Thrombophilias	Therapeutic anticoagulation
Environmental factors	Limit exposure to tobacco or alcohol

Source: Adapted from Ford HB, Schust D. Recurrent pregnancy loss: etiology, diagnosis and therapy. Rev in Obstet Gynecol. 2009;2(2): 76-83.
(APS: antiphospholipid syndrome; IVF: in vitro fertilization; LMWH: low-molecular-weight heparin; PCOS: polycystic ovarian syndrome; SLE: systemic lupus erythematosus)

- *Karyotyping*:
  - Cytogenetic analysis on products of conception of the third and subsequent consecutive miscarriages.
  - Blood karyotyping of both parents in couples with recurrent miscarriages.
- *Anatomical evaluation*: All women with RPL in the first trimester and one or more second-trimester miscarriages should undergo pelvic ultrasound. Suspected anomalies require confirmatory tests such as hysteroscopy, laparoscopy, or three-dimensional pelvic ultrasound.
- *Thrombophilia:* In women with second-trimester miscarriages, thrombophilia evaluation such as factor V Leiden, prothrombin gene mutation, and protein S should be done.

Treatment of Recurrent Pregnancy Loss

- *APS*: Pregnant women with APLA syndrome should be treated with low-dose aspirin and heparin to prevent RPL. This combination decreases the risk of miscarriage rate by 54%. There are no adverse fetal outcomes noted with low-dose aspirin. Corticosteroids or intravenous immune globulin (IVIG) do not improve outcomes **(Table 3)**.
- *Genetic factors*: Parental karyotype abnormalities should be promptly referred to a clinical geneticist. Preimplantation genetic diagnosis with in vitro fertilization is proposed as a treatment option in couples who are carriers of translocation. However, it is not useful for routine unexplained recurrent miscarriages.
- *Anatomical factors*: There are insufficient data to assess the role of septal resection in women with recurrent miscarriage with uterine septum.

Women with a history of second-trimester miscarriage and suspected cervical weakness should be offered serial cervical sonography. If a cervical length of 25 mm or less is detected by a transvaginal scan before 24 weeks of gestational age, cerclage should be offered.

STILLBIRTH

Stillbirth is defined as fetal death occurring before birth after a selected, predefined duration of gestation. The timing of stillbirth could be antenatal or intrapartum. Since the gestational age of viability is varied across various countries, the definition is quite varied.

A single stillbirth can meet the definition of BOH.

Incidence of Stillbirth

Globally, the stillbirth rate (SBR) is 18.4 per 1,000 total live births (2015). 98% of all stillbirths occur in low- and middle-income countries. India has the highest number of stillbirths in the whole world. However, the numbers have been consistently decreasing over years. The current rate of SBR is 13.9 per 1,000 live births (2019). The Government of India has developed an Indian Newborn Action Plan (INAP) which includes efforts to reduce stillbirths to <10 per 1,000 births by 2030.

Causes of Stillbirth

The cause of death of a fetus is often unknown but is usually attributed to various origins. In about 25-60% of cases, the cause is unknown.

Risk Factors

Maternal Causes

- *Maternal infections*: These are the most important causes of stillbirth. Common ascending infections due to *Escherichia coli*, Group B Streptococci, *Mycoplasma*, etc., are the causative agents. In developing nations, the common other infections of note are malaria, syphilis, and HIV. Viral causes are parvovirus and CMV.
- *Maternal disorders*: Maternal diabetes is an important cause of late third-trimester sudden fetal deaths. Thyroid abnormalities, hypertensive disorders, SLE, renal diseases, cholestasis of pregnancy, and sickle cell diseases are other noted risk factors.
- Anemia and nutritional deficiencies are also long studied causes of stillbirths.

Fetal Causes

- Poor fetal growth is the most frequent cause of stillbirth. This is usually due to placental dysfunction.
- Other cited causes are multiple gestation, congenital anomalies, genetic abnormalities, fetal infections, and postmaturity.

Placental Causes

The cited causes of stillbirth in relation to placenta and membranes are placental abruption, premature rupture of membrane, vasa previa, vascular malformations, umbilical cord accidents, and chorioamnionitis.

External Causes

- Antepartum maternal injuries/trauma
- Labor incidents resulting in prolonged intrapartum asphyxia are a noted cause of stillbirth in developing countries.

Epidemiological Factors

Factors associated with increased risk are body mass index (BMI) > 30 kg/m^2, smoking, substance abuse, and multiple gestations.

Diagnosis of Stillbirth

Clinical Signs

Antepartum: Lack of fetal movements, maintained or decreased maternal weight, and absent fetal heart sounds (though not a sensitive method to ascertain the presence or absence of viable fetus). Real-time ultrasonography is the gold standard to diagnose stillbirth.

Postpartum: Death is confirmed by APGAR score of 0 at 1 and 5 minutes and absent vital signs. The degree of maceration can determine the time of death.

Recurrence of Stillbirth

There is a four-fold increase in SBR after a previous stillbirth. Rates of recurrence of stillbirth are higher in women with medical complications such as diabetes or hypertension. In those with an obstetric cause of stillbirth, the patients with placental abruption are at significantly higher risk for recurrence **(Table 4)**.

RECURRENT PRETERM BIRTH

Prematurity is the most common cause of neonatal mortality in India and the developed world. About 30% of all neonatal deaths in India are due to prematurity. This, therefore, contributes to poor obstetric outcomes when recurrent.

Recurrent preterm birth is defined as two or more deliveries before 37 completed weeks of gestational age.

Preterm birth is usually preceded by one of the three reasons: Preterm labor (PTL), preterm prelabor rupture of membranes (PPROM), or "indicated" preterm termination of pregnancy.

Studies have shown that with each preterm delivery, the risk of prematurity increases in subsequent pregnancies. The more preterm the previous delivery, the greater are the

TABLE 4: Management of pregnancy after previous stillbirth.

Prepregnancy or first visit: • Detailed medical/obstetric workup • Evaluation and workup of previous stillbirth • Determination of recurrence risk • Smoking cessation • Weight loss in obese women (prepregnancy only) • Genetic counseling if family history of genetic condition • Diabetic screening • Acquired thrombophilia testing • Support and reassurance	*First trimester:* • Dating sonography • *First-trimester screening*: Pregnancy associated plasma protein A, TIFFA scan for nuchal translucency or cell free fetal DNA testing • Support and reassurance *Second trimester:* • Fetal anatomical survey at 18–20 weeks • Offer genetic screening • Support and reassurance
Third trimester: • Sonographic evaluation for fetal growth restriction after 32 weeks • Antepartum fetal surveillance after 32 weeks or 1–2 weeks earlier than the previous stillbirth • Support and reassurance	*Delivery:* • Planned delivery at $39^{0/7}$ weeks of gestation or as dictated by obstetric indications • If severe parental anxiety, after shared decision making exercise, can deliver at early term gestation

(TIFFA: targeted imaging for fetal anomalies)

odds of recurrence of prematurity. The chance of recurrence, therefore, depends on the cause of the prematurity and the gestation of delivery.

PPROM and Recurrence

Preterm prelabor rupture of membranes contributes to 30-40% of all preterm deliveries. The risk of recurrence of PPROM could be as high as 13-32% in subsequent deliveries as opposed to just 4% among pregnancies which were not complicated by PPROM. The only consistently associated risk factor for PPROM is short cervical length.

Cervical Insufficiency and Recurrent Prematurity

Cervical insufficiency is traditionally suspected in women with midtrimester abortions or recurrent early preterm deliveries. On ultrasound, the shorter the cervix, the greater are the chances of preterm delivery. There is no single consensus on the length of cervix, but a length <25 mm at 24 weeks of gestational age is considered short.

Indicated Preterm Birth and Prematurity

This includes deliveries necessitated by risk posed to the mother or fetus due to complications from obstetric or medical conditions. Gestational hypertension is the most common cause that could result in fetal growth restriction or impending symptoms in the mother prompting delivery.

There is a two-fold increased risk of recurrence in prematurity in this group in subsequent pregnancies.

Management

Prevention of preterm birth:
- *Progesterone administration*: Patients with a previous history of one or more spontaneous preterm birth showed significant reduction in prematurity with the use of progesterone. The number needed to treat in the progesterone group is as small as 4.7 women to avoid one preterm birth below 34 weeks. There is no benefit noted with prematurity due to multiple gestations.
- *Cerclage*: Since a short cervix is associated with PPROM and preterm birth, cervical cerclage is considered a treatment modality to prevent prematurity. Available evidence suggests that patients with clinical evidence of acute cervical insufficiency and those with history of cervical insufficiency and progressive shortening of cervix benefit most with cerclage.

EARLY NEONATAL DEATH

Early neonatal deaths are defined as death of a newborn in the first 7 days of life and they account for 73% of all postnatal deaths worldwide. In India, about 40% of all stillbirth and neonatal deaths occur during labor or on the day of birth. India is gearing up to achieve its target to single digit neonatal mortality rate (NMR) by the year 2030 as per India Newborn Action plan; however, there has not been much improvement in the END rates as opposed to late neonatal and postneonatal deaths.

Incidence

In India, the NMR is about 22 per 1,000 live births with over 72% of them occurring in the first week of life. There is a considerable difference between urban and rural population. There is also wide variation among various states in the same.

Etiology

Important risk factors include the following:
- *In developed nations*: Prematurity, congenital anomalies, and sudden infant death syndrome.
- *In developing nations*: Perinatal events such as asphyxia and infections.
- *In India*: Prematurity (35%), asphyxia (20%), pneumonia (16%), sepsis (15%), and malformations (9%).

Role in Recurrence

Any END should prompt the treating clinician to look at the possibility of recurrence. While common causes, such as prematurity and intrauterine growth restriction (IUGR), resulting in low birth weight are known to repeat in the subsequent pregnancies and contribute to neonatal mortality and morbidity, less frequent causes of END such as malformations and inborn errors of metabolism (IEM) can also recur.

Management of Pregnancies with Previous Early Neonatal Deaths

- Detailed obstetric history and ascertain the cause of previous END
- Recurrence risk is evaluated
- Support the current pregnancy with the available data
- Antenatal testing where possible, such as fetal anatomical survey and genetic testing where relevant.
- Prematurity preventive strategies

For families with a history of END due to suspected IEM, subsequent neonates are evaluated even if asymptomatic. Babies are kept in observation and started on minimal breast feeds. The feeds are slowly increased over the next 24-48 hours. Metabolic evaluation is done and if negative, full feeds are established over the next 2-3 days. Families are counseled about the need for repeat evaluation if there are any clinical signs.

WORKUP OF A PREGNANCY WITH BAD OBSTETRIC HISTORY

- *Ascertain the nature of "BOH"*: Recurrent first-trimester pregnancy loss or previable second-trimester pregnancy loss or preterm birth or stillbirth or END.

- Baseline risk:
  - Maternal age
  - Paternal age
  - Marital life
  - Obesity
  - Prepregnancy genital tract procedures
  - *Maternal medical history*: Immunological/infections (tuberculosis)/geneti/IEM
  - *Maternal lifestyle history*: Smoking, alcohol, or substance abuse
- Previous obstetric history:
  - *Detailed account of every conception*: Natural or assisted, planned or unplanned
  - *Gestation of termination*: Delivery or abortion
  - Obstetric complications during pregnancy
  - Medical complications during pregnancy
  - Treatment of each complication
  - *In the event of pregnancy loss*: Cause, tests performed to ascertain
  - Interpregnancy interval
- Workup to be done for:
  - Previous recurrent pregnancy losses
  - Previous stillbirth
  - Previous preterm delivery
  - Previous END
- Workup in between pregnancies
- END: Complete details of birth gestation, birth weight, any history of asphyxia, timing of neonatal death, probable cause of neonatal death, evaluation of the neonatal death along with autopsy report if available.

CHAPTER AT A GLANCE

Bad Obstetric History—Any pregnancy at risk for a poor outcome due to previous obstetric history

RPL
- Two or more unplanned miscarriages
- Majority of couples—cause is unknown
- Immunological/Endocrine/Anatomical causes—measures can be taken for prevention
- Antiphospholipid antibody syndrome is an important cause of RPL
- Genetic causes—can be treated with IVF with donor ovum/sperm
- Thrombophilias—anticoagulation is used

Recurrent stillbirth
- The definition of stillbirth is linked to the definition of viability and hence it changes from country to country
- Maternal infections and gestational diabetes are important causes of stillbirth
- Poor fetal growth is an important cause of stillbirth
- Fetal surveillance is the key to avert recurrance of stillbirth

Recurrent preterm
- Causes: PPROM, preterm labor, and indicated preterm (for fetal or maternal reasons)
- Short cervical length and previous prematurity strongly predict recurrence in prematurity
- Progestrone and cervical cerclage are offered to prevent prematurity

Recurrent END
- Death in the first 7 days of life is called early neonatal death (END)
- Most common causes: Prematurity, asphyxia and sepsis
- In developed nations: Congenital anomalies contribute significantly to END
- Prematurity, anomalies and IEM can recur and need to be carefully monitored and evaluated during pregnancy as well as postnatally

(IEM: inborn errors of metabolism; IVF: in vitro fertilization; PPROM: preterm prelabor rupture of membranes; RPL: recurrent pregnancy loss)

KEY POINTS

- BOH describes a pregnancy wherein the previous obstetric performance by the woman is more likely to result in unfavorable outcome in the current pregnancy.
- It can be recurrent miscarriages, recurrent preterm births, stillbirths, or END.
- While a vast majority of pregnancy losses are due to unexplained reasons, it is important to evaluate the couples where there are recurrent losses. Potential causes with good response to therapy are immunological, endocrine, or anatomical reasons.
- For pregnancies with previous stillbirth, careful evaluation, monitoring and constant support throughout pregnancy are needed to avert any complications.
- In pregnancies with previous preterm birth, use of progesterone and cervical cerclage are shown to be effective.
- END forms major part of neonatal death in India. Prevention of asphyxia and sepsis is the key to bring down this number.
- In families with history of previous END, careful escalation of feeds under supervision and investigation for IEM will avert sudden postnatal collapse due to IEM-related complications.

SUGGESTED READING

1. El Hachem H, Crepaux V, May-Panloup P, Descamps P, Legendre G, Bouet PE. Recurrent pregnancy loss: current perspectives. Int J Womens Health. 2017;9:331-45.
2. Kapoor M, Kim R, Sahoo T, Roy A, Ravi S, Shiva Kumar AK, et al. Association of Maternal History of Neonatal Death with Subsequent Neonatal Death in India. JAMA Netw Open. 2020;3(4):e202887.
3. Lamont K, Scott NW, Jones GT, Bhattacharya S. Risk of recurrent stillbirth: systematic review and meta-analysis. BMJ. 2015;350:h3080.
4. Lehtonen L, Gimeno A, Parra-Llorca A, Vento M. Early neonatal death: a challenge worldwide. Semin Fetal Neonatal Med. 2017;22(3):153-60.
5. RCOG Practice Guidelines. Recurrent pregnancy loss: Update on investigation and management. Updated 2017.
6. Yang J, Baer RJ, Berghella V, Chambers C, Chung P, Coker T, et al. Recurrence of preterm birth and early term birth. Obstet Gynecol. 2016;128(2):364-72.

CHAPTER 30

Chorioamnionitis

Deepti Thandaveshwar, KB Suma

INTRODUCTION

Chorioamnionitis or intra-amniotic infection refers to an acute inflammation of the membranes and chorion of the placenta. This occurs due to ascending bacterial infection and is frequently associated with premature rupture of the membranes. Chorioamnionitis is a dreaded complication of pregnancy resulting in maternal, fetal, and neonatal complications. The incidence varies from 2-4% to approximately 40-70% in term and preterm deliveries, respectively. Chorioamnionitis can be defined both clinically and histologically. Maternal symptoms like fever, abdominal pain, foul-smelling vaginal discharge, and leukocytosis are clinical clues while histologically, inflammation and necrosis throughout the chorionic plate and amnion are apparent. Diagnosis and management of subclinical chorioamnionitis is often challenging.

OBJECTIVES

- To define chorioamnionitis and its epidemiology
- To summarize the pathophysiology of chorioamnionitis
- To discuss the clinical features and diagnosis
- To outline the maternal and neonatal management in a setting of chorioamnionitis
- To briefly discuss the prevention strategies of chorioamnionitis

DEFINITION AND EPIDEMIOLOGY

Definition

Chorioamnionitis, or intra-amniotic infection, is an infection with resultant inflammation of any combination of the amniotic fluid, placenta, fetus, fetal membranes, or decidua. The two main varieties of chorioamnionitis are clinical and histological chorioamnionitis. Clinical chorioamnionitis can further be subclassified as acute and subclinical. Acute chorioamnionitis is strongly related to early-onset sepsis while the subclinical variety may increase the risk of chronic lung disease and brain injury in the neonate.

Histologic chorioamnionitis is described by the presence of acute histological changes on examination of the amniotic membrane and chorion of the placenta. The hallmark of funisitis is leukocyte infiltration of the umbilical vessel wall or Wharton's jelly. These changes can be seen in subclinical as well as clinical chorioamnionitis. Histologic chorioamnionitis is thrice more common than clinical chorioamnionitis.

The National Institute of Child Health and Human Development (NICHD) expert panel have recommended to use the word "Triple I" instead of chorioamnionitis. "Triple I" refers to intrauterine infection, inflammation, or both. Its use however, has not been universally accepted.

Epidemiology

Premature rupture of membranes, prolonged labor, nulliparity, invasive fetal monitoring, epidural anesthesia, multiple vaginal examinations, alcohol, smoking, bacterial vaginosis, colonization with certain pathogens like group B streptococcus and ureaplasma are the common risk factors.

Recently, gene studies have revealed single nucleotide polymorphisms in immunoregulatory genes that may influence the susceptibility to chorioamnionitis.

PATHOPHYSIOLOGY OF CHORIOAMNIONITIS

Mechanism of Infection

During pregnancy, the main role of the cervical mucus plug, fetal membranes, and placenta is to protect the developing fetus from bacterial invasion. The cervical mucus plug is particularly important because it not only acts as an anatomic barrier but also contains numerous antibacterial peptides with bactericidal activity against pathogens that commonly colonize the vaginal tissues. Chorioamnionitis is an ascending infection originating from the lower genitourinary tract and culminating in the amniotic cavity. After the ascent into the amniotic cavity through the cervical part of membranes, the bacteria replicate locally, then invade the amnion and its connective tissue, and advance into the chorion and decidua. The probable sites of pathogen spread include the choriodecidual space (between maternal tissues and the fetal membranes), the fetal membranes, the placenta, the amniotic fluid, the umbilical cord, and the fetus. Infrequently infection can occur through the hematogenous spread and following invasive procedures like amniocentesis or chorionic villous sampling **(Fig. 1)**.

Bacterial infection releases endotoxins and exotoxins, which in turn stimulate the release of cytokines from the decidua and fetal membranes. The inflammatory response may induce clinical chorioamnionitis and lead to prostaglandin release, ripening of the cervix, membrane rupture, and labor. Preterm prelabor rupture of membranes (PPROM) that persists for more than 24 hours before the onset of labor augments the incidence of histological chorioamnionitis and the risk of neonatal sepsis.

Additional to the risk of sepsis in the fetus, the infection also triggers a fetal inflammatory response syndrome (FIRS) characterized by elevation of circulating cytokines (IL-6) in the fetal circulation ultimately leading to detrimental effects on multiple fetal organs.

Causative Organisms

Etiology is most often polymicrobial and can be due to bacterial, fungal, or viral agents. *Ureaplasma urealyticum* and *Mycoplasma hominis* are the most commonly isolated organisms in culture-proven chorioamnionitis (47% and 30%, respectively). Anaerobes, such as *Gardnerella vaginalis* (25%) and *Bacteroides* (30%), and aerobes including Group B streptococcus (15%) and *Escherichia coli* (8%) are few other known causative pathogens. *Listeria monocytogenes* infection is postulated to be a hematogenous spread. *Candida* species are also seldom the cause of chorioamnionitis.

CLINICAL FEATURES

Chorioamnionitis commonly presents with fever, uterine tenderness, maternal tachycardia (>100/min), fetal tachycardia (>160/min) and purulent or foul-smelling vaginal discharge.

Maternal fever is the most vital clinical sign of chorioamnionitis seen in almost 95–100% of cases. Temperature >100.4°F persisting for more than 1 hour or any fever ≥101°F should be investigated and managed appropriately. Maternal tachycardia (>100 BPM) and fetal tachycardia (>160 BPM) are also significant clinical signs. When maternal fever and maternal and/or fetal tachycardia are present, then a strong suspicion of intrauterine infection should be considered.

Subclinical chorioamnionitis however does not present with any of the above clinical signs but may be apparent as preterm labor or more often, as PPROM.

Classically, the presence of fever >100.4°F along with two other signs (uterine tenderness, maternal or fetal tachycardia, and foul/purulent amniotic fluid) is required to make a clinical judgment. The presence of three clinical signs together in the absence of other etiologies is of high value to make a diagnosis. The presence of risk factors of chorioamnionitis, especially membrane rupture, further strengthens the finding. However, it should be noted that isolated maternal fever does not always mean chorioamnionitis.

The recommendation from the NICHD expert panel for the diagnosis of Triple I include presence of maternal fever and the presence of at least one of the following **(Table 1)**:
- Fetal tachycardia
- Maternal leukocytosis in the absence of steroids
- Purulent fluid from cervical os
- Biochemical or microbiologic evidence of infection in amniotic fluid or placenta

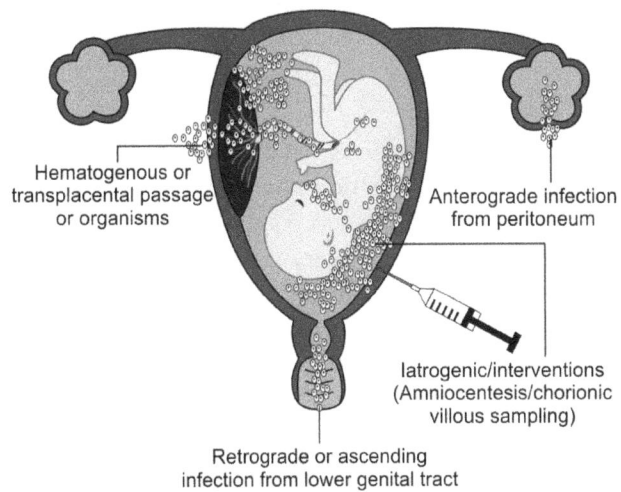

Fig. 1: Routes of spread of infection.
Source: Illustration by Dr Venkat Reddy Kallem.

TABLE 1: Classification of isolated fever and Triple I based on recommendations from the NICHD expert panel.

Terminology	Features
Isolated maternal fever (not Triple I)	• Even a single episode of oral temperature of at least 39°C • Persistent temperature of at least 38–38.9°C
Suspected Triple I	*Fever plus any of the following*: Fetal tachycardia/leukocytosis/purulent fluid from cervical os
Confirmed Triple I	*All of the above plus*: Amniocentesis proven infection through a positive gram stain or low glucose or positive culture, or placental pathology showing features of infection

(NICHD: National Institute of Child Health and Human Development)

EVALUATION
Laboratory Tests

Laboratory testing may help in confirming the diagnosis of chorioamnionitis, particularly when the clinical signs are ambiguous.

Complete Blood Count

Maternal leukocytosis (WBC >15,000/mm^3) or a shift to left often tips toward chorioamnionitis. Leukocytosis is seen in nearly 70–90% of cases of clinical chorioamnionitis. However, isolated leukocytosis in the absence of other signs or symptoms is not of much significance.

Other Blood Tests

Laboratory parameters like elevated levels of C-reactive protein (CRP), lipopolysaccharide-binding protein (LBP), soluble intercellular adhesion molecule 1 (sICAM 1), and interleukin 6 correlate with an increased risk of chorioamnionitis in the presence of PPROM or preterm delivery.

Amniotic Fluid Testing

Several amniotic fluid markers like Gram stain, low glucose levels (<15 mg/dL), elevated white blood cell counts, leukocyte esterase, matrix metalloproteinase, cytokines [e.g., tumor necrosis factor-alpha (TNF-α), interleukins-6 and -8, matrix metalloproteinase-8] and qualitative assessment of amniotic proteins (proteomics) can be useful for the diagnosis of chorioamnionitis. However, obtaining amniotic fluid sample is mainly by amniocentesis, which is usually avoided. A recent Cochrane analysis found that the value of evidence for the utility of these biomarkers was low. Few studies have also revealed that levels of these proteins particularly interleukins may be raised in certain conditions of pregnancy, like preeclampsia thus making their precision in diagnosis questionable.

The amniotic fluid culture is the gold standard but its utility in clinical practice is limited since the growth is more often absent due to treatment with antibiotics and the difficulty of isolating fastidious organisms. Moreover, culture results may not be available for up to 3 days.

Placental and Umbilical Cord Pathology

Postpartum histopathologic examination of the placenta is indicated when an infection is suspected to establish the presence and severity of infection. The staging of chorioamnionitis to know the severity and extent is done by documentation of polymorphonuclear leukocyte location, density, and degeneration. Increased neutrophil infiltration and necrosis, thickening of the amnion basement membrane, and chorionic micro-abscesses are present in advanced infection. In addition, the fetal inflammatory response may advance from chorionic/umbilical vasculitis (neutrophil infiltration in the chorionic or umbilical vessels) to necrotizing funisitis (inflammation of the connective tissue of the umbilical cord). The pathologic finding of funisitis is more serious than chorioamnionitis alone as it indicates a fetal response to infection.

Differential Diagnosis

Low-grade fever in an intrapartum patient with an epidural catheter in the absence of tachycardia (maternal or fetal) or other clinical signs of intrauterine inflammation is labeled as epidural-associated fever. Extrauterine infections like urinary tract infection (pyelonephritis), influenza, appendicitis, and pneumonia may mimic chorioamnionitis. Noninfectious conditions associated with abdominal pain (usually in absence of fever) like thrombophlebitis, round ligament pain, colitis, connective tissue disorders, and placental abruption should be ruled out.

MANAGEMENT
Obstetric Management

Antibiotics

The most crucial step in the prevention of maternal and fetal complications in chorioamnionitis is the early initiation of antibiotic therapy. Administration of broad-spectrum antibiotics and prompt delivery of the fetus in acute clinical chorioamnionitis reduces both fetal and maternal morbidity. Ampicillin and gentamicin are the recommended antibiotics for intra-amniotic infection as per the American College of Obstetrics and Gynecology (ACOG) **(Table 2)**. Clindamycin (or metronidazole) can be considered for anaerobic coverage, if a cesarean section is performed. Ideally, a single additional dose of intravenous antibiotics should be administered after delivery. However, persistent fever or bacteremia in the postpartum period may require the continuation of antibiotic therapy. Treatment with oral antibiotics might not be beneficial.

Mode of Delivery

Clinical chorioamnionitis is not an absolute indication for cesarean delivery. Induction and trial of labor should be done unless contraindicated. Vaginal delivery is a better option and cesarean delivery should be done only for standard obstetric indications. There is no evidence to prove the benefit of cesarean section in improving neonatal outcomes and may only increase maternal complications.

Antenatal Corticosteroids

The literature available on trials to support the efficacy and safety of antenatal corticosteroids (ACS) in clinical chorioamnionitis is limited. The administration of ACS to

TABLE 2: Recommended antibiotic regimens for treatment of intra-amniotic infection.

Antibiotics		Dose
First choice	Ampicillin	2 g IV q 6 hours
	Gentamicin	2 mg/kg IV loading dose followed by 1.5 mg/kg q 8 hours; or 5 mg/kg IV q 24 hours
Mild penicillin allergy	Cefazolin	2 g IV q 8 hours
	Gentamicin	Same as above
Severe penicillin allergy	Clindamycin	900 mg IV q 8 hours
	Vancomycin	1 g IV q 12 hours
	Gentamicin	Same as above
Alternative drugs	Ampicillin-sulbactam	3 g IV q 6 hours
	Piperacillin-tazobactam	3.375 g IV q 6 hours or 4.5 g IV q 8 hours
	Cefotetan	2 g IV q 12 hours
	Cefoxitin	2 g IV q 8 hours
	Ertapenem	1 g IV q 24 hours

Source: Adapted from American College of Obstetricians and Gynecologists, 2017/08. ACOG committee opinion No. 712.
Postcesarean delivery: One additional dose of the chosen regimen is recommended. Add at least one additional dose of clindamycin 900 mg IV or metronidazole 500 mg IV.

augment fetal lung maturity in the setting of chorioamnionitis in preterm babies is controversial because it is presumed that the immunosuppressive effects of steroids may aggravate maternal or neonatal infectious complications. However, antenatal steroids may reduce neonatal complications like respiratory distress syndrome, severe intraventricular hemorrhage, and periventricular leukomalacia. As delivery is almost imminent in chorioamnionitis, the present evidence recommends that the administration of at least a single dose of ACS to patients with clinical chorioamnionitis is advantageous to the preterm neonate without causing any adverse outcomes.

Supportive Care

Other supportive measures include the use of IV fluids and antipyretics (acetaminophen). The combination of intrapartum fever and fetal acidosis is associated with a high incidence of neonatal encephalopathy.

Neonatal Management

Acute chorioamnionitis is a risk factor for early-onset sepsis (EOS), one of the most common causes of neonatal morbidity and mortality. The risk of a neonate getting infected in utero is inversely proportional to the gestational age. The affected newborn may present with lethargy, hypothermia, refusal to feed, apnea, and cyanosis, or may be even asymptomatic. Fever is a rare presentation in EOS. In severe cases, the neonate may be symptomatic at birth and present with respiratory distress and pneumonia. Group B streptococcus and *E. coli* are the most common organisms responsible for EOS. A few of the less common pathogens are *Staphylococcus aureus, Klebsiella, Pseudomonas, Enterobacter* spp, and *Listeria monocytogenes*.

Febrile illness in the mother with evidence of bacterial infection within 2 weeks before delivery, foul-smelling liquor, prolonged labor, rupture of membranes for >18 hours, single unclean or >3 sterile vaginal examinations and use of internal fetal monitoring devices during labor are a few of the maternal risk factors leading to EOS. Prematurity/low birth weight, congenital anomalies and perinatal asphyxia contribute to sepsis in neonates.

The presence of foul-smelling liquor or any three of the above-mentioned risk factors requires starting antibiotics in the neonate. Suspected neonates should undergo a sepsis screen consisting of total and differential counts, C-reactive protein, procalcitonin, and blood culture. Cytokines like interleukins and TNF-α, molecular methods such as multiplex polymerase chain reaction and DNA microarrays, are gaining popularity. Other additional investigations like chest X-ray and lumbar puncture are done based on symptoms.

Symptomatic neonates should be managed in the neonatal intensive care unit and treated with supportive management like IV fluids and respiratory support. The neonates with suspected EOS are recommended to be started empirically on a combination of ampicillin and gentamicin. Third-generation cephalosporins (e.g., cefotaxime, ceftriaxone, ceftazidime) are used at times due to increasing resistance of ampicillin and gentamicin-resistant *E. coli* strains. Vancomycin the drug of choice for Coagulase-negative staphylococcal and methicillin-resistant *S. aureus* (MRSA) infections while methicillin-sensitive

S. aureus (MSSA) is treated with oxacillin and nafcillin. When the sepsis screen is negative and blood culture does not yield any growth, antibiotics should be stopped by 36–48 hours unless site-specific infection requires treatment. Blood culture positive cases should undergo a lumbar puncture to rule out meningitis. Duration of antibiotic therapy depends on type of organism isolated and the site of infection.

There is growing evidence to suggest that close observation, rather than empiric antibiotic therapy, is the preferred strategy for the management of asymptomatic full-term and late preterm infants exposed to chorioamnionitis. These babies should be observed in the hospital for at least 48 hours.

COMPLICATIONS

Chorioamnionitis can lead to life-threatening complications in the mother, fetus, and neonate.

Maternal complications: Increased risk of preterm and operative delivery, postpartum uterine atony with hemorrhage, endometritis, pelvic abscess, thromboembolism, bacteremia, sepsis, subcutaneous wound infections, acute respiratory distress syndrome, and rarely, death may occur.

Fetal and neonatal complications: Increased risk of stillbirth, prematurity, and fetal brain injury subsequently leading to cerebral palsy and other neurodevelopmental disabilities. The neonates are at high risk for development of bronchopulmonary dysplasia (BPD) and retinopathy of prematurity (ROP). Pneumonia, meningitis, sepsis, and death may also occur in the neonate.

PREVENTION

Chorioamnionitis may be prevented by the following strategies:
- Regular antenatal check-ups
- Screening for bacterial vaginosis in the second trimester of pregnancy
- Screening for group B streptococcal infection at 35–37 weeks of pregnancy
- Reducing the number of vaginal examinations performed during labor
- Avoiding invasive intrapartum monitoring
- Appropriate antibiotics in cases of PROM

CHAPTER AT A GLANCE

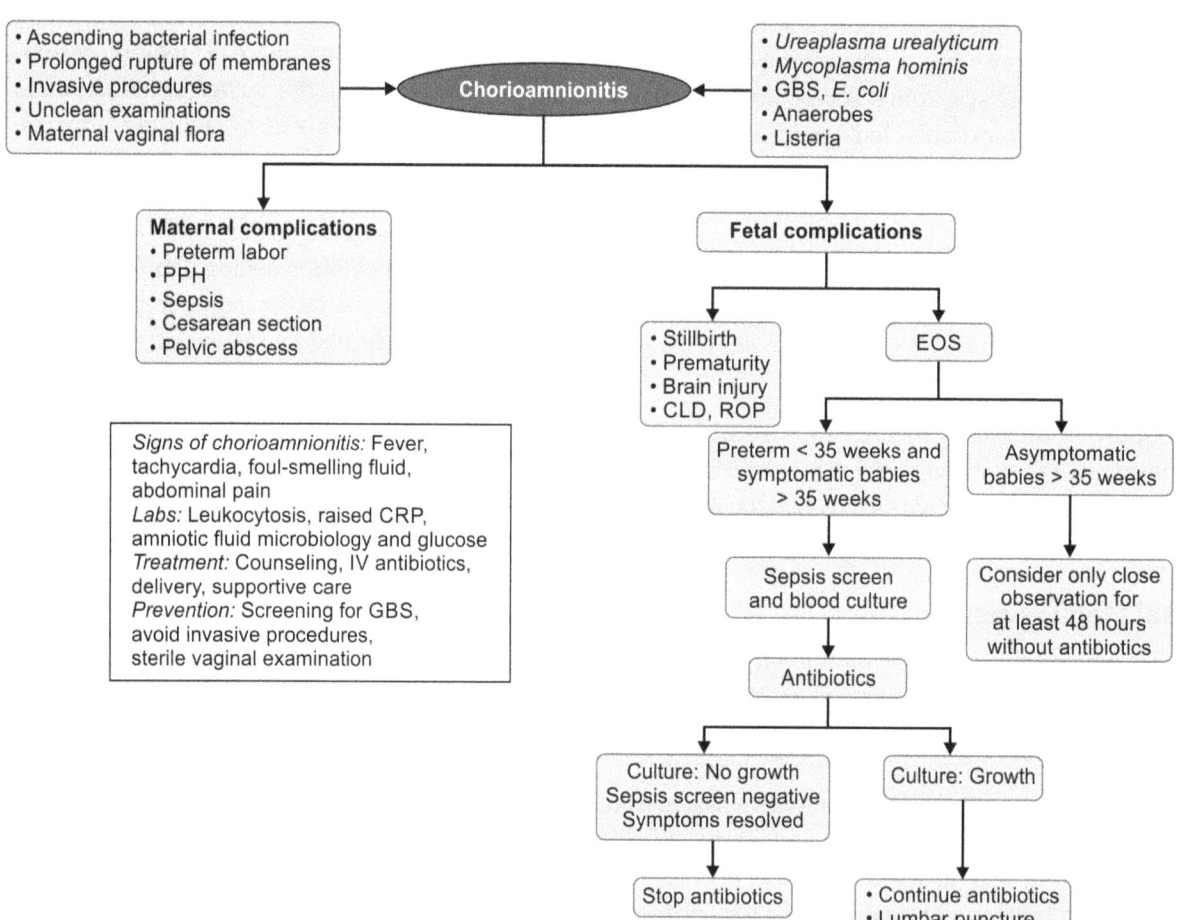

(CLD: chronic lung disease; CRP: C-reactive protein; EOS: early-onset sepsis; GBS: Group B streptococcus; PPH: post-partum hemorrhage; ROP: retinopathy of prematurity)

KEY POINTS

- Chorioamnionitis is an infection during pregnancy, commonly associated with prolonged membrane rupture or labor.
- Diagnosis is based on clinical signs and symptoms such as maternal fever, foul-smelling liquor, abdominal pain and leukocytosis.
- Chorioamnionitis results in detrimental fetal complications like premature birth, neonatal sepsis, BPD, ROP and cerebral palsy.
- Prophylactic antibiotics to women with preterm premature rupture of membranes can be preventive.
- Antibiotic therapy and delivery are the ideal management strategies.
- Symptomatic neonates exposed to chorioamnionitis should be screened for sepsis and treated with empirical antibiotics.

SUGGESTED READING

1. ACOG (2017). Intrapartum Management of Intraamniotic Infection [online]. Available from https://www.acog.org/en/clinical/clinical-guidance/committee-opinion/articles/2017/08/intrapartum-management-of-intraamniotic-infection. [Last accessed November, 2021].
2. Conde-Agudelo A, Romero R, Jung EJ, Garcia Sánchez ÁJ. Management of clinical chorioamnionitis: an evidence-based approach. Am J Obstet Gynecol. 2020;223(6):848-69.
3. Kim CJ, Romero R, Chaemsaithong P, Chaiyasit N, Yoon BH, Kim YM. Acute chorioamnionitis and funisitis: definition, pathologic features, and clinical significance. Am J Obstet Gynecol. 2015;213(4):S29-52.
4. Peng C-C, Chang J-H, Lin H-Y, Cheng P-J, Su B-H. Intrauterine inflammation, infection, or both (Triple I): A new concept for chorioamnionitis. Pediatr Neonatol. 2018;59(3):231–7.
5. Polin RA, Committee on fetus and newborn. Management of neonates with suspected or proven early-onset bacterial sepsis. Pediatrics. 2012;129(5):1006-15.
6. Simonsen KA, Anderson-Berry AL, Delair SF, Davies HD. Early-onset neonatal sepsis. Clin Microbiol Rev. 2014;27(1):21-47.
7. Tita ATN, Andrews WW. Diagnosis and management of clinical chorioamnionitis. Clin Perinatol. 2010;37(2):339-54.

SECTION 5

Congenital Infections

Shilpa Kalane, Ashish Jain

- **Approach to a Neonate with Suspected Congenital Infection**
  Shilpa Kalane, Ashish Jain
- **Toxoplasmosis—Perinatal Perspective**
  Ruchi Nimish Nanavati, Anahita Chauhan
- **Rubella—Perinatal Perspective**
  Girija Wagh, Sandeep Kadam
- **Cytomegalovirus—Perinatal Perspective**
  Mayur A Thosar, Tushar B Parikh
- **Herpes Simplex Virus—Perinatal Perspective**
  Vandana Bansal, Anish Pillai, Nandkishor Kabra
- **Syphilis—Perinatal Perspective**
  Gopal Agrawal, Ritu Sethi
- **Other Viral Infections such as Zika Virus, Dengue Virus, Chikungunya Virus, Varicella Virus, H1N1 Influenza Virus**
  Amanpreet Sethi, Seema Grover Bhatti
- **Tuberculosis—Perinatal Perspective**
  Rohit Sasidharan, Neeraj Gupta
- **HIV—Perinatal Perspective**
  Prakash V, Deviprasadh PM
- **Viral Hepatitis—Perinatal Perspective**
  Ramani Ranjan, Manju Gupta
- **SARS-CoV-2 Infection—Perinatal Perspective**
  Shikha Rani, Deepak Chawla

31 Approach to a Neonate with Suspected Congenital Infection

Shilpa Kalane, Ashish Jain

INTRODUCTION

Available optimal antenatal surveillance, early diagnosis, treatment, and implementation of immunoprophylaxis have resulted in remarkable progress in preventing nonbacterial congenital infections. Despite recent advances in fetal medicine and perinatology, it is not uncommon for a neonatologist to be called on to identify unusual, infected neonate. One of the most difficult decisions to make is when to affirmatively pursue a diagnosis of congenital infection. A high index of suspicion as well as awareness of the prominent features of congenital infections, always aid in early diagnosis and assist in tailoring an appropriate diagnostic evaluation. For many of the nonbacterial congenital infections, a timely diagnosis is critical to ensure that an appropriate therapy is initiated well in time. This also allows for family counseling about the prognosis so that an appropriate care and follow-up can be planned.

OBJECTIVES

- To know the spectrum of nonbacterial causes of congenital infection
- To understand their pathogenesis
- To identify the clinical manifestations of these infection in neonates
- To understand the step-by-step approach of evaluating a case of suspected congenital infection

Nonbacterial Causes of Congenital Infections

Viral infections are a major cause of morbidity and mortality in fetuses and newborns. The cumulative frequency of viral infections in the fetus or newborn infant may be as high as 6–8% of all live births, whereas systemic bacterial disease affects only 1–2% of newborns.

The pathogens most commonly associated with intrauterine infections are syphilis, toxoplasmosis, rubella, cytomegalovirus (CMV), and herpes simplex virus (HSV)—commonly referred to as STORCH. A more comprehensive acronym, CHEAP TORCHES, has also been proposed to include chicken pox, hepatitis (B, C, and E), enterovirus, AIDS (acquired immunodeficiency syndrome), and parvovirus. The list of "other" infections is ever growing with newer etiologies being discovered, such as dengue, chikungunya, H1N1, zika, and most recently SARS-CoV-2 (severe acute respiratory syndrome coronavirus 2) infection. Often malaria and tuberculosis are faced as challenges due to resurgence.

Pathogenesis

These infections may be divided into congenital, perinatal or natal, and postnatal based on time periods of acquisition (**Table 1**). Congenital infections are transmitted to the developing fetus during a maternal infection. The majority of these are caused by primary maternal infections, but some may be transmitted during a recurrent (reactivation or reinfection) of a maternal infection.

The spectrum of manifestations varies. It can cause embryo resorption, spontaneous abortion or miscarriage, stillbirth, congenital malformation, prematurity, intrauterine growth restriction (IUGR) or acute disease apparent in utero, at birth, or shortly after birth (**Fig. 1**). Certain infections (e.g., CMV) may be silent in early life, causing sequelae later, or they may be asymptomatic with no long-term sequelae (**Fig. 1**).

Suspicion of a Congenital Infection

Intrauterine infection may be suspected antenatally based on prenatal ultrasonography findings or laboratory results obtained during pregnancy. In the absence of suggestive maternal laboratory results, suspicion is strong when a newborn exhibits certain clinical manifestations or combinations of clinical manifestations as illustrated in **Figure 2** (but not limited to). These clinical features may have significant overlap across the various etiologies (**Table 1**). Certain clinical findings in selected congenital infections can suggest specific diagnosis (**Table 2**). Sick neonates with culture-negative sepsis, unexplained intrauterine growth restriction with or without polyhydramnios and

TABLE 1: Period of transmission of selected viruses to the fetus or newborn infant.

Viruses	Congenital	Natal	Postnatal
Adenovirus (HAdV)	+	+	+
Chikungunya (CHIKV)	++	+	−
Cytomegalovirus (CMV)	++	++	++
Dengue (DENV)	++	−	−
Ebolavirus (EBOV)	++	+	+
Echoviruses	+	+	+
Epstein–Barr virus (EBV)	+	−	+
Hepatitis A (HAV)	−	++	+
Hepatitis B (HBV)	+	++	+
Hepatitis C (HCV)	+	++	−
Herpes simplex virus (HSV)	+	++	+
Herpesvirus 6 (HHV 6)	+	−	+
Human enterovirus (HEV)	−	+	+
Human immunodeficiency virus (HIV)	+	++	+
Parvovirus B19 (B19V)	+	−	−
Influenza (H1N1)	(+)	−	+
Lymphocytic choriomeningitis virus (LCMV)	++	−	−
Measles	+	−	+
Mumps	+	−	−
Parechovirus (HPeV)	−	+	+
Poliovirus	+	+	+
Rubella	++	−	−
SARS–CoV–2	(+)	+	++
Smallpox	+	+	+
St Louis encephalitis virus (SLEV)	(+)	−	(+)
Type B coxsackieviruses (CVB)	+	+	+
Vaccinia virus (VACV)	+	+	+
Varicella Zoster virus (VZV)	++	+	+
West Nile virus (WNV)	+	−	+
Western equine encephalitis virus (WEEV)	+	−	+
Zika virus (ZIKV)	++	?	(+)

(++: major demonstrated route; +: minor demonstrated route; (+): suggested route, few supporting data; −: route not demonstrated)

bronchopulmonary dysplasia with atypical presentation should be evaluated for underlying congenital infections.

Ocular Manifestations in Infants with Congenital Infection

The most characteristic eye finding of a prenatal, and thus congenital, infection is a chorioretinal scar or active chorioretinitis, as seen in congenital toxoplasmosis, CMV, HSV, lymphocytic choriomeningitis virus, or varicella zoster virus (VZV) infections. Congenital cataracts are suggestive, but not specific for congenital infection. They may be a rare finding in rubella, syphilis, and varicella zoster and Epstein-Barr virus infections. They are linked to extensive eye involvement in congenital toxoplasmosis, HSV, and CMV. Ocular manifestations of specific congenital infections have been thoroughly discussed in other chapters in this section.

Evaluation of Mother

History: Routine testing for congenital infection in an infant with only prematurity or intrauterine growth retardation is unlikely to yield positive results and is thus not advised. To identify those newborns in whom further clinical

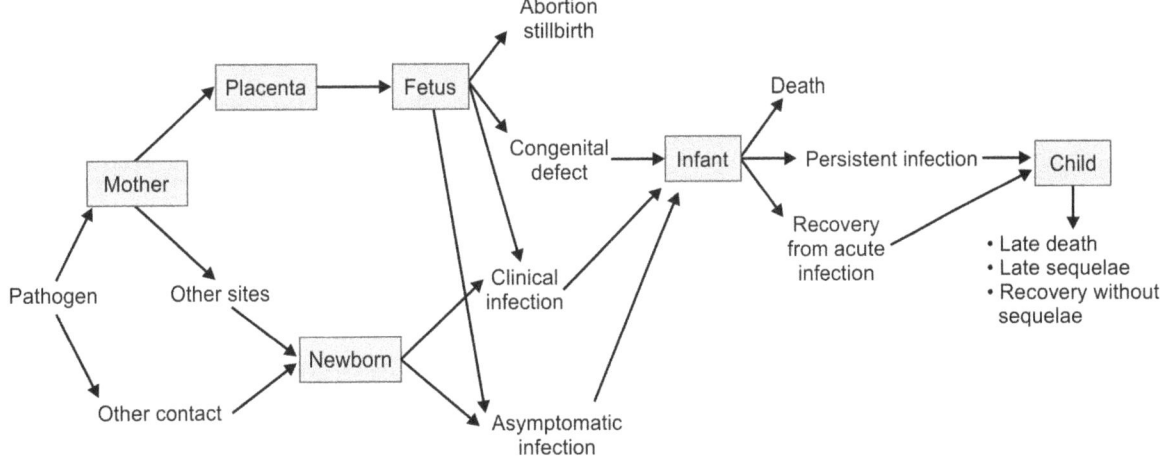

Fig. 1: Pathogenesis of infections in the fetus and newborn.

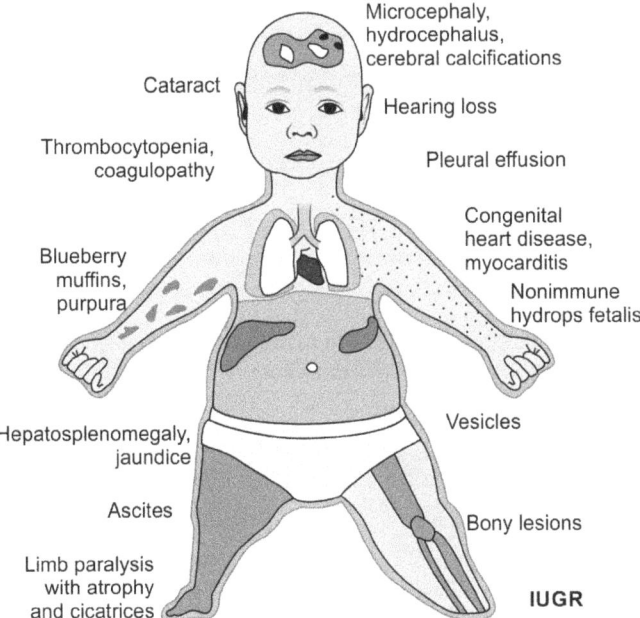

Fig. 2: Clinical findings in neonates with congenital infection. (IUGR: intrauterine growth restriction)

evaluation [i.e., cranial computed tomography (CT) scan or ophthalmology examination] or laboratory investigations it may be worthwhile, reviewing maternal history **(Table 3)**.

MATERNAL TORCH SCREENING AND ITS INTERPRETATION

A TORCH screen is a set of tests that can be used to diagnose infections in pregnant women.

Indications for TORCH Screening during Pregnancy

- TORCH panel screening is recommended in pregnancies that are suspected of being complicated by congenital infections, such as those with:
  - Fetal hydrops
  - Fetal brain lesions
  - Unexplained IUGR
  - Other sonographic markers of fetal infection.
- Pregnant women with nonvesicular rash and other symptoms of systemic infection should be screened for rubella and parvovirus B19.
- Pregnant women who have had significant contact with a person with such illness should be tested for rubella and parvovirus B19 infection, whether or not they develop a rash.

Interpretation of TORCH Screening Results

Enzyme-linked immunoassay (ELISA) is the most common modality among the many available tests. The sensitivity and specificity of each test vary; hence, when interpreting test results, one must exercise caution. Paired serological tests are most useful when the first sample is obtained while the patient is ill. The second sample is drawn 4 weeks later, and any increase in titer or other factor is used to interpret the test results and diagnose infection. Maternal serum samples are collected and stored during the first antenatal visit can be very useful later on if there is a suspicion of CHEAP STORCH during the pregnancy.

The timing of maternal infection can be found by avidity test for the particular infection. The test measures the binding affinity of IgG postinfection. The affinity increases over time. Thus low avidity would mean recent infection (within 3 months) and high avidity means past infection (before 3 months). **Flowchart 1** depicts an overview of the interpretation of the TORCH report.

Maternal TORCH Screening and Fetal Implications

Fetal infection can be suspected if maternal infection has been diagnosed during the pregnancy or fetal ultrasound suggests infection. Definitive diagnosis of fetal infection is

TABLE 2: Clinical findings in specific congenital infections indicating the diagnosis.

Congenital infection	Specific-related clinical findings
Rubella	Cloudy cornea, cataracts, pigmented retinopathy, petechiae with "blueberry muffin" rash, bone defects with longitudinal bands of demineralization ("celery stalking"), cardiovascular malformations (patent ductus arteriosus, peripheral pulmonary artery stenosis), sensorineural hearing loss (SNHL)
CMV	Microcephaly with periventricular calcifications, chorioretinitis, petechiae with thrombocytopenia, jaundice, SNHL, hepatosplenomegaly, bone abnormalities, abnormal dentition, hypocalcified enamel
HSV	Skin vesicles (ulceration, scarring), keratoconjunctivitis, micropthalmia, central nervous system findings (seizures, hydranencephaly, microcephaly), hepatitis, pneumonitis
VZV	Limb hypoplasia, dermatomal scarring in a cicatricial pattern, gastrointestinal tract atresia, microcephaly
ZIKV	Microcephaly, intracranial calcifications, arthrogryposis, hypertonia/spasticity, ocular abnormalities—retinitis, sensorineural hearing loss
Parvovirus B19	Hydrops, ascites, hepatomegaly, ventriculomegaly, hypertrophic myocardiopathy, anemia
HEV/HPeV	Fever, rash, irritability, poor feeding, gastrointestinal symptoms (vomiting, diarrhea), respiratory symptoms (cough, wheezing, rhinorrhea, tachypnea, and herpangina), aseptic meningitis, sepsis, encephalitis or meningoencephalitis, myocarditis, pneumonia, and/or hepatitis
LCMV	Hydrocephalus, chorioretinitis, intracranial calcifications
CHIKV	Fever, hyperalgesia syndrome, diffuse inflammatory lower limb edema, centrofacial hyperpigmentation
DENV	Fever, diffuse erythematous blanchable rash
Toxoplasma	Intracranial calcification, hydrocephalus, chorioretinitis, otherwise unexplained mononuclear CSF pleocytosis or elevated CSF protein
Syphilis	Maculopapular rash (predominantly on palms and soles), persistent rhinitis, pseudoparalysis, skeletal abnormalities (osteochondritis, periostitis)
Tuberculosis	Failure to thrive, hepatosplenomegaly

(CHIKV: chikungunya; CMV: cytomegalovirus; CSF: cerebrospinal fluid; DENV: dengue virus; HEV/HPeV: human enterovirus/parechovirus; HSV: herpes simplex virus; LCMV: lymphocytic choriomeningitis virus; VZV: varicella zoster virus; ZIKV: zika virus)

TABLE 3: Important pointers of congenital infection from maternal history.

Maternal history	Probable infection
History of exposure	
Season	Parvovirus B19 (winter, spring), rubella (winter, spring), enterovirus (summer, autumn)
Ongoing pandemic	SARS-CoV-2 (COVID 19 pandemic), H1N1 (flu pandemic)
Handling or ingestion of raw meat that has never been frozen or handling animal or kitty litter or gardening	Toxoplasmosis
Contact with diapered children in daycare, household or school	Cytomegalovirus (CMV), parvovirus
Exposure in travel to certain geographic regions	SARS-CoV-2, toxoplasmosis, tuberculosis, malaria, trypanosomiasis, Ebola
Multiple sex partners, commercial sex workers, illicit drug use	HIV, HBV, HSV, CMV
Unimmunized	Rubella, varicella
Illness	
Rash	Rubella, syphilis, parvovirus B19, enterovirus, dengue
Arthritis/arthralgia	Rubella, parvovirus B19, chikungunya
Mononucleosis like fatigue, lymphadenopathy	CMV, toxoplasmosis, HIV
Screening in pregnancy	HIV, HBV, syphilis
Fetal ultrasonography	Variable

(COVID 19: coronavirus disease; HBV: hepatitis B virus; HIV: human immunodeficiency virus; HSV: herpes simplex virus; SARS-CoV-2: severe acute respiratory syndrome coronavirus 2)

Flowchart 1: Overview of interpretation of TORCH report.

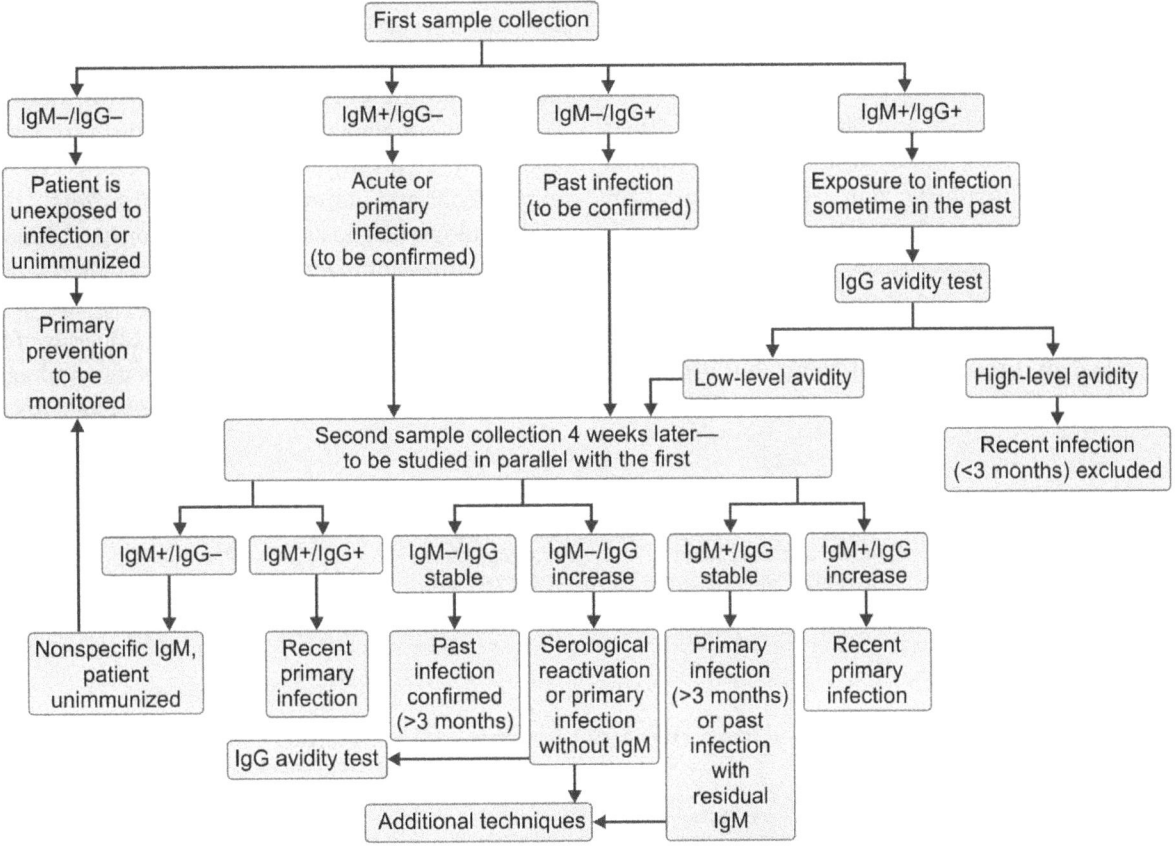

(TORCH: toxoplasmosis, rubella, cytomegalovirus, and herpes simplex virus)

only possible by amniotic polymerase chain reaction (PCR). The amniotic fluid PCR will become positive only after 4 weeks from the maternal infection. Thus the amniocentesis needs to be timed accordingly. Evidence of fetal infection does not necessarily mean fetal affection. The fetus may not have structural anomalies in spite of getting infected. Long-term fetal sequelae are not predictable.

Differential Diagnosis

In a neonate with a suspected congenital infection, the differentials should include, but is not limited to:
- Bacterial sepsis
- Fungal sepsis
- Erythroblastosis fetalis
- Inborn errors of metabolism
- Genetic chromosomal abnormalities

WORKUP OF A SUSPECTED CASE

Initial Workup (Box 1)

Specific Evaluation

The results of the initial evaluation may aid in determining whether further testing for a specific pathogen (or pathogens) is required.

BOX 1: Initial clinical investigations for suspected congenital infections.

Detail maternal history **(Table 3)**

Assessment of the neonate

Physical examination:
- Gestational age, birth weight, total length, head circumference, ponderal index
- Liver, spleen size
- Skin lesions
- Ophthalmological examination

Laboratory:
- Complete blood count, peripheral blood smear
- Liver function test (LFT)
- Cerebrospinal fluid (CSF) examination
- Maternal and infant sera for microbiological tests
- Pretransfusion blood for additional tests

Other investigations:
- Brain computer tomography (CT) scan with contrast
- Long bone X-ray (if D/D syphilis or rubella)
- Placental pathology

Follow up:
- Auditory assessment
- Serology

(D/D: differential diagnosis)

Testing amniotic fluid for viral culture and PCR or fetal blood for viral-specific immunoglobulin IgM and PCR tests can be used to make a prenatal diagnosis of fetal viral infection. Histopathologic examinations of the placenta may also be performed.

In neonates, urine, saliva, and blood should be tested for CMV; throat, cataracts, and occasionally cerebrospinal fluid (CSF) or urine for rubella; skin vesicles, blood, CSF, conjunctivae, throat, stool, and urine for HSV; throat, stool, urine, CSF, or blood for enteroviruses; and skin vesicles and blood for VZV; stool, blood, and urine for diagnosing human enterovirus and human parechovirus (HeV and HpeV); nasopharyngeal or oropharyngeal swab, endotracheal secretions, bronchoalveolar lavage for SARS-Cov-2.

Furthermore, pathogen isolation or molecular identification by PCR from biopsy or autopsy materials can be attempted. Electron microscopy of vesicle fluid or tissue can show typical herpes virus particles in both HSV and VZV infection but cannot differentiate between the two. Retrospective diagnosis of congenital CMV can be made by retrieving dried blood spots archived after completion of newborn screening for metabolic and immunodeficiency disorders.

A serologic diagnosis of viral infection can be made using one of the three approaches: (1) By testing paired sera (mother and her infant) at birth and at 5–6 months of age for antiviral antibody (predominantly IgG activity); (2) assay of neonatal serum for IgM antibody against a specific viral agent, and (3) assay of neonatal serum for quantitative IgM assay.

CHAPTER AT A GLANCE

```
  Antenatal abnormal blood       Clinical stigmata of        Sepsis mimic – not
  investigations for            intrauterine infection       responding to
  CHEAP TORCHES                                              conventional management
                                                                    │
                                                                    ▼
                                                            Investigate for bacterial/
  Sonography markers     →  Suspect congenital infection ←─-ve─ fungal or tropical viral infections,
  of fetal infection                                         IEM, erythroblastosis fetalis,
                                                             hemophagocytosis, genetic
                                                             chromosomal abnormalities
                                                                    │ +ve
                                                                    ▼
        Investigate:                                         Initiate cause
        • Initial work up—CBC, peripheral                    specific treatment
          smear, LFT, CSF, neuroimaging,         ─+ve→
          echocardiography, etc.
        • Specific evaluation—Long bone X-ray,
          cranial CT scan with enhancement,
          maternal and infant serology, etc.
                    │ -ve                                    Long-term follow-up—
                    ▼                                        Auditory evaluation,
             Refer to infection                              developmental follow
             disease specialist                              up ± serology
```

(TORCH: toxoplasmosis, rubella, cytomegalovirus, and herpes simplex virus)

KEY POINTS

- In summary, an appropriate index of suspicion, a reasonable clinical evaluation, and prudent microbiological evaluation are the current best efforts to identify infants with congenital infection at an early age.
- Intrauterine and perinatal infections are a major cause of fetal and neonatal death, as well as a major contributor to childhood illness.
- The ability to recognize the key clinical signs of TORCH and other intrauterine/perinatal infections is critical for timely diagnosis and treatment.
- Intrauterine infection may be suspected in neonates with particular clinical signs or combinations of clinical signs, including hydrops fetalis, microcephaly, seizures, cataract, and hearing loss, congenital heart disease, hepatosplenomegaly, jaundice, and/or rash, in the absence of maternal laboratory results associated with intrauterine infection.

SUGGESTED READING

1. Karen EJ. (2021). Overview of TORCH infections. [online] Available from https://somepomed.org/articulos/contents/mobipreview.htm?5/23/5489?source=see_link. [Last accessed November, 2021].
2. Neu N, Duchon J, Zachariah P. TORCH infections. Clin Perinatol. 2015;42(1):77-103.
3. Yvonne AM, Victor N, Jerome OK, Jack SR, Christopher BW. Remington and Klein's Infectious Diseases of the Fetus and Newborn Infant. Current Concepts of Infections of the Fetus and Newborn Infant,. 8th edition. Philadelphia: Saunders/Elsevier; 2016. pp. 3-23.

CHAPTER 32

Toxoplasmosis—Perinatal Perspective

Ruchi Nimish Nanavati, Anahita Chauhan

INTRODUCTION

Toxoplasmosis is an infection caused by *Toxoplasma gondii (T. gondii)*, an intracellular protozoan parasite that is distributed globally. Most infections are asymptomatic or subclinical and are acquired by ingesting food contaminated by felines (cats), who are the natural reservoir of *T. gondii*. Toxoplasmosis in pregnancy can be vertically transmitted to the fetus with manifestations including neurological and ocular diseases and anomalies of the cardiac system.

OBJECTIVES

- To learn about the pathogenesis of fetal toxoplasma infection
- To learn how to manage pregnant women infected with toxoplasmosis
- To learn about the manifestations of congenital toxoplasma infection
- To learn the current recommendations for diagnosis, prevention, and management of congenital toxoplasma infection.

ETIOPATHOGENESIS OF TOXOPLASMA INFECTION

Epidemiology

Toxoplasma is a significant public health problem, estimated to infect one-third of the world's population. Felines are the definitive hosts of *T. gondii*. Three predominant clonal lineages of *T. gondii* have been identified, with varied geographic distribution. Seroprevalence varies widely between countries, from as low as 10% to as high as 80%. In India, seroprevalence is around 20% but is geographically heterogeneous. North India has an average prevalence of 9–20%; a higher prevalence of 40% has been found in Kerala.

Etiology and Risk Factors

Humans are infected by ingesting infected meat (pork/lamb), food, or water contaminated with oocysts from the environment. Less frequently, food or water can be contaminated with cat feces. Solid-organ transplantation can also transmit toxoplasma infection from the donor to the recipient, as certain organs may harbor persistent cysts such as the muscle. Patients who have undergone heart transplants are thus more likely to acquire toxoplasmosis than liver or kidney transplant recipients.

Moist environment increases the survival of oocyst, which may account for the high prevalence in tropical countries. Oocysts are also resistant to freezing and high-water temperatures and are unaffected by chlorination and ozone treatment of water. Other risk factors include immune-compromised persons, older people, and poor hygiene.

Primary maternal infection during pregnancy or just before conception can result in fetal infection. This is the most common cause of transmission, seen in about 30% of cases. Rarely, there may be a reactivation of past toxoplasma infection in immune-compromised pregnant women. Travel and infection with a different strain may also be responsible for new infection.

Clinical Manifestation of Toxoplasma Infection in Adults

Primary infection with toxoplasma results in subclinical or asymptomatic infection in the majority of immune-competent individuals. Symptomatic patients have nonspecific flu-like illness, myalgia, or fatigue may occur. Cervical lymphadenopathy may be the only feature seen. In immune-compromised patients, life-threatening encephalitis may be seen.

Clinical presentation in pregnancy is also mild, with less than one-third showing any signs or symptoms. Primary infection in pregnancy may cause spontaneous abortion in the index pregnancy. However, toxoplasma is not an etiological factor for recurrent pregnancy loss (RPL). Hence, there is limited value to evaluating patients of RPL with TORCH (Toxoplasma, Syphilis, Rubella, Cytomegalovirus, and Herpes Simplex) titers. Rarely, visual changes as a result of toxoplasma chorioretinitis may be seen.

TOXOPLASMA INFECTION IN PREGNANCY

History, physical signs, symptoms, and clinical examination do not help diagnose toxoplasmosis. The diagnosis in the mother is generally made retrospectively based on maternal antibody testing. Vertical transmission can be confirmed antenatally by amniocentesis and polymerase chain reaction (PCR) testing of the amniotic fluid, as well as by ultrasonography; and postnatally by serology for antibodies.

Diagnosis in Pregnancy

The maternal serum is tested for *T. gondii* IgM and IgG antibodies. After primary infection, IgM antibodies may be detected for up to 2 years. *T. gondii* IgG antibody avidity testing allows for the timing of maternal infection. Maternal serology testing is also done when a neonate with suspected features of toxoplasmosis is noted (hydrocephalus, cerebral calcifications, or chorioretinitis). History of fever or lymphadenopathy, other risk factors, or suspicious sonographic features in the fetus should prompt testing. The interpretation of serological tests in pregnancy is shown in **Flowchart 1**.

Diagnosis of Fetal Toxoplasma Infection

History of fever or lymphadenopathy, other risk factors, or suspicious sonographic features in the fetus should prompt testing. Serological tests should be interpreted as follows:

Fetal infection is diagnosed by
- PCR of *T. gondii* by amniocentesis
- Presence of IgM antibodies in amniotic fluid (amniocentesis) or fetal blood (cordocentesis)

Amniocentesis should be offered to women with serological results suggesting acute toxoplasma infection in pregnancy, and the procedure is done at 18 weeks of gestation. Performing amniocentesis before 18 weeks has been associated with a higher fetal risk and poorer sensitivity and specificity.

Ultrasonography should be repeated every month, if the mother has been diagnosed with toxoplasmosis during pregnancy. Features suggestive of fetal toxoplasmosis infection are:
- Hyperechogenic lesions in the brain parenchyma or periventricular region and ventricular dilatation.
- Intracranial, hepatic, and splenic calcification.
- Hyperechogenic intestine, hepatosplenomegaly, ascites, pleural effusion, and placentomegaly may be noted.

Management of Toxoplasma Infection in Pregnancy

The main aim of therapy is to prevent vertical transmission. The management of toxoplasma infection in pregnancy is given in **Table 1**.

CONGENITAL TOXOPLASMA INFECTION

Risk of vertical transmission and the severity of fetal affectation depend on the gestational age when the mother is infected. The placental barrier plays a major role by acting both as a barrier as well as the location of parasite multiplication. As the placental barrier is more efficient in earlier gestations, transmission to the fetus is least in the first trimester (<10%), which rises significantly in the second and third trimesters to about 30% and 60%, respectively.

Conversely, fetal consequences are inversely correlated to gestation age. Severe affectations of the fetus, mainly neurological and ocular consequences, are seen, if infection occurs in early gestation as compared to later gestation.

The risk of these major complications is 0.8, if maternal seroconversion occurs in the first 5 weeks of gestation, which reduces to <0.2, if maternal seroconversion occurs later in pregnancy. Cumulatively, the maximum risk of developing

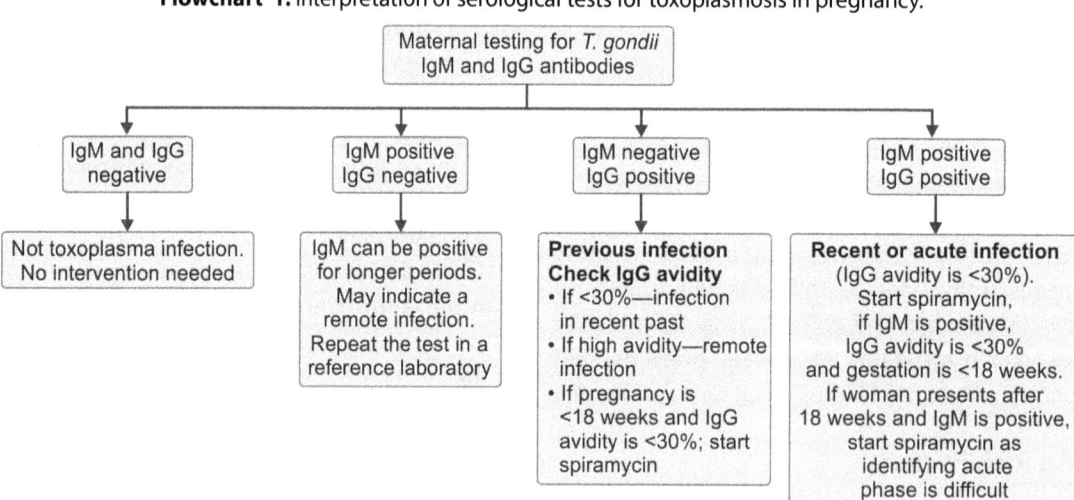

Flowchart 1: Interpretation of serological tests for toxoplasmosis in pregnancy.

TABLE 1: The management of toxoplasma infection in pregnancy.

Maternal seroconversion status	Management
In pregnant women, fetus is infected during gestation and gestational age is <18 weeks	- Spiramycin (macrolide antibiotic) - Spiramycin is concentrated in the placenta and decreases the risk of fetal infection by 50%. If fetus is already infected severity of disease is not altered by spiramycin treatment - *Dose*: 1 g three times per day - *Duration*: Continue till term, if fetal infection is ruled out by amniocentesis at 18 weeks' gestation and fetus does not have any clinical findings by ultrasound
In pregnant women, fetus found infected after 18 weeks or if fetal infection confirmed	- Pyrimethamine-Sulfadiazine and Leucovorin (folinic acid) - Severity of fetal disease is reduced by maternal treatment with combination chemotherapy - Pyrimethamine is contraindicated in the first 14 weeks of gestation due to teratogenic effects. Pyrimethamine, a folic acid antagonist, is the most effective drug against toxoplasmosis. However, it can cause bone marrow suppression, thrombocytopenia, and pancytopenia, hence regular monitoring of blood counts should be done and folinic acid should be given concomitantly - *Dose:* Pyrimethamine 50 mg twice daily for 2 days followed by 50 mg/day orally - *Sulfadiazine*: 1.5–2 g per day in two divided doses with eight glasses of water (to reduce the risk of nephrolithiasis) - *Folinic acid (leucovorin)*: 10–20 mg daily (during and 1 week after completion of pyrimethamine therapy) - *Duration:* Till term

symptomatic congenital toxoplasmosis peaks at 24–30 weeks of gestation.

Factors (any or a combination) associated with an increased risk of mother-to-child transmission (MTCT) are as follows: (1) acute *T. gondii* infection during pregnancy, (2) immunocompromising conditions, (3) lack of antepartum treatment, (4) high *T. gondii* strain virulence, and (5) high-parasite load.

Clinical Features of Congenital Toxoplasma Infection

The four recognized subtypes of presentation are described as.

1. *Subclinical or asymptomatic infection*: Described in 70–90% of infants at birth. If untreated, these infants may later (several months to years) develop visual (retinal lesions, often consisting of unilateral macular retinal scars) and neurological deficits including small, focal cerebral calcifications, elevated cerebrospinal fluid (CSF) protein with or without CSF mononuclear pleocytosis, hearing impairment, learning disabilities, or mental retardation.
2. *Neonatal symptomatic disease*: Approximately 10–30% of infants will have clinically apparent signs and symptoms at birth or in early infancy. Signs at birth include maculopapular rash, lymphadenopathy, splenomegaly, hepatomegaly, jaundice (liver damage, hemolysis, or both), pneumonia, hypothermia, anemia, petechiae, thrombocytopenia. Central nervous system (CNS) spectrum ranges from a massive acute encephalopathy to a subtle neurologic syndrome. Internal obstructive hydrocephalus (often present at birth or appears shortly thereafter and usually progressive), seizures, meningoencephalitis, cerebral calcifications, spinal or bulbar involvement (manifested by paralysis of the extremities, difficulty in swallowing, and respiratory distress), CSF abnormalities (xanthochromia, mononuclear pleocytosis, elevated protein content > 1 g/dL). Occular manifestations include chorioretinitis (macular scars, optic atrophy, and congenital cataract). A history of "dancing eyes" should always raise the possibility of a bilateral congenital central chorioretinitis—a typical ocular lesion of CT. Classic triad of chorioretinitis, cerebral calcifications, and hydrocephalus is the most severe form seen in small percentage of infants (occurs in <10% of cases).
3. *Delayed onset*: Mostly seen in preterm infants manifesting in the first 3 months of age in whom severe CNS and eye lesions appear. In the full-term infant with delayed onset of disease, manifestations arise mainly during the first 2 months of life. Clinical signs may be related to generalized infection (e.g., hepatosplenomegaly, delayed onset of icterus, lymphadenopathy), CNS involvement (e.g., encephalitis or hydrocephalus), or eye lesions, which may develop months or years after birth.
4. *Relapse or sequelae in infancy through adolescence of a previously untreated infection*: Focal necrotizing chorioretinitis, retinal scars, convulsions, cerebral calcifications, and neurologic relapse (late obstruction of the aqueduct).

Differential Diagnosis of Congenital Toxoplasma Infection

Other congenital infections: CMV, rubella, syphilis, herpes simplex, and HIV.

Other diseases: Bacterial sepsis, hemolytic diseases, metabolic disorders, immune thrombocytopenia, congenital leukemia.

Diagnosis of Congenital Toxoplasmosis

Indications for Toxoplasma Testing

- History of maternal toxoplasmosis
- Clinical manifestations suggestive of toxoplasmosis in a neonate.

Tests Available for Diagnosis

Several methods have been used for decades for the diagnosis of CT such as detection of toxoplasma-specific humoral immune responses, amplification of toxoplasma DNA, identification of toxoplasma-specific antigen in tissues, and isolation of the parasite.

- *Toxoplasma-specific humoral responses*: For *toxoplasma* IgG detection, the dye test is remains the gold standard. Other methods more commonly used are ELISA and ELISA-like assays, agglutination, and indirect immunofluorescence. For *toxoplasma* IgM detection, in addition to the above methods used, IgM immunosorbent agglutination assay (ISAGA) is used, which has higher sensitivity compared to ELISA and ELISA-like assays (e.g., 81.1% vs. 64.8%). The IgM ISAGA is the method of choice for the detection of *toxoplasma* IgM in infants younger than 6 months of age. ISAGA IgM and IgA increase sensitivity and specificity to almost 100%. Western blotting has been shown to establish diagnosis up to 3 months earlier than conventional serological methods. The diagnostic criteria for congenital toxoplasmosis based on serological tests are shown in **Box 1**.
- *Toxoplasma nucleic acid amplification (DNA PCR)*: Positive result in any body fluid (e.g., CSF, blood, urine) particularly helpful when antenatal screening program is not available.
- *Other investigations*:
  - *CSF analysis*: Highly increased proteins, eosinophilia
  - *Complete blood count*: Thrombocytopenia
  - *Liver function test*: Increased direct bilirubin, increased transaminases
  - *T. gondii specific immunoperoxidase tissue staining*: Presence of extracellular antigens and inflammatory response.

BOX 1: Diagnostic criteria for congenital toxoplasmosis based on serological tests.
- Positive IgM after 5 days of life and in the absence of blood transfusions
- Positive IgA after 10 days of life
- *Persistence of toxoplasma IgG beyond 1 year of age*: The gold standard to establish a diagnosis of CT. The standard to rule out the diagnosis is the decrease of IgG titers until its disappearance at ≤12 months of age in the absence of treatment
- *IgG, IgM, and IgA to specific toxoplasma antigens using western blot*: Presence of specific bands only seen in the newborn or bands with higher intensity than maternal ones for IgG and/or IgM and/or IgA in a reference laboratory
- IgG, IgM, and IgA should always be tested since having a combination of IgM and IgA test results, in addition to IgG, has greater sensitivity than either test alone

- *Tissue samples from the placenta*: PCR for parasite detection.
- *Neuroimaging*: Small (1–3 mm) round calcifications are the most specific finding. They may occur singly or in larger numbers. They are diffuse but predominate in the periventricular regions of the parietal-occipital or temporal lobes. Hydrocephalus: usually due to periaqueductal stenosis. Massive hydrocephalus may develop within 7 days.

In the absence of comprehensive clinical history and previous laboratory test results, diagnosis of CT after the first year of life is confounded by the possibility of the child acquiring infection in the postnatal period. For this reason, all reasonable efforts should be undertaken to diagnose or exclude CT during gestation or the infancy.

Treatment of Congenital Toxoplasmosis

Symptomatic Infants

A combination treatment of pyrimethamine, sulfadiazine, and folinic acid is given for 12 months (**Table 2**). The combination drug therapy can result in adverse effects and monitoring is essential. Folinic acid dose should be increased if the absolute neutrophil count (ANC) drops below 1,000/mm^3 and pyrimethamine should be temporarily withheld, if the ANC falls below 500. Sulfadiazine can cause neutropenia, liver and renal dysfunction. Monitor serum alanine transaminase (ALT) and creatinine every 3 months.

The combination therapy of 1 year duration is associated with a decrease incidence of neurologic, cognitive, auditory, and retinal sequelae. Ventricular shunting for hydrocephalus is recommended when necessary. Early shunt placement before 25 days of life was associated with better cognitive and motor outcomes.

TABLE 2: Drug therapy for management of congenital toxoplasma infection.

Drug	Dose	Monitoring
Pyrimethamine	1 mg/kg twice daily for 2 days, then 1 mg/kg once daily for 6 months, then 1 mg/kg three times a week (every other day) to complete 1 year of therapy (maximum 25 mg/dose)	Monitor for pancytopenia, monitor complete blood count (CBC) weekly. Stop drug if absolute neutrophil count (ANC) < 500 and restart after improvement
Sulfadiazine	50 mg/kg every 12 hours for 1 year	Hemolysis can occur in infants with glucose-6-phosphate dehydrogenase (G6PD) deficiency. Risk of bone marrow suppression, renal failure, and hypersensitivity. Alternative therapy for infants who develop allergy to sulfadiazine includes clindamycin
Folinic acid	*Dose*: 10 mg three times a week, administered until 1 week after completing pyrimethamine	Administered to prevent the potentially toxic side effects of pyrimethamine
Prednisone [If cerebrospinal fluid (CSF) protein >1 g/dL or active chorioretinitis with lesions very close to macula]	*Dose*: 0.5 mg/kg every 12 hours till above indication subsides followed by tapering and discontinuation	Start steroids after 72 hours of anti-toxoplasma therapy. Check weight weekly and adjust dose accordingly for all medications

TABLE 3: Follow-up schema for infants with congenital toxoplasma infection.

Evaluation	Schedule
Complete blood counts to monitor drug toxicity	Once a week while on daily pyrimethamine and once a month while on alternate day pyrimethamine
Neurodevelopmental follow-up	Periodically including developmental assessment
Ophthalmology exam	At birth and every 3 months until 18 months of age followed by every 6–12 months until 18 years old
Hearing evaluation	Auditory brainstem response by 3 months of age. Full audiological evaluation by 24 months of age

Asymptomatic Infection

Use same regimen as used for symptomatic infants for 3 months.

Follow-up of Infants Diagnosed with Congenital Toxoplasmosis

Follow-up for infants diagnosed with congenital toxoplasma infection is provided in **Table 3**.

Outcomes of Congenital Toxoplasma Infection

The National Collaborative Congenital Toxoplasmosis (NCCT) study has reported the outcomes of 120 children with congenital Toxoplasmosis who were treated for 1 year with pyrimethamine and sulfadiazine. This study observed that all infants who were asymptomatic or had mild disease at birth and received treatment have normal cognitive, neurological, and auditory outcomes. A majority (70%) of infants with moderate or severe neurological disease (focal calcifications in brain, seizures, motor abnormalities, hydrocephalus, microcephaly, elevated CSF protein levels, macular scarring, optic atrophy, visual, or hearing impairment) who receive treatment for 1 year also have normal neurological and cognitive outcomes. This study showed that treatment of congenital toxoplasmosis results in significant and long-lasting benefits, even for children with milder disease.

PREVENTION OF CONGENITAL TOXOPLASMA INFECTION

Pregnant women should observe the following precautions:
- Cooking meat thoroughly
- Hygiene measures—wash hands, avoid touching mucus membranes, clean kitchen surfaces and utensils after coming in contact with raw meat.
- Avoid contact with cat feces, and use gloves when cleaning cat litter box and disinfect with boiling water.
- Wash fruits and vegetables before consumption.
- Avoid drinking water potentially contaminated with oocysts.
- Avoid pregnancy for at least 6 months after a documented infection.
- Routine serological screening with IgG and IgM antibodies of all pregnant women in early gestation, ideally in the first trimester. Some countries like France and Australia have effective screening programs. However, in India this is not feasible or practical.

Chapter at a Glance

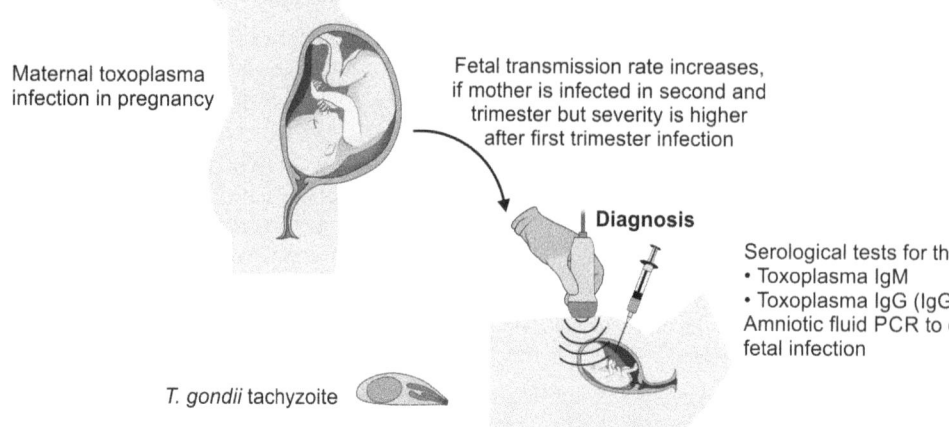
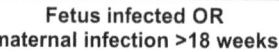

(PCR: polymerase chain reaction)

KEY POINTS

- The risk of mother to fetal transmission of toxoplasma infection depends on the gestational age at which maternal infection occurs. The risk of transmission is higher in second and third trimesters but severity of infection is higher when fetus is infected early in pregnancy.
- Maternal treatment with spiramycin can decrease fetal infection. If fetus is already infected, maternal treatment with combination chemotherapy decreases the severity of infection.
- The common manifestations of congenital toxoplasma infection are related to CNS and eyes in two-thirds; one-third have systemic findings. CNS manifestations include intracranial calcifications, hydrocephalus, chorioretinitis, and seizures.
- Treatment of infants with congenital toxoplasma with combination drug therapy for 12 months results in good outcomes.

SUGGESTED READING

1. Ahmed M, Sood A, Gupta J. Toxoplasmosis in pregnancy. Eur J Obstet Gynecol Reprod Biol. 2020;255:44-50.
2. Maldonado YA, Read JS; Committee on infectious diseases. Diagnosis, treatment, and prevention of congenital toxoplasmosis in the United States. Pediatrics. 2017;139(2): e20163860.
3. McLeod R, Boyer K, Karrison T, Kasza K, Swisher C, Roizen N, et al. Toxoplasmosis Study Group. Outcome of treatment for congenital toxoplasmosis, 1981-2004: the National Collaborative Chicago-Based, Congenital Toxoplasmosis Study. Clin Infect Dis. 2006:15;42(10):1383-94.
4. Pomares C. Montoya JG. Laboratory diagnosis of congenital toxoplasmosis. J Clin Microbiol. 2016;54(10):2448-54.
5. Robert-Gangneux F, Dardé ML. Epidemiology of and diagnostic strategies for toxoplasmosis. Clin Microbiol Rev. 2012;25(2):264-96.

CHAPTER 33

Rubella—Perinatal Perspective

Girija Wagh, Sandeep Kadam

INTRODUCTION
Rubella or German measles is a viral infection of relevance due to its teratogenic potential. The rubella virus can easily cross the placenta and leads to many effects, including miscarriage and heart, eye, and ear defects.

OBJECTIVES
- To review the epidemiology and risk of transmission of rubella virus
- To discuss the issues related to rubella during pregnancy
- To review the risk of rubella associated congenital defects
- To understand the preventive aspects, including rubella immunization

PATHOGENESIS

Rubella Virus
Rubella virus is a single-stranded RNA virus belonging to the Togaviridae family transmitted via airborne droplets and infected secretions. Humans are the only known host.

Rubella is a vaccine-preventable disease. Screening for Rubella antibodies is done in women planning pregnancy or pregnant women presenting with fever and rash or as a screening prenatal test. The antibodies protect the fetus against intrauterine infection. Rubella vaccine should be important preconceptional measure administered to all potential mothers and proactively done, so in women seeking preconceptional guidance and before embarking on fertility treatments.

Epidemiology
The Ministry of Health and Family Welfare, the Government of India, is committed to eliminating rubella by 2023. In a recent serosurvey from six sentinel sites in India, it was estimated that 14,000–50,000 neonates were born with congenital rubella syndrome (CRS).

Clinical Manifestations in the Mother
Rubella infection is an asymptomatic or mild, self-limiting illness in pregnancy. A quarter to half may experience fever, myalgia, throat ache, headache, and cough 15–21 days after exposure. A characteristic erythematous maculopapular rash with mild pruritus may occur. Rarely complications such as polyarthritis, polyarthralgia, and thrombocytopenia may occur.

Routine Screening to Identify Rubella Susceptible Women
Some countries routinely screen women of childbearing age for rubella antibodies. If rubella-specific IgG titer is greater than 10 IU/mL, it indicates immunity. Susceptible women should be vaccinated before pregnancy is planned. Countries also do rubella serology at the first antenatal visit in women without documented evidence for two doses of rubella vaccine. If the initial serology is negative, the test is repeated at 20 weeks of pregnancy, and susceptible women are offered vaccination after delivery. Routine screening is not done in India.

Diagnosis of Maternal Rubella Infection
Which test? Since fever with a rash can occur with other viral infections, laboratory diagnosis is essential to confirm a recent rubella infection. Serological tests measure rubella virus (RV) IgM, RV-IgM, and RV-IgG avidity. Testing for RV in nasopharyngeal secretions by reverse transcription-polymerase chain reaction (RT-PCR) is not done. The RV-IgM antibodies appear a few days after the onset of rash and disappear by 4–12 weeks, while RV-IgG appears a week after the rash and persist throughout life. The RV-IgG avidity test can be used to date the primary infection; in recent infections (<3 months), the IgG avidity is low; while a high avidity excludes a recent infection. However, this test should be interpreted with caution if the RV-IgG titer is low.

The following features characterize acute rubella infection:

- A fourfold increase in the IgG titer between acute and convalescent serum specimens.
- The presence of rubella IgM antibodies.

When to test? A pregnant woman with recent contact with a suspected rubella case should be tested (RV-IgM and RV-IgG) as soon as possible (preferably before 12 days). Other indications for testing include suspected rubella-like illness in the mother or fetal malformations in ultrasonography.

Test interpretation: The interpretation of the test and further action is provided in **Flowchart 1**.

Maternal-fetal Transmission of Rubella

Mother-to-baby transmission of rubella infection is transplacental. The virus spreads through the vascular system of the developing fetus and causes cytopathic damage to the blood vessels in various organs. The rate of infection and the risk of congenital malformation are dependent on gestational age **(Flowchart 2)**.

Management of Maternal Rubella

Management is symptomatic. Acetaminophen is used for fever and pain relief. Maternal complications such as thrombocytopenia or encephalopathy may need specific treatment (platelet transfusion and glucocorticoids). Counsel regarding the risk of infection and fetal malformation **(Flowchart 2 and Table 1)**.

Prenatal Diagnosis

Chorion villus sampling (11–13 weeks), amniotic fluid testing (16 weeks), and fetal blood sampling (18–20 weeks) can be done to detect rubella virus RNA and antibodies against rubella. However, these are difficult to translate in a regular antenatal clinical practice. Sonographic evaluation of the fetus for malformations, cardiac septal defects, cataracts, microphthalmia, microcephaly, and hepatosplenomegaly can be done. However, the features are not diagnostic, and the sensitivity of ultrasound is poor.

CONGENITAL RUBELLA INFECTION

Congenital rubella infection (CRI) has a varied presentation in neonates ranging from miscarriage, stillbirths, fetal growth restriction, prematurity, and triad of CRS (deafness, cardiac defect, and cataract).

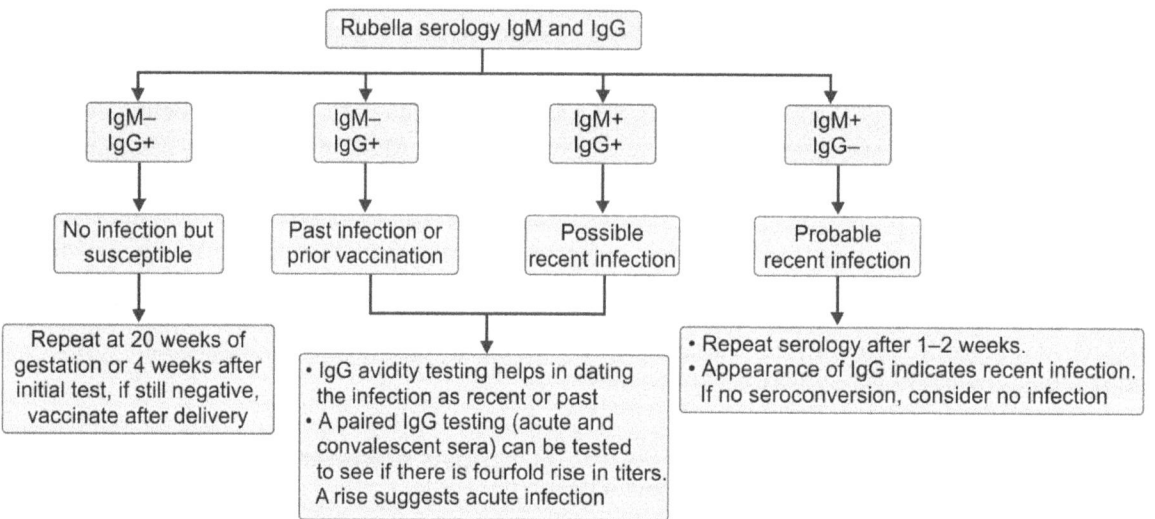

Flowchart 1: Rubella testing in pregnancy and interpretation.

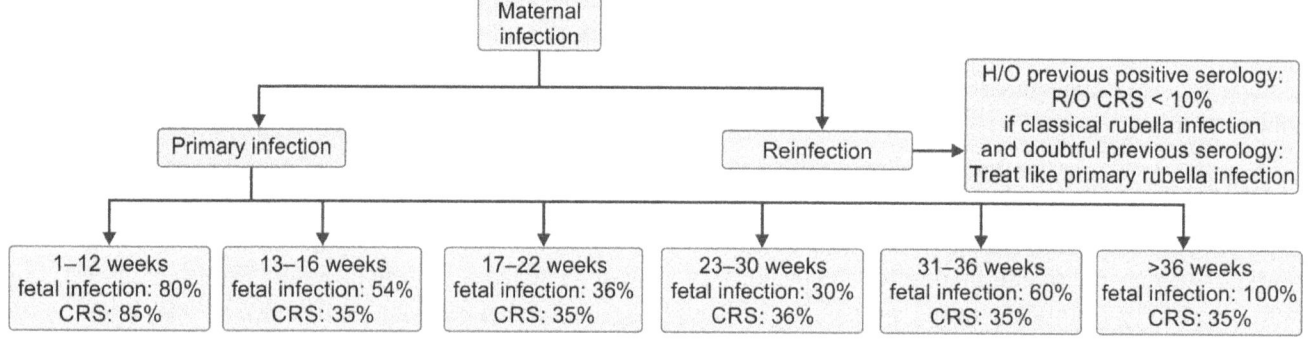

Flowchart 2: The risk of fetal infection and congenital rubella syndrome (CRS) following maternal rubella.

TABLE 1: Management of maternal rubella infection.

Maternal immune status	Management in a confirmed maternal rubella infection
Vaccinated and immune	• Possible maternal reinfection • *Before 12 weeks*: The risk of congenital rubella syndrome (CRS) is 8%. Offer counseling and shared decision making • *After 12 weeks*: Reassure. CRS is not documented
Nonimmune or unknown immune status	• Before 16 weeks, if the maternal infection is confirmed, termination of pregnancy can be offered (especially for gestations below 12 weeks) based on local legal guidelines • Between 16 and 20 weeks, the risk of CRS is <1%. Continue pregnancy and follow-up with fetal ultrasonography for malformations and growth. Testing of amniotic fluid for rubella virus RNA or serology can be offered • Beyond 20 weeks, reassure mother as the risk of CRS is negligible

CRI— is the broader term, encompassing the full spectrum of outcomes from intrauterine rubella infection, ranging from miscarriage or stillbirth to combinations of birth defects to asymptomatic infection.

CRS—is a subcategory of CRI that refers to a variable constellation of birth defects (e.g., sensorineural hearing loss, congenital heart disease, cataracts, congenital glaucoma).

Clinical manifestations of congenital rubella

- *Hearing defects (60–75%)*: Sensorineural deafness
- *Cardiac defects (10–20%)*: Peripheral pulmonary artery stenosis, patent ductus arteriosus, ventricular septal defect
- *Eye (10–25%)*: Pigmentary retinopathy, cataracts, microphthalmia, and congenital glaucoma **(Figs. 1 and 2)**
- *Central nervous system defects (10–25%)*: Microcephaly, meningoencephalitis, developmental delay
- *Others*: Hepatosplenomegaly, jaundice thrombocytopenia, radiolucent bone disease **(Fig. 3)**, and blueberry muffin skin rash

Late manifestations (childhood and adult): Diabetes mellitus, thyroiditis, growth problems, and behavioral disorder

Laboratory diagnosis:
- Rubella-specific IgM
- Rising IgG titers over a period of time
- Polymerase chain reaction for rubella virus
- Isolation of virus

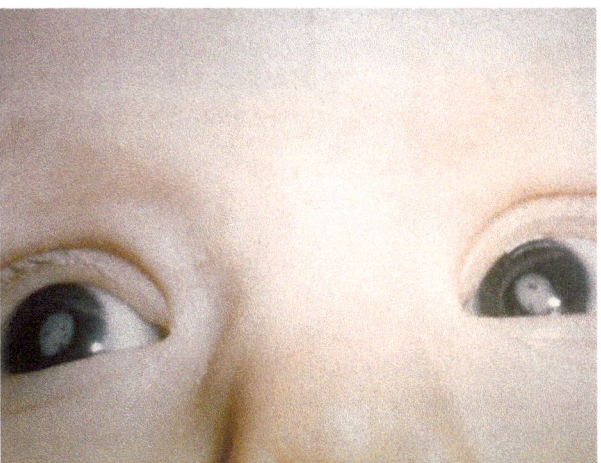

Fig. 1: Congenital rubella cataract.

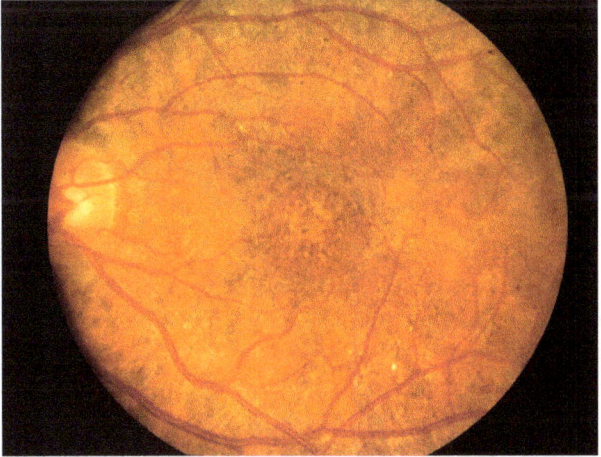

Fig. 2: Salt and pepper retinopathy of congenital rubella syndrome.

Evaluation

Re-evaluate maternal history to ascertain rubella infection and vaccination status. Lack of a history or previous vaccination does not preclude CRS in the neonate. Neonatal assessment includes:
- *Eye examination*: Glaucoma, cataracts, chorioretinitis
- *Cardiac*: clinical and echocardiography
- Evaluation for jaundice, thrombocytopenia, purpuric spots, and hepatosplenomegaly
- Neurological examination
- Hearing evaluation
- Skeletal X-ray (radiolucent bone disease)

Investigations

Laboratory evaluation should be done before the age of 1 year.

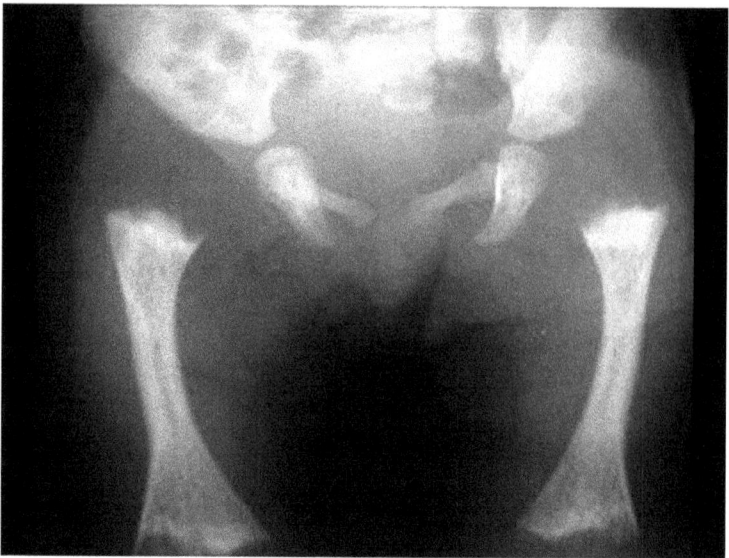

Fig. 3: Osseous manifestations of congenital rubella syndrome—Celery stalk metaphysis.

Serological Tests

Rubella-specific IgM: The test should be done before 3 months of age and a sensitive IgM-capture assay is preferable as this is more sensitive for the diagnosis of CRI than indirect IgM enzyme immune assays. For IgM test done between 3 and 18 months, IgM-capture EIAs should be preferred. A negative IgM at birth and up to 3 months of life rules out CRS. Beyond 18 months rubella, IgM levels wane away.

Rubella-specific IgG: The interpretation is IgG levels is influenced by transplacentally transferred maternal antibodies and infant vaccination (generally given by 9 months). The crux lies in serial testing and demonstration of persistently elevated antibodies (present on at least two occasions between 6 and 12 months of age). Hence, IgG testing is considered when IgM is negative or testing for rubella virus is not feasible.

Isolation of rubella virus: by nucleic acid amplification tests or rubella virus isolation. Throat swab is preferred. Other samples include nasal swabs, blood, urine, or cerebrospinal fluid. Infected infants may continue to excrete rubella virus for longer periods up to 2 years or more.

Management

The treatment of CRS is supportive care. There is *no role of anti-viral drugs* in CRI. The management of CRS is multidisciplinary, early intervention, growth monitoring, and correction of hearing, and cardiac problems.

Outcome

Majority of cases of CRS survive. However, the long-term outcomes of these babies need to be monitored for intellectual disability, speech, and visual assessment. Growth and developmental outcomes need to be monitored.

PREVENTION OF RUBELLA INFECTION

Rubella is a vaccine preventable disease. The vaccine available in India is a live attenuated RA 27/3 strain of rubella virus propagated in human diploid cells. Vaccination results in a high rate of seroconversion (95%) and life-long protection. Initially, the rubella vaccination as part of measles-mumps-rubella (MMR) vaccine is recommended for children at 12–15 months and with booster doses in childhood (4–7 years) and adolescence (12–18 years). The measles-rubella (MR) campaign was introduced by the Government of India in 2017 in a phased manner initially in five states namely Karnataka, Tamil Nadu, Goa, Lakshadweep, and Puducherry followed by expansion.

The MR program and campaign was introduced to eradicate measles and to control rubella and CRS by 2020. In the routine program, MR vaccine will be administered in two doses; the first between 9 and 12 months of age (the MR vaccine replaces the measles vaccine) and a second dose is given at 16–24 months of age. The campaign is a mass vaccination drive targeting a wide age group of children (9 months to 15 years) irrespective of previous immunization status or history of measles or rubella disease with a planned follow-up campaign at a periodicity of every 3–5 years.

Women should avoid becoming pregnant for 1 month postvaccination. In case of an inadvertent vaccination or immediate pregnancy, the risk of CRS is negligible and women can be reassured to continue pregnancy. In susceptible women, vaccination is advised after delivery.

CHAPTER AT A GLANCE

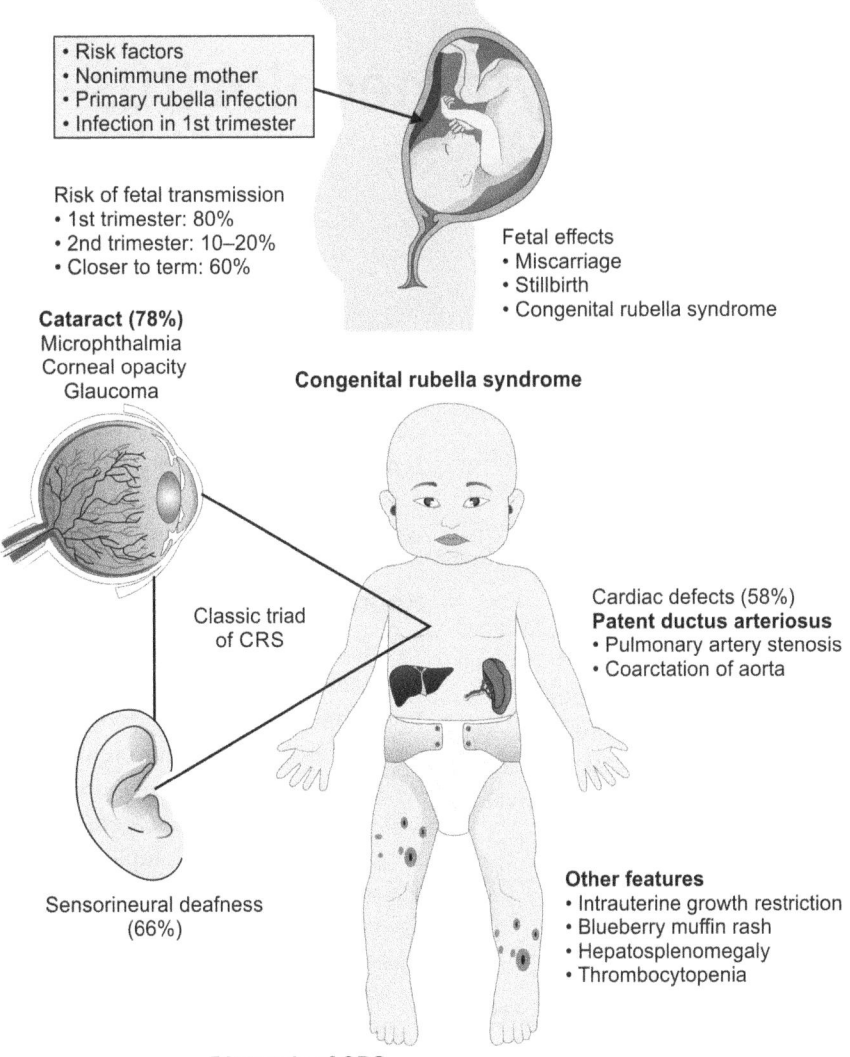

(PCR: polymerase chain reaction)

KEY POINTS

- The clinical spectrum of CRI is variable and ranges from miscarriage or stillbirth, to a combinations of birth defects called CRS.
- The risk of CRS is high with maternal primary infection before 12 weeks of gestation.
- Diagnosis of rubella infection in pregnancy is based on serological tests (rubella-specific IgM, IgG and IgG avidity testing).
- Diagnosis of rubella infection in the infants is based on detection of rubella-specific IgM by immunocapture ELISA and persistence of rubella-specific IgG levels in infancy.
- Infants with suspected rubella infection should undergo cardiac, ophthalmologic and audiologic evaluation and enrolled in follow-up program.
- Preventive measures include immunization in early childhood and documenting rubella immunity in pregnant women.

SUGGESTED READING

1. American Academy of Paediatrics. Rubella. In: Kimberlin DW, Brady MT, Jackson MA, Long SS (Eds). Red Book: 2018 Report of the Committee on Infectious Diseases, 31st edition. Itasca, IL: American Academy of Paediatrics; 2018. p. 705.
2. Best JM. Rubella. Semin Foetal Neonatal Med. 2007;12(3):182-92.
3. Muliyil DE, Singh P, Jois SK, Otiv S, Suri V, Varma V, et al. Seroprevalence of Rubella among pregnant women in India, 2017. Vaccine. 2018;36(52):7909-12.
4. Murhekar M, Verma S, Singh K, Bavdekar A, Benakappa N, Santhanam S, et al. Epidemiology of congenital rubella syndrome (CRS) in India, 2016-18, based on data from sentinel surveillance. PLoS Negl Trop Dis. 2020;14(2):e0007982.
5. Reef SE, Plotkin S, Cordero JF, Katz M, Cooper L, Schwartz B, et al. Preparing for elimination of congenital rubella syndrome (CRS): summary of a workshop on CRS elimination in the United States. Clin Infect Dis. 2000;31:85.

CHAPTER 34

Cytomegalovirus—Perinatal Perspective

Mayur A Thosar, Tushar B Parikh

INTRODUCTION

Cytomegalovirus (CMV) is a ubiquitously found DNA virus a member of the human herpes virus family. Hence, it retains distinct characteristic of becoming dormant after primary infection followed by reactivation and viral shedding after prolonged period of time.

Cytomegalovirus is the most common congenital viral infection with incidence of 0.2–2.2% of all live births as well as leading nongenetic cause of neurological disability or sensorineural hearing loss (SNHL). Though most infected infants are asymptomatic at birth, 10–15% will become symptomatic at birth, while same proportion will develop symptoms later in childhood.

OBJECTIVES

- To understand the epidemiology and transmission of CMV
- To know the signs and clinical features to suspect CMV in pregnancy or peripartum period
- To understand serological diagnosis and importance of avidity testing
- To know treatment modalities and follow up in antenatal or perinatal infection
- To know importance of preventive strategies

EPIDEMIOLOGY

Prevalence

Cytomegalovirus infection in children and adult is highly prevalent in developed as well as developing world. Though congenital infection is found in 0.2–2% of neonates, seropositivity in adult ranges from 45% to even up to 100%.

Seropositivity of CMV in pregnant women as reported by various studies range from 56.8% in Australia or 84% in Spain to 39–94.7% in the USA and 84.5–95% in Turkish population. Seroprevalence in Indian general population ranges variedly. Studies from northern most state of Kashmir shows CMV IgM positivity of 15.98% in general population and while Delhi and Punjab shows positivity rate of 12.9% and 22.03%, respectively. While similar studies from southern India shows seropositivity rate of 92% while IgM positivity of 4–6% in high-risk pregnancies. The seroprevalence in infants is reported from 5 to 7.4%.

Routes of Transmission

Cytomegalovirus infection to expectant mother may be acquired first time as primary infection or it can be reactivation from previously acquired dormant virus in salivary glands or monocytes. CMV has been cultured from multiple body fluids including saliva, urine, nasopharyngeal secretions, cervical and vaginal secretions, semen, blood, as well as breast milk. Though there can be multiple ways to acquire CMV infection, the most common mode of transmission in reproductive age group is exposure to urine and saliva of young children specially those attending day care.

Vertical transmission may occur to in utero fetus as placental cytotrophoblasts are permissive to CMV replication. Intrapartum or perinatal infection can occur due to contact with cervicovaginal secretions and blood, or postnatally through breastfeeding. The transmission can also occur in neonatal care units via blood transfusion or via breast milk especially in cases of preterm neonates.

Vertical transmission is more likely with primary maternal infection causing congenital infection in up to 30% cases compared to just 1–2% with reactivation of CMV. Risk of vertical transmission increases with gestational age of acquiring primary infection. Though incidence of transmission to fetus is lower with primary infection acquired in early pregnancy; for those who get infected chances of neurological involvement or severe fetal infection increases significantly.

CLINICAL PRESENTATION

In Pregnancy

Primary infection with CMV is mostly asymptomatic. Few women may develop prodrome similar to infectious mononucleosis including fever, malaise, myalgia, lymphadenopathy, and rarely hepatitis or pneumonia. About one-third of primary cases of CMV are associated with dermatologic manifestations including macular, popular, rubelliform and scarlatiniform eruptions.

Nonprimary maternal infection includes reactivation of previously dormant virus or reinfection with another strain in presence of previous antibodies. Nonprimary maternal infection is mostly asymptomatic and is suspected in case of suggestive ultrasound features like such as ventriculomegaly, microcephaly, calcifications, intraventricular synechiae, intracranial hemorrhage, periventricular cysts, cerebellar hypoplasia, cortical abnormalities, echogenic bowel, growth restriction, pericardial effusion, ascites, and hydrops fetalis. Diagnosis of reactivation or nonprimary infection is done mainly by serological tests. In absence of routine screening, true incidence of nonprimary infection and risk of vertical transmission in such cases is difficult to ascertain.

Clinical Presentation of Congenital CMV Infection

With better diagnostic modalities, it is now clear that most congenital infections in the fetus remain asymptomatic. Up to 10% neonates may have symptomatic disease at birth while additional 10% though asymptomatic at birth develop neurological sequelae such as SNHL, microcephaly, mental retardation, development delay, seizure disorders, and cerebral palsy. In fact congenital CMV is the leading nonhereditary cause of SNHL in the newborns. It has been recognized that congenital CMV infection causes more long-term disabilities in a year than other common causes such as fetal alcohol syndrome, Down's syndrome, spina bifida, HIV, invasive *Haemophilus influenzae* B infection or congenital rubella syndrome.

Symptomatic Neonate

Symptomatic at Birth

Approximately, 10% neonates with congenital CMV are symptomatic at birth. One-third neonates are born premature and 50% neonates are small for gestation. Common features **(Figs. 1A and B)** at birth include petechiae/thrombocytopenia (77%), hepatosplenomegaly (60%), jaundice (67%), purpura/blue-berry muffin rash (13%) and neurologic manifestations such as, microcephaly (53%), lethargy/hypotonia/poor suck (20%), and seizures (7%). Almost 30–50% of symptomatic CMV have SNHL, which is commonly progressive during first 2 years. Overall mortality among symptomatic neonates is 4–8% during first year of life. Common cause of death includes severe end organ disease involving, lungs, liver, bone marrow, central nervous system (CNS) or viral associated hemophagocytic syndrome. Babies who survive, neurologic sequelae are permanent.

The acute fulminant presentation: A small subset of symptomatic neonates present with life-threatening severe illness in neonatal period with high mortality to the tune of 30%. These babies may have hydrops, severe pneumonia, hepatitis, severe thrombocytopenia, and seizures.

The primary neurophenotype presentation: Some babies have subtle symptoms at birth with only mild microcephaly without other somatic abnormalities like hepatosplenomegaly, thrombocytopenia, petechiae, etc. The microcephaly becomes pronounced with time along with other neurologic signs like, abnormal tone, global developmental delay, and seizures. Neuroimaging may demonstrate calcification, polymicrogyria, or other cortical dysplasia.

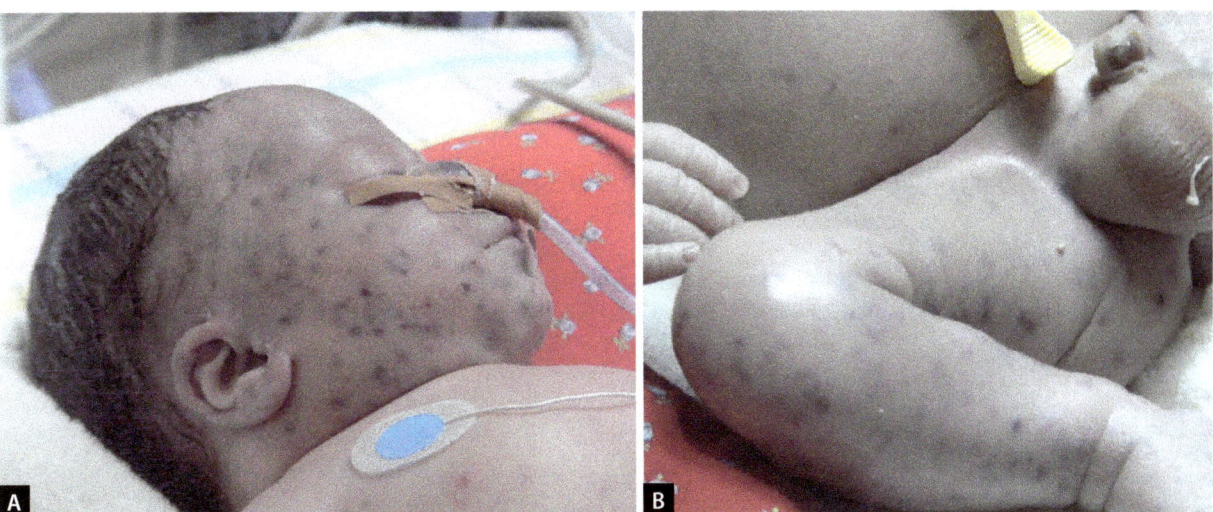

Figs. 1A and B: Baby with symptomatic congenital CMV at birth. Note the blue berry muffin rashes. (Photographs taken with permission).

Asymptomatic at Birth

Almost 90% babies born with congenital CMV are completely asymptomatic at birth. About 15% of these babies develop SNHL during first 2 years. Therefore, these babies should be closely monitored for isolated SNL and treatment offered as needed. Some babies are also at risk of mental retardation, motor spasticity, and microcephaly. Some babies may have dental enamel production defects evident later in life.

Postpartum Infection (Term and Preterm)

Some babies acquire CMV infection postpartum, commonly from their mother through breast milk. CMV seropositive women also secrete virus in the birth canal, saliva and urine. Rarely, CMV is transmitted through blood products, especially if they are not leucodepleted or irradiated. Term neonates are usually asymptomatic but babies born at <32 weeks/<1,500 g may develop symptomatic disease during second or third month of life in the form of sepsis, pneumonia, neutropenia, thrombocytopenia, hepatitis, colitis, and recurrent apnea. Commonly, CMV infection is considered in diagnosis when there is no improvement after first line antibiotic treatment and negative blood culture reports. Thrombocytopenia, raised liver enzymes, and direct hyperbilirubinemia are diagnostic clues to postnatal CMV infection. To call it postnatally acquired, it should be demonstrated after 21 days of life, with negative CMV viral tests in the first 3 weeks. Multiple population-based studies have failed to show any association between postnatal CMV and SNHL. Data on developmental outcomes showed conflicting results with some studies showing lower cognitive and motor scores while others showing no difference in those outcomes.

DIAGNOSTIC EVALUATION IN PREGNANCY

Settings of Primary Infection

Confirming diagnosis of CMV in pregnancy is based on serological tests. IgM after primary infection may persist for months or may also be raised in secondary infections. IgM can also be raised due to cross reactivity with other viruses or due to nonspecific immune reaction. As rise in IgM levels in absence of previous negative tests is not reliable to confirm diagnosis, IgG avidity test is necessary to define timing of infection (**Table 1**).

Hence, a primary infection is confirmed by either CMV specific IgG in previously seronegative woman or detection of CMV IgM with low IgG avidity index. As IgG levels may increase due to nonspecific immune reaction, suspected secondary infection can be confirmed only with invasive testing, and polymerase chain reaction (PCR) of amniotic fluid.

The commercially available test kits for CMV IgG and IgM utilize either enzyme immune assay or chemiluminous immunoassay. The cutoff of both differs depending on manufacturer and is reported as negative—borderline—positive. In suspected cases with borderline results retesting can be done after interval of 10–15 days.

Role of Invasive Testing

With maternal infection with CMV or ultrasound suspicious with CMV infection, invasive testing is indicated to rule out fetal infection. Confirmation of fetal infection can be done with real time polymerase chain reaction (RT-PCR) of amniotic fluid. Fetal infection occurs in steps as placental infection and replication—transmission to fetus—replication in kidneys—excretion in urine which usually

TABLE 1: Interpretation of cytomegalovirus (CMV) serological tests in pregnancy.

CMV antibodies	IgG avidity	Interpretation	Implications
IgM– and IgG–	Not applicable	Uninfected or very early infection	Counsel about behavioral measures to reduce risk of acquiring infection
IgM+ and IgG–	Not applicable	May be false positive (90%) due to another virus, autoimmune disease, laboratory methods	Repeat in 2 weeks. Positive IgM and IgG in repeat sample indicates recent primary infection
IgM+ and IgG+	Low	Recent infection seroconversion is diagnostic of primary infection	Counsel about likelihood of fetal infection, possible sequelae, and options for prenatal diagnosis and management
IgM+ and IgG+	High	• Past infection versus recurrent infection • As a significant rise (at least double) in serial IgG titers suggests reactivation or reinfection	Counsel about low possibility of fetal infection, but if infected possible sequelae
IgM– and IgG+	High	• Past infection • Absence of a significant rise in serial IgG titers suggests absence of reactivation or reinfection	• Counsel about low risk of fetal infection and possible sequelae • No need for further testing
IgM– and IgG+	Low	Unclear as avidity tests have been validated only in the setting of true positive IgM	

TABLE 2: Ultrasound detectable abnormalities in cytomegalovirus (CMV).

Cerebral abnormality	Extra cerebral abnormality compatible with fetal CMV infection
• Periventricular calcifications • Ventriculomegaly (>15 mm) • Cerebral calcification • Intraventricular adhesion • Lenticulostriate vasculopathy • Microcephaly • Large cisterna magna • Polymicrogyria • Cerebellar hypoplasia	• Fetal growth restriction • Abnormal amniotic fluid volume • Ascites and/or pleural effusion • Hydrops • Placentomegaly > 40 mm • Hyperechogenic bowel • Hepatomegaly > 40 mm • Splenomegaly > 30 mm • Liver calcifications

takes 6-8 weeks. Hence, amniocentesis should preferably be planned 8 weeks after primary maternal infection.

Fetal blood sampling for confirming CMV disease is not recommended now. As platelet count, liver enzyme levels and beta 2 microglobulin levels may help to predict severity of disease, in specific conditions fetal blood sampling can be done for above investigations. The decision of fetal blood sampling should be taken case to case basis with opinion from fetal medicine specialist.

Role of Imaging—Ultrasound versus MRI

Normal ultrasound features before and on follow up are reassuring but is not sensitive enough to rule out symptomatic neonate at birth or in later childhood.

Ultrasound is most common modality for suspecting CMV in asymptomatic mothers as well as for follow up. Presence of bilateral periventricular calcifications is supposed to be most characteristic finding. A serial ultrasound examination 2-4 weeks apart is useful to detect development of abnormalities as these can appear 12 weeks or more after maternal primary infection **(Table 2)**.

Fetal magnetic resonance imaging (MRI) in suspected or diagnosed case of fetal CMV infection is generally considered complimentary investigation to ultrasound. MRI may diagnose neurological abnormalities in up to 6% of fetus with no detectable abnormality on ultrasound. MRI may be advocated in doubtful findings on ultrasound requiring better clarity. Absence of no detectable ultrasound or MRI abnormality in third trimester generally points to favorable outcomes, though cannot negate congenital infection.

TREATMENT IN PREGNANCY
Role of Antiviral

In immunocompetent pregnant women with CMV infection routine treatment with antiviral is rarely indicated. The treatment mainly consists of supportive medications like acetaminophen. In immunocompromised nonpregnant women, many drugs are available for treatment of CMV infection, but due to high teratogenicity of ganciclovir, valganciclovir, cidofovir, and foscarnet only valaciclovir (prodrug of acyclovir) can be used in pregnancy.

There are limited studies suggesting use of high dose oral valaciclovir in fetal infection with high viral load but no detected CNS abnormalities with favorable outcomes. But due to small sample size of those studies, further randomized trials need to generate evidence before recommending routine use.

Role of Hyperimmune Globulin

Use of hyperimmune globulin (HIG) was hypothesized to decrease the transmission, reduce the immunological reactions elicited by virus and reduce development of the neurological abnormalities. But studies failed to elicit any of above expected beneficial effect. Rather use of HIG was found to have poor obstetrical outcomes like increased risk of preterm labor, growth restriction, and development of preeclampsia. Hence, HIG use is not recommended at present.

DIAGNOSTIC EVALUATION OF SUSPECTED CONGENITAL CMV INFECTION

Cytomegalovirus infection can be asymptomatic in the neonates and hence a universal screening approach has been advocated by some experts. PCR-based test on dried saliva spot has potential for reliable large scale screening program. Until that happens, infants who show clinical signs suggestive of Congenital CMV are screened for CMV infection. Infants who have confirmed fail unilateral or bilateral hearing screening test also should undergo testing for congenital CMV.

Laboratory Clues to Diagnosis of Congenital CMV

Typically congenital CMV has multisystem affection. Laboratory abnormalities pertaining to hematologic, gastrointestinal, liver, and brain are seen **(Table 3)**.

Other less common findings include hemolytic anemia, neutropenia, lymphopenia/lymphocytosis, thrombocytosis or leukemoid reaction.

Neuroimaging

Seventy percent of symptomatic neonates will show abnormalities on neuroimaging. MRI is imaging modality of choice, however, first modality invariably is bedside ultrasound due to ease of access. Findings on neuroimaging

SECTION 5 | Congenital Infections

TABLE 3: Common laboratory abnormalities.

Laboratory abnormality	Frequency (%)
Elevated liver enzymes (SGPT)	83
Thrombocytopenia:	
• $<100 \times 10^3/mm^3$	77
• $<50 \times 10^3/mm^3$	53
Conjugated hyperbilirubinemia:	
• Direct bilirubin >2 mg/dL	81
• Direct bilirubin >4 mg/dL	69
Hemolysis	51
Increased CSF protein (>120 mg%)	46

Source: Adapted from Boppana SB, Pass RF, Britt WJ, Stagno S, Alford CA. Symptomatic congenital cytomegalovirus infection: neonatal morbidity and mortality. Pediatr Infect Dis J. 1992;11:93.
(CSF: cerebrospinal fluid)

include; intracranial calcification, usually periventricular in location (34–70%), lenticulostriate vasculopathy—calcification along blood vessels in basal ganglia seen in 27–68% cases, ventriculomegaly (10–53%), white matter disease (22–57%), neuronal migration disorders including focal polymicrogyria, pachygyria, and lissencephaly (10–38%) and occasionally periventricular leukomalacia and cystic abnormalities (11%). Primary neuropathic type congenital CMV, typically have neuronal migration disorders with polymicrogyria and other cortical dysplasias. Asymptomatic neonates with congenital CMV 5–20% have punctate calcifications and ventriculomegaly. Babies with postnatal CMV, Head Ultrasound studies are typically normal but some babies may show lenticulo-striatal vasculopathy or germinolytic cysts.

Laboratory Diagnosis

The laboratory diagnosis of CMV is made if the virus is identified in urine, saliva, blood, or respiratory secretions in the baby. Identification of the virus within first 3 weeks of life confirms congenital nature of the CMV infection. Saliva sample is sometimes contaminated with breastmilk (False positive) or too little sample (False negative), so most prefer urine sample.

Viral culture, modified viral culture (shell viral assay), and PCR are methods to identify virus. All these three methods have near 100% sensitivity and specificity. PCR methods are preferred for high-sensitivity, accuracy, cost-effectiveness and rapid turnaround. In addition, PCR provides quantitative result which can help monitor the progress of disease.

Serological Evaluation

Serologic tests (IgG and IgM) are not recommended in neonate as IgG reflects maternal level and CMV IgM antibody level is insensitive and has high falsely negative rate (>50%) in infected newborns. Negative immunoglobulin G (IgG) titers in both maternal and infant sera are sufficient to exclude congenital CMV infection. Transplacentally acquired anti CMV IgG wanes off over period of first 4–9 months.

TREATMENT OF CONGENITAL OR PERINATALLY ACQUIRED CMV

Postdiagnosis Evaluation

Baby with congenital CMV is evaluated for the extent of involvement and prognostication.

- Detailed anthropometry
- Laboratory evaluation—Hemogram, liver function tests, renal function tests and coagulation studies
- Hearing evaluation at baseline once the baby is stabilized and then once in 6 months during follow up
- Ophthalmic evaluation for chorioretinitis
- *Neuroimaging*: MRI brain is preferred modality
- Chest X-ray for interstitial pneumonia
- *Cerebrospinal fluid (CSF) examination*: CSF-CMV PCR test is recommended, if there is any doubt about CNS involvement. If CSF CMV PCR is positive, infant should be classified to have CNS disease.

Antivirals

Ganciclovir

Ganciclovir is the drug of choice for CMV infection for nearly last four decades. It is synthetic acyclic nucleoside analogue which phosphorylases in presence of viral proteins and exerts its antiviral effect on CMV infected cell. *Indications*: symptomatic neonates with either CNS involvement or severe end-organ disease such as hepatitis, pneumonia or refractory thrombocytopenia. Multiple randomized controlled trials have demonstrated benefit of Ganciclovir therapy in these category of patients in improving survival and neurodevelopmental outcome especially SNHL. Ganciclovir is not recommended for asymptomatic CMV infected neonates at present due to lack of any proven benefits. *Dose*: Ganciclovir is used in a dose of 6 mg/kg twice a day intravenously. Ganciclovir is given intravenously only as it has poor oral bioavailability. Babies who are able to take oral medications, valganciclovir is a reasonable alternative to intravenous (IV) ganciclovir. *Side effects*: Even though ganciclovir is regarded as fairly safe and well-tolerated; in animal models ganciclovir has been shown to be carcinogenic, teratogenic, and gonadal toxic however no such association has shown in humans. *Duration*: Traditional recommended duration of therapy for congenital CMV was 42 days; however recent reports suggest that longer duration of therapy for 6 months, with oral valganciclovir improves neurodevelopmental outcomes and reduces chances of

SNHL. *Monitoring*: During ganciclovir therapy one should monitor for Neutropenia and thrombocytopenia. Granulocyte monocyte colony stimulating factor (GM-CSF) can be given for severe neutropenia.

Valgancyclovir

Alternative to intravenous ganciclovir is use of its prodrug, *valganciclovir* is well-absorbed following oral administration and rapidly metabolized. Oral medicine obviates need for central venous catheter and patient can be discharged early. Dose of oral valganciclovir is 16 mg/kg/dose every 12 hourly. Duration of therapy is for 6 months for congenital CMV.

For postnatal/acquired CMV, ganciclovir or valganciclovir are used in 2 weekly blocks. Blood CMV DNA viral loads are checked weekly and therapy is stopped once the CMV DNA is negative. Treatment duration is generally less than 8 weeks. There are no proven benefits of using it more than 42 days in postnatal CMV.

Situations where symptomatic disease does not respond, underlying immunodeficiency disorder should be considered (e.g., HIV or severe combined immune deficiency, etc.).

Use of antivirals does not completely eliminate virus from the body. The mucosal shedding in saliva or urine may rebegin after the course of antiviral has stopped.

Foscarnet and cidofovir are other antivirals tried in congenital CMV with very little experience. They are reserved for special situation of poor response to ganciclovir or known resistance to ganciclovir.

PROSPECTS OF PREVENTION

CMV Vaccine

As there is no clinically effective and approved vaccine for CMV, the corner stone for prevention lies with behavioral modification. Simple hygiene measures like hand washing after touching nasal/oral secretions or diapers by reproductive age women is found to significantly reduce rates of seroconversion. As pregnant women are more likely to be receptive for information and adhere to behavioral modifications, there should be program to provide them with adequate information and counseling.

Prevention in Day Care Setting

Day care workers are one of high-risk groups to contact CMV and should be well-educated about mode of transmission and possible effects in pregnancy. Pregnant women working in care of young children are to be educated about hygiene measures to reduce exposure. Routine serological screening of day care workers is not recommended. Healthcare workers are not found to have increased risk of transmission of CMV infection likely due to adherence of universal precautions while handling body fluids.

In women with recent CMV infection, presence of CMV virus is documented in blood or body fluids for period even up to 6 months. Though there is no standard recommendation or evidence, many experts are of opinion to avoid conception for 3-6 months to reduce chances of transmission to fetus.

Use of Breastmilk from CMV Seropositive Mother

Almost 80% seropositive mothers will excrete CMV in breastmilk. Colostrum to a great extent is CMV free but later, CMV DNA is detected in breastmilk by 4-8 weeks of lactation. Therefore, most European Neonatology associations recommend pasteurization of breastmilk from CMV-positive mothers for babies <1,500 g and <32 weeks corrected gestation. Pasteurization reduces energy, fat, and lactose content of milk besides it inactivates beneficial immunological components of human milk (lactoferrin, defensins, leukocytes, and immunoglobulin). Also studies have shown that pasteurization of breastmilk or Freezing breastmilk (–20°C for 24 hours) substantially reduced, but did not eliminate risk of postnatal CMV transmission from breast milk. American academy of Pediatrics (AAP) recommends fresh breastmilk to all preterm babies to preserve nutritional benefits as risk of milk-acquired severe CMV infections and "sepsis-like" episodes were estimated to be very low. Routine CMV sero-status screening of pregnant women or that of mothers of VLBW/ELBW infants is not recommended at present. However, this needs further research and recommendations from peak professional bodies.

Blood Transfusion in Neonates

Blood transfusion can be a potential source of CMV infection for a premature neonate. To reduce this risk, RBC transfusion should be CMV negative (Seronegative or CMV DNA negative blood) and leucodepleted to reduce risk of transfusion associated CMV infection. CMV resides in white blood cells. Leucodepletion decreases the number of white cells from 1×10^8 to less than 5×10^6 per unit. Studies have shown that this approach can considerably reduce chances of transfusion related CMV infection, if not completely eliminate the problem. The Canadian National Advisory Committee on blood transfusion has recommended that CMV safe (leukoreduced) and CMV IgG seronegative products be considered equivalent *except* for intrauterine transfusion. Blood transfusions in neonate for exchange transfusion or in very low birth weight neonate should be irradiated to reduce risk of transfusion associated graft versus host disease.

CHAPTER AT A GLANCE

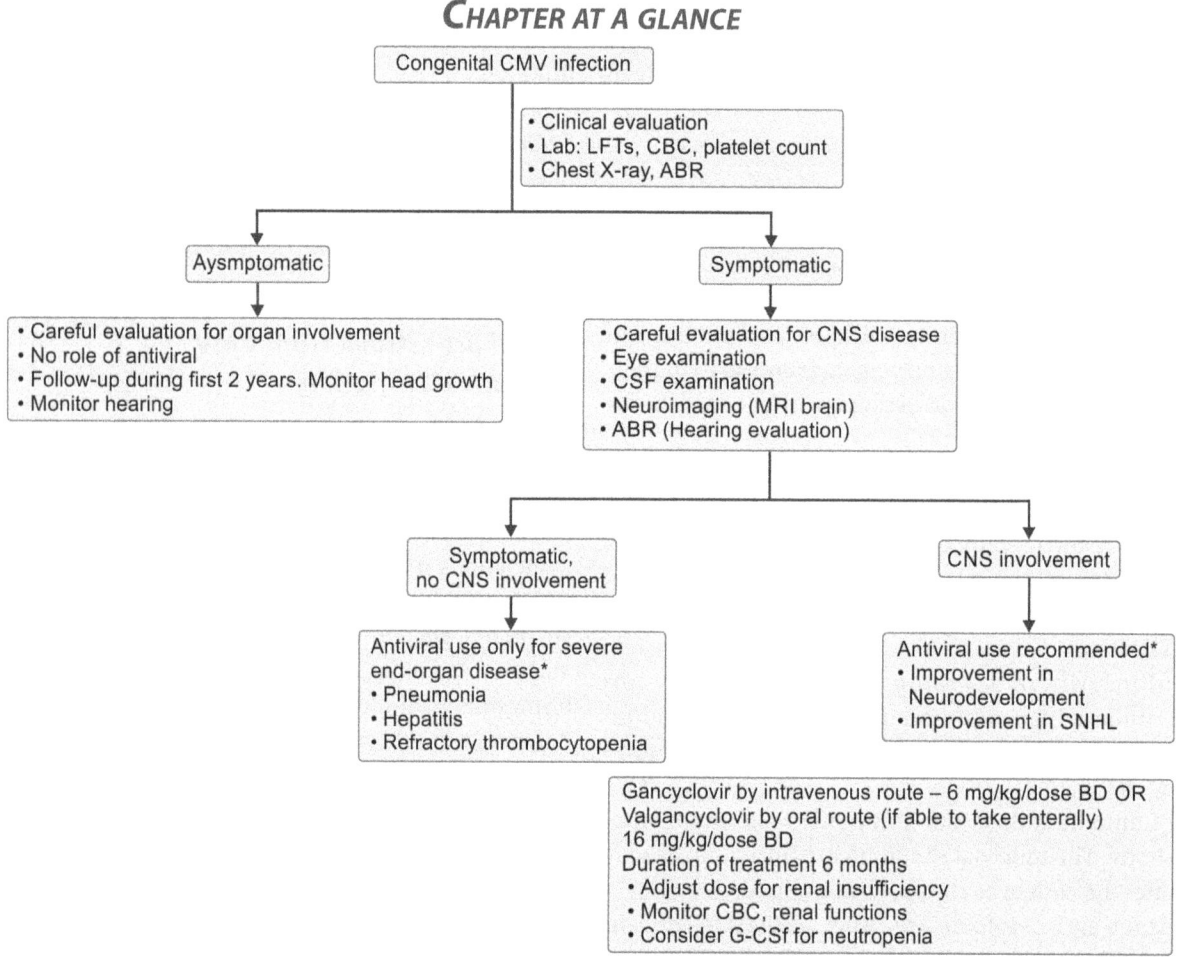

(ABR: auditory brainstem response; CBC: complete blood count; CMV: cytomegalovirus; CNS: central nervous system; G-CSF: granulocyte cerebrospinal fluid; LFT: liver function test; MRI: magnetic resonance imaging; SNHL: sensorineural hearing loss)

KEY POINTS

- Congenital CMV infection is one of leading non genetic cause of neurodevelopmental disabilities and SNHL.
- Most cases of CMV infection in pregnancy are asymptomatic or may present with mild febrile illness.
- Diagnosis of primary infection versus recurrent infection is mainly based on serological tests along with avidity testing.
- The gestational age at primary infection is important determinant of vertical transmission. Though absolute risk of transmission is more in third trimester than first, the risk of developing neurological or SNHL is more in early infections.
- Invasive testing with amniocentesis with RT-PCR is most reliable test to confirm fetal infections.
- A serial ultrasound examination is most useful tool to monitor affected fetus, with MRI or cord blood test to be used in specific circumstances.
- Maternal therapy with antiviral drugs or immunoglobulins is not recommended.
- Prevention of CMV infection with simple hygiene methods is most important to reduce disease burden.
- Congenital CMV affects approximately 1% neonates, however only 10% of those infected are symptomatic at birth.
- Hepatosplenomegaly, thrombocytopenia and blue berry muffin rash are typical presentations of symptomatic CMV at birth.
- Asymptomatic CMV infection are at risk of developing SNHL during first 2 years, hence periodic assessment for hearing is recommended during first 2 years.

SUGGESTED READING

1. Bialas KM, Swamy GK, Permar SR. Perinatal cytomegalovirus and varicella zoster virus infections: epidemiology, prevention, and treatment. Clin Perinatol. 2015;42(1):61-75.
2. Boppana SB, Pass RF, Britt WJ, Stagno S, Alford CA. Symptomatic congenital cytomegalovirus infection: neonatal morbidity and mortality. Pediatr Infect Dis J. 1992;11(2):93-9.
3. Cannon MJ, Davis KF. Washing our hands of the congenital cytomegalovirus disease epidemic. BMC Public Health. 2005;5:70.
4. Kadambari S, Whittaker E, Lyall H. Postnatally acquired cytomegalovirus infection in extremely premature infants: how best to manage? Arch Dis Child Fetal Neonatal Ed. 2019;0:F1-6.
5. Khalil A, Heath P, Jones C, Soe A, Ville YG. On behalf of the Royal College of Obstetricians and Gynaecologists. Congenital Cytomegalovirus Infection: Update on Treatment. Scientific Impact Paper No. 56. BJOG. 2018;125:e1-11.
6. Practice bulletin no. 151: Cytomegalovirus, parvovirus B19, varicella zoster, and toxoplasmosis in pregnancy. Obstet Gynecol. 2015;125(6):1510-25.
7. Swanson EC, Schleiss MR. Congenital cytomegalovirus infection: new prospects for prevention and therapy. Pediatr Clin North Am. 2013;60(2):335-49.

35
Herpes Simplex Virus—Perinatal Perspective

Vandana Bansal, Anish Pillai, Nandkishor Kabra

INTRODUCTION

Herpes simplex virus (HSV) is a large double-stranded DNA virus belonging to the family herpesviridae and subfamily alpha-herpesvirinae. Based on the glycoprotein in their envelope, HSV is differentiated as HSV type 1 (glycoprotein G1) and HSV type 2 (glycoprotein G2). HSV-1 causes herpes labialis and gingivostomatitis. HSV-2 is sexually transmitted and causes most cases of genital herpes. Although a majority of infections in adults are asymptomatic, HSV infection in neonates can result in significant morbidity and mortality.

OBJECTIVES

- Review the epidemiology of perinatal HSV
- Understand the pathophysiology and transmission
- Describe the clinical features and diagnosis
- Discuss the management and prevention

EPIDEMIOLOGY

As per estimates by the World Health Organization (WHO), over 60% of the people under the age of 50 years have HSV-1 infection and 13% have HSV-2 subclinical infection globally. The seroprevalence of HSV varies by country and ethnicity, with a higher incidence in girls and the Black population. The prevalence of genital herpes infection in pregnant women is around 10–65%, however, the majority of women are asymptomatic. Studies from India have shown that the prevalence of HSV in pregnant women is around 6–10%. Transmission of HSV from mother to baby can occur via various routes, such as transplacental (5%), intrapartum (85%), or postnatal (10%). The incidence of neonatal HSV, defined as infection within 28 days of birth, is variable in different parts of the world. The incidence of neonatal HSV in the UK is around 1.6 per 100,000 live births, in Canada around 6 per 100,000 live births, in the US it is higher at 12–60 per 100,000 live births. HSV infections can be fatal in neonates if untreated.

PATHOPHYSIOLOGY

Transmission: Factors that increase the risk of HSV transmission from mother to baby include the type of maternal infection (first episode primary infection), vaginal delivery, prolonged rupture of membranes, and instrumentation during delivery. Types of maternal infection can be any of the following:

- Newly acquired:
  - First episode primary infection (new infection with no serum HSV antibodies)
  - First-episode nonprimary infection (new infection with one HSV type in the presence of antibodies to the other HSV type); or
- Previously acquired (mother has antibodies to the type of HSV that she is infected with):
  - Reactivation of latent disease
  - Asymptomatic viral shedding

The neonatal transmission rate is the highest in the case of first-episode primary infection during pregnancy (30–50%), followed by first episode nonprimary infection (25–35%), and least for recurrent/reactivation of latent infection (1–3%). Clinically, it is difficult to distinguish whether genital HSV infection is primary or recurrent, as many suspected first episode HSV infections may not be true primary.

Herpes simplex virus enters the body via breaks in the mucus membranes or skin and attaches to the epithelial cells. During the incubation period of 3–14 days, the virus replicates in the epidermis/dermis. The virus is transported from the sensory nerve endings in the dermis to the sensory ganglia where it persists lifelong. It periodically reactivates, as asymptomatic shedding or recurrent ulcers. Antibody response occurs after 3–4 weeks and persists lifelong. However, these protective antibodies do not prevent local recurrences.

CLINICAL MANIFESTATION

- *Maternal outcomes*: Most maternal HSV infections are asymptomatic. Around 75% of women with a neonate infected with HSV do not have any history of genital

HSV. Thus, clinical history may be unreliable and there must be a high index of suspicion. In the case of primary infection, symptoms include tender vesicles that may rupture and ulcerate. Local manifestations such as pain, dysuria, itching, vaginal discharge, and lymphadenopathy may be present. Constitutional symptoms such as fever, headache, nausea, and myalgia are due to viremia. Symptoms associated with recurrent disease are milder. Pregnant women with untreated genital herpes have a greater chance of preterm delivery, compared to the general population. Rarely, severe manifestations including fulminant hepatitis, maternal viral sepsis, pneumonitis, or encephalitis may be seen.

- *Congenital infection*: Intrauterine HSV infections are uncommon. The manifestations are similar to other intrauterine infections causing growth restriction, skin lesions (vesicles and scarring), neurologic injury (intracranial calcifications, microcephaly, hypertonicity, and seizures), and eye involvement (microphthalmia, cataracts, chorioretinitis, blindness, and retinal dysplasia). These manifestations probably result from the destruction of normally formed organs, rather than defects in organogenesis, mostly by HSV-2 infections.
- *Neonatal infection*: Most neonatal HSV infections present in the initial 2-4 weeks of life, however, it may occasionally present up to 6 weeks. The clinical features can fit in any of the following subtypes, or may even have overlapping features (**Table 1**).

Outcomes

The outcome depends on the type of disease and the timing of initiation of treatment.

- *Disseminated*: Mortality in infants with the disseminated disease is 85% without timely treatment with acyclovir and around 40-50% survivors have abnormal neurodevelopment with treatment. With timely initiation of parenteral acyclovir therapy, mortality has decreased to 29%, with over 80% of infants having normal neurodevelopment at 1 year.
- *Central nervous system (CNS) disease*: Mortality in babies with CNS herpes has reduced from 50% (without treatment) to under 10% following antiviral therapy. Despite treatment, around 50-70% of survivors have developmental delay, epilepsy, blindness, and cognitive disabilities.
- *SEM (skin, eye, mouth) disease*: Infants with isolated SEM disease usually recover well. However, it should be noted that SEM disease also requires parenteral antiviral therapy and testing to rule out CNS/dissemination. Around 98% of infants with SEM disease have normal development at 1 year.

DIAGNOSIS

Maternal Work-up

Routine HSV screening of all pregnant women is not recommended. For women without a known history of genital herpes, maternal HSV screening could reduce neonatal transmission by offering them suppressive antiviral therapy near term. HSV culture has historically been considered as the gold standard for diagnosis of HSV infection, with a sensitivity of 70% and a specificity of nearly 100%. However, the culture report takes a few days and its sensitivity may be variable based on HSV type, stage of disease, and location of the disease. HSV polymerase chain reaction (PCR) has become increasingly popular, as test results are faster (1 day) and it is more sensitive than viral culture. For patients who have a clinical history suggestive of HSV, but no active genital lesions or negative PCR, serologic tests (antibody test) can be performed. Antibody tests can differentiate type 1 and type 2 HSV, and inform regarding past infection. However, antibodies take a few weeks to develop, and repeat testing may be needed during pregnancy to document seroconversion. The Tzanck smear is performed after unroofing and scraping of the base of a lesion. After spraying with a fixative and staining, light microscopy will show the presence of multinucleated giant cells.

Diagnosis of neonatal HSV is challenging and may be delayed due to nonspecific clinical presentation (lethargy, poor feeding, irritability), and absence of skin lesions in many cases of disseminated or CNS disease. If a diagnosis is delayed, there is a high risk of mortality and sequelae despite antiviral therapy. The diagnostic tests for neonatal HSV are described in **Table 2**.

TABLE 1: Clinical features of HSV infections in neonates.

SEM (skin, eye, mouth)	CNS	Disseminated
• Most common, 45% presentation • Skin: Coalescing or clustering vesicular lesions with erythematous base • Eyes: Watery eyes, conjunctival erythema • Mucosa: Localized ulcers • Does not cause mortality, however, can progress to CNS/disseminated • Needs systemic treatment	• 35% of neonatal HSV • Retrograde spread to CNS from nasopharynx/olfactory nerves or through hematogenous spread • Presents in second or third week of life • Clinical features: Poor activity, irritability, abnormal tone, poor feeding, seizures, full anterior fontanelle	• 20–25% of neonatal HSV • Multiorgan involvement with sepsis-like picture • Lungs: Pneumonitis • Liver: Hepatitis (raised enzymes, coagulopathy) • CNS: Meningoencephalitis • Heart: Myocarditis • Adrenals, bone marrow, coagulation system, kidneys, GIT can also be involved

(CNS: central nervous system; GIT: gastrointestinal tract; HSV: herpes simplex virus)

TABLE 2: Diagnosis of neonatal HSV.

Antigen detection	Antibody detection	Supportive tests
• Viral culture: Swabs from conjunctive, nasopharynx, rectum, skin lesions. Can be falsely positive on the first day due to contamination due to intrapartum exposure • PCR: Can be performed in blood, CSF, or skin lesions. Plasma PCR is positive in 78% of neonates with SEM, 65% in CNS, and 100% in disseminated HSV. CSF PCR has the highest sensitivity in CNS disease • Tzank smear—used in the acute setting to differentiate from other skin conditions. Best if a sample is taken from a fresh blister. Multinucleated giant cells will be seen in HSV. Does not differentiate type 1 from type 2	• IgG: Tests to detect IgG cannot differentiate maternally transferred IgG from infant IgG, so it does not inform regarding new infection • IgM: Infants with severe illness may not produce an antibody response. Commercial assays for HSV IgM have limited reliability • Direct immunofluorescent antibody skin test—skin scraping from ulcer base or vesicle can be stained with a direct fluorescent antibody. It is a rapid test and can distinguish HSV-1 from HSV-2. However, PCR is more sensitive	• Sepsis workup, including CBC, CRP, and blood culture to rule out bacterial infection • CSF will show pleocytosis, with lower sugar and higher protein • Liver function—raised transaminases to fulminant liver failure • Eye examination—keratoconjunctivitis to chorioretinitis • MRI—parenchymal brain edema, hemorrhage, or destructive lesions in temporal lobe or brainstem • EEG—focal/multifocal discharges epileptiform discharges from frontotemporal lobes

(CBC: complete blood count; CNS: central nervous system; CRP: C-reactive protein; CSF: cerebrospinal fluid; EEG: electroencephalogram; HSV: herpes simplex virus; IgG: immunoglobulin G; MRI: magnetic resonance imaging; PCR: polymerase chain reaction; SEM: skin, eye, mouth)

TABLE 3: Maternal herpes simplex virus infection treatment.

Indication	Acyclovir
Primary or first-episode infection	400 mg orally thrice daily for 7–10 days. May extend treatment if healing is incomplete after 10 days
Symptomatic recurrent disease	400 mg orally, thrice daily for 5–7 days
Daily suppression	400 mg orally, thrice daily from 36 weeks estimated gestational age up to delivery
Severe or disseminated disease	5–10 mg/kg intravenously, thrice daily for 5–7 days, followed by oral therapy

MANAGEMENT

Maternal Treatment

Pregnant women with an HSV outbreak should be started on acyclovir to reduce the duration and the severity of the symptoms as well as decrease viral shedding as described in **Table 3**.

Neonatal Treatment

Management pathways vary as per maternal status (primary or recurrent), neonatal symptoms (asymptomatic or symptomatic), and results of testing (PCR positive or negative). The mainstay of therapy is an antiviral medication. The algorithms for approach to neonate born to mother with primary or recurrent herpes are summarized in **Flowcharts 1 and 2**.

Intravenous acyclovir is the first-choice drug for treating neonatal HSV. It is given as 20 mg/kg/dose administered every 8 hours. Renal function should be monitored and adequate hydration must be maintained. Duration of therapy is 2 weeks for SEM disease and 3 weeks for CNS or disseminated disease. Potential adverse effects are neutropenia (reversible), renal impairment, toxicity (seizures), and drug extravasation. Periodic monitoring for renal functions, urine output, and complete blood count is recommended.

For infants with ocular disease, topical agents (e.g., 1% trifluridine, 0.15% ganciclovir) may be used along with parenteral acyclovir. Detailed ophthalmic examination by an ophthalmologist is a must in cases of eye involvement. Ganciclovir may be used as a second-line agent if acyclovir is unavailable. Trials have shown that suppressive therapy with oral acyclovir (300 mg/m^2/dose three times a day) is given for 6 months following completion of IV acyclovir treatment reduces cutaneous recurrences and is associated with improved neurologic outcomes in infants with CNS disease.

Supportive Management

- Maintain fluid/electrolyte balance, adequate hydration, sugar monitoring
- Respiratory support as needed to maintain oxygenation/ventilation
- In the case of CNS disease, antiseizure medications
- If there is coagulopathy, platelet or fresh frozen plasma transfusions based on laboratory reports
- Broad-spectrum antibiotics for secondary bacterial infections

PREVENTION

- Take a detailed history of the woman and her sexual partner regarding HSV during the first prenatal visit. Pregnant women with no previous history should be counseled regarding prevention strategies and safe sexual practices.

Flowchart 1: Approach to neonate born to mother with first episode genital herpes in pregnancy. Treatment for SEM disease is 2 weeks and for disseminated/CNS disease is 3 weeks.

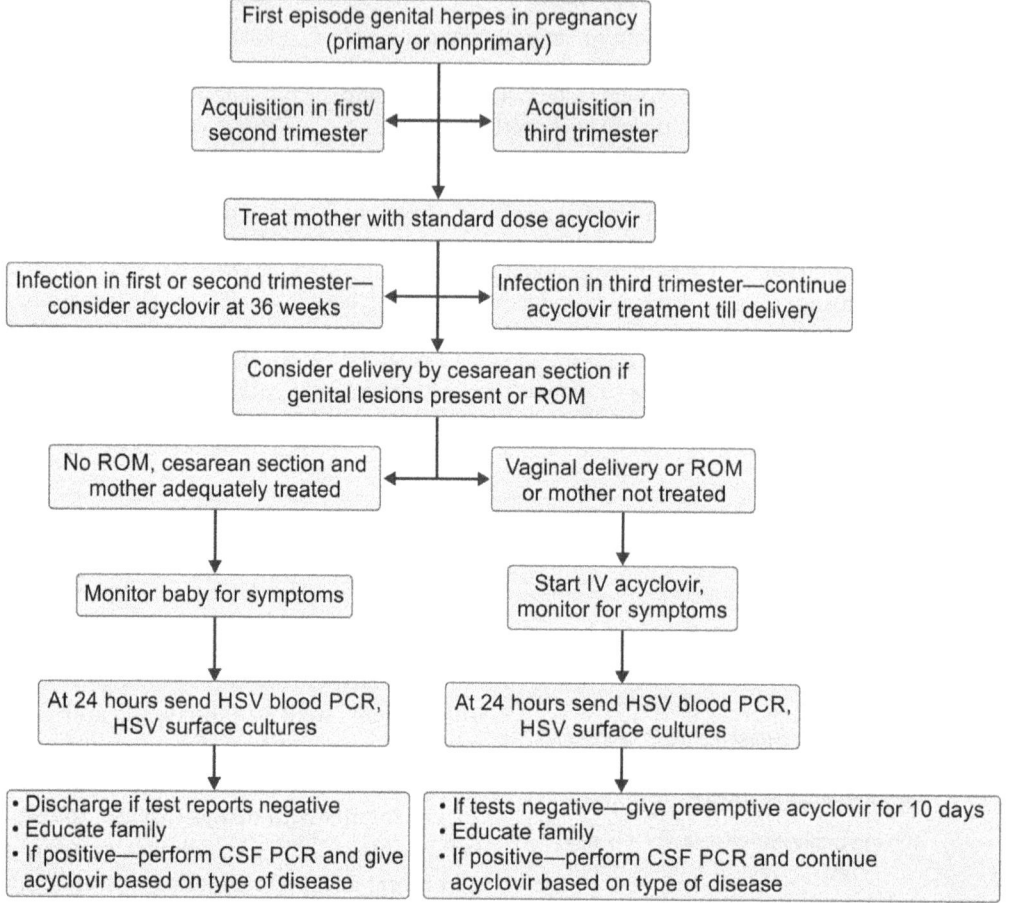

(CNS: central nervous system; CSF: cerebrospinal fluid; HSV: herpes simplex virus; IV: intravenous; PCR: polymerase chain reaction; ROM: rupture of membranes; SEM: skin, eye, mouth)

Flowchart 2: Approach to neonate born to mother with recurrent herpes in pregnancy.

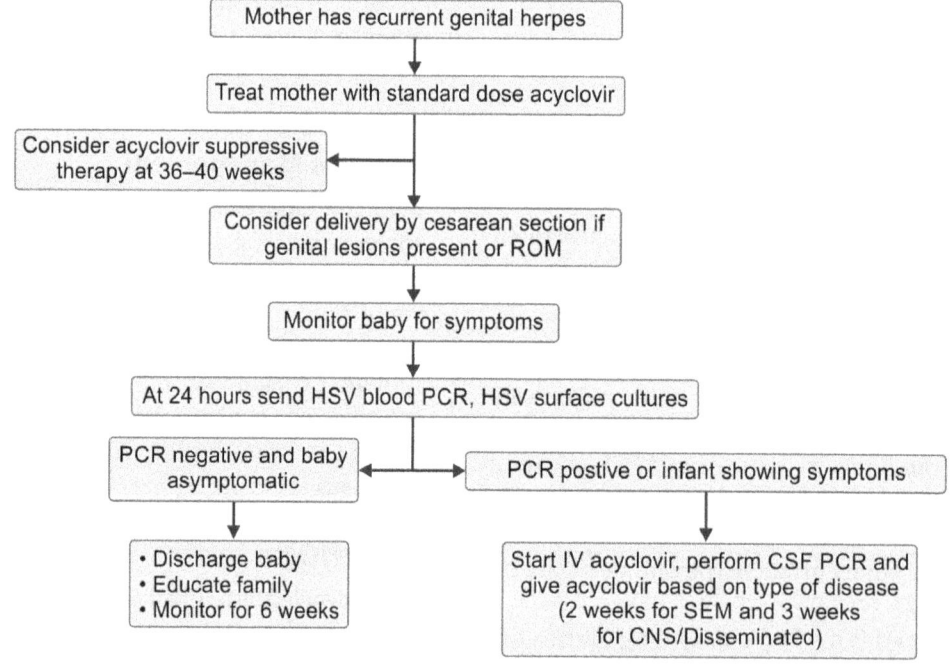

(CNS: central nervous system; CSF: cerebrospinal fluid; HSV: herpes simplex virus; IV: intravenous; PCR: polymerase chain reaction; ROM: rupture of membranes; SEM: skin, eye, mouth)

- If there is active genital herpes infection near delivery, acyclovir therapy must be given and delivery should be performed by cesarean section.
- Prophylactic acyclovir suppression should be considered in the third trimester for women with frequent genital HSV outbreaks.
- Avoid invasive fetal monitoring (scalp electrode) and instrumentation use during delivery.
- Neonates with confirmed or suspected HSV should be managed in neonatal intensive care unit (NICU) using contact precautions.
- Mothers with herpes should practice contact precautions, wear a mask, and cover lesions while caring for their neonates.
- Breastfeeding is considered safe unless there are herpetic lesions on the breast.
- Staff with skin lesions due to HSV must practice meticulous hand hygiene, wear a surgical mask, and cover their lesions. Direct care of neonates and immunocompromised patients may be avoided.

CHAPTER AT A GLANCE

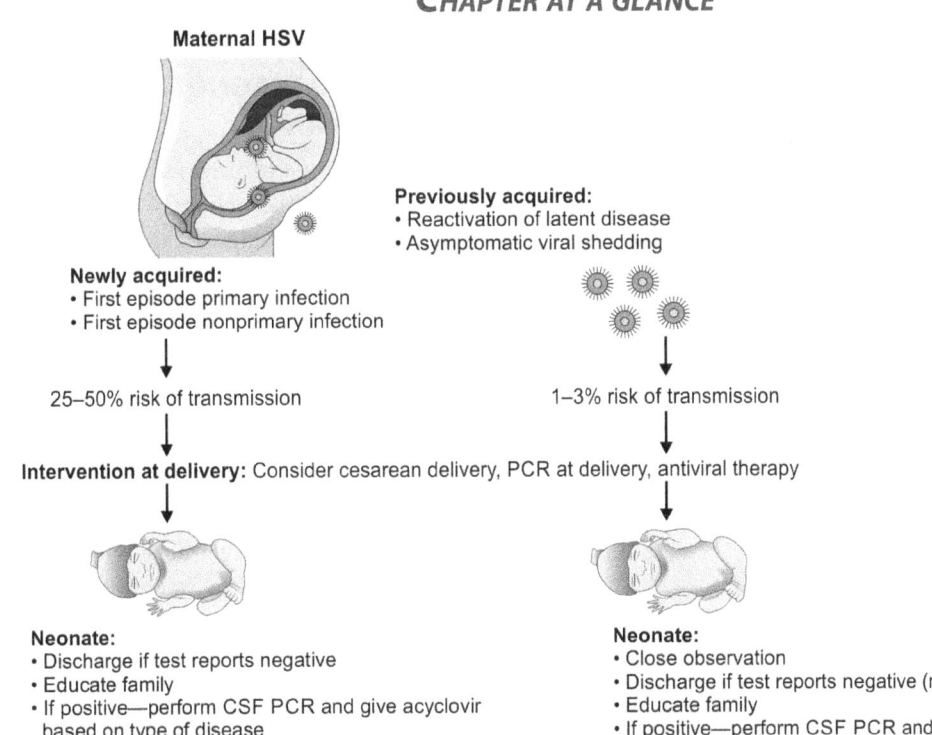

(CSF: cerebrospinal fluid; PCR: polymerase chain reaction; HSV: herpes simplex virus ROM: rupture of membranes

KEY POINTS

- Herpes simplex virus has a high seroprevalence in pregnant women.
- Most mothers of neonates with confirmed HSV infection do not have a history of symptomatic herpes disease during pregnancy.
- Diagnosis can be made by strong clinical suspicion, confirmatory tests are DNA PCR from blood, CSF, and skin lesions or viral culture.
- Early diagnosis and treatment are crucial to prevent mortality and adverse long-term outcomes in neonates.
- Preventive measures include treating active lesions in the mother, delivery by cesarean section, and adequate contact precautions.

SUGGESTED READING

1. Allen UD, Robinson JL; Canadian Paediatric Society, Infectious Diseases and Immunization Committee. Prevention and management of neonatal herpes simplex virus infections. Paediatr Child Health. 2014;19(4):201-12.
2. Corey L, Wald A. Maternal and neonatal HSV infections. N Engl J Med. 2009;361(14):1376-85.
3. Foley E, Clarke E, Beckett VA, Harrison S, Pillai A, FitzGerald M, et al. (2014). Management of genital herpes in pregnancy. Royal College of Obstetricians and Gynecologists. Date of review: by 2018. NICE accredited. [online] Available from https://www.rcog.org.uk/globalassets/documents/guidelines/management-genital-herpes.pdf [Last accessed November, 2021].
4. Management of Genital Herpes in Pregnancy. ACOG Practice Bulletin. 2007.

36
Syphilis—Perinatal Perspective

Gopal Agrawal, Ritu Sethi

INTRODUCTION

Syphilis is a systemic infection caused by *Treponema pallidum*, which is of particular concern during pregnancy because of the risk of transplacental transmission to the fetus. Syphilis remains an important health concern for pregnant women despite the availability of effective treatment.

OBJECTIVES

- To understand the epidemiology of syphilis
- To know the signs and clinical features of neonatal syphilis
- To understand serological diagnosis
- To know treatment modalities and follow up in antenatal and perinatal infection

EPIDEMIOLOGY AND BURDEN OF SYPHILIS

The World Health Organization (WHO) estimates that more than 2 million pregnant women suffer from syphilis each year. High-risk factors are pregnant women who lack antenatal care, use illicit drugs, are infected with other sexually transmitted diseases (STDs) and being a sex worker. The estimated congenital syphilis rate is nearly 5 per 1,000 live births. Adverse pregnancy outcomes are 12 times more likely in women with syphilis as compared to seronegative women. Adverse outcomes in pregnancy occur in 80% of women with active syphilis, including still birth, perinatal death, and serious neonatal infection.

SCREENING AND DIAGNOSING SYPHILIS DURING PREGNANCY

Clinical manifestations in pregnant women are similar to those of acquired syphilis. A chancre may be overlooked due to its location inside the vagina, on the cervix, or on the labia. Systemic disease presents 4-8 weeks after the appearance of the initial chancre. They may present with constitutional symptoms such as fever, weight loss, anorexia, fatigue, and arthralgias. Because of the protean clinical manifestations, syphilis has been described as one of the "great imitators". Thus, a high index of suspicion is needed for the clinician to consider syphilis in a pregnant female. Clinical features may vary as per clinical staging **(Table 1)**.

Universal antepartum screening is widely recommended because screening followed by treatment with appropriate antibiotics usually prevents adverse maternal, fetal, and neonatal outcomes. Serologic testing to diagnose syphilis should include the use of both treponemal and nontreponemal tests **(Box 1)**. Biologic false positive and false negative tests are common with these serologic tests. False positive nontreponemal tests could be due to transient biologic reaction due to pregnancy, acute febrile illness or recent immunization whereas false negative result could be due to prozone phenomenon. False positive treponemal tests could be due to biologic reaction due to pregnancy, advanced age, tumor, dialysis, or autoimmune conditions. All cases of suspected false positive results should undergo repeat testing at least 4-6 weeks after delivery.

TABLE 1: Clinical stages of syphilis.

Stage	Timeline	Clinical features
Primary	2–4 weeks	Chancre (painless ulcer) at the site of inoculation
Secondary	4 weeks to 6 months	Fever, disseminated rash, generalized lymphadenopathy, weight loss, mucositis, condyloma lata, hepatitis, arthritis
Latent	6 months to 5 years	Usually, asymptomatic
Tertiary	5–20 years	*Skin:* Granulomatous lesions of the skin, bones *CVS:* Aortic aneurysm *CNS:* Seizures, psychiatric features, tabes dorsalis, dementia

A diagnosis of syphilis is made when both treponemal and nontreponemal tests are reactive. In 2011, CDC affirmed that nontreponemal test should be used for "screening" and treponemal test should be used for "confirmation" of syphilis (traditional approach). Recently, "reverse sequence" screening has been tested (treponemal test for screening and nontreponemal test for confirmation). In view of high-discordant results, CDC recommends traditional approach for diagnosis of syphilis during pregnancy.

TREATMENT OF SYPHILIS DURING PREGNANCY AND OUTCOMES

Penicillin is the gold standard for the treatment of syphilis in both pregnant and nonpregnant individuals **(Table 2)**. For non-penicillin treatment of late syphilis, WHO recommends treatment with erythromycin 500 mg orally four times daily for 30 days. Erythromycin and azithromycin do not cross the placental barrier completely, so the fetus is not effectively treated. Therefore, WHO also recommends that infants born to women who were treated during pregnancy with nonpenicillin regimens receive a 10-15 days course of penicillin treatment. Women treated for early syphilis should have a titer checked at the time of treatment to establish a baseline against which to monitor response to treatment. A fourfold decline in the titer (e.g., from 1:16 to 1:4 or from 1:32 to 1:8) is considered to be an acceptable response to syphilis therapy.

Treatment of syphilis may precipitate the Jarisch-Herxheimer reaction, an acute febrile reaction accompanied by headache, myalgia, rash, and hypotension. The Jarisch-Herxheimer reaction may also precipitate uterine contractions, preterm labor, and/or nonreassuring fetal heart rate tracings in pregnant women treated in the second half of pregnancy.

Penicillin therapy in pregnancy is effective for treating maternal disease, preventing transmission to the fetus, and treating established fetal disease. Congenital infection has been diagnosed in 1-2% of offspring of women adequately treated during pregnancy. The WHO estimates that treatment reduces early fetal deaths or stillbirths by 82%, preterm or low-birth weight by 65%, neonatal deaths by 80%, and clinical disease in infants by 98%.

Impact on the Offspring (Fig. 1)

Treponema pallidum readily infects the placenta. Transplacental transmission to the fetus can start from 8 to 10 weeks' of gestation and can occur at any stage of maternal disease. The frequency of vertical transmission increases with increasing gestational age at acquisition of maternal infection and the duration of maternal syphilis. If untreated, the risk of congenital infection is 50% for primary and secondary syphilis, 40% for early latent syphilis, and 10% for late syphilis. After the placenta is infected, transplacental passage of spirochetes to the fetal circulation leads to fetal hepatic infection and dysfunction, followed by amniotic fluid infection, fetal hematologic abnormalities (anemia, thrombocytopenia), ascites, hydrops, and fetal immunoglobulin M (IgM) production. Findings on ultrasound are nonspecific and include: Hepatomegaly, placentomegaly, anemia, polyhydramnios, ascites or hydrops. So, at least one ultrasound examination after 20 weeks of gestation should be performed to look for signs of congenital infection. Findings on ultrasound are nonspecific and include:

BOX 1: Nontreponemal and treponemal tests during pregnancy.

Nontreponemal test:
- Rapid plasma reagin and venereal disease research laboratory (VDRL)
- A sustained fourfold decrease in titer of the nontreponemal test with treatment demonstrates adequate therapy

Treponemal tests:
- Fuorescent treponemal antibody absorption, microhemagglutination test for antibodies to *T. pallidum* (MHA-TP), *T. pallidum* particle agglutination assay and *T. pallidum* enzyme immunoassay
- The treponemal tests correlate poorly with disease activity and usually remain positive for life, even after successful therapy, and therefore should not be used to assess treatment response

TABLE 2: Stages of maternal syphilis and appropriate treatment.

Stage of syphilis	Treatment
Primary/Secondary/Early latent	Benzathine penicillin—2.4 million units IM single dose
Late latent/Tertiary	Benzathine penicillin—2.4 million units IM weekly for 3 weeks
Neurosyphilis	Aqueous penicillin G—3-4 million units IV every 4 hourly for 10-14 days OR Procaine penicillin G—2.4 million units IM once daily for 10-14 days

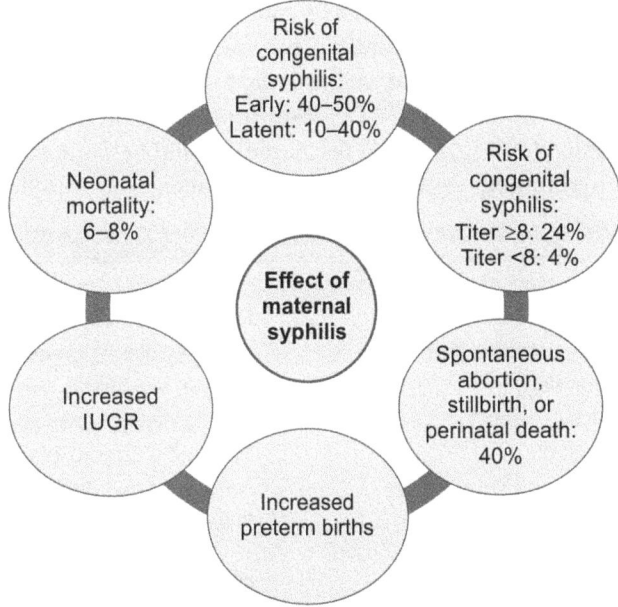

Fig. 1: Impact of maternal syphilis on the fetus and neonate. (IUGR: intrauterine growth restriction)

- Hepatomegaly, defined as liver length >95th percentile for gestational age
- Placentomegaly, defined as placental thickness >2 standard deviations above mean for gestational age
- Anemia, based on Doppler middle cerebral artery peak systolic velocity >1.5 multiples of the median
- Polyhydramnios
- Ascites or hydrops

Congenital syphilis in affected infants can be early congenital syphilis or late congenital syphilis. Early congenital syphilis signs manifest in the first 2 years of birth and are due to active infection and inflammation while late congenital syphilis signs appear in the first two decades of life and are due to malformations or stigmata induced by initial lesions of early congenital infection or the result of chronic inflammation **(Table 3)**.

DELIVERY

Late preterm delivery for neonatal treatment is warranted when there is a high risk of fetal treatment failure (e.g., progressive worsening signs of congenital syphilis on ultrasound examination, hydrops). At delivery, pediatric providers should be notified about maternal syphilis stage and treatment, and fetal ultrasound findings.

POSTNATAL DIAGNOSIS AND MANAGEMENT OF NEONATES

The diagnosis of congenital syphilis should be suspected in all infants whose mothers have reactive nontreponemal and treponemal tests for syphilis. The nontreponemal test [Venereal disease research laboratory (VDRL) or rapid plasma reagin (RPR)] that is performed on the infant should be the same as that which was done on the mother, so that the infant's titers can be compared with the mother's titers. Physical examination for evidence of congenital syphilis, and darkfield microscopic examination or direct fluorescent antibody (DFA) staining of suspicious lesions or body fluids (e.g., nasal discharge) should be done along with pathologic examination of the placenta or umbilical cord with specific fluorescent antitreponemal antibody staining (if available).

Isolation with standard precautions should be followed for infants with suspected or proven congenital syphilis. Gloves should be worn when caring for patients with congenital, primary, and secondary syphilis with skin and mucous membranes lesions until 24 hours of treatment has been completed because moist open lesions, secretions, and possible blood are contagious in all patients with syphilis.

CDC guidelines and American Academy of Pediatrics (AAP) have proposed the following four scenarios in managing neonates with history of maternal syphilis enumerated in **Figure 2**.

Infant VDRL or RPR nonreactive: The neonate who has a normal physical examination and nonreactive VDRL or RPR does not require additional evaluation.

In case of nonavailability of penicillin, inj. Ceftriaxone can be considered, although there is insufficient evidence to support this recommendation. Ceftriaxone should be used with caution in neonates with significant jaundice.

Long-term Follow-up

Infants who have reactive serologic tests for syphilis or were born to mothers who were seroreactive at delivery should undergo evaluation for manifestations of congenital syphilis during regularly scheduled well-child care visits during the first year and beyond (for manifestations of late congenital syphilis). Nontreponemal tests (VDRL or RPR) should be repeated every 3 months until the test becomes negative or the titers decline four-fold. If adequately treated or the infant is noninfected, the titers decline by 3 months of age and turns negative by 6 months of age. If the titers fail to decline or increases by 6–12 months of age, this indicates treatment failure. Such infants should undergo further detailed evaluation and be treated with parenteral penicillin for 10 days (irrespective of previous treatment status). Treponemal tests should not be used to evaluate treatment response. Evaluation for hearing loss, ophthalmologic abnormalities, and neurodevelopmental problems should occur yearly.

TABLE 3: Clinical features of congenital syphilis.

Early congenital syphilis (<2 years)	
Systemic signs	Fever, generalized lymphadenopathy, failure to thrive, organomegaly, pneumonia
Muco-cutaneous features	Snuffles (rhinitis), generalized maculopapular rash (including palms and soles), condylomata lata
Hematology	Anemia, leukopenia, thrombocytopenia, jaundice
Musculo-skeletal	Pseudo-paralysis, periostitis
Neurologic	Meningitis, cerebrospinal fluid abnormalities
Radiological signs	Periostitis (Irregular periosteal thickening), Wimberger sign (osteolytic lesions in the tibia, upper end), Wegner sign (irregular metaphyses)
Late congenital syphilis (>2 years)	
Facial, ophthalmologic	Frontal bossing, saddle nose, interstitial keratitis
Oral	Hutchison teeth, mulberry molars
Musculo skeletal	Saber shins, clutton joints, general paresis

Scenario I	Scenario II	Scenario III	Scenario IV
Proven or highly probable	**Possible**	**Less likely**	**Unlikely**
An abnormal physical examination OR VDRL or RPR titer ≥ fourfold the maternal titer OR A positive darkfield test of body fluid, placenta or umbilical cord	Normal physical examination AND VDRL or RPR < fourfold the maternal titer AND Mother was not treated, was inadequately treated or had evidence of relapse	Normal physical examination AND VDRL or RPR < fourfold the maternal titer AND Mother was treated adequately DURING pregnancy, was treated > 4 weeks before delivery and had no evidence of relapse	Normal physical examination AND VDRL or RPR < fourfold the maternal titer AND Mother was treated adequately BEFORE pregnancy and had no evidence of relapse
Evaluation*	Evaluation*	No evaluation	No evaluation
Aqueous penicillin G 50,000 units/kg/dose IV 12 hourly (for ≤7 days of age) and 8 hourly (for >7 days of age) for a total of 10 days	Procaine penicillin G 50,000 units/kg IM once daily for 10 days	Benzathine penicillin G 50,000 units/kg IM single dose	No treatment

* Evaluation:
- Complete blood count (CBC) with differential and platelet count
- CSF examination for cell count, protein, and VDRL
- Additional tests as clinically indicated: Long-bone radiographs, chest radiograph, liver function tests, cranial ultrasound, ophthalmologic examination, and auditory brainstem response

Fig. 2: Approach to the management of a neonate born to mother with history of syphilis.
(CSF: cerebrospinal fluid; RPR: rapid plasma reagin; VDRL: venereal disease research laboratory)

CHAPTER AT A GLANCE

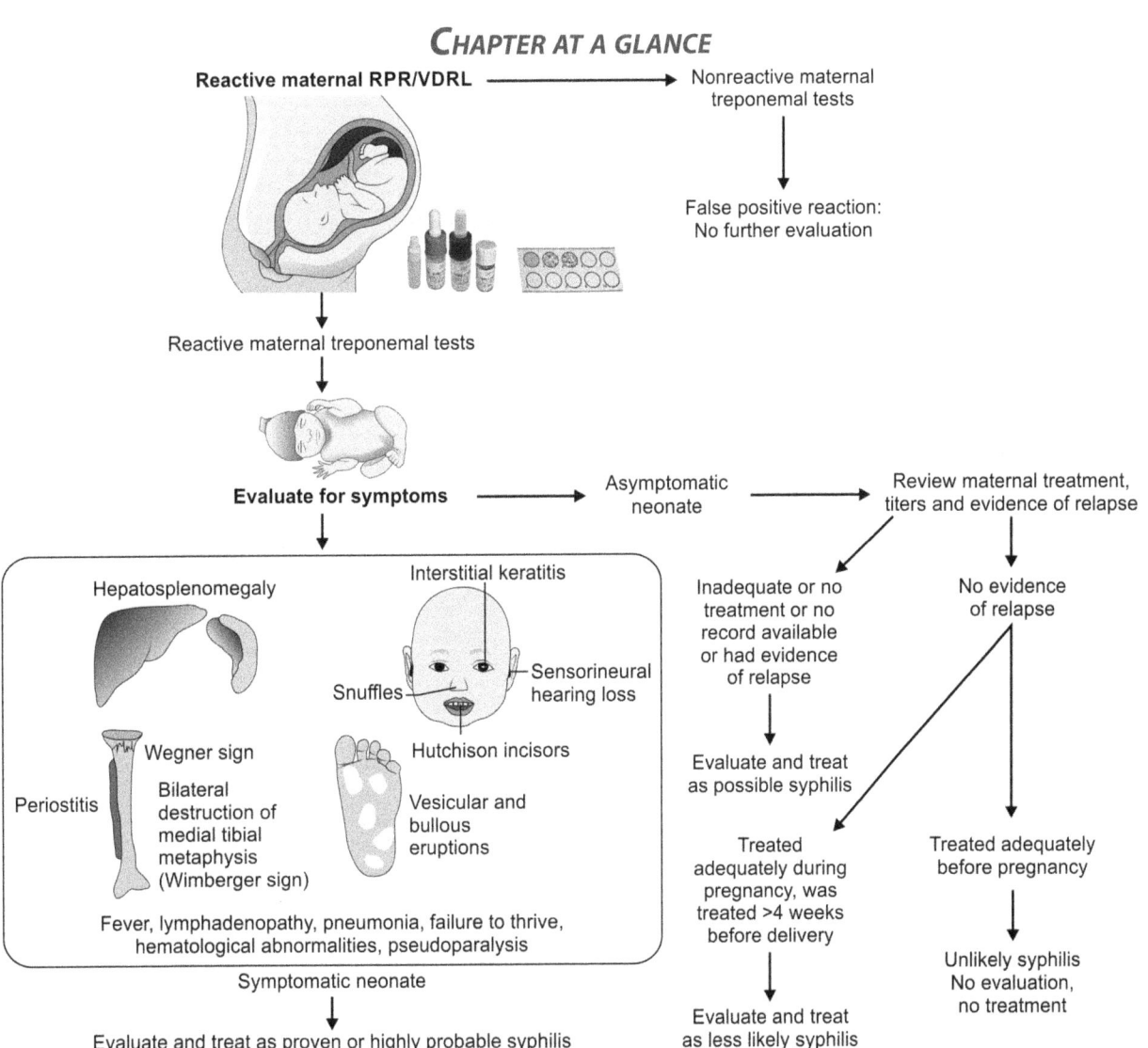

(RPR: rapid plasma reagin; VDRL: venereal disease research laboratory)

KEY POINTS

- Syphilis remains an important health concern for women despite the availability of effective and inexpensive treatment.
- Penicillin therapy is effective for treating maternal disease, preventing transmission to the fetus, and treating established fetal disease.
- The diagnosis of congenital syphilis should be suspected in all infants born to women who have reactive nontreponemal and treponemal tests for syphilis and infants/children with clinical findings compatible with congenital syphilis.
- For infants with proven or highly probable congenital syphilis, treatment with 10 days of parenteral penicillin is recommended.
- Infants born to women with syphilis or a history of syphilis remain at risk for syphilis even if the infant has a normal physical examination and VDRL or RPR, i.e., nonreactive or less than fourfold the maternal titer.

SUGGESTED READING

1. American Academy of Paediatrics. Syphilis. In: Kimberlin DW, Brady MT, Jackson MA, Long SS (Eds). Red Book: 2018 Report of the Committee on Infectious Diseases, 31st edition. Itasca, IL: American Academy of Paediatrics; 2018. p. 773.
2. Blencowe H, Cousens S, Kamb M, Berman S, Lawn JE. Lives saved tool supplement detection and treatment of syphilis in pregnancy to reduce syphilis related stillbirths and neonatal mortality. BMC Public Health. 2011;11(Suppl 3):S9.
3. Kilpatrick SJ, Papile L (Eds); American Academy of Paediatrics Committee on Foetus and Newborn and American College of Obstetricians and Gynaecologists Committee on Obstetric Practice. Guidelines for Perinatal Care, 8th edition. Itasca, IL: American Academy of Pediatrics and American College of Obstetricians and Gynecologists; 2017.
4. Korenromp EL, Rowley J, Alonso M, Mello MB, Wijesooriya NS, Mahiané SG, et al. Global burden of maternal and congenital syphilis and associated adverse birth outcomes-Estimates for 2016 and progress since 2012. PLoS One. 2019;14:e0211720.
5. Wendel GD Jr, Sheffield JS, Hollier LM, Hill JB, Ramsey PS, Sánchez PJ. Treatment of syphilis in pregnancy and prevention of congenital syphilis. Clin Infect Dis. 2002;35:S200.
6. Workowski KA, Bolan GA, Centers for Disease Control and Prevention. Sexually transmitted diseases treatment guidelines, 2015. MMWR Recomm Rep. 2015;64:1.

CHAPTER 37

Other Viral Infections such as Zika Virus, Dengue Virus, Chikungunya Virus, Varicella Virus, H1N1 Influenza Virus

Amanpreet Sethi, Seema Grover Bhatti

INTRODUCTION

This topic will review the epidemiology of relatively common neonatal viral infections, which pose challenges in clinical management. Epidemiology and clinical manifestations have been discussed briefly. Additional details on specific viral pathogens are presented in separate chapters.

Objectives

To provide the practicing clinician with an overview of the perinatal aspect of varicella zoster virus (VZV), dengue (DENV), chikungunya (CHKV), HIN1, and zika virus (ZIKV) infection, as well as to discuss the investigation plan and management of these infections in neonates.

VARICELLA-ZOSTER VIRUS

Varicella (chickenpox) is a highly communicable disease caused by infection with VZV. It is a DNA herpes virus also known as human herpes virus 3. After infection, the latent virus continues in the dorsal spinal root ganglia and may lead to dermatomal-specific herpes zoster later in the life.

Epidemiology and Transmission

The only known reservoirs of VZV are humans. After infection the immunity is usually life-long with a very rare recurrence of chickenpox in immunocompetent and seropositive individuals. Most of the times the reinfection is mild but in pregnant women due to decreased T-cell immunity infections can be severe along with more incidence of recurrence.

The reported incidence of primary varicella infection in pregnancy is 2-3/1,000 pregnancies/year in countries where universal immunization is followed. There is no universal immunization against varicella in India, so it is assumed that the rate will be much higher in India. In a recent study from Karnataka in 430 pregnant women, it was found that around 23% of all pregnant women were seronegative for varicella antibodies. Pregnant women in the age group of 21-25 years had the highest susceptibility of 47% to varicella during pregnancy. So, this data again reiterates the importance of inclusion of varicella vaccine in national immunization schedule.

The most common modes of transmission of virus are airborne droplet spread and direct contact with the vesicular lesions. The incubation period is usually 10-21 days but it can be delayed for 28 days, if a person has received varicella zoster-specific immunoglobulins. The maximum infectivity is 1-2 days before the onset of rash. The index case remains infective till all the vesicular lesions are crusted and dried (usually 6 days after the onset of rash). A pregnant mother developing vesicular rash any time between 2 days before the delivery and 5 days after delivery has the highest chance of infecting the new born. The virus after entry into the nasopharynx invades the local lymph nodes. After some time, there is a transient viremia, which seeds the visceral organs and skin. Subsequently viremia episodes lead to formation of crops of vesicles leading to the activation of T-cell immunity, which is responsible for further limiting the infection. The virus then develops a latent infection in the dorsal root ganglia.

Varicella in Pregnancy

Varicella in pregnancy presents with a short episode of fever, malaise, and headache followed by generalized rash starting from the face and trunk and proceeding centripetally. There are recurrent crops of vesicles for 2-6 days. After that the vesicles begin to crust and scab leading to healing without scarring. The secondary opportunistic bacterial infection of the vesicles can lead to various complications of sepsis, meningitis, and pneumonia. Pneumonia caused by varicella is the most common cause of mortality in these patients.

Varicella zoster is because of reactivation of the latent infection in the dorsal root ganglia characterized by bunch of vesicles in 2-3 sensory dermatomes. These vesicles are extremely painful and pruritic and may lead to postherpetic neuralgia for months. In the pregnancy, the maximum risk of severe infection is in the second and third trimester. The studies have not reported increased risk of abortions, intrauterine growth retardation (IUGR), and prematurity with varicella in pregnancy unless the fetus develops congenital varicella syndrome (CVS). Oral acyclovir therapy is recommended for the treatment in second and third trimester. Any susceptible pregnant women exposed to varicella should be given varicella-zoster immune globulin (VZIG) as soon as possible or within 4 days of exposure to decrease the risk of mortality. It has been noted in some case reports that administering VZIG to pregnant women may not prevent fetal varicella infection. So, the fetus should be monitored for varicella related complications throughout the pregnancy.

Congenital Varicella Syndrome

Congenital varicella syndrome is the most dreaded complication of maternal varicella infection. It results from the hematogenous spread across the placenta. The lowest risk of CVS is in the first trimester of pregnancy that is around 0.55%. The risk of CVS almost triples between 12 and 20 weeks of pregnancy that is around 1.4% and almost nonexistent thereafter. Only few case reports of CVS are there after 20 weeks of gestation. The complication rate is also less after a late maternal infection.

The typical clinical presentation of CVS consists of intrauterine growth restriction, cicatricial skin lesions (which may be depressed and pigmented in a dermatomal distribution), limb abnormalities (which often include hypoplasia of bone and muscle), ocular defects (such as cataracts, chorioretinitis, Horner syndrome, microphthalmos, and nystagmus), central nervous system abnormalities (such as cortical atrophy, seizures, and intellectual disability).

The real problem arises while counseling pregnant women with varicella. As the incidence of CVS is very low so routine recommendation of abortion following maternal infection is not followed. The risk of fetal infection is 25% after maternal infection but it does not tell us about the risk of CVS. Level one and level two ultrasound usually helps us to ascertain fetal affection but sometimes abnormalities are detected, so late that medical abortion is not recommended. Presence of limb abnormalities carries a 50% risk of brain involvement and early mortality. Other abnormalities like hydrocephalus, hydrops, liver calcifications and polyhydramnios can also be detected on fetal ultrasound.

Perinatal and Postnatal Chickenpox

Maternal varicella in the high-risk period as mentioned above can result in severe varicella pneumonia leading to high neonatal mortality. Newborns born to mothers who are exposed to VZV or have clinical chickenpox within 2 weeks of delivery are at the greatest risk for infection. Nosocomial acquisition of VZV also can occur. The case fatality rate is high if the mother develops varicella symptoms from 5 days before to 2 days after delivery as no protective antibodies are transferred from mother to fetus during this time. During this time, the infection attack rate is around 24–50% with 20–30% neonatal mortality. Premature infants are at increased risk for nosocomial acquisition of VZV due to lack of maternal protective antibodies which occurs primarily during third trimester of pregnancy. Neonatal chickenpox presenting within 10 days of birth is also known as congenital varicella. The incubation period in the neonates is also shorter that is between 9 and 15 days from the onset of maternal rash. Clinical features vary from mild illness to a disseminated infection. Fever may develop within the first day after birth, followed by a generalized vesicular eruption (**Fig. 1**). Generalized rash with the lesions appearing in different stages of development is the characteristic of varicella rash. It starts as macules and rapidly progresses to papules and then to characteristic vesicular lesions before crusting. It usually appears first on the head and then generalizes. In mild cases, the lesions heal within 7–10 days. However, disseminated disease may present, with varicella pneumonia, hepatitis, and meningoencephalitis. Reports of neonatal herpes zoster in neonates born to mothers with varicella during pregnancy are rare.

Diagnosis

The diagnosis can be made clinically based upon the characteristic varicella rash, i.e., appearance of generalized vesicular skin lesions in various stages of development and healing in a neonate born to a mother exposed to VZV or with clinical symptoms close to the time of delivery.

In uncertain cases the diagnosis can be made by isolating virus by polymerase chain reaction (PCR). PCR can detect VZV from vesicular swabs or scrapings, scabs from crusted lesions, tissue from biopsy samples, and/or cerebral spinal fluid. Direct fluorescent antibody (DFA), viral culture, and serological testing (IgM/IgG) are not used in lieu of PCR

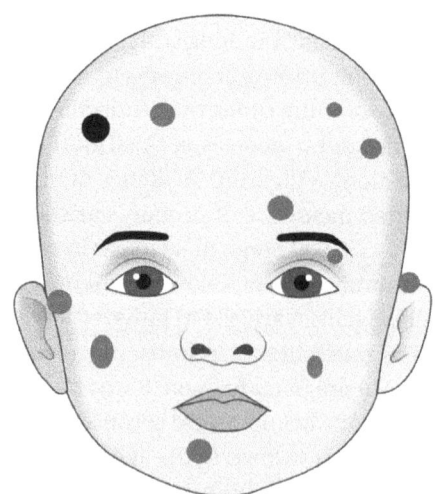

Fig. 1: Congenital varicella.

testing. DNA PCR of the scrapings from the scab or vesicular fluid is the preferred investigation of choice. Viral culture and serologic tests are not much reliable.

Prenatal diagnosis of fetal varicella can be made by doing PCR testing of fetal blood or amniotic fluid for VZV DNA in conjunction with ultrasonography for detection of fetal abnormalities.

Varicella Prevention

Active Immunization

With availability of a live vaccine, the strategy should be to prevent this deadly disease in mothers. The published literature has shown that vaccine is around 85% effective in preventing the infection. The general guidelines are to vaccinate the susceptible population in the child age group. But in India, varicella vaccine is not in the National Immunization schedule. So, adolescent girls and women in child age group are at high risk of acquiring varicella. If at an individual level, one decides to vaccinate this age group then care should be taken to avoid pregnancy for at least 1 month after vaccination. Though, there has been no case report of CVS even if pregnant women are inadvertently given the vaccine but a theoretical risk of giving a live vaccine is always there. The vaccine can be administered to expose lactating women as vaccine virus strain has not been detected in the mother's breast milk.

Isolation

Isolation for the mother and infant depends upon whether there is active disease or the timing of exposure. A mother with active varicella lesions must be isolated. The infant is isolated from the mother until she is not infectious. A seronegative mother exposed to VZV 6–21 days before hospital admission should be isolated from other patients and the nursery because she may develop varicella while hospitalized.

Postexposure Prophylaxis

The American Academy of Pediatrics (AAP), Centers for Disease Control and Prevention (CDC), and the Advisory Committee on Immunization Practices (ACIP), recommend administration of VZIG to newborns who have had a significant exposure to VZV plus one or more of the following:

- *Maternal symptoms:* Neonates whose mothers have signs and symptoms of varicella around the time of delivery (within 5 days before or 2 days after).
- *Preterm infants ≥ 28 weeks of gestation:* Hospitalized preterm infants born at ≥28 weeks of gestation who have had a significant exposure to VZV and whose mothers do not have documented immunization, serologic immunity, or prior documented history of varicella infection.
- *Preterm infants <28 weeks of gestation:* Hospitalized premature infants born at <28 weeks of gestation or who weigh <1,000 g at birth who have had a significant exposure to VZV regardless of maternal history of varicella or vaccination.

After exposure, the VZIG should be administered within 96 hours. The dose of VZIG is 62.5 IU and 125 IU intramuscularly (IM) for neonates ≤ 2 kg and > 2 kg, respectively. If VZIG is not available then intravenous immune globulin (IVIG) or acyclovir prophylaxis can be considered.

Treatment

Acyclovir (A synthetic nucleoside analog) is the drug of choice for neonatal varicella. It acts by inhibiting viral DNA polymerase by competing with deoxyguanosine triphosphate (dGTP) thus resulting in premature chain termination. Newborns with severe disseminated VZV infection (e.g., pneumonia, encephalitis, thrombocytopenia, severe hepatitis) are treated with intravenous acyclovir (30 mg/kg per day in three divided doses) for 10 days.

Antiviral treatment must be started as soon as possible after the onset of symptoms.

Breastfeeding—is encouraged in newborns exposed to or infected with varicella because antibody in breast milk may be protective. The approach to the management of varicella in neonates is shown in **Flowchart 1**.

INFLUENZA VIRUS (H1N1 VIRUS)

H1N1 is a Type A influenza virus which is an RNA virus of orthomyxoviridae family. Type A virus is characterized by the presence of two glycoprotein antigens on the surface that is Hemagglutinin (H) and Neuraminidase (N) antigens. Hemagglutinin antigen is required for binding to the cellular receptor and Neuraminidase antigen releases virus from the cell after replication. The production of antibodies against these antigens is largely responsible for protection against these viruses. Minor changes in these antigens can lead to Antigenic drifts but sometimes there is a complete change in H and N antigen leading to Antigenic shifts responsible for epidemics and pandemics across the world. H1N1 influenza A virus caused 2009 flu pandemic leading to four times increased case fatality rate among children as compared to the earlier flu infections.

Epidemiology and Transmission

Influenza is a highly infectious disease with a high-secondary attack rate. It can spread by droplet infection or by contact with the infected fomites. The large aerosol droplet particles can travel up to six feet only. The patient can spread infection 24 hours prior to the onset of symptoms till the symptoms persist. A virus can survive in the external environment without host for 2–8 hours. So, to prevent the spread of infection social distancing, wearing masks, and using frequent hand washing is necessary. There has been no case report of vertical transmission of H1N1 flu to the neonate as the virus is not able cross the placenta.

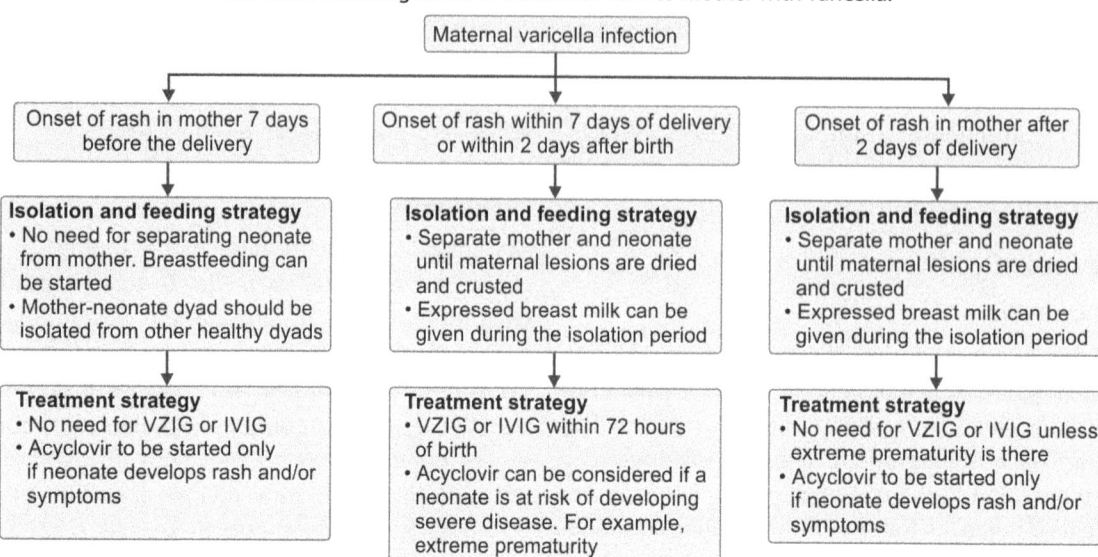

Flowchart 1: Management of a neonate born to mother with varicella.

(VZIG: varicella-zoster immune globulin; IVIG: intravenous immune globulin)

Clinical Features

H1N1 influenza infection is usually characterized by rapid onset high-grade fever with chills along with headache, malaise, severe myalgia, red watering eyes, running nose, sore throat and otitis media. The course of infection is usually 4–5 days. Sometimes it can present as vomiting and diarrhea. Life-threatening complications or red flag signs can also manifest in otherwise healthy kids as myocarditis, pneumonia leading to shock, and hypoxic respiratory failure. Central nervous system complications like encephalitis with seizures can also occur. There can be secondary bacterial infections leading to deterioration and increased mortality in these patients.

In the neonatal population, most of the flu infections are asymptomatic. This can be because of transfer of protective antibodies from the mother. Breast milk is also protective against flu infection. The protection may last up to 6 months of age. The symptoms in the first year of life consist of high-grade fever, prodrome of upper respiratory tract infection, which in due course of time may progress to bronchiolitis like presentation. Some infants may present with features of apnea, feeding difficulty, and irritability.

2009 H1N1 influenza virus had increased rates of hospitalization and death among pregnant women resulting in increased perinatal complications. Obesity, multiparity, asthma, and twin/triplet pregnancy were the most important risk factors for severe disease among pregnant women.

PREVENTION

To prevent severe disease among pregnant women, they should be vaccinated during prenatal visits with the seasonal flu vaccine, which also prevents severe disease among infants less than 6 months of age. The caregivers and the hospital staff caring for young infants should also be vaccinated. As per 2020 Indian Academy of Pediatrics (IAP) guidelines on immunization, inactivated influenza vaccine in a dose of 15 μg (0.5 mL) should be administered after 6 months of age. A total of two doses 4 weeks apart should be covered before the rainy season. IAP also recommended using the most recently available strain for vaccination. After primary vaccine coverage, annual flu vaccination till 5 years of age should be continued. After 5 years of age, vaccination is recommended only in high-risk children with comorbidities. A recent multinational randomized trial in children between 6 months and 35 months of age across multiple influenza seasons has shown that the quadrivalent vaccine in a dose of 0.5 mL demonstrated a protective efficacy of 63% against moderate to severe disease.

Diagnosis and Treatment

As the case fatality rate among susceptible young infants is very high so in case of suspected H1N1 infection, it is highly recommended to start treatment soon after sending nasopharyngeal swabs. Reverse transcriptase-polymerase chain reaction (RT-PCR) of the nasopharyngeal swab is the diagnostic test of choice with very good sensitivity and specificity.

The drug of choice for H1N1 infection is Oseltamivir, which is a neuraminidase inhibitor thus it stops the release of virus in the respiratory tract and other tissues. It has got very good tolerability with most common side effects of vomiting and diarrhea. It is available freely in public health care setting as an oral suspension with a concentration of 12 mg/mL. The Pediatric dosage guidelines as per age of the child by Ministry of Health and Family Welfare Government of India are shown in **Table 1**. Oseltamivir can also be used in preterm infants as benefits of treatment are more as compared to the risks involved in treatment. The dose recommended is lower that is 1 mg/kg/day as compared to 3 mg/kg/day in preterm neonates. Aspirin containing products should be avoided in patients suspected to have H1N1 infection to prevent Reye syndrome. The management approach to H1N1 infection in the Pediatric age group is shown in **Flowchart 2**.

DENGUE VIRUS

Dengue is one of the most dangerous mosquito vector-borne viral diseases with a 30-fold increase in worldwide incidence over a period of 50 years. The causative agent dengue virus (DEN) is an RNA virus belonging to family Flaviviridae. It consists of four different serotypes (DEN 1, DEN 2, DEN 3, and DEN 4). Primary infection with one serotype results in life-long immunity to that infecting serotype only. Moreover, in a Dengue endemic area all four DEN serotypes are circulating simultaneously as immunity to one serotype cannot protect the host from another serotype. Secondary infection with a different serotype can increase the risk of severe disease. The most common reason being cited is that Dengue virus has a unique ability to utilize preexisting heterotypic antibodies to enhance viral replication in the body thus leading to an enhanced immunological response. In India, all four serotypes are commonly isolated.

Transmission

Aedes aegypti (Female) mosquito is the main vector in the urban areas. In some states, female *Aedes albopictus* is also active in the transmission of Dengue virus. Aedes mosquito mostly breeds in the urban areas where water is artificially stored or gets collected after the rain. These mosquitoes usually bite during the day time. After 8–10 days of acquiring the virus (extrinsic incubation period), Aedes mosquito is able to transfer the virus to other healthy hosts. Although the most common cause of transmission is through the bite of infected mosquito, there are case reports of viral transmission through blood transfusion and organ transplantation. There are also case reports of vertical transmission of dengue virus from the mother to fetus, which we will be covering in detail in the subsequent section.

Dengue Viral Infection in Pregnancy

As the infection is endemic in India, so pregnant women are quite susceptible to contract this deadly disease. The most common presentation of dengue in pregnancy is high-grade fever, myalgia, arthralgia, malaise, and rash similar to nonpregnant patients. Severe dengue infection may progress to dengue hemorrhagic fever (DHF) and shock (DSS). Dengue infection in pregnancy can transmit vertically with an estimated rate of 20%. A recent prospective study from a tertiary care center in India involving 44 pregnant women with

TABLE 1: Infant dosage guidelines of Oseltamivir as per Ministry of Health and Family Welfare, India.

Postnatal age	Dose
Treatment	
<3 months	12 mg per orally twice daily for 5 days
3–5 months	20 mg per orally twice daily for 5 days
6–11 months	25 mg per orally twice daily for 5 days
Chemoprophylaxis	
<3 months	Not recommended unless treating doctor strongly considers
3–5 months	20 mg per orally once daily for 10 days
6–11 months	25 mg per orally once daily for 10 days

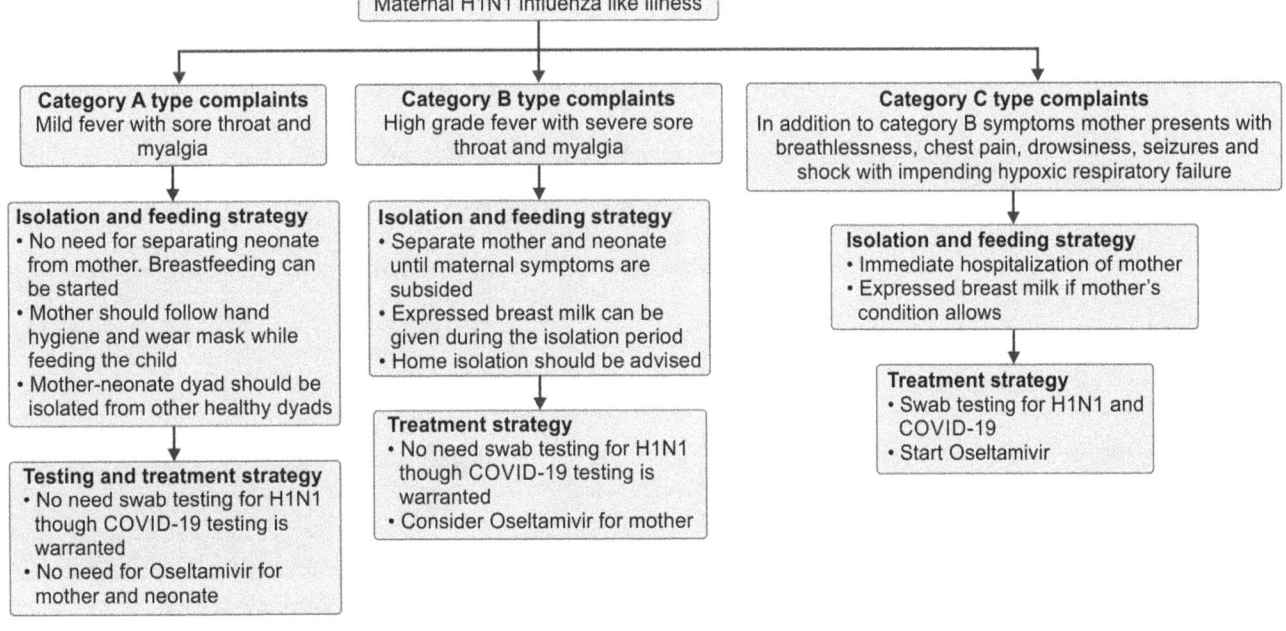

Flowchart 2: Approach to the neonate born to mother with H1N1 influenza like illness.

confirmed dengue infection demonstrated increase in worse pregnancy outcomes like premature labor, preeclampsia, intrauterine growth retardation, and still births. There was also increase in maternal complications like thrombocytopenia, acute kidney injury, postpartum hemorrhage, and acute respiratory distress syndrome (ARDS).

Neonatal Dengue

The maximum risk of neonatal Dengue is there when the expecting mother develops high grade fever within 10 days of delivery. The mode of delivery has no effect on the transmission rates. The literature review suggests that the median time of presentation between neonatal symptoms and maternal fever is 7 days (with a range of 5-13 days). The most common symptoms in the neonatal population are fever, maculopapular rash **(Figs. 2A and B)** and thrombocytopenia with petechiae. There is a lack of prospective studies on the clinical presentation of neonatal dengue. A recent retrospective study involving 32 confirmed neonatal cases from a tertiary care hospital in Vietnam demonstrated that almost 25% and 12.5% cases were initially wrongly diagnosed as neonatal sepsis and immune thrombocytopenia, respectively. The major clinical presentation included fever (100%), petechiae (87.5%), mucosal hemorrhage (6.3%), and hepatomegaly (75%). Neonates may not manifest with the clinical phases of dengue as seen in adults. The febrile phase (day 1-3), the critical phase (day 4-6), and the convalescent phase may overlap in neonates. When there is rapid deterioration and decrease in platelet count. Severe neonatal disease is rare and can present with sepsis and encephalitis.

Laboratory Diagnosis

Dengue should be suspected in any neonate presenting with fever, rash, and thrombocytopenia especially in the peak dengue season. As in adult and pediatric population, diagnosis can be confirmed by direct tests that are positive viral antigen nonstructural protein one rapid test (NS1) and positive IgM antibody test by enzyme linked immunosorbent assay (ELISA). Low level of viremia can give rise to false negative diagnostic results first 2 days after birth. In the initial 4-5 days of presentation, NS1 antigen test is more sensitive and after that antibody tests are more useful. More specific tests like viral culture and PCR tests are also available but are less frequently employed because of their high cost. Cerebrospinal fluid (CSF) study should be performed in case of neurological manifestations.

Treatment

The treatment of neonatal dengue is largely supportive with timely fluid therapy.

Presence of persistent ductus arteriosus and the ensuing fluid overload status complicates the management of dengue in a neonate due to the contradicting needs of the two pathologies. Point of care ultrasonography can be used to tailor the fluid therapy. The prognosis is good in dengue fever. The outcome varies with the severity of clinical presentation.

CHIKUNGUNYA VIRUS

Chikungunya (CHIKV) is a single-strand (SS) positive-sense RNA virus with an envelope. It also causes Aedes mosquito linked vector-borne viral disease. The most common vectors are *Aedes aegypti* and *Aedes albopictus*. CHIKV was first isolated in Tanzania in the year 1952. After that there have been numerous sporadic outbreaks and isolated case reports in Africa till 2004. In 2005-2006, there was a large-scale outbreak of CHIKV in India with most of the cases reported from South Indian states namely Andhra Pradesh, Tamil Nadu, and Karnataka. Initially, this disease was often misdiagnosed as dengue-like illness but now with the wide spread availability of the diagnostic tools; CHIKV infection is also commonly diagnosed.

Clinical Presentation

Chikungunya presents with high-grade fever, which is rapid in onset followed by headache, myalgia, arthralgia,

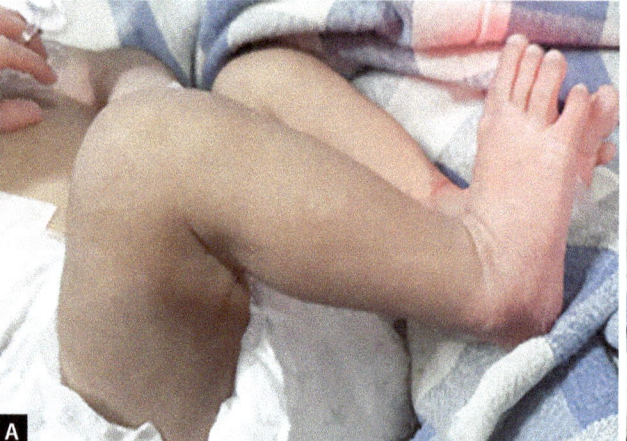
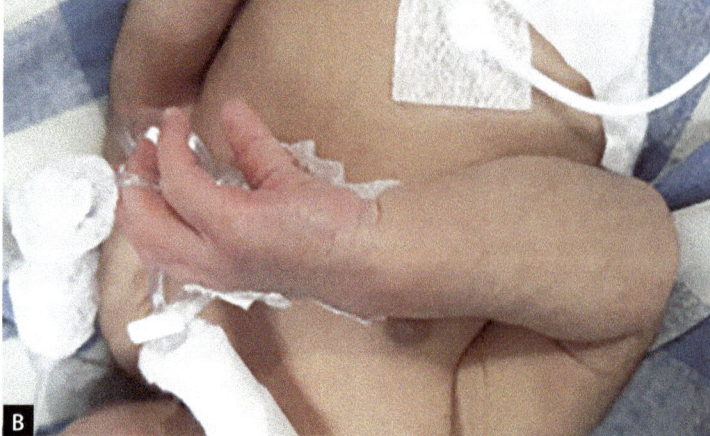

Figs. 2A and B: (A) Maculopapular rash over lower limbs; (B) Maculopapular rash on forearm and hand.

and maculopapular rash. The presence of symmetric severe debilitating arthralgia across all the large joints is a pathognomonic sign of CHIKV infection present in almost 90% of all the cases. CHIKV is rarely fatal. The mean incubation period is very short which is approximately 3 days. A large proportion of infected people recover fully with supportive treatment but symptoms of joint pain and swelling may persist for months. Rarely, severe complications like myocarditis and encephalitis can occur.

Chikungunya in Pregnancy

As per the available literature, there is no increased risk of pregnancy-related complications like still birth, premature birth, intrauterine growth retardation, and congenital anomalies as compared to noninfected mothers. However, CHIKV infections prior to 20 weeks of gestation have been associated with increased fetal loss. Congenital malformations have not been reported. The reported vertical and perinatal transmission rate is around 50% in symptomatic mothers. The reported vertical transmission rate is 27.2–48.2%. The risk of maternal-fetal transmission is highest when pregnant women are symptomatic during the intrapartum period (2 days before delivery to 2 days after delivery). During this period, vertical transmission occurs in approximately half of cases.

Chikungunya in Neonates

As per the available literature, almost 100% of neonates with CHIKV infection are symptomatic. Encephalopathy is one of the most dangerous complications in the neonatal period present in approximately 50% of all the cases. The usual presentation of the perinatally acquired infection is high-grade fever, incessant cry, joint swelling, arthralgia, poor feeding, lethargy, and maculopapular rash along with severe hepatic and hematologic abnormalities. This usually happens after 3–5 days of birth. Sometimes, the clinical presentation is similar to bacterial sepsis with multiorgan dysfunction syndrome (MODS). 89% of neonates will have thrombocytopenia. Centrofacial pigmentation, also known as "Brownie-nose pigmentation" in the perioral region 3–4 days after the onset of fever is common **(Fig. 3)**. The long-term prognosis varies with the severity of presentation and presence of encephalopathy. Neurologic sequalae in the form of neurocognitive impairment, microcephaly, and cerebral palsy has been reported.

Diagnosis

In a CHIKV outbreak setting, any pregnant women presenting with fever and joint pain should be evaluated for CHIKV infection. The hallmark of neonatal CHIKV fever is hyperalgesia syndrome, diffuse inflammatory lower limb edema and skin rash. There are two major diagnostic methods for CHIKV infection:

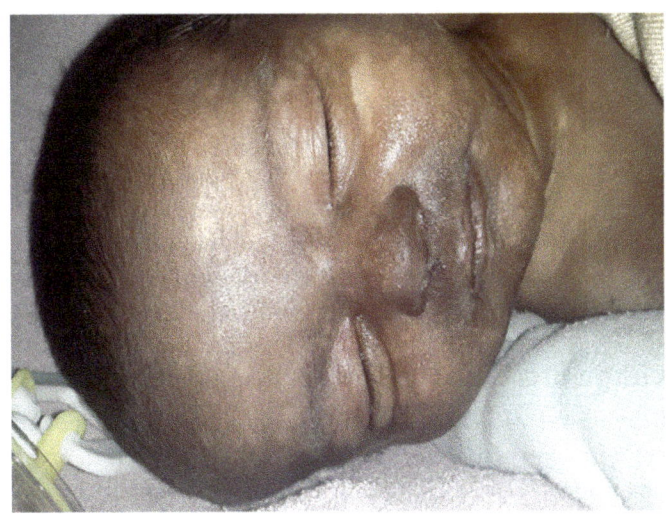

Fig. 3: Centrofacial pigmentation (brownie nose pigmentation).

1. *Serological tests:* Antibody capture ELISA demonstrates IgM and IgG CHIKV antibodies. IgM should be done 5 days after the fever onset. The peak IgM anti-CHIKV antibody levels are formed 3–4 weeks after the infection and usually persist for 2 months.
2. *Virus isolation:* Nucleic acid amplification of viral RNA by RT-PCR. This test is more sensitive and specific in the first week.

Treatment

The treatment of neonatal CHIKV is largely supportive. Long-term multidisciplinary follow up is required.

ZIKA VIRUS

Zika virus like dengue virus belongs to the family Flaviviridae. It is an enveloped SS RNA virus transmitted predominantly by *Aedes aegypti* mosquitoes and ticks. ZIKV infection can also spread by blood transfusion, organ transplantation and unprotected sex.

Epidemiology

In the year 1947, ZIKV was first isolated from a Rhesus monkey of the Zika forest in Uganda. Ever since, ZIKV was circulating among monkeys and other nonhuman primates with occasional human transmission in the rural areas. In the year 2007, there were reports of virus outbreaks in the urban areas of Micronesia and France. In the year 2015, the Health Ministry of Brazil reported a cluster of cases of congenital microcephaly associated with in-utero maternal ZIKV infection. In the year 2017, first four cases of ZIKV were isolated from India followed by outbreaks in the states of Rajasthan and Madhya Pradesh. Fortunately, in the Indian outbreak, the rates of neurological complications were not high with no reported case of congenital microcephaly.

Clinical Presentation

Zika virus infection has an incubation period ranging from 3 to 14 days. Most infections are asymptomatic. The usual presentation is mild-grade fever, conjunctivitis, arthralgia, myalgia, and rash. Sometimes, rare complications like meningoencephalitis, Guillain-Barre syndrome (GBS), myocarditis and thrombocytopenia are also reported. Similarly, ZIKV infection in pregnancy is mostly asymptomatic with no increased risk of pregnancy-related complications.

Congenital Zika Virus Infection

Congenital ZIKV syndrome (CZS) is the most dreaded complication of maternal infection. Maternal infection in the first trimester carries the highest risk of CZS. Overall, the risk of birth defects is around 10% with confirmed maternal ZIKV infection anytime during the pregnancy. Symptomatic ZIKV infection in mother carries a more risk of microcephaly than asymptomatic infection.

Zika virus because of its neurotropism causes direct damage to the developing fetal brain resulting in severe volume loss and microcephaly. This microcephaly results in a typical presentation of overlapping sutures, hanging skin over the scalp, occipital bone prominence, craniofacial asymmetry at birth. MRI brain generally reveals intrinsic abnormalities like intracranial calcifications, ventriculomegaly, cortical atrophy, reduced brain volume, delayed myelination, simplified gyral patterns (e.g., polymicrogyria, pachygyria, lissencephaly), thinning or hypoplasia of the corpus callosum, hypoplasia of the brainstem and cerebellum, enlargement of the cisterna magna, increased extra-axial fluid spaces. Sometimes, these MRI findings are seen in normocephalic neonates at birth and microcephaly ensues after birth. The clinical presentation usually consists of severe microcephaly, intrauterine growth retardation, arthrogryposis, hyper-reflexia, and early hypertonia with evidence of extrapyramidal involvement, seizures and irritability. Ophthalmological abnormalities like macular atrophy, optic disk hypoplasia, microphthalmia, retinal pigmentation, iris colobomas, and lens subluxation are also commonly seen. Sensorineural hearing loss is also found in around 7% neonates with CZS.

Evaluation

Infants who warrant ZIKV laboratory testing include either of the following:
- Newborns of mothers with laboratory evidence for ZIKV infection during pregnancy.
- Newborns who have clinical or neuroimaging findings suggestive of CZS and a maternal epidemiologic link suggesting possible transmission (which includes paternal exposure), regardless of maternal ZIKV test results. A normal head circumference does not exclude the possibility of CZS.

Laboratory Investigations

Serum and urine for ZIKV RNA via rRT-PCR.

Serum ZIKV IgM ELISA [The plaque reduction neutralization test (PRNT) should be used to rule out false positive IgM results].

Interpretation

Confirmed Congenital Zika Virus Infection

The presence of ZIKV RNA in infant serum, urine, or CSF collected within the first few days of life confirms the diagnosis of congenital ZIKV infection.

Probable Congenital Zika Virus Infection

A negative rRT-PCR with positive ZIKV IgM indicates probable congenital ZIKV infection.

Unlikely Congenital Zika Virus Infection

If both rRT-PCR and IgM are negative, congenital infection is unlikely.

Neuroimaging

All neonates with suspected or probable congenital zika infection should undergo neuroimaging—brain ultrasonography and MRI or CT scan.

If CSF is available, test CSF for ZIKV RNA (via rRT-PCR) as well as ZIKV IgM. CSF specimens need not be collected for the sole purpose of ZIKV testing.

Diagnosis

A definitive diagnosis of congenital ZIKV infection is confirmed by the presence of ZIKV RNA in infant serum, urine, or CSF collected within the first 2 days after birth.

Postnatal ZIKV infection should be suspected in an infant or child with relevant epidemiologic exposure in the last 2 weeks and ≥2 of the following manifestations: fever, rash, conjunctivitis, or arthralgia.

Management

Zika virus infection is usually self-limiting so the supportive care is the main stay for managing this infection in adults. Neonates with CZS should be managed by a multidisciplinary team consisting of neonatologist, developmental supportive care specialist, audiologist, ophthalmologist, orthopedic surgeon and physiotherapist. The detailed evaluation of a neonate with possible congenital ZIKV infection is shown in **Flowchart 3**.

Prevention

Vector control is the most important intervention to control this deadly disease. There is no vaccine against ZIKV. Prevention efforts are aimed at reducing zika infection during pregnancy.

Flowchart 3: Approach to a neonate with possible congenital zika virus (ZIKV) infection and congenital zika virus syndrome (CZS).

Possible ZIKV exposure

Possible ZIKV exposure AND clinical findings suggestive of CZS

- Detailed physical examination at birth, eye examinations and audiological assessment
- ZIKV RT PCR with serum and urine sample within few days of birth
- ZIKV IgM serology within few days of birth
- CSF ZIKV RT PCR and IgM should also be considered
- Head ultrasound (USG) and MRI brain before discharge
- BERA test before discharge or by 1 month of age
- Multidisciplinary follow up, developmental supportive care and early intervention

Possible ZIKV exposure AND clinical findings not suggestive of CZS but confirmed ZIKV infection in mother

- Detailed physical examination at birth, eye examinations and hearing screening
- ZIKV RT PCR with serum and urine sample within few days of birth
- ZIKV IgM serology within few days of birth
- Head USG by 1 month of age
- BERA test by 1 month of age

→
- Initial evaluation positive for ZIKV infection
- Detailed evaluation and high risk follow up as mentioned for CZS

→
- Initial evaluation negative for ZIKV infection
- Routine follow up

Possible ZIKV exposure AND clinical findings not suggestive of CZS with no confirmed ZIKV infection in mother

- Routine physical examination at birth with no further testing
- If during routine follow up findings suggestive of CZS are there then detailed evaluation as mentioned for CZS

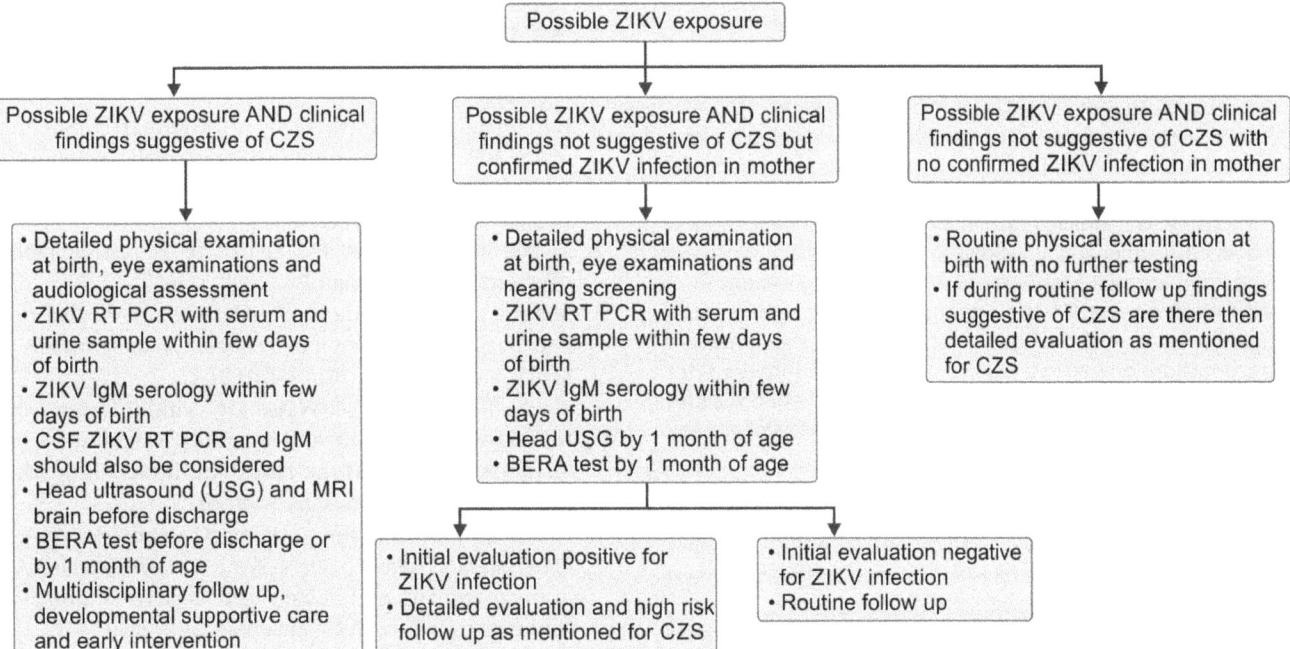

(BERA: Brain Evoked Response Auditory; CSF: cerebrospinal fluid; MRI: magnetic resonance imaging; RT PCR: reverse transcription polymerase chain reaction)

CHAPTER AT A GLANCE

Other viral infections in pregnancy

Varicella zoster

- Risk of transmission is more if onset of rash within 7 days of delivery or within 2 days after birth
- The risk of CVS is more in the second trimester (12–20 weeks)

→
- **Varicella in pregnancy:** Usually presents with short episode of fever, malaise with typical rash and very rarely as pneumonia
- **Varicella in neonates:** Can be dangerous with pneumonia as a dangerous complication especially in preterm infants
- **Treatment:** Acyclovir is drug of choice in neonates if indicated

Zika virus (ZIKV)

- Maternal infection in the first trimester carries the highest risk of CZS
- Overall, the risk of birth defects is 10% with confirmed maternal ZIKV infection anytime during the pregnancy

→
- **ZIKV in pregnancy:** Mostly asymptomatic with no increased risk of pregnancy-related complications
- **CZS in neonates:** Microcephaly is the most dangerous complication. IUGR and macular atrophy is also prominent.
- **Treatment:** Multidisciplinary follow-up with early stimulation

Dengue virus

- The risk of vertical transmission is 20%
- The risk is high, if mother develops high grade fever within 10 days of delivery

→
- **Dengue in pregnancy:** Can be dangerous with more chances of dengue and pregnancy related complications like PPROM, preterm labor and still birth
- **Dengue in neonates:** Median time of neonatal presentation is 7 days after maternal fever. Fever, maculopapular rash and thrombocytopenia is the most common presentation. Severe disease is rare in neonates
- **Treatment:** Supportive care

Chikungunya (CHIKV)

- The risk of vertical transmission rate is around 27–48%
- The highest risk is in symptomatic mothers 2 days before delivery to 2 days after delivery

→
- **CHIKV in pregnancy:** There is no increased risk of pregnancy related complications
- **CHIKV in neonates:** Almost 100% neonates are symptomatic. Usual presentation is 3 to 5 days after birth. High-grade fever, incessant cry, joint swelling, arthralgia, poor feeding, lethargy, and maculopapular rash along with severe hepatic and hematologic abnormalities. Encephalopathy is the most dangerous complication
- **Treatment:** Supportive care

H1N1

- The mode of transmission is usually by droplet spread (Horizontal transmission)
- Vertical transmission not reported

→
- **H1N1 in pregnancy:** Can be dangerous with more incidence of severe complications thus affecting neonatal outcomes
- **H1N1 neonates:** Infection mostly asymptomatic with viral URI like symptoms in infancy
- **Treatment:** Drug of choice is Oseltamivir

(CVS: congenital varicella syndrome; CZS: congenital zika virus syndrome; IUGR: intrauterine growth retardation; PPROM: preterm prelabor rupture of membranes; URI: upper respiratory infections)

KEY POINTS

- Viral infections in pregnancy are major causes of maternal and fetal morbidity and mortality. Infections can develop in the neonate transplacentally, perinatally (from vaginal secretions or blood), or postnatally (from breast milk or other sources).
- Detail maternal and epidemiological history helps in narrowing down the differentials. The clinical manifestations of neonatal infections vary depending on the viral agent and gestational age at exposure. Generalized rash in different developing stage is characteristic of neonatal varicella infection. Fever, hyperalgesia syndrome, diffuse limb edema with hyperpigmentation is hallmark of neonatal CHKV infection. Fever, diffuse erythematous macular rash with flushed peripheries is the common presentation of neonatal DENV infection. Neonates with microcephaly, neurological abnormalities, ocular abnormalities or hearing loss in the setting of a maternal epidemiological link should be evaluated for ZIKV infection.
- Postexposure prophylaxis with VZIG can prevent varicella in exposed neonates or ameliorate the disease course in patients in whom the infection was not fully prevented. Oseltamivir remains the drug of choice for H1N1 infection and the treatment of neonatal DENV, CHKV, and ZIKV remains supportive.
- Viral infections in neonate need multidisciplinary management and long-term follow-up.

SUGGESTED READING

1. Brar R, Sikka P, Suri V, Singh MP, Suri V, Mohindra R, et al. Maternal and fetal outcomes of dengue fever in pregnancy: a large prospective and descriptive observational study. Arch Gynecol Obstet. 2012;304:91-100.
2. de St Maurice A, Ervin E, Chu A. Ebola, Dengue, Chikungunya, and Zika infections in neonates and infants. Clin Perinatol. 2021;48(2):311-29.
3. Inbaraj LR, Chandrasingh S, Arun Kumar N, Suchitra J, Manesh A. High susceptibility to varicella among urban and rural pregnant women in South India: a brief report. Epidemiol Infect. 2021;149:e63.
4. Kalane SU, Gokhale AN, Kalane UD. Dengue Encephalitis in a newborn. Indian J Pediatr. 2021;88(7):716.
5. Maria A, Vallamkonda N, Shukla A, Bhatt A, Sachdev N. Encephalitic presentation of Neonatal Chikungunya: A Case Series. Indian Pediatr. 2018;55(8):671-4.
6. Martin RJ, Fanaroff AA, Walsh MC. Viral infections in the Neonate. In: Fanaroff and Martin's Neonatal-Perinatal Medicine Diseases of the Fetus and Infant, 11th edition. Amsterdam, Netherlands: Elsevier; 2020.
7. Pomar L, Vouga M, Lambert V, Pomar C, Hcini N, Jolivet A, et al. Maternal-fetal transmission and adverse perinatal outcomes in pregnant women infected with Zika virus: prospective cohort study in French Guiana. BMJ. 2018; 363:k4431.
8. World Health Organization (2016). Screening, assessment and management of neonates and infants with complications associated with Zika virus exposure in utero—rapid advice guideline. [online] Available from http://apps.who.int/iris/bitstream/10665/204475/1/WHO_ZIKV_MOC_16.3_eng.pdf?ua=1. [Last accessed October, 2021].

CHAPTER 38

Tuberculosis—Perinatal Perspective

Rohit Sasidharan, Neeraj Gupta

INTRODUCTION

Perinatal tuberculosis (TB) is an underdiagnosed condition with high mortality, if left untreated. TB in the neonate can be either congenital (acquired in-utero) or postnatal (acquired early after birth from untreated mother or caretakers) in origin. Congenital TB is due to either transplacental IU infection of the fetus by *Mycobacterium tuberculosis* or aspiration/ingestion of contaminated amniotic fluid/infected vaginal secretions in-utero or intrapartum. Postnatal TB in the neonates is more common and can occur via horizontal transmission from infected mother or caregivers. As it is often difficult to identify the exact route of transmission, "Perinatal Tuberculosis" is preferred to "congenital" or "post-natal" TB in clinical practice. The best way to prevent "Perinatal TB" is through early diagnosis and treatment of maternal TB infection.

With most available literature on perinatal TB derived from case studies, the estimated vertical transmission from a TB infected mother could be as high as 16%. As, the current incidence of maternal TB among reproductive age is around 100 cases per 1 lakh population, it is estimated that 20,000–40,000 Indian pregnant women are likely to have active TB each year and may contribute to as high as 3,200–6,400 cases of congenital TB per year. Hence, the reported literature grossly underestimates the exact prevalence of TB in pregnancy and congenital TB.

Tuberculosis in pregnancy not only leads to an increased risk of perinatal TB but is also associated with significant adverse maternal and perinatal outcomes. Pregnancy complicated with active TB infection is associated with significantly increased risks of overall maternal morbidity (OR 2.8), miscarriage (OR 9), maternal anemia (OR 3.9), and cesarean section (OR 2.1). The maternal mortality rate is up to 40–100%, with higher mortality associated with delayed diagnosis and inappropriate treatment. It is also associated with two-fold increase in the risk of fetal distress (15.2% vs. 6.3%; $P < 0.01$), prematurity (22.8% vs. 11.1%; $P < 0.01$), low-birth weight (LBW) neonates (34.2% vs. 16.5%; $P < 0.01$), small for gestational age (SGA) (20.2% vs. 7.9%), and six-fold increase in perinatal deaths (10.1% vs. 1.6%; $P < 0.001$).

Furthermore, advances in artificial reproductive techniques (in those having infertility secondary to undiagnosed genital TB), a resurgence of TB in pregnant mothers with HIV disease, and the emergence of multidrug resistant and extreme-drug resistant TB has made perinatal TB an area of recent concern.

OBJECTIVES

The reader will be able to learn:
- What is the pathophysiology of perinatal tuberculosis?
- When to suspect perinatal tuberculosis?
- How to diagnose?
- How to manage?
- How to do a follow-up?

PATHOPHYSIOLOGY OF PERINATAL TB INFECTION

The pathophysiology of TB in pregnancy is similar to that of a nonpregnant woman. Though pregnancy does not alter the course and outcome of TB, few studies reported an increased incidence of extrapulmonary, miliary, and disseminated TB during pregnancy. The mothers who transmit TB to the neonates usually have active TB during pregnancy or in the postnatal period. The majorities of these mothers are asymptomatic or have mild symptoms during pregnancy and often get missed. Moreover, a high index of suspicion is required as the signs and symptoms of the infection may be attributed to the pregnancy itself. Other reasons include its insidious onset, protean, and nonspecific manifestations, overlapping presentation common to other tropical infectious diseases, and the reluctance of the physicians to get chest radiography even in symptomatic patients to avoid fetal exposure to radiations. A pregnant woman who gets primary TB infection during pregnancy or develops reactivation of latent infection can have placental dissemination and is at

Flowchart 1: Types of perinatal TB infection.

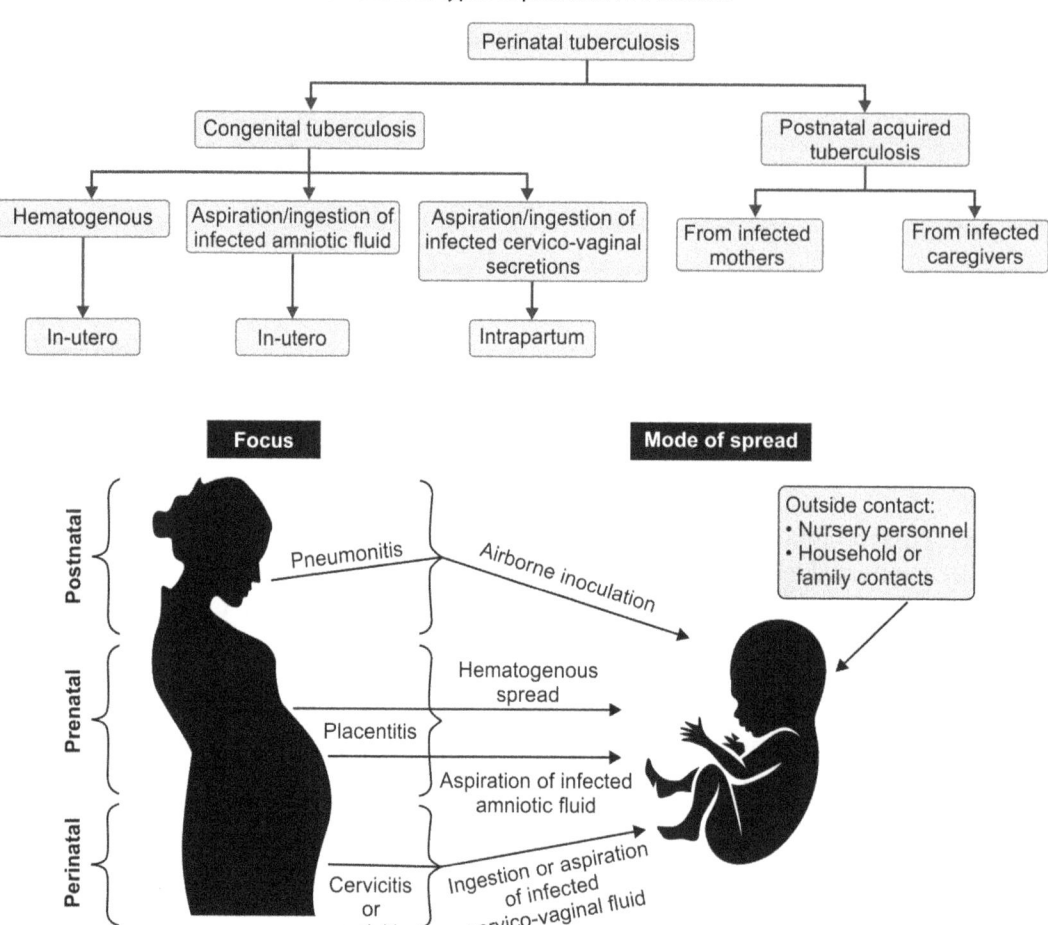

Fig. 1: Potential modes of transmission of TB from mother to newborn infant.
Source: Adapted from Collaborative framework for the management of tuberculosis in pregnant women, MOHFW, GOI, 2020.

risk of transmission to the fetus. Congenital TB secondary to primary infection in the mother is more severe than that due to reactivation disease. Extrapulmonary, miliary disease, and genital TB in the mother are associated with increased risk for perinatal TB. **Flowchart 1 and Figure 1** illustrate the types of perinatal TB and its potential modes of transmission from the mother to the infant.

Congenital TB

Congenital TB can be acquired by two distinct mechanisms. Transplacental transmission can be by hematogenous spread from an infected placenta via the umbilical vein leading to a primary tuberculous lesion in the liver and sometimes lung. Hepatic involvement is more common in this route of transmission, but pulmonary involvement may also be seen secondary to systemic dissemination. The presence of a hepatic primary complex and a caseating hepatic granuloma is a hallmark of congenital TB.

Another transmission mechanism is via aspiration or ingestion of the infected amniotic fluid by the fetus either in-utero or during delivery, which can lead to primary infection in the lungs or gastrointestinal tract. This occurs when a caseous lesion of the placenta ruptures into the amniotic cavity. Unlike transplacental transmission, liver involvement is rare, but middle ear involvement is not uncommon because the eustachian tubes in the newborn permits direct access to the pharyngeal fluids. Rarely, direct infection from established primary genitourinary TB in the mother, such as ovaries, Fallopian tubes, uterus, and cervix, can transmit the infection to the fetus directly. As most of these infection results in infertility, this is a less common mechanism for fetal infection but is increasing due to in-vitro fertilization.

Congenital TB may secondarily disseminate to other organs such as bone marrow, bones, lymph nodes, middle-ear, gastrointestinal tract, spleen, kidneys, meninges, or the skin. In intrauterine infection, the risk of disseminated disease in the fetus is likely to be high as the fetal immune system is immature. The presence of maternal miliary TB or tuberculous endometritis increases the risk of congenital infection. The histologic lesions are similar in appearance to those of older children or adults. The placental lesions in perinatal tuberculosis include chronic necrotizing granuloma in the decidua or endometrium of the uterus. The placenta may often show acute or chronic villitis, often accompanied by intervillitis and an acute neutrophilic histiocytic (nongranulomatous) lesion in the acute phase. Demonstration of caseating hepatic granuloma in the periportal area and hepatic lobules may be feasible by a percutaneous liver biopsy in suspected cases. The majority of cases of congenital TB present within 3 weeks, though diagnosis made as late as 148 days has been reported in the literature.

Postnatal TB

The postnatal infection of the neonate can occur via respiratory transmission from untreated mothers or other family members having TB. This is more commonly seen than congenital TB. Often, it is difficult to differentiate this from congenital infection, but it is crucial for epidemiological reasons. Appropriate antenatal treatment of the mother for 2-3 weeks reduces the risk of postnatal infection. HIV in pregnancy is a risk factor for maternal TB and modifies the type of disease to more severe forms such as cavitary pulmonary, extrapulmonary, and miliary TB, which in turn increases the risk of vertical transmission of TB to the infant. The symptoms of postnatally acquired TB are similar to that of congenital infection. Still, they typically present later, at the age of 1-4 months, and lack the primary hepatic focus seen in congenital TB.

WHEN TO SUSPECT PERINATAL TB?

The clinical diagnosis of perinatal TB is often challenging and requires a high index of suspicion because of:
- Nonspecific signs and symptoms
- Clinical presentation mimics more common conditions such as sepsis and other intrauterine infections (TORCH)
- The majority of the mothers with TB during pregnancy are asymptomatic, and as many as half to two-thirds of mothers remain undiagnosed till their infants' diagnosis.

However, one should suspect perinatal TB early in the following situations:
- Infants with respiratory distress, hepatosplenomegaly, and fever during the first 3 months after birth.
- The infant is not responding to multiple antibiotic treatments, and other congenital viral infections have been ruled out.
- Chest imaging shows a picture of miliary pattern, especially after 4 weeks of postnatal age.
- Abdominal imaging shows multiple focal lesions in the liver and spleen.
- Mothers had active TB during pregnancy.

TABLE 1: Common signs and symptoms of perinatal TB.

System	Symptoms	Percentage
Nonspecific	• Fever	70
	• Hepatosplenomegaly	64
	• Lethargy/irritability	40
	• Jaundice	14
	• Lymphadenopathy	14
Respiratory	• Respiratory distress	70
	• Cough	42
	• Wheeze/rales	36
Gastrointestinal	• Poor feeding	36
	• Failure to thrive	26
	• Abdominal distention	21
	• Vomiting	8
Neurologic	• Lethargy/irritability	40
	• Meningitis	–
	• Seizures	4
	• Apnea	<10
Others	• Skin rash	10
	• Ear discharge	5
	• Facial paralysis	6
	• Bone deformity	–
	• Hemophagocytic syndrome	–

CLINICAL FEATURES

The symptoms of perinatal TB may appear during the first days of life, but the majority of the infected newborns are asymptomatic at birth and more frequently become overtly symptomatic at 2-3 weeks of postnatal age when they develop respiratory problems, hepatosplenomegaly, or lymphadenopathy. Postnatally acquired TB also has similar manifestations but tends to present a little later.

The most common clinical symptoms are nonspecific and may mimic neonatal bacterial sepsis or other congenital infection and include fever, poor feeding, lethargy or irritability, failure to gain weight, cough, and respiratory distress. Hepatic involvement with altered liver functions and respiratory symptoms are the two major systems involved in congenital TB. Other less common presentation includes lymphadenopathy, abdominal distention, chronic ear discharge, osteomyelitis, parotitis, meningitis, vertebral cold abscess, and papular skin lesions. In less than 10% of the cases, the infants may present as apnea, vomiting, jaundice, seizures, cyanosis, and petechiae. The risk of disseminated disease, including meningeal involvement, is also high due to an immature immune system. **Table 1** shows the typical manifestations of perinatal TB.

As neonates tend to present with atypical signs, the diagnosis of TB must be considered in the presence of sepsis-like illness not responding to typical antibiotics. Sometimes, the clinical signs of congenital or postnatally acquired TB may be typically occult and delayed in presentation because of the immaturity of the newborn.

DIAGNOSIS

Diagnostic evaluation should be initiated when the clinical features are suggestive of perinatal TB disease or when the neonate is exposed to a source with active TB disease, such as the mother, any other close contact, or a healthcare worker. Active communication between the physician caring for the pregnant or postpartum woman with TB and the pediatrician caring for the exposed or infected newborn is essential.

Historically, the original diagnostic criteria for congenital TB were proposed by Beitzke in 1935. It included the presence of proven tuberculous lesions in the infant and one of the following:
- Lesions in the first few days of life
- A primary hepatic complex
- Exclusion of postnatal transmission by separation of the infant at birth from mother and other sources of infection.

Since, the criteria included the demonstration of a primary hepatic complex either by an open surgical procedure or autopsy to confirm liver and regional lymph node involvement, Cantwell in 1994 proposed revised criteria to increase the sensitivity of antemortum diagnosis of congenital TB. Accordingly, congenital TB may be diagnosed in the presence of a proven tuberculous disease such as positive smear or culture, AND any one of the following conditions such as:
- Lesions in the newborn within the first week of life.
- Primary hepatic complex or caseating hepatic granulomas.
- TB infection of the placenta or maternal genital tract.
- Exclusion of the possibility of postnatal transmission by investigation of contacts, including hospital staff.

However, there are certain limitations of Cantwell's criteria that should be taken into consideration, such as:
- Late clinical presentation in neonates beyond 2–3 weeks is not uncommon.
- Difficulty in demonstration of acid fast bacilli (AFB) in neonates from sites other than gastric aspirates.
- Inadequate opportunities or facilities for the examination of the placenta and endometrium.
- Difficulty in performing a percutaneous liver biopsy in sick newborns with multiple comorbidities.
- Incomplete evaluation of the mother for active TB, especially when the symptoms are not florid.
- Inadequate evaluation of contacts, including hospital healthcare workers, to rule out active TB.

The laboratory findings of congenital tuberculosis can get easily confused with that of general bacterial infections. The

TABLE 2: Common laboratory findings of perinatal TB.

Tests	Percentage
Leukocytes counts ≥ 12,000/μL	64
Neutrophil ≥ 50%	79
Hemoglobin <10 g/dL	60
Thrombocytopenia (<1 lakh/μL)	80
Elevated ESR > 20 mm/hour	61
Elevated C-reactive protein	95
Positive tuberculin skin test	13

(ESR: erythrocyte sedimentation rate)

total counts are elevated with a neutrophil predominance in the majority of the cases. Thrombocytopenia, deranged liver enzymes, and elevated C-reactive protein are other common findings. **Table 2** present the common laboratory findings in perinatal TB.

The commonly available TB specific tests are tuberculin skin test (TST), interferon gamma release assay (IGRA), AFB smear, culture, microscopic observed drug susceptibility (MODS) testing, and molecular methods such as nucleic acid amplification tests (NAATs), line probe assays and histological examination. The interpretation of these TB-specific tests in neonates is rather complicated due to decreased sensitivity and specificity.

The TST is universally negative in neonates. Hence, infants younger than 3 months are likely to give a false negative result. Even after infection, it may take several months for TST to become positive. Moreover, Bacille Calmette-Guérin (BCG) vaccination interferes with its specificity while its sensitivity is lowered in the neonates due to coexisting prematurity, growth retardation, and immunodeficiency. Revised National Tuberculosis Control Program (RNTCP) 2019 Updated Pediatric TB guidelines also highlights the limited role of TST in neonates and young infants and does not recommend it.

Interferon-γ release assays (IGRAs) measure interferon-γ production from T lymphocytes in response to antigens specific to *M. tuberculosis*. IGRA is almost always negative in newborns due to immature T-lymphocyte activity. The advantage of IGRA is that BCG vaccination will not interfere with the results, and it does not require a follow-up visit to read the TST results. It is generally not recommended for use in children less than two years by the American Academy of Pediatrics (AAP). The National Tuberculosis Elimination Program (NTEP) by the Government of India does not recommend the use of TST or IGRAs for the diagnosis of tuberculosis in adults or children, though there is a limited role in latent tuberculosis infection (LTBI).

Acid fast bacilli smear detection of gastric washings, tracheal aspirates, bronchoalveolar lavage fluids, pleural fluids, cerebrospinal fluid (CSF), urine, or other body fluids/tissues provides the first definitive evidence of mycobacteria. Neonatal gastric fluid is easy and rapid to collect and provides good results. The sample should be collected in the morning before feeding on three separate days and has an overall diagnostic yield of 30-50%. Fluorescent staining methods may be used to increase the yield.

Culture for *M. tuberculosis* in neonates seldom yields positive results due to the paucibacillary nature of the neonatal infection. Blood, CSF, endotracheal or bronchial aspirates, gastric aspirates, stool, ear wax, and biopsy specimens of lymph nodes, liver, and skin are commonly used for culture testing. Low bacterial loads in infants make it challenging to isolate mycobacteria, especially in smear-negative cases. Liquid media culture facilitates the growth of mycobacteria but still takes an average of 3-6 weeks to grow. Mycobacteria growth indicator tube system (MGIT-B) is an automated culture system that detects the growth of mycobacteria. The culture results are usually available for up to 42 days.

Nucleic acid amplification tests using polymerase chain reaction (PCR) offer a rapid technique for the detection of MTB, especially in neonates with low bacterial loads, and are also helpful for detecting the presence of putative resistance genes. Previous studies have shown up to 88% sensitivity and 98% specificity with DNA amplification techniques.

Chest imaging may show normal findings initially, with abnormal findings appearing by 4-8 weeks postnatal age. The abnormal findings in chest X-ray may be nonspecific or show characteristic miliary TB, multiple pulmonary nodules, cystic lesions, pneumonia, mediastinal lymphadenopathy, lobar opacification, compression of large airways, primary pulmonary complex, pleural effusion or pleuritis. The common abdominal imaging findings are multiple focal lesions in the liver and spleen, hepatosplenomegaly, primary liver complex, or ascites.

Histologic examination of the placenta, liver, lymph nodes, or any other affected organ can aid in the diagnosis. The presence of a caseating granuloma in the liver or evidence of tubercular infection of the placenta is diagnostic of congenital TB.

MANAGEMENT AND FOLLOW-UP

Neonatal management depends on the nature and classification of maternal infection and whether there is a clinical suspicion of perinatal TB in symptomatic infants. **Flowchart 2** provides an algorithmic approach to infants with suspected perinatal TB.

Symptomatic Infant with Clinical Suspicion of TB Infection

Any infant who is symptomatic and features suggestive of TB should undergo a complete diagnostic evaluation, and if found to be suggestive of perinatal TB, should be started on treatment. At the same time, the mother and other family members should be screened actively for evidence

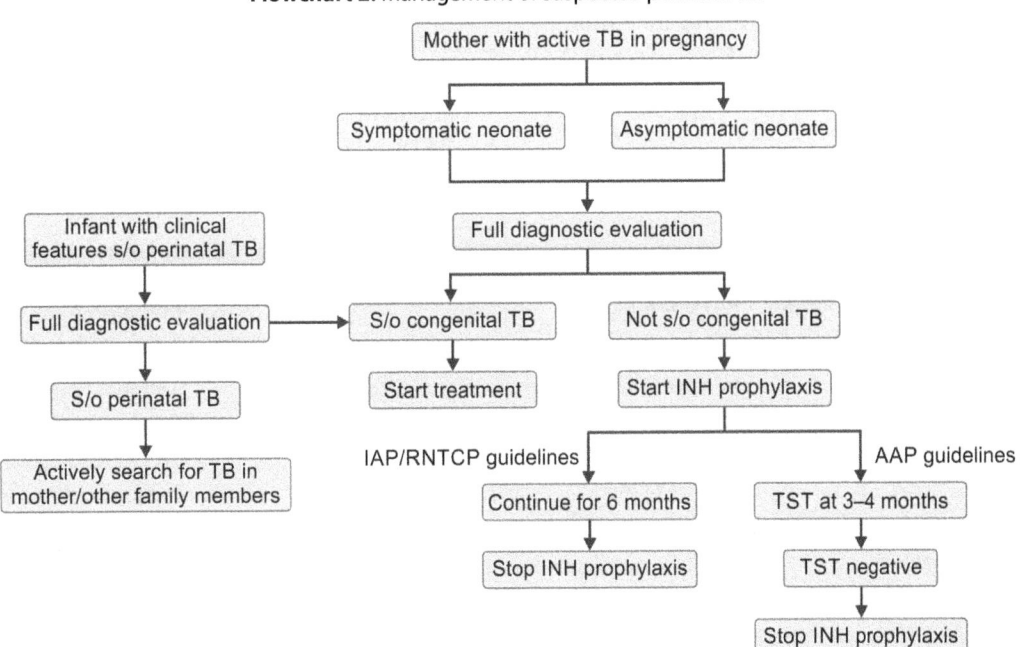

Flowchart 2: Management of suspected perinatal TB.

(AAP: American Academy of Pediatrics; IAP: Indian Academy of Pediatrics; INH: isoniazid; RNTCP: Revised National Tuberculosis Control Program; TB: tuberculosis; TST: tuberculin skin test)

of active TB. A diagnosis of congenital TB may be made, if they are fulfilling Cantwell's criteria though there are some limitations of these criteria as highlighted in the "diagnosis" section.

Infant Born to a Mother with Latent TB Infection during Pregnancy

The mother is asymptomatic with a positive TST and a normal chest X-ray. The neonate need not be separated from the mother or worked up for TB infection; breastfeeding should be continued. All other family members need to be screened for active infection. The mother should be considered for isoniazid (INH) preventive therapy during pregnancy if there is a recent TST conversion, a recent contact with a contagious person, or immunocompromised. In other situations, the treatment can be delayed until after delivery. Infant should receive BCG vaccination at birth.

Infant Born to a Mother with Active Maternal Infection during Pregnancy

In cases where the maternal physical examination, chest radiograph, and other workup suggest active TB, the mother should be promptly started on treatment, and other family members should undergo screening. The infant, once born, should be promptly worked up, and if active TB has been ruled out, the neonate should be started on INH prophylaxis. The 2019 RNTCP Updated Pediatric TB guidelines recommend preventive therapy for all neonates whose mother has any form of active TB, whether pulmonary or extrapulmonary detected in pregnancy. INH preventive therapy should be given in a dose of 10 mg/kg for 6 months. Pyridoxine may be given along with. However, the AAP recommends INH prophylaxis for 3-4 months followed by a TST. If TST is negative, INH can be stopped. If TST is positive, the infant should be reevaluated for active TB disease, and if found to be absent, INH prophylaxis should be continued for 9 months (**Flowchart 2**). Chemoprophylaxis is not recommended in MDR contacts since the efficacy of 2nd line drugs in preventing TB is not unequivocally established and also because these drugs can be fairly toxic. The mother and baby should stay together, and the baby should continue to breastfeed regardless of the mother's status of TB.

Treatment of Perinatal TB

If the infant has features of active perinatal TB, start treatment promptly with INH, pyrazinamide, rifampicin, and ethambutol for 2 months during the intensive phase (2 HRZE). Some guidelines recommend an aminoglycoside instead of ethambutol. Pyrazinamide should be stopped in the continuation phase, but rests of the drugs are to be continued for an additional period of 4 months (4 HRE). This regimen of 2 HRZE plus 4 HRE is recommended for pulmonary, miliary, and disseminated TB. In special situations such as central nervous system TB and skeletal TB, the continuation phase may be extended to 10 months, and the recommended regimen is 2 HRZE plus 10 HRE. Corticosteroids should be added in a confirmed case of TB meningitis at 2 mg/kg/day of prednisolone for the first 4 weeks and then tapered slowly over the next 4 weeks. They may also be considered in endobronchial disease and miliary TB. The recommended drug doses are shown in **Table 3**.

The current Indian RNTCP guidelines (2019), NTEP training modules (2020), as well as the World Health Organization (WHO) recommend the usage of a fixed-drug combination (FDC) for infants more than 4 kg weight. According to the guidelines, pediatric anti-TB drug formulations are available as FDC:
- *3 FDC*: H50, R75, Z150 (INH 50 mg, rifampicin 75 mg, and pyrazinamide 150 mg)
- *2 FDC*: H50, R75 (INH 50 mg and rifampicin 75 mg)

TABLE 3: First line drugs used in the treatment of perinatal TB.

Drug	Dose (range) mg/kg/day	Adverse effects	Monitoring
Rifampicin	15 (10–20)	Hepatotoxicity, red color of urine and other body fluids	Liver function tests
Isoniazid	10 (7–15)	Hepatotoxicity, flu-like syndrome, cutaneous hypersensitivity, peripheral neuropathy	Liver function tests
Pyrazinamide	35 (30–40)	Gastrointestinal intolerance, hepatotoxicity, hyperuricemia	Liver function tests, serum uric acid
Ethambutol	20 (15–25)	Optic neuritis	Visual assessment
Streptomycin	20 (15–20)	Renal impairment, ototoxicity	Renal function tests

Ethambutol is available as a single drug formulation of 100 mg (E 100) as the drug may be required to be stopped, if the infant develops optic neuritis as a side effect. Pyridoxine should be given to all infants beyond the neonatal period at a dose of 10 mg once a day who are on INH containing regimen because of the risk of INH-induced peripheral neuropathy. For infants weighing 4–7 kg, the schedule is a single tab "3 FDC" + single tab E100 in the intensive phase and a single tab "2 FDC" + single tab E100 in the continuation phase.

The response to treatment is assessed in terms of clinical improvement. The clinical response is usually seen within 2–3 weeks of starting therapy. In case of a lack of clinical improvement or worsening despite 6–8 weeks of therapy, the following possibilities need to be ruled out:
- Lack of compliance to therapy
- Possibility of drug-resistant TB (DR TB)
- Underlying immunodeficiency conditions including HIV

Tuberculosis and Breastfeeding

Exclusive breastfeeding is the healthiest choice that a mother can make for her newborn. It not only provides nutrition but also protects the infection from infections and provides long-term health benefits to both the child and the mother. So, in most situations of perinatal infection, the benefits of breastfeeding far exceed the risk of perinatal transmission. The same rules are applicable to perinatal TB too.

In case of latent TB infection in the mother, who is asymptomatic and having normal chest X-ray, no separation of the infant or restriction of breastfeeding is required. Even in case of active maternal infection, baby and mother should stay together, and the baby should continue to breastfeed regardless of the mother's TB status. In the case of maternal smear-positive active TB shortly before delivery, there is an increased chance of the infant acquiring perinatal TB. The mother should be started promptly on anti-tubercular treatment, and the infant screened for congenital TB and development of TB in infancy. Regardless of the severity of the active disease, patients become noninfectious within two weeks of starting therapy and the number of viable bacilli get greatly reduced after 24 hours of treatment. Therefore, separation of the mother-infant dyad is no longer considered mandatory however; hand hygiene and cough hygiene measures should be advised for the mother. Separation is also not warranted once the infant is receiving INH prophylaxis or started on treatment for perinatal TB. Separation of the mother-infant dyad should only be considered if the mother is ill enough to require hospitalization, if she has been or is expected to become non-adherent to her treatment, or if she is infected with a drug-resistant strain of *M. tuberculosis*. In a situation where mother and newborn infant are separated, expressed breast milk by cup or pallade should be fed. Formula milk and bottle feeding must be avoided for quality survival.

If the mother is on first-line anti-tubercular treatment, it is safe to continue exclusive breastfeeding as only a minimal amount of the drugs is secreted in the breastmilk, and the risk of side effects in the neonate is considered minimal. Caution is advised if the mother had multi-drug resistant TB and is on second like anti-tubercular treatment, as limited data is available regarding their concentration in the breastmilk and the risk of side effects in the neonate.

Monitoring and Follow-up

Infants with perinatal TB would require regular follow-up in high-risk newborn clinics especially, for assessing compliance to anti-tubercular therapy (ATT), proper dosages, clinical response to ATT, and any adverse events. Serial blood counts, liver function test, serum creatinine, hearing assessment, and visual assessment by a pediatric ophthalmologist and should be done periodically.

Infants with perinatal TB also need growth monitoring, nutritional assessment, development, and neurological assessment. All routine vaccinations should be given as per the normal schedule. BCG vaccine is not required for infants diagnosed with perinatal TB. However, all infants born to mothers with active TB should receive BCG vaccination after ruling out congenital TB. It may be given at the end of INH prophylaxis as recommended by WHO. However, the RNTCP Revised Updated Pediatric Guidelines 2019 recommends that the BCG vaccine should be given at birth, even if infants are receiving INH prophylaxis. Similarly, the AAP also supports BCG vaccination at birth if follow-up of the patients cannot be ensured.

Prognostic Factors

The following factors have been found to be associated with poor outcomes:
- Age of onset of symptoms less than 3 weeks
- Intracranial involvement
- Miliary pattern and multiple pulmonary patterns in chest X-ray
- Elevated leukocyte counts < 12,000/μL
- Lack of treatment

SECTION 5 | Congenital Infections

CHAPTER AT A GLANCE

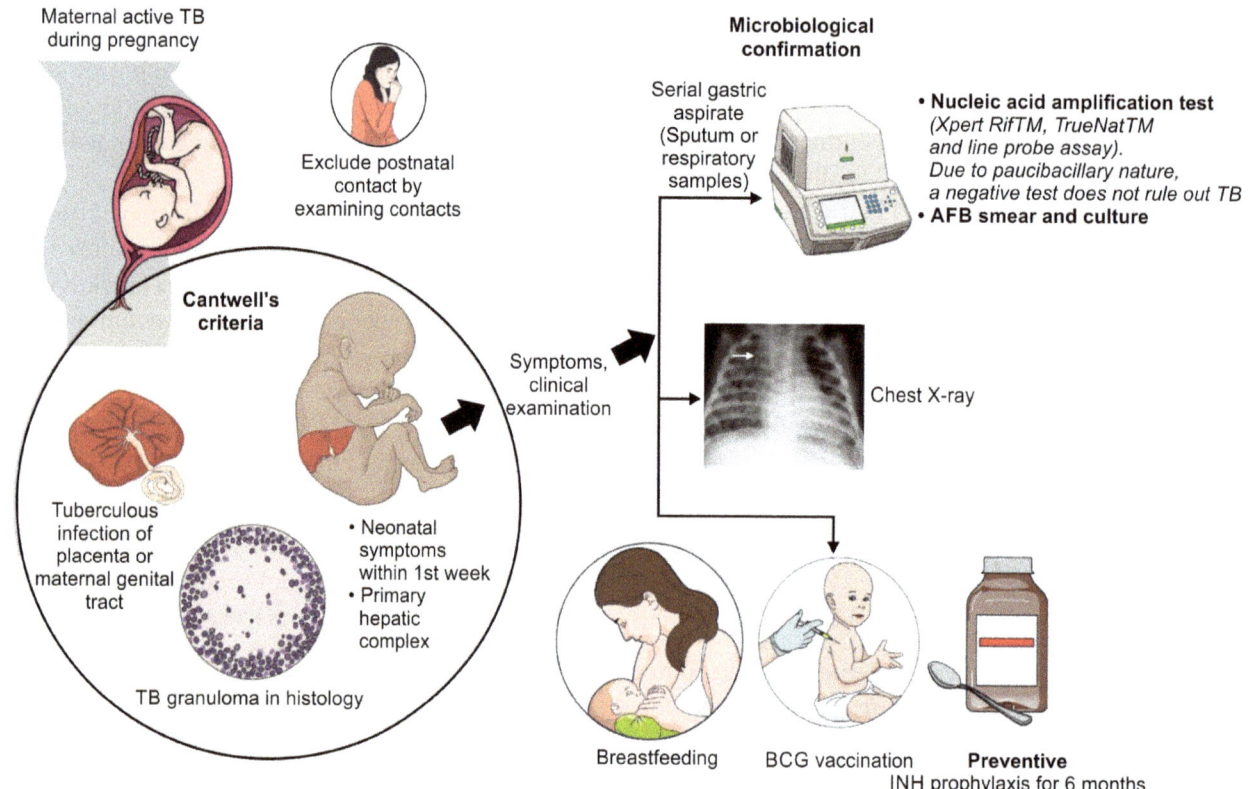

Transmission, diagnosis and management of perinatal tuberculosis
(AFB: acid-fast bacillus; INH: isoniazid; HRZE: rifampicin, pyrazinamide, ethambutol; BCG: Bacille Calmette-Guérin)

KEY POINTS

- Perinatal TB may be acquired either transplacentally, through aspiration or ingestion of infected amniotic fluid, or via respiratory transmission after birth.
- Perinatal TB is an underdiagnosed entity associated with high morbidity and mortality, especially if there is a delay in diagnosis, and inappropriate treatment is initiated.
- A high index of suspicion is required as the clinical manifestations are nonspecific and may mimic neonatal sepsis and other congenital viral infections.
- More than 50% of the mothers are asymptomatic and remain undiagnosed until a diagnosis is made in the infant.
- All at-risk and suspected neonates should undergo extensive evaluation to rule out perinatal TB.
- Diagnosis is difficult due low yield of AFB and the poor sensitivity and specificity of a diagnostic test in infants.
- Chemoprophylaxis with INH is recommended for high-risk exposure after ruling out perinatal TB.
- Active neonatal infection may require prolonged treatment, corticosteroids, and regular follow up and monitoring.
- Mother and infant should not be separated, and breastfeeding should be continued.

SUGGESTED READING

1. Alene KA, Adane AA, Jegnie A. Impact of multidrug-resistant tuberculosis and its medications on adverse maternal and perinatal outcomes: protocol for a systematic review and meta-analysis. BMJ Open. 2019;9(12):e034821.
2. Jana N, Barik S, Arora N, Singh AK. Tuberculosis in pregnancy: The challenges for South Asian countries: Tuberculosis in pregnancy in South Asia. J Obstet Gynaecol Res. 2012;38(9):1125-36.
3. Li C, Liu L, Tao Y. Diagnosis and treatment of congenital tuberculosis: a systematic review of 92 cases. Orphanet J Rare Dis. 2019;14(1):131.
4. Ministry of Health and Family Welfare, Government of India. Collaborative Framework for Management of Tuberculosis in Pregnant Women. New Delhi: Ministry of Health and Family Welfare; 2020. p. 46.
5. Mittal H, Das S, Faridi MM. Management of newborn infant born to mother suffering from tuberculosis: current recommendations & gaps in knowledge. Indian J Med Res. 2014;140(1):32-9.
6. Newberry DM, Robertson BT. Congenital tuberculosis: A new concern in the neonatal intensive care unit. Adv Neonat Care. 2018;18(5):341-9.
7. Peng W, Yang J, Liu E. Analysis of 170 cases of congenital TB reported in the literature between 1946 and 2009: Analysis of Congenital TB. Pediatr Pulmonol. 2011;46(12):1215-24.

CHAPTER 39

HIV—Perinatal Perspective

Prakash V, Deviprasadh PM

INTRODUCTION

Human immunodeficiency virus (HIV) is one of the most common diseases affecting millions worldwide and presents a unique opportunity for its prevention of transmission to subsequent generations with a few targeted measures. In India, every year, around 22,000 pregnancies occur in HIV-infected women. Babies can acquire infection during all stages of pregnancy, childbirth, or through breastfeeding. The older term mother-to-child transmission (MTCT) is replaced with prevention of parent to child transmission (PPTCT) emphasizing the part played by both parents in transmitting the disease to their babies.

OBJECTIVES

- To review the risk of transmission and various obstetric measures
- To discuss the intrapartum management of an HIV-infected mother
- To discuss the role of antiretroviral therapy (ART) in the mother and the baby
- To discuss the continuum of care postpartum for the mother–infant dyad

TRANSMISSION RISK

Risk of Perinatal Transmission

The maternal HIV RNA level is directly linked to the risk of perinatal HIV transmission, so viral load testing 4–6 weeks before delivery helps to determine the risk of perinatal transmission.

In a study from United Kingdom and Ireland, observed MTCT rates were as follows:

- Mother with HIV RNA copies between 50 and 1,000/mL near delivery, transmission risk is 1–2%.
- Mother with HIV RNA copies < 50/mL near delivery, transmission risk is <1%.

Timing of HIV Transmission from Mothers to their Infants

More than 90% of pediatric HIV cases result from perinatal transmission. This can occur during pregnancy (in utero), at labor/delivery (intrapartum), or postdelivery (postnatal) through breastfeeding. In nonbreastfeeding settings, one third of transmission have been thought to have occurred in utero and the remaining two third intrapartum. In breastfeeding settings in the era of nonavailability of antiretroviral (ARV) interventions, about 25–40% of infant infections were estimated to occur during pregnancy, about 50% intrapartum or through very early breastfeeding, and the remainder during the breastfeeding period.

Other Factors Affecting Perinatal Transmission Risk

- Premature rupture of the membranes (PROM) >4 hours
- *Placental disruption*: Abruptio placenta, chorioamnionitis
- ARV intervention and risk of HIV transmission
  - *No ARV and breastfeeding*: 30–45%
  - *No ARV and no breastfeeding*: 20–25%
  - *Short course with one ARV with breastfeeding*: 15–25%
  - *Short course with one ARV without breastfeeding*: 5–15%
  - *Short course with two ARVs and breastfeeding*: 5%
  - *ARVs (ART) with breastfeeding*: 2%
  - *ARVs (ART) with no breastfeeding*: 1%

OBSTETRIC MANAGEMENT STRATEGIES

Antenatal Period

At the first antenatal visit, for all antenatal mothers, HIV testing should be done on an OPT-OUT basis, and if positive, appropriate health information should be provided and triple-drug ART should be started and adherence ensured. Screening for other sexually transmitted diseases should also be undertaken in consult with a venereologist. The use of ARV agents by pregnant women and their children is a critical component of prevention of MTCT during the antepartum and peripartum periods as well as throughout the duration of breastfeeding. ART should be initiated as early as possible in all pregnant women with HIV and continued lifelong.

Serodiscordant Couples

Attempt viral load suppression before conception (<50 copies/mL). Two RCTs on this topic *HPTN 052 (HIV Prevention Trials Network trial 052)* have shown that initiating ART earlier led to a 93% reduction in the rate of sexual transmission of HIV to the partner, and *PARTNER [Partners of People on ART-A New Evaluation of the Risks]* study showed that out of 1,166 couples of differing HIV statuses (both heterosexual couples and men who have sex with men) in which the partner with HIV was on suppressive ART and had unprotected sex, no cases of transmission were reported after a median follow-up of 1.3 years.

National Program Guidelines

The efficacy of combination ART in reducing perinatal transmission has also been demonstrated in several observational studies in resource-limited settings. In these studies, ART was associated with MTCT rates at birth and in the early postpartum period of <5%, comparable to the low transmission rates achieved in resource-rich settings.

All pregnant and breastfeeding women living with HIV will receive a "single-pill" triple-drug ART regimen [Tenofovir disoproxil fumarate + Lamivudine + Efavirenz (TDF + 3TC + EFV)] lifelong therapy, regardless of CD4 count or clinical stage **(Table 1)**.

Intrapartum Management

- Minimal vaginal examinations
- Shorten labor by using oxytocin infusion
- Avoid all invasive interventions—artificial rupturing of membranes, no routine episiotomies, avoid assisted extractions (vacuum, forceps), and avoid invasive fetal scalp PH monitoring.

Preterm Labor in HIV Positive Mother

- With threatened preterm labor, antenatal corticosteroids should be given when appropriate to accelerate fetal lung maturity.
- Women with early labor or spontaneous rupture of membranes (ROM) occurs >34 weeks of gestation with HIV copies (≤1,000/mL); intervention to decrease the delivery interval should be considered (oxytocin admin).
- But with copies <1,000 mL, preterm labor, or spontaneous ROM at <34 weeks of gestation, the decision of timing and mode of delivery is based on considering the risk of prematurity and HIV transmission.

Recommendation on Mode of Delivery

Although scheduled cesarean section is associated with reduced rates of MTCT among women who have received either no ARV drugs or zidovudine (AZT) alone, this recommendation is not practical in resource-limited regions and may increase maternal morbidity; thus, the presence and status of HIV infection in the mother do not affect decisions on delivery mode in resource-limited settings.

If HIV positive status is first identified in a woman presenting with labor, the triple-drug regimen (TDF + 3TC + EFV) should be given at least 4 hours before the delivery. In women who have been receiving ART for several weeks and virally suppressed (<50 copies/mL) at near delivery, vaginal delivery can be undertaken. So, women should be informed that cesarean section is not routinely recommended for

TABLE 1: Antiretroviral therapy (ART) regimen for pregnant women with HIV.

Category	Drug regimen
• Pregnant and breastfeeding • Women with HIV ("Not-already" receiving ART)	TDF (300 mg) + 3TC (300 mg) + EFV (600 mg)—to be given 2 hours after low-fat or fat-free dinner
Pregnant and breastfeeding women with HIV already receiving ART	The same ART regimen must be continued
ART regimen for pregnant women having prior exposure to NNRTI for PPTCT	FDC of TDF (300 mg) + 3TC (300 mg) - 1-tab OD and FDC of LPV (200 mg)/r (50 mg) 2-tab BD
Presenting in active labor, no prior ART	• Initiate TDF (300 mg) + 3TC (300 mg) + EFV (600 mg) and continue postpartum also • If the mother has not received any ART antenatally, the minimum duration of nevirapine prophylaxis for the infant is 12 weeks • If HIV-positive status is first identified in a woman presenting with labor, the triple-drug regimen (TDF + 3TC + EFV) should be given at least 4 hours before the delivery

(PPTCT: prevention of parent to child transmission; NNRTI: non-nucleoside reverse transcriptase inhibitor; FDC: fixed dose combination; EFV: efavirenz; HIV: human immunodeficiency virus; TDF: tenofovir disoproxil fumarate)

those with low HIV viral load and is not beneficial. The mode of delivery is decided based on obstetric indications only.

International Recommendations

- As per National AIDS Control Organization (NACO) and World Health Organization (WHO) guidelines:
  - Normal vaginal delivery is recommended unless a woman has an obstetric indication. The American College of Obstetricians and Gynecologists (ACOG) recommends:
    - For HIV copies >1,000/mL, elective cesarean delivery at 38 weeks of gestation to decrease the likelihood of spontaneous onset of labor or rupture of membranes.
    - For HIV RNA copies <1,000/mL, labor should not be induced at 38 weeks for prevention of perinatal transmission during vaginal delivery (as there is no difference in transmission in who delivered vaginally at 38 weeks and between 38 and 40 weeks of gestation).
- *British HIV Association guidelines*: If the viral load is >400 HIV RNA copies/mL at 36 weeks, a scheduled cesarean section should be offered.

NEONATAL MANAGEMENT

Immediately after Birth

- Universal aseptic precautions should strictly be adhered to.
- Resuscitation should be performed as per the updated 2020 guidelines.
- Delayed cord clamping should be performed for all the vigorous babies.
- Alert the ART center/NACO counselor of the delivery.
- Physical examination for signs/symptoms of HIV infection. If asymptomatic, administer all birth dose vaccines.
- Start ARV prophylaxis as per the following guidelines.

ARV Prophylaxis for Infant

For mothers with viral load <1,000 copies/mL:
- All infants born to people living with HIV/AIDS (PLWHA) mother should be started on nevirapine (NVP) prophylaxis immediately after birth and continued for minimum 6 weeks. Duration of NVP prophylaxis will depend upon how long the mother had received ART prior to delivery.
- *ARV prophylaxis for HIV-exposed infants* **(Table 2)**
- If infants exposed to HIV-2 (or combined HIV-1 and HIV-2):
  Then start syrup AZT and not NVP
  - Body weight >2,500 g: 15 mg/dose/twice daily
  - Body weight <2.5 kg: 10 mg/dose/twice daily

TABLE 2: Antiretroviral prophylaxis for HIV-exposed infants.

Baby birth weight	NVP daily dose in mg	NVP daily dose in mL (10 mg/mL suspension)	Duration
<2,000 g	2 mg/kg once daily	0.2 mL/kg once daily	Minimum 6-week duration
2,000–2,500 g	10 mg once daily	1 mL once daily	
>2,500 g	15 mg once daily	1.5 mL once daily	

(HIV: human immunodeficiency virus; NVP: nevirapine)

TABLE 3: Cotrimoxazole prophylaxis in HIV-exposed infants.

Dose (200-mg/5-mL syrup)		
Up to 6 kg	2.5 mL	Once a day
6–9.9 kg	5 mL	Once a day

- *If mother has viral load >1,000 copies/mL:*
  - Asymptomatic neonate—start two-drug regimen (AZT + NVP) in the above doses
  - Symptomatic/sick neonate—start triple-drug regimen (AZT + NVP + 3TC)
- *Indication for 12 weeks' NVP infant prophylaxis:*
  - Mother had not received ART in pregnancy/received ART for <24 weeks continuously prior to delivery.
  - If the mother decides only to give exclusive replacement feeding, this can be reduced to 6 weeks' duration, after consulting with the ART consultant medical officer.

Cotrimoxazole Prophylaxis (Table 3)

Start for all HIV-exposed infants starting at 6 weeks of age and continue till 6 months irrespective of DNA polymerase chain reaction (PCR) status; thereafter, continue if PCR is positive.

- If PCR is negative at 6 months and the infant has not been breastfed before 6 months, stop cotrimoxazole.
- If PCR is negative at 6 months, but the infant has been breast fed before 6 months, continue cotrimoxazole and stop only after doing PCR after 6 weeks of stopping breastfeeding.

Feeding the HIV-exposed Infants

- Recommendations on infant feeding must balance the risk of HIV transmission through breast milk with the risk of malnutrition and serious infections through unsafe feeding practices. The WHO recommends that for mothers known to have HIV, public health authorities should focus either on promoting breastfeeding and providing ARV interventions to prevent transmission or on avoiding all breastfeeding and providing alternate sources of safe nutrition.

- *Exclusive breastfeeding for the first 6 months is recommended.* The healthcare workers should motivate and assist the mother for the same and ensure it on regular intervals.
- Whenever exclusive feeding is not possible, reassure the mother that ART is protective even in the context of mixed feeding and not to switch over to exclusive replacement feeding.
- Mothers living with HIV should breastfeed for at least 12 months and may continue breastfeeding for up to 24 months or beyond while being fully supported for ART adherence.
- The choice of breastfeeding should be the decision of woman based on proper information; counseling on breastfeeding should begin during the antenatal period itself.
- Mothers when opt for exclusive replacement feeding should fulfill the AFASS criteria—*Affordable* and *Feasible* to provide sufficient replacement feeds, family members are *accepting* of it and can *sustain* it for 6 months without interruption. *Safe* water and sanitation assured at household levels to prepare clean feeds.

Workup of Newborn

- DNA PCR testing for HIV can be done postnatally, before 6 weeks. If positive, start ART irrespective of the CD4 count in all infants.
- HIV DNA PCR sensitivity is increased to 95% at 4 weeks and 99% at 6 months. If the PCR is positive at birth, it means infected in utero; if the PCR is negative at birth and positive later, intrapartum or postpartum transmission is suspected.
- Confirm it by the second test on a separate sample repeated after 2–4 weeks of the first.
- Repeat the HIV DNA PCR test at 6 months if the child is symptomatic.
- Get the test done after 6 weeks of complete cessation of breastfeeding.
- Confirmation test for HIV has to be done in all at 18 months using three rapid tests.
- Follow routine well baby visits and immunization schedule.

Interpretation of Tests

- HIV infection can be reasonably excluded if the infant had at least two negative virologic results with at least one performed at ≥4 months of age.
- Two or more negative Ab tests performed 1 month apart in absence of hypogammaglobulinemia and clinical evidence of HIV disease excludes HIV infection in a >18-month child.

IMMUNIZATION (TABLE 4)

- Routine immunization is given to all asymptomatic newborns.
- Newborns HIV DNA PCR positive *along with immunosuppressive* symptoms—avoid bacille Calmette-Guerin (BCG), live oral polio vaccine, MMR (measles, mumps, and rubella), and varicella.
- Varicella and MMR can be given in not severely immunocompromised children.
- The infant of an HIV mother must be vaccinated with *Haemophilus influenzae type* b (Hib) and Pneumococcal conjugate (PCV) vaccines.

TABLE 4: Recommended immunization for children with HIV infection.

Vaccine	Asymptomatic	Symptomatic
BCG	Yes (at birth)	No
Measles	Yes, at 9 months	Yes, if CD4+ count >15%
MMR	Yes, at 15 months and 5 years	Yes, if CD4+ count >15%
Hepatitis B	Yes, at 0, 1, and 6 months	Yes, four doses, double dose, check for seroconversion and give regular boosters
Hepatitis A vaccine	Yes	Yes, check for seroconversion, boosters if needed
Varicella vaccine	Yes, 2 doses at 1–3 months interval	• Yes if CD4 count >200/mm^3 for more than 6 months • Two doses 1–3 months apart
DTwP/DTaP/TT/Td/Tdap	Routine—6, 10, 14 weeks, 18 months, 5 years	
Polio vaccines	IPV at 6, 10, 14 weeks, 12–18 months, 5 years IPV to household contacts also	
Pneumococcal vaccines PPSV	• Routine— 6, 10, 14 weeks, and 12–15 months • Two doses—one dose 2 months post-PCV, second dose 5 years after the first dose	
Inactivated influenza vaccine	Routine—begin at 6 months; annually revaccinate	
Rotavirus	The ACIP/WHO recommends to give in asymptomatic infants only	
Vi-typhoid/Vi-conjugate vaccine	TCV 9–12 months	
HPV vaccine	Start at 10 years, 3 doses—0 dose at 10 years, second dose 2 months later, third dose— 6 months later from the first dose	

(ACIP: The Advisory Committee on Immunization Practices; BCG: bacille Calmette-Guerin; HIV: human immunodeficiency virus; IPV: inactivated poliovirus vaccine; MMR: measles, mumps, and rubella; PPSV: pneumococcal polysaccharide vaccine; WHO: World Health Organization)

BCG Vaccination

In all symptomatic infants born to HIV positive mother, do not give BCG.

The WHO guidelines for BCG vaccination in asymptomatic infants are based on risk versus benefit, pending strong evidence.

Maternal status HIV positive, baby asymptomatic, and early virological testing unavailable, give BCG and keep a close follow-up to provide early identification and treatment of any BCG-related complication.

Maternal status HIV positive, baby asymptomatic:
- Early virological testing available—do virological testing. If the result of test is negative, give BCG.
- Asymptomatic baby—early virological testing. If the result of the test is positive, do not give BCG.

CHAPTER AT A GLANCE

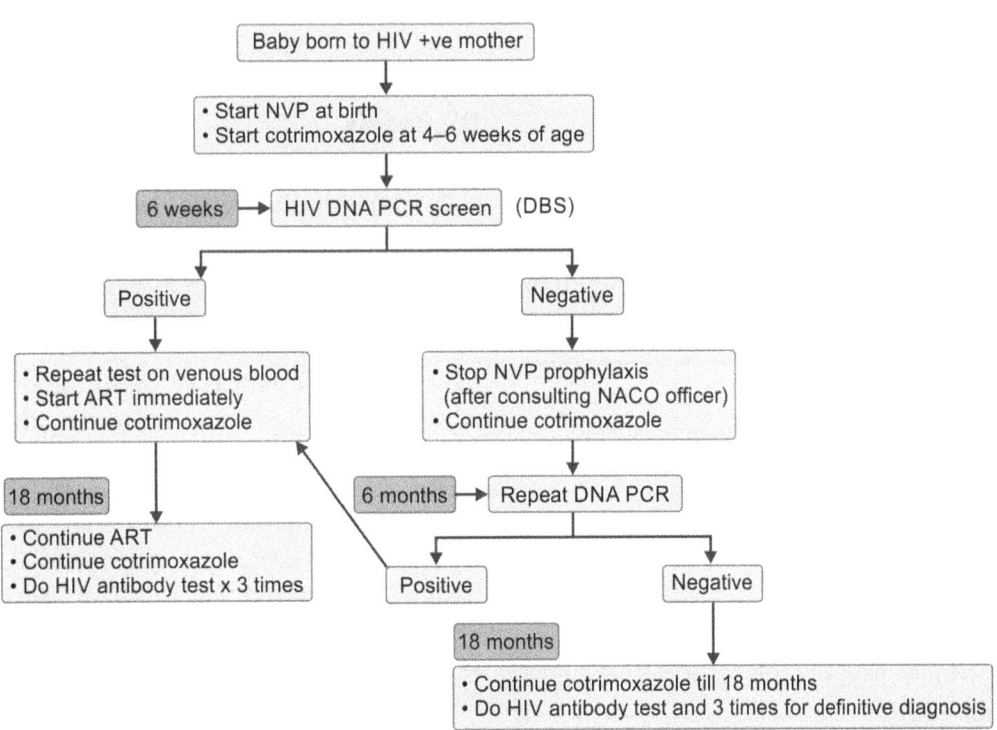

(ART: antiretroviral therapy; DBS: dried blood spot; NACO: National Aids Control Organization; PCR: polymerase chain reaction; HIV: human immunodeficiency virus; NVP: nevirapine)

KEY POINTS

- Health providers should identify all the HIV-positive mothers during the antenatal period at the earliest and start ART.
- Risk of perinatal transmission is negligible if ART is initiated early in pregnancy.
- Goal is to maximally reduce viral load prior to delivery.
- Mode of delivery is decided purely based on the obstetric indication.
- In neonates born to an HIV-positive mother, ARV prophylaxis should be started soon after birth and continued for 6 weeks.
- Cotrimoxazole prophylaxis should be initiated from 6 weeks and continued till HIV can be excluded.
- Routine immunization along with Hib and PCV should be done for all asymptomatic neonates.

SUGGESTED READING

1. National AIDS Control Organization. (2018). National technical guidelines on antiretroviral treatment. [online] Available from http://naco.gov.in/sites/default/files/NACO%20-%20National%20Technical%20Guidelines%20on%20ART_October%202018%20%281%29.pdf [Last accessed November, 2021].
2. UNAIDS. (2016). UNAIDS factsheet. [online] Available from https://www.unaids.org/sites/default/files/media_asset/2016-AIDS-data_en.pdf [Last accessed November, 2021].
3. UNAIDS. (2016). UNAIDS global AIDS update. [online] Available from https://www.unaids.org/en/resources/documents/2016/Global-AIDS-update-2016 [Last accessed November, 2021].
4. World Health Organization. WHO Consolidated Guidelines on Use of Antiretroviral Drugs for Treating and Preventing HIV Infection. Geneva: World Health Organization; 2016.
5. World Health Organization. WHO Guidelines on Cotrimoxazole Prophylaxis for HIV Related Infections Among Children. Geneva: World Health Organization; 2014.

40. Viral Hepatitis—Perinatal Perspective

Ramani Ranjan, Manju Gupta

INTRODUCTION

Neonatal infections with the hepatitis viruses occur as a result of perinatal or vertical transmission from infected mothers. The risk of perinatally or neonatal-acquired infection and its clinical implications vary depending on the hepatotropic virus.

OBJECTIVES

By the end of this chapter, the learner should be able to:
- Understand perinatal transmission of individual viruses.
- Know the investigation(s) for diagnosis and anticipated clinical picture in affected neonates.
- Appreciate the importance and ways to prevent mother-to-child transmission (MTCT).
- Formulate a care plan as applicable for at risk newborns.

HEPATITIS A

Hepatitis A virus (HAV) is a nonenveloped, positive, single-stranded RNA virus in the genus Hepatovirus of the Picornavirus family.

Epidemiology and Transmission

The incidence of HAV infection is inversely related to the sanitation facilities available in a country as the virus spreads through fecal–oral route. HAV infection is usually self-limiting in pregnant women. HAV infection during pregnancy is not associated with congenital deformities, stillbirths, intrauterine growth restriction, or spontaneous abortions; however, it has been implicated in many pregnancy-related complications such as premature contractions, placental abruption, preterm rupture of membranes, and per vaginal bleeding. There are case reports of vertical transmission of HAV weeks before or at delivery; however, the risk of perinatal transmission is low. There is negligible risk of transmission of HAV via breast milk hence breastfeeding is not contraindicated for HAV-infected mothers. Neonatal-acquired HAV infection is rare.

Diagnosis

Immunoglobulin M antibody to the hepatitis A virus (anti-HAV IgM) is the diagnostic marker in pregnant women and the fetus/newborn. Polymerase chain reaction assays for hepatitis A are also available.

CLINICAL MANIFESTATIONS

Most newborns with HAV infection are asymptomatic; however, in the rare case where mother-to-child HAV infection occurs, it can be associated with fetal ascites, meconium peritonitis, neonatal icteric HAV infection, and distal ileal perforation. There are few rare case reports of HAV-associated symptoms in neonates. Fever, difficulty in feeding, and recurrent vomiting have been reported in these babies. Hepatomegaly and biochemical evidence of mild hepatitis during course of disease followed by complete recovery and no long-term sequelae were seen in most of the affected newborns. Fulminant hepatitis resulting from infection with HAV is rare in children and has never been reported in the newborn infant.

Treatment

The treatment for newborn infants with HAV infection is supportive. Experts in developed countries have advocated use of serum immune globulin as postexposure prophylaxis in infants; however, the efficacy of immune serum globulin in these circumstances has not been fully established and immunoprophylaxis may be less effective in newborn infants than in older children. HAV-positive babies may remain infectious for long; hence, strict infection control is necessary.

Prevention

Clean water, hygienic food, improved sanitation, hand washing, and hepatitis A vaccine are the most important steps in preventing HAV infection in mother and hence subsequent perinatal transmission in the newborns. As per the current recommendations, hepatitis A vaccine is given at 1 year of age and above.

HEPATITIS B

Hepatitis B virus (HBV) is a member of the Hepadnaviridae family and is an enveloped virus.

Epidemiology and Transmission

Perinatal exposure from an HBV-infected mother is the most common route of neonatal infection. Hepatitis B infection is transmissible from an infected pregnant woman to her baby at birth and this may happen during a vaginal delivery or during C-section. Hepatitis B surface antigen (HBsAg) seroprevalence in India is 3–7% with over 40 million carriers. The prevalence of hepatitis B infection in Indian pregnant women is variable depending on the geographical area and ranges from 1 to 9%. Hepatitis B e antigen (HBeAg) prevalence in our country is nearly 60% indicating high risk of transmission. Neonates born to HBV-infected mothers have high chance of contracting the disease if they are not offered prophylaxis soon after birth and this infection often leads to devastating chronic sequelae later in adulthood. There is 70–90% likelihood of infants acquiring perinatal HBV infection who are born to mothers known to be HBsAg and hepatitis B "e" antigen (HBeAg) positive and 85–90% of those infected tend to become chronic HBV carriers.

The most significant risk factor for MTCT is positive HBeAg and/or a high HBV DNA level in the mother. Transmission via placenta or during obstetrical procedure is infrequent but there is a 10–16% risk of intrauterine transmission. Procedures such as amniocentesis do not seem to increase the risk of intrauterine transmission; similarly, instrumental delivery does not seem to increase the risk of transmission. Breastfeeding does not seem to pose substantial risk and is considered safe in maternal HBV infection.

Clinical Manifestations

Newborn babies with HBV infection are rarely symptomatic at birth with most showing biochemical features of hepatitis (raised liver enzymes) beginning 2 months of age. Fulminant hepatitis has also been reported in few infants around the same age. Most affected infants become chronically infected which inturn might lead to cirrhosis and hepatocellular carcinoma later on in adulthood.

Diagnosis

HBsAg may be detected in infants by 1–2 months of age secondary to vertical transmission however HBsAg may be transiently positive in neonates up to 21 days following hepatitis B vaccination. It is therefore prudent to measure HBsAg and anti-HBs (hepatitis B surface antibody) levels at 6–12 months (1–2 months after completing the primary vaccination course) in infants born to mothers with chronic hepatitis B infection.

Adequate anti-HBs levels (≥10 mIU/mL) and HBsAg negativity mean that infant is protected. For anti-HBs level is <10 mIU/mL, revaccination and further testing have to be considered with involvement of a gastrointestinal expert.

Prevention of Mother-to-child Transmission

To reduce global burden of chronic HBV infection prevention of MTCT is a crucial step. Immunoprophylaxis to newborn is highly effective in blocking natal transmission; however, in minority of cases infection may have occurred prenatally.

Maternal Prophylaxis

Hepatitis B immune globulin (HBIG) during pregnancy was shown to reduce MTCT but almost all the trials have originated from China and high risk of bias was noted in almost all the studies. Further well-conducted RCTs are needed before it can be considered as a therapeutic strategy to reduce MTCT.

Neonatal Prophylaxis

The standard prophylaxis regimen consists of both passive and active immunization. HBV vaccine and HBIG are given simultaneously at two different sites. HBIG is given by intramuscular injection in the dose of 100 IU. A higher dose of 200 IU has also been used in few countries. Infants should receive HBIG immediately afterbirth—ideally within 12 hours of birth and certainly within 48 hours. The efficacy of HBIG decreases significantly if given >48 hours after birth; however, utmost can be given no later than 1 week of age **(Box 1, Flowchart 1)**.

Hepatitis B monovalent vaccine dose should preferably be given within 24 hours of birth and certainly within 7 days. Vaccination must not be delayed as this sole intervention is quite effective in preventing infection if given early enough. Infants should receive three more doses

---

BOX 1: Immunoprophylaxis of newborns born to mothers with hepatitis B infection.

Hepatitis B vaccination of all newborn at birth
- For neonates born to hepatitis B infected mothers:
  - Hepatitis B vaccine 0.5 mL IM as soon as possible and within first 24 hours
  - HBIG 0.5 mL (100–200 IU) IM as soon as possible within first 12 hours
- For unknown HBsAg status of mothers:
  - Hepatitis B vaccine 0.5 mL IM as soon as possible and within first 24 hours
  - HBIG 0.5 mL (100–200 IU) IM as soon as mother is diagnosed HBsAg positive ideally within 72 hours
  - Vaccination of at-risk adults who have not been vaccinated earlier

(HBIG: hepatitis B immune globulin; HBsAg: hepatitis B surface antigen)

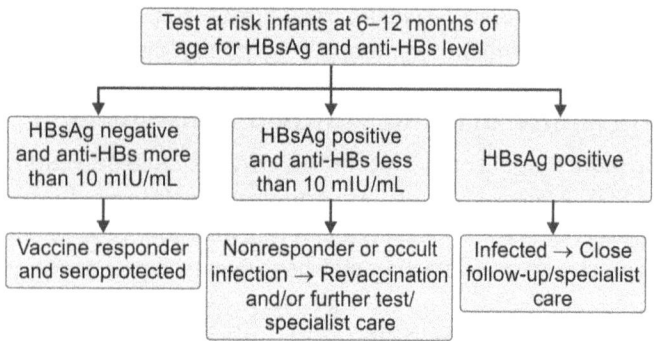

Flowchart 1: Follow-up care plan of newborns at-risk for hepatitis B infection.

(anti-HBs: Hepatitis B surface antibody; HBsAg: hepatitis B surface antigen)

> **BOX 2:** Hepatitis B vaccination and antibody response.
>
> - Testing is recommended at least 4–8 weeks after last hepatitis B vaccination and no earlier than 6 months of age. Test done earlier than 9 months may indicate passively transferred antibody so should be inferred with caution.
> - The threshold of protection is defined as anti-HBs level > 10 mIU/mL. Infants who are HBsAg-negative but with anti-HBs < 10 mIU/mL should be advised for HBV DNA levels testing to rule out occult HBV infection.
> - Chronic hepatitis B infection is diagnosed if persistence of HBsAg is for 6 months or more.

if receiving combination vaccine (6-10-14 weeks schedule) to make a total of four doses of hepatitis B-containing vaccines. In preterm/low birth weight babies weighing less than 2 kg, HBV vaccine should be given even though the immunogenicity is known to be less in preterm and low birth weight neonates and this should be followed by further three doses beginning at 6 weeks of age. HBIG should also be given along with vaccine even in preterm and low birth weight neonates.

About 5–10% of neonates acquire infection despite immunoprophylaxis usually due to high maternal HBV DNA and HBeAg positivity. Antivirals during last trimester of pregnancy to decrease the maternal DNA load seem to be effective in reducing the transmission. Lamivudine or tenofovir (TDF) in the last trimester has shown to reduce immunoprophylaxis failure in the neonates and should be considered in mothers with high viral DNA load.

It is not unusual to find women presenting in labor without documentation of HBsAg test. It is recommended to draw blood for tests as soon as possible and while results are pending, baby should receive first dose of hepatitis B vaccine (without HBIG) within 24 hours or less after birth, irrespective of birth weight. If mother is found to be HBsAg-positive, the infant should receive HBIG as soon as possible.

HEPATITIS C

Hepatitis C virus (HCV) is single-stranded, small, enveloped RNA virus and is a member of the Flaviviridae family. HCV is now considered to be the leading cause of chronic viral hepatitis in children because of robust hepatitis B vaccination program in most nations across the globe.

Epidemiology and Transmission

Vertical transmission is the most common source of infection in pediatric age group. The perinatal transmission risk associated with HCV is less than that of HBV and HIV but currently there is no available vaccine that can prevent or reduce its transmission. Almost 33% of the infected babies acquire infection during intrauterine period and up to 50% get it intrapartum. High maternal viral load at delivery, high maternal liver enzymes 12 months before pregnancy and/or at the time of delivery, rupture of membranes >6 hours, prolonged and/or difficult deliveries, concomitant HIV infection, and invasive fetal monitoring increase the risk of HCV perinatal transmission. Multivariable analysis has confirmed the link between maternal intravenous drug use and HCV transmission. Cesarean section does not seem to decrease the risk of transmission.

Rarely transmission may occur through breast milk as HCV RNA is detectable in colostrum; however, discouraging breastfeeding in HCV-infected mothers is not recommended. There is no significant evidence to suggest increase in the risk of HCV transmission with breastfeeding although multiple expert groups recommend that HCV-infected women should avoid breastfeeding if the nipples are cracked or bleeding. The American College of Obstetricians and Gynecologists and the American Academy of Pediatrics support breastfeeding by HCV-infected mothers.

Clinical Manifestations

Newborn babies born to HCV-infected mothers are largely asymptomatic at birth and remain free of symptoms for years. The disease advances more rapidly in adults as compared to children. Mild-to-moderate intermittent increased liver enzymes may be noticed in first two decades of life. Histological changes in liver are minimal and there is uncertainty in predicting as to how many of infected infants would progress to serious sequelae such as cirrhosis and hepatocellular carcinoma in adulthood.

Diagnosis

Hepatitis C virus infection is primarily diagnosed by detecting antibodies to HCV (anti-HCV). Perinatal transmission is confounded by passive transfer of maternal antibody till up to 13-18 months of age; hence, anti-HCV testing is not recommended in infancy.

Presence of HCV RNA is considered a marker of infection if found positive two or more times. In infants, it is advisable to do HCV RNA test at 10-14 weeks of age so that it coincides with routine immunization visits. Negative tests need to be repeated after 6-12 months. HCV RNA positive signifies infection and hence needs referral to gastroenterology team. In children with HCV infection, annual ultrasound and alpha-fetoprotein (AFP) level estimation is recommended to monitor for progression of liver disease and to pick sinister sequelae like hepatocellular carcinoma at an early stage.

Prevention

No single intervention has been found to substantially decrease the risk of MTCT of HCV. Avoidance of measures which facilitate transmission (listed under "transmission" above) might be considered for HCV-infected mothers. An effective strategy to curtail the likelihood of vertical HCV transmission is by identifying and treating HCV-infected women prior to conception. It is recommended that children infected with HCV should be immunized against both hepatitis A and B.

Treatment

The treatment of chronic HCV infection has changed dramatically since the development of direct-acting antiviral agents (DAAs) and combination drug regimens. These therapies represent a major milestone in the treatment of HCV in adults, adolescents, and children as young as 6 years of age and are likely to be available for younger children in near future. For children younger than 3 years of age with HCV infection treatment is mostly deferred.

HEPATITIS E

Hepatitis E virus (HEV) is structurally similar to Calicivirus and is a single-stranded positive-sense RNA virus. Infection with HEV usually is self-limiting with features similar to acute hepatitis caused by HAV though fulminant hepatitis can occur. HEV infection in pregnancy carries an unfavorable prognosis for mothers. In severely affected cases, this may lead to fulminant hepatic failure and even death. Maximum number of deaths occurs in resource-poor countries where fecal contamination of water results in sporadic cases and frequent outbreaks.

Vertical Transmission and Clinical Manifestations

Although information regarding perinatal transmission is limited, there are several case series of vertical transmission of HEV. Mother-to-infant transmission of HEV mainly HEV-1 occurs frequently and accounts for substantial fetal loss and perinatal mortality but its contribution to overall disease burden appears to be small. Mild disease in pregnant women may cause abortion, intrauterine death, stillbirth, or preterm delivery.

There are reports of vertical transmission in >50% infants born to HEV-infected women who were viremic antenatally. Every affected infant had derangement in liver function tests with mortality up to 33% in different series. Icteric or anicteric hepatitis may be present from birth in a majority of neonates born to HEV-infected mothers. Those who survive have good prognosis with liver function tests returning to normal by 3 months. HEV infection does not lead to chronic hepatitis.

Diagnosis

Hepatitis E virus infection diagnosis is based on detection of IgM antibodies. These antibodies appear with onset of symptoms. The use of recombinant DNA technology has led to detection of antibodies to HEV particles. IgM and IgG assays are now available to differentiate between acute and old infections.

Treatment

Supportive care is the only available treatment as specific treatments for infected infants do not exist.

HEPATITIS D

Hepatitis D virus (HDV) is a unique RNA virus dependent on HBV. Infection with HDV occurs in HBsAg positive persons either as a coinfection (infection with HBV and HDV occurring together) or as a superinfection (infection of a chronic HBV carrier additionally with HDV).

Vertical transmission of HDV is uncommon. Interventions to prevent perinatal acquisition of HBV in infants born to HBsAg-positive mothers also prevent transmission of HDV. As HDV cannot be transmitted independently, routine immunization of newborns with the hepatitis B vaccine also gives protection against HDV. The symptoms of hepatitis D infection are similar but tend to be more severe than those of the other hepatic viruses. HDV-circulating antigen has not been recognized. Antibody to HDV (IgM) is the marker of infection and the diagnostic test.

CHAPTER AT A GLANCE

Prenatally acquired neonatal viral hepatitis

Hepatitis A	Hepatitis B	Hepatitis C	Hepatitis D	Hepatitis E
• HAV infection during pregnancy is not associated with congenital deformities but may be implicated in pregnancy related conditions • **Diagnosed by:** IgM antibody to hepatitis A (anti-HAV IgM) • **Prevention:** Improved sanitation and hepatitis A vaccine starting 1 year of age	• High risk of perinatal transmission in India due to relatively high HBeAg prevalence • **Diagnosed by:** HBsAg and anti-HBs levels at 6–12 of age in infants born to affected mothers • **Prevention:** Hepatitis B vaccination of all newborns at birth. In babies of affected mothers hepatitis B vaccination within 24 hours of birth and HBIG immediately afterbirth—ideally within 12 hours of birth should be given	• Vertical transmission is the most common source of infection • **Diagnosed by:** HCV RNA if found positive on two or more occasions→ advisable to do HCV RNA test at 10–14 weeks of age Negative tests need to be repeated after 6–12 months • **Prevention:** No vaccine available. Cutting down vertical HCV transmission by identifying and treating HCV-infected women prior to conception is most effective strategy	• Vertical or independent transmission of HDV is rarity. Mostly presents as coinfection or superinfection with HBV • **Diagnosed by:** IgM antibodies hepatitis D • **Prevention:** Measures same as for HBV prevention	• HEV infection in pregnancy carries an unfavorable prognosis for mothers. HEV infection does not lead to chronic hepatitis. • **Diagnosed by:** IgM antibodies hepatitis E • **Prevention:** Improved sanitation practices. No vaccine available

For anti-HBs level is <10 mIU per mL, revaccination and further testing has to be considered with involvement of a gastrointestinal expert

Prevention of mother-to-child transmission (MTCT) is a crucial step and effective in blocking perinatal transmission of virus.

(HAV: hepatitis A virus; HBIG: hepatitis B immune globulin; HCV: hepatitis C virus; HEV: hepatitis E virus)

KEY POINTS

- Hepatotropic viruses vary in their clinical implications in the perinatal period. Most common cause of neonatal infection is vertical transmission from mother.
- Hepatitis A infection is mostly asymptomatic in neonatal age group and most affected babies have good outcome.
- Hepatitis B virus is highly transmissible from affected mother to baby; however, timely immunoprophylaxis with hepatitis B vaccine (within 24 hours) and HBIG (within 12 hours) is highly effective in reducing the likelihood of neonatal infection. Postvaccination serologic testing (PVST) is recommended in infants born to seropositive mothers to identify nonresponders and catch hold of those who are infected.
- Hepatitis C is now leading cause of pediatric chronic viral hepatitis globally with a subset of infected children developing complications in adulthood. Currently, there is no available immunoprophylaxis available to prevent MTCT with HCV infection.
- Hepatitis E may run a fulminant course in pregnant women with mortality as high as 33% in affected newborns.
- Breastfeeding is considered safe in all perinatally acquired hepatic viral infections.

SUGGESTED READING

1. Baker CJ (Ed.). Red Book Atlas of Pediatric Infectious Diseases, 3rd edition. Elk Grove Village, IL: American Academy of Pediatrics; 2017.
2. Fanaroff A, Martin R, Walsh M. Fanaroff and Martin's Neonatal-Perinatal Medicine, 9th edition. St. Louis, MO: Elsevier Mosby; 2011.
3. Jonas M. Hepatitis B and pregnancy: an underestimated issue. Liver Int. 2009;29:133-9.
4. Khuroo MS, Khuroo MS, Khuroo NS. Hepatitis E: discovery, global impact, control, and cure. World J Gastroenterol. 2016;22:7030-45.
5. Kimberlin DW, Barnett E, Sawyer MH, Lynfield R. Red Book, 32nd edition. Elk Grove Village, IL: American Academy of Pediatrics; 2021. p. 805.
6. Kliegman RM, Stanton B, Geme J, Schor NF, Behrman RE. Nelson Textbook of Pediatrics, Vol 2, 20th edition. Philadelphia, PA: Elsevier - Health Sciences Division; 2016. pp. 1950-51.
7. Rennie J. Chapter 39, Part 2: Infection in the newborn. Rennie & Roberton's Textbook of Neonatology, 5th edition. Edinburgh: Churchill Livingstone; 2012.
8. Schillie S, Vellozzi C, Reingold A, Harris A, Haber P, Ward J, et al. Prevention of hepatitis B virus infection in the United States: recommendations of the Advisory Committee on Immunization Practices. MMWR Recomm Rep. 2018;67(1):1-31.
9. Slowik M, Jhaveri R. Hepatitis B and C viruses in infants and young children. Semin Pediatr Infect Dis. 2005;16(4): 296-305.

CHAPTER 41

SARS-CoV-2 Infection—Perinatal Perspective

Shikha Rani, Deepak Chawla

INTRODUCTION

Severe acute respiratory syndrome coronavirus-2 (SARS-CoV-2) is a RNA virus with glycoprotein spikes. After the appearance of the first case in Wuhan, China in December 2019, SARS-CoV-2 has spread rapidly worldwide and was declared pandemic by WHO on March 11, 2020. The disease caused by SARS-CoV-2 has been named Coronavirus disease 2019 or COVID-19. SARS-CoV-2 infection may be asymptomatic or have a spectrum of presentation from mild features like fever, sore throat and body aches to lethal form with acute respiratory distress syndrome (ARDS) and multiorgan failure. Till date, SARS-CoV-2 has infected 178 million people across the globe. India is the second worst affected country with 2.97 million cases and 0.38 million deaths. With ongoing pandemic, various mutant strains of the virus have emerged. Some of the variants have been labeled as "variants of concern" due to increased capability to spread and/or higher probability of severe disease and death. One such variant is the "delta" variant responsible for the second wave in India.

Pregnant women are as likely to be infected with SAR-CoV-2 as the nonpregnant individuals but have higher risk of developing severe forms of disease and obstetric complications. This chapter outlines the approach to diagnosis, prevention, and management of SARS-CoV-2 infection in pregnant women and neonates.

OBJECTIVES

- SARS-CoV-2 infection in pregnancy:
  - Incidence and testing strategy
  - Effect on pregnant woman and fetus
  - Management of COVID-19 in pregnancy
- SARS-CoV-2 infection in neonates:
  - Incidence and testing strategy
  - Effect on neonate
  - Management of COVID-19 in neonates

SARS-COV-2 INFECTION IN PREGNANCY

Incidence in Pregnant Women and Testing Strategy

Incidence of SARS-CoV-2 infection in pregnancy is similar to the general population. Studies have reported varying degrees of positivity depending on the testing strategy (universal vs. targeted testing) and incidence in the source population. In the first wave of pandemic, the test positivity rate in the hospitalized settings was 5–12%. Of these only 5–10% were symptomatic and severe COVID-19 was uncommon (1–2% of positive cases). Higher positivity rates of up to 20% with greater proportions of symptomatic and severe disease have been reported in the second wave of pandemic in India (April-May, 2021). This change in epidemiological pattern has been ascribed to a mutant strain of the virus (the "delta" variant). Classification of disease severity in pregnant women suggested by the Society of Maternal and Fetal Medicine (SMFM) is given in **Table 1**.

Testing Strategy in Pregnant Women

Testing for the COVID-19 is guided by the recommendations of Indian Council of Medical Research (ICMR) and various professional organizations. Following group of pregnant women can be tested:

- When they present to hospital for delivery or any other obstetric procedure. However, admission or emergency

TABLE 1: Classification of disease severity in pregnant women.

Severity	Criteria
Asymptomatic	Only test positive; no signs, and symptoms
Mild	Upper respiratory tract symptoms and/or fever, no shortness of breath or hypoxia
Moderate	Breathlessness or RR > 24/min OR SpO_2 90% to < 93% on room air
Severe	Breathlessness, RR > 30/min OR SpO_2 < 90% on room air

procedures (e.g., emergency cesarean section) should not be delayed while awaiting the test report.
- For pregnant women who do not need admission in the hospital for obstetric indication, the testing strategy recommended for nonpregnant individuals can be followed. This includes:
  - Individuals with symptoms suggestive of COVID-19, direct contact with a laboratory-confirmed case and returning after travel into an area with high test positivity (>10%), containment zone or an area with transmission of "variant of concern".

The gold standard test is real-time polymerase chain reaction (RT-PCR). However, it may take 18–36 hours to get the results. If available, tests like TrueNat and Cartridge-based Nucleic Acid Amplification Test (CBNAAT) are considered equivalent to RT-PCR. If a facility for RT-PCR or similar test is not available, a rapid antigen test (RAT) can be performed. RAT has also been found useful for quick identification of infected individuals before OPD consultation and before emergency procedures while awaiting the results of RT-PCR.

Testing should not be repeated as a discharge criterion. For individuals who are hospitalized, testing should not be done more than once a week. No emergency procedure or delivery should be delayed due to lack of test. Also, no referral should be done for non-availability of tests. Arrangements should be made for the collection and transfer of samples to testing centers.

Effect on Pregnancy and Fetus

Pregnant women with COVID-19 are at increased risk of not only severe infection but also various pregnancy complications, e.g., preeclampsia/eclampsia, gestational diabetes, and thrombosis. These conditions increase the risk of hospitalization, admission to the intensive care unit, and death. These adverse effects are more pronounced in symptomatic women and in the third trimester. Increased maternal age, obesity, any pre-existing maternal comorbidity, chronic hypertension, pre-existing diabetes and preeclampsia have been associated with severe COVID-19 in pregnancy. Fetal effects of COVID-19 in pregnancy include increased risk for stillbirth, intrauterine growth restriction, and preterm birth. These fetal complications are also more likely among symptomatic than asymptomatic women. At present, most reports of fetal outcome are from infection during the second or third trimester of the pregnancy. Sparse data available does not support teratogenic effects of SARS-CoV-2 infection. However, further studies are needed to evaluate the fetal effects of the infection during the first trimester. In addition, certain drugs used in treatment of COVID-19 have teratogenic potential and careful evaluation of risk-benefit ratio is needed before their use.

Management of COVID in Pregnancy

Admission to Hospital

The Government of India has defined different levels of healthcare facilities for management of COVID positive persons. These include COVID care centers (CCC), dedicated COVID health centers (DCHC) and dedicated COVID hospitals (DCH). The designated health facilities where SARS-CoV-2 positive pregnant women are admitted should be equipped with obstetrics and neonatal care. In large facilities, three demarcated zones—(1) clean, (2) potentially contaminated, and (3) contaminated, each housing all the required equipment and services should be organized for the management of non-COVID, suspected and confirmed COVID-19 pregnancies. Referral pathway for admission of pregnant women with complications like preterm labor, obstructed labor or eclampsia should be identified.

Indications of admission: Asymptomatic and mild infections can be managed at home. However, due to higher risk of complications as described above, home quarantined pregnant women need to be monitored. For this they should be enrolled in a teleconsultation monitoring program with active surveillance of their condition. In case of moderate or severe disease or presence of pregnancy complications, admission to an appropriate level of health facility may be needed. Following are indications of admission of a pregnant women with COVID-19:
- Labor or need of termination of pregnancy (based on obstetric indications)
- Obstetric complications needing admission
- Moderate or severe COVID illness
- Mild COVID-19 illness but monitoring by teleconsultation is not available
- Socioeconomic conditions do not allow appropriate monitoring and management at home

Mode and Timing of Delivery

During the initial phase of the pandemic, cesarean section was the most common mode of delivery in women with COVID-19. However, accumulating evidence shows that mode of delivery should be guided not by COVID status but by obstetric indications and physiological stability (cardiorespiratory status and oxygenation). COVID status itself is not an indication for induction of labor or cesarean section. If a critically ill pregnant woman is having refractory hypoxemia, cesarean section may be indicated for better management of respiratory failure.

Timing of delivery should be individualized and based on the disease severity, pregnancy complications, medical comorbidities, and the gestation. In asymptomatic and mild disease, delivery should not be delayed or advanced just due to SARS-CoV-2 positive status. In severe and critical disease, a multi-disciplinary team consisting of obstetrician, intensivist, pulmonologist, internist and neonatologist should assess and to make a decision along with the family. Termination of pregnancy may be indicated, if it is expected that it may improve respiratory status of the woman. On the other hand, pregnancy may be continued, if there is no imminent threat to maternal and fetal life.

Management of COVID in Pregnancy

Based on guidelines of the Government of India, SMFM and NNF-FOGSI-IAP, the medical management of COVID in pregnancy is summarized in **Table 2**.

Use of corticosteroids:
- *If indicated for fetal lung maturity*: Dexamethasone 6 mg IM every 12 hours for four doses, irrespective of maternal COVID-19 status.
- *If indicated for management of COVID in pregnant women but not for fetal lung maturity*: Methylprednisolone or Prednisolone or Hydrocortisone in equivalent doses indicated for COVID for 10 days or until discharge, whichever is earlier.
- *If indicated for both management of COVID in pregnant women and for fetal lung maturity*: Dexamethasone 6 mg IM every 12 hours for four doses (2 days) followed by methylprednisolone or prednisolone or hydrocortisone in equivalent doses for 8 more days or until discharge whichever is earlier.

TABLE 2: Medical management of COVID in pregnancy.

Disease severity	Suggested management

Asymptomatic or mild illness	• Home isolation
	• Home care comprises supportive measures, e.g., hydration, adequate rest, and frequent ambulation with physical activity as tolerated
	• No role of hydroxychloroquine, chloroquine, ivermectin, or azithromycin
	• Enrolment in teleconsultation program
	• Delay next antenatal physical visit till completion of the mandated quarantine period
	• Monitor fetal well-being by daily fetal movement count
	• Look for following warning signs
	  – Unremitting fever >39°C despite appropriate use of paracetamol
	  – Inability to tolerate liquids
	  – Persistent pleuritic chest pain
	  – Confusion
	  – Any obstetric complications
	  – Respiratory rate ≥20–24 breaths/min
	  – Heart rate >100 beats per minute
	  – Oxygen saturation less than 95%

Moderate or severe illness	• *Admit*: Admission in dedicated COVID hospital having adult HDU/ICU with a multidisciplinary team including obstetrician, critical care experts, infectious disease specialists, and trained nursing team • *Blood and radiological investigations* as indicted for maternal illness. Do not withhold for risk to fetus if needed for management of the woman • *Monitor fetal well-being* by weekly biophysical profile and twice a week non-stress test in stable patients • *Oxygen therapy*: Maintain SpO$_2$ ≥ 95% • *Prone position*: Awake prone positioning can be performed in the left lateral decubitus position or the fully prone position. Padding above and below the gravid uterus >24 weeks to offload the uterus and avoid aortocaval compression • *Antipyretics*: Paracetamol • *Venous thromboembolism prophylaxis*: Prophylactic-dose anticoagulation is recommended for pregnant patients hospitalized for moderate to severe COVID-19 and continued for 10 days following hospital discharge, if there are no contraindications to its use. Women with persistent morbidity should be reassessed for a longer duration of thromboprophylaxis • *Remedesivir*: Use as per GoI guidelines in "select moderate/severe hospitalized COVID-19 patients on supplemental oxygen" • *Interleukin-6 receptor antagonist (anti-IL6) Tocilizumab*: Do not withhold if indicated combination. Discuss potential benefits and risks with family • *Convalescent plasma*: No role • No role of hydroxychloroquine, chloroquine, ivermectin, or azithromycin • *Monoclonal antibody (bamlanivimab-etesevimab and casirivimab-imdevimab)*: Do not withhold, if indicated combination. Discuss potential benefits and risks with family • *Corticosteroids*: Refer to detailed recommendation in text

SARS-COV-2 INFECTION IN NEONATES

Incidence and Testing Strategy

A neonate may get SARS-CoV-2 infection from following sources:
- Vertical transmission through hematogenous route (transplacental intrauterine infection)
- Vertical transmission from exposure to maternal body fluids at the time of delivery (intrapartum infection).
- Horizontal transmission through aerosols or direct contact with body fluids in postnatal period from mother, family, community or healthcare providers.

Transmission of infection through breast milk has not been proven.

NNF-FOGSI-IAP guidelines recommend following classification to differentiate between horizontal and vertical transmission:
- *Vertical transmission*: Positive nasopharyngeal virological test (RT-PCR or RAT) in a neonate during the first 72 hours after birth. This includes intrauterine and intrapartum transmission. Testing may be avoided in the first 12 hours to minimize detection of false positives due to superficial colonization.
- *Horizontal transmission*: Negative virological test within the first 72 hours AND positive virological test any time after 72 hours of birth, irrespective of the mother's SARS-CoV-2 status.

Incidence of vertical transmission to the fetus is very low. Overall incidence of neonatal infection varies from 0.5 to 13% (median 2%). However, true incidence of infection may be higher as not all neonates in the reported studies were tested in the later neonatal period (when horizontal transmission occurs) and most of infected neonates are asymptomatic.

Testing strategy in neonates: Testing for the COVID-19 is guided by the recommendations of ICMR and various professional organizations. Following neonates can be tested:
- *Suspected perinatal transmission*: Neonates born to women with COVID-19 detected within 14 days before or within 2 days after delivery should be tested between 24 and 48 hours of age.
- *Postnatal history of exposure to persons with COVID-19*: Neonates exposed to a SARS-CoV-2 positive person should be tested once between day 5 and 10 of coming in contact.
- *Symptomatic neonates*: Neonates presenting with symptoms or signs suggestive of COVID-19 (see Effect on Neonate next) should be tested at the time of presentation.

RT-PCR for SARS-CoV-2 is the test of choice. However, if RT-PCR is not available, point of care tests including TruNat/CBNAAT or RAT can be used for triaging and rapid diagnosis.

Effect on Neonate

Most neonates are likely to be asymptomatic or develop mild illness. A proposed classification of disease severity is presented in **Table 3**. As bacterial pneumonia-sepsis-meningitis is more common than COVID-19 in neonates, it is important to investigate and manage the systemic sepsis till it is ruled out in neonates presenting with symptoms or signs of moderate to severe disease in neonates.

Multisystem inflammatory syndrome-neonatal (MIS-N): MIS-N is a rare effect of maternal COVID-19 infection and is hypothesized to result from neonatal hyper-immune response to the SARS-CoV-2 specific maternal IgG antibodies transferred across the placenta. Manifestation of MIS-N can vary from mild to severe and may include severe multiorgan dysfunction, including myocarditis, pericardial effusion, disseminated intravascular coagulation, hypoxemia, acute kidney injury, diarrhea, necrotizing enterocolitis like illness and skin ulceration. World Health Organization's definition of MIS-N includes the following:
- Children and adolescents 0–19 years of age with fever > 3 days
  AND
- Two of the following:
  - Rash or bilateral nonpurulent conjunctivitis or mucocutaneous inflammation signs (oral, hands, or feet).
  - Hypotension or shock.
  - Features of myocardial dysfunction, pericarditis, valvulitis, or coronary abnormalities (including ECHO findings or elevated Troponin/NT-proBNP).
  - Evidence of coagulopathy (by PT, PTT, elevated d-Dimers).
  - Acute gastrointestinal problems (diarrhea, vomiting, or abdominal pain).

TABLE 3: Classification of neonatal COVID-19 severity.

Severity	Criteria
Mild	Fever, rhinorrhea, cough, diarrhea, vomiting AND No tachypnea or respiratory distress or hypoxia
Moderate	Tachypnea (respiratory rate >60/minute) OR hypoxia (SpO$_2$ 90–94%) in room air) AND No signs of severe disease
Severe	Any of the following: • *Pneumonia with any of these*: SpO$_2$ < 90%, grunting or chest retractions • *CNS features*: Lethargy, refusal to feed or seizures • Severe diarrhea and/or vomiting leading to dehydration • Critical disease if any of the following is present • ARDS • Shock • Multiorgan dysfunction syndrome • Acute thrombosis

(CNS: central nervous system; ARDS: acute respiratory distress syndrome)

AND
- Elevated markers of inflammation such as ESR, C-reactive protein, or procalcitonin.
AND
- No other obvious microbial cause of inflammation, including bacterial sepsis, staphylococcal or streptococcal shock syndromes.
AND
- Evidence of COVID-19 (RT-PCR, antigen test, or serology positive) or likely contact with patients with COVID-19.

Resuscitation and Immediate Postnatal Care

Resuscitation and immediate postnatal care of neonates born to SARS-CoV-2 positive pregnant women should adhere to the following guidelines:
- The neonatal resuscitation should be conducted following the standard neonatal resuscitation program (NRP) guidelines.
- The team attending neonatal resuscitation should wear full PPE including full face shield or goggles and N95 mask.
- Delayed cord clamping has not been associated with increased risk of infection transmission to the neonate and therefore should be practiced, if indicated as per NRP.
- Risk-benefit ratio favors performing immediate skin-to-skin contact.
- If mother and baby are stable breastfeeding should be initiated within 30 minutes of birth.

Place of Care and Breastfeeding

Breastfeeding has not been associated with increased risk of transmission of COVID from mother to baby. Rooming-in is an important intervention to initiate and sustain breastfeeding.
- *If both mother and baby are stable and gestation at birth is > 33 weeks*: The neonate should be roomed-in with the mother. The mother-baby dyad must be isolated from uninfected mothers and neonates. When roomed-in, exclusive breastfeeding must be promoted. Formula feeding and mixed feeding must be avoided. Mother should wash hands frequently including before breastfeeding and wear an appropriate mask. Kangaroo mother care can be provided to stable low-birth-weight neonates.
- *If the mother is sick but the baby is stable and gestation at birth is > 33 weeks*: The neonate should be shifted to a "Well baby COVID postnatal ward" or similar designated area in SNCU. Such a neonate can be cared for by a healthy uninfected family member. If possible due to maternal condition, expressed breast milk can be given.
- *If the baby is sick or gestation at birth is < 34 weeks*: Baby should be shifted to a COVID SNCU/NICU. Symptomatic neonates with suspected SARS-CoV-2 infection should be isolated from other healthy mothers and neonates. Further, if possible neonates with confirmed and suspected infection should be kept in separate areas. Based on neonatal and maternal conditions, expressed breast milk can be given.

Management of COVID in Neonates

Based on NNF-FOGSI-IAP guidelines, the medical management of COVID in neonates is summarized in **Table 4**.

Discharge, Immunization, and Follow-up

Stable neonates exposed to SARS-CoV-2 infection and roomed-in with their mothers can be discharged along with their mothers. Stable neonates in whom rooming-in is not possible because of the sickness in the mother and who are being cared for by a trained family member, may be discharged from the facility by 24–48 hours of age. Early discharge to home should be followed by telephonic follow-up or home visit by a designated healthcare worker. Mothers and family members should be counseled regarding the danger signs. If the neonate develops any danger signs during home isolation, he/she should be taken to a designated hospital. Mothers and family members should wear a triple-layered

TABLE 4: Management of COVID in neonates.

Severity	Management
Asymptomatic or mild	• No laboratory testing or specific management • Monitor vitals • Continue routine care as for an uninfected neonate
Moderate or severe COVID-19 illness	• Blood and radiological investigations as indicated to monitor the disease's progression. These investigations include chest X-ray, complete blood counts, C-reactive protein (CRP), procalcitonin, IL-6, ferritin, and coagulation profile. Interpret test reports based on gestation and postnatal age based normative data • No role of remdesivir, lopinavir/ritonavir, chloroquine/hydroxychloroquine, ivermectin, or interferon • *Corticosteroids*: If severe disease: Dexamethasone: 0.15 mg/kg once daily for 5–14 days (alternates with equivalent doses include: 3.75 mg/kg hydrocortisone or 0.8 mg/kg methylprednisolone or 1 mg/kg prednisolone)

mask, follow respiratory etiquettes and wash their hands frequently including before touching and feeding the baby. Routine immunization policy should be followed in healthy neonates born to mothers with suspected/confirmed COVID-19. In neonates with suspected/confirmed infection, vaccination should be completed before discharge from the hospital. Administration of IVIG or corticosteroids is not a reason to delay the vaccination.

CHAPTER AT A GLANCE

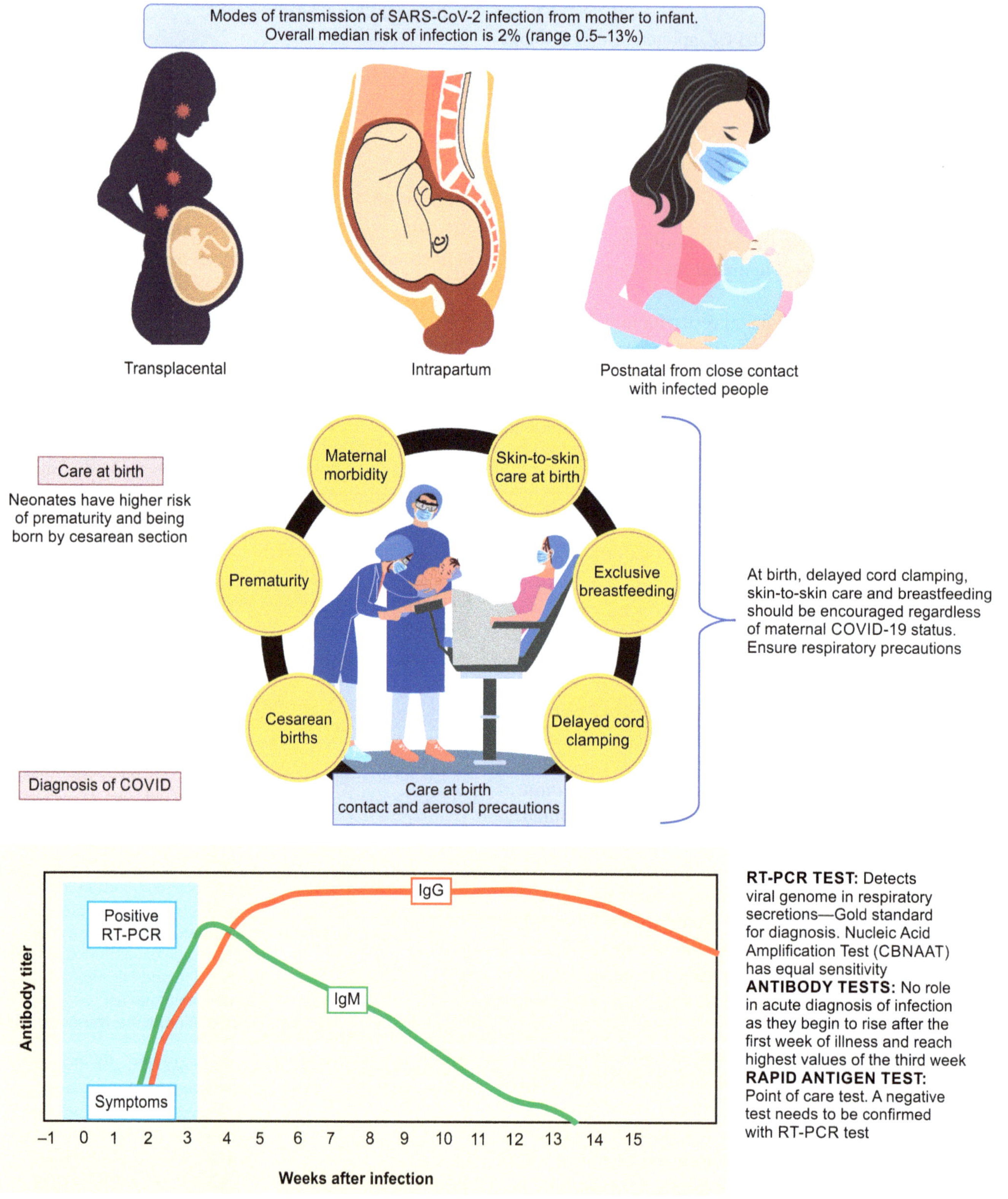

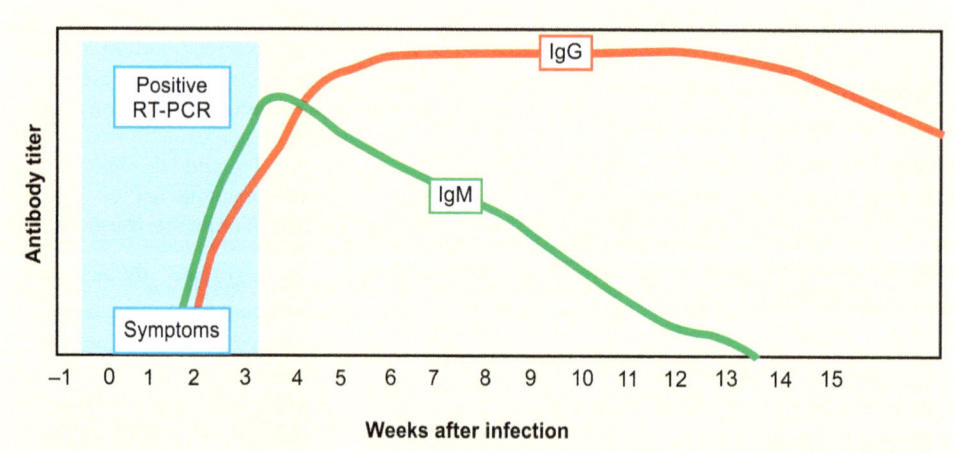

KEY POINTS

- SARS-CoV-2 infection is usually mild or asymptomatic in pregnant women. However, in comparison to noninfected women, infected women are at higher risk of severe disease and obstetric complications including preterm birth.
- SARS-CoV-2 positive pregnant women under home-isolation should be actively monitored by a tele-consultation program.
- Disease severity should be classified and appropriate management should be followed in pregnant women with SARS-CoV-2 infection.
- Vertical transmission from mother to neonate is rare. Risk of horizontal transmission after birth can be minimized by following droplet and contact precautions.
- Resuscitation of neonates born to SARS-CoV-2 positive women should follow standard NRP. Delayed cord clamping and early skin-to-skin contact can be practiced.
- Stable healthy neonates born to SARS-CoV-2 positive women should be roomed in with their mothers. Exclusive breastfeeding should be promoted.
- Neonates born to SARS-CoV-2 positive women should be tested once by RT-PCR at 24–48 hours of birth, before discharge from the hospital.

SUGGESTED READING

1. Allotey J, Stallings E, Bonet M, Yap M, Chatterjee S, Kew T, et al. Clinical manifestations, risk factors, and maternal and perinatal outcomes of coronavirus disease 2019 in pregnancy: Living systematic review and meta-analysis. BMJ (Clinical Research Ed.). 2020;370:m3320.
2. Chawla D, Chirla D, Dalwai S, Deorari AK, Ganatra A, Gandhi A, et al. National Neonatology Forum, India, Federation of Obstetric & Gynaecological Societies of India and Indian Academy of Pediatrics. Perinatal-Neonatal Management of COVID-19 Ver.3.0. Indian Pediatr. 2020;57(6):536-48.
3. Indian Council of Medical Research. Advisory on strategy for COVID-19 testing in India. Available from https://www.icmr.gov.in/cteststrat.html. [Last accessed June, 2021].
4. Ministry of Health and Family Welfare Government of India. Clinical management protocol for COVID-19 (In Adults). Version 6. Dated: May 24, 2021. Available from https://www.mohfw.gov.in/pdf/UpdatedDetailedClinicalManagementProtocolforCOVID19adultsdated24052021.pdf. [Last accessed November, 2021].
5. More K, Chawla D, Murki S, Tandur B, Deorari AK, Kumar P, et al.; National Neonatology Forum (NNF) COVID-19 Registry Group. Outcomes of neonates born to mothers with coronavirus disease 2019 (COVID-19) - National neonatology forum (NNF) India COVID-19 registry. Indian Pediatr. 2021;58(6):525-31.
6. Sivanandan S, Chawla D, Kumar P, Deorari AK. COVID-19 in neonates: A call for standardized testing. Indian Pediatr. 2020;57(12):1166-71.
7. Society for Maternal-Fetal Medicine. Management Considerations for Pregnant Patients With COVID-19. Version 2.2.21. Dated: February 02, 2021. Available from https://s3.amazonaws.com/cdn.smfm.org/media/2734/SMFM_COVID_Management_of_COVID_pos_preg_patients_2-2-21_(final).pdf. [Last accessed November, 2021].

SECTION 6
Delivery Room Management

Sindhu Sivanandan, Anish Keepanasseril

- **Neonatal Resuscitation**
  Aparna Chandrasekaran, Pujitha Devi Suraneni

- **Umbilical Cord Management**
  Sindhu Sivanandan, Yavana Suriya Venkatesh

- **Perinatal Asphyxia**
  Rajendra Prasad Anne, Avantika Gupta

- **Care at Birth**
  Manikumar S, Thenmozhi G

- **Postnatal Care and Discharge Planning**
  Tanushree Sahoo, Abhishek S Aradhya, Monica Gupta

- **Surgical Conditions Presenting at Birth**
  Srishti Goel, Vikram Khanna

- **Birth Trauma**
  Chanchal Kumar, S Thanigainathan, Charu Sharma

- **Ethical and Medicolegal Issues in the Perinatal Period**
  Niharika Allu, Femitha Pournami

CHAPTER 42

Neonatal Resuscitation

Aparna Chandrasekaran, Pujitha Devi Suraneni

INTRODUCTION

Approximately 10% of neonates will need some assistance at birth, and 1% may need extensive resuscitation at birth. Perinatal asphyxia, currently rephrased as intrapartum-related events, remains one of the three leading causes of neonatal mortality. This chapter elaborates on the current best evidence-based recommendations for neonatal resuscitation, based on the 7th edition of the International Liaison Committee on Resuscitation (ILCOR) guidelines published in 2015 and the American Heart Academy (AHA) update in 2020.

OBJECTIVES

To understand the following:
- Steps of preparation at birth
- Routine care
- Placental transfusion
- Initial steps
- Positive pressure ventilation
- *Advanced steps*: Intubations, chest compressions, and medications
- Special situations
- Postresuscitation care

STEPS OF PREPARATION AT BIRTH

Assessment of Maternal Risk Factors

Readiness for neonatal resuscitation requires assessing perinatal risk factors (**Table 1**), a system to assemble the appropriately trained personnel based on that risk, an organized method for ensuring immediate access to supplies and equipment coupled with a checklist and standardization of behavioral skills to ensure effective teamwork and communication.

The questions that must be asked before every delivery are:
- What is the gestational age at delivery?
- Is the amniotic fluid clear?
- Is it multiple pregnancies? If so, how many babies are expected?
- Are there any additional risk factors?

The question on "Umbilical cord management plan?" has replaced the number of babies expected in the NRP, 8th edition. The additional risk factors are summarized in **Table 1**. Every birth should be attended by at least one person who is trained in the initial steps of newborn resuscitation and positive-pressure ventilation (PPV). In the presence of significant perinatal risk factors, additional personnel trained in performing advanced steps such as chest compressions, endotracheal (ET) intubation, and umbilical vein catheter insertion should be immediately available. The risk factors are summarized in **Table 1**.

Team Preparation

Once the required number of skilled personnel has been assembled, they must plan the following steps:

TABLE 1: Perinatal risk factors.

Antepartum risk factors
- Gestational age < $36^{0/7}$ weeks
- Gestational age ≥ $41^{0/7}$ weeks
- Preeclampsia or eclampsia
- Maternal hypertension
- Multiple gestation
- Fetal anemia
- Polyhydramnios
- Oligohydramnios
- Fetal hydrops
- Fetal macrosomia
- Intrauterine growth restriction
- Significant fetal malformations or anomalies
- No prenatal care

Intrapartum risk factors
- Emergency cesarean delivery
- Forceps or vacuum-assisted delivery
- Breech or other abnormal presentation
- Category II or III fetal heart rate pattern
- Maternal general anesthesia
- Maternal magnesium therapy
- Placental abruption
- Intrapartum bleeding
- Chorioamnionitis
- Narcotics administered to mother within 4 hours of delivery
- Shoulder dystocia
- Meconium-stained amniotic fluid
- Prolapsed umbilical cord

TABLE 2: Equipment checklist for neonatal resuscitation.		
Thermal care	• Preheated warmer switched on at least 20 minutes before delivery • Warm towels or blankets (at least 2) • Temperature sensor and sensor cover for prolonged resuscitation • Hat • Plastic bag or plastic wrap (<32 weeks' gestation) • Thermal mattress (<32 weeks' gestation)	
Airway	• 10 F or 12 F suction catheter attached to wall suction, set at 80–100 mm Hg • 6 F and 8 F suction catheters for endotracheal suction • Meconium aspirator	
Assessment	Stethoscope and pulse oximeter with sensor and cover	
Ventilation	• Oxygen blender set to 21% (21–30% if <35 weeks' gestation) • Positive-pressure ventilation (PPV) device – self-inflating bag or T-piece resuscitator • Term- and preterm-sized masks • 8 F feeding tube and a large syringe	
Oxygenation	• Oxygen flow meter with tubings/nasal cannula • Target oxygen saturation table	
Intubation	• Laryngoscope with size-0 and size-1 straight blades (size 00, optional) • Endotracheal tubes (sizes 2.5, 3.0, 3.5) • Measuring tape and endotracheal tube insertion depth table • Waterproof tape or tube-securing device • Scissors • Laryngeal mask (size 1) and 5-mL syringe	
Medication	• 1:10,000 (0.1 mg/mL) epinephrine • Normal saline • Umbilical venous catheter, three way stop cock, blade, cord tie, skin scrub solution • Electronic cardiac (ECG) monitor leads and ECG monitor	
Miscellaneous	Cord clamp, scissors, ID tag	

- *Identify the team leader, assign roles and responsibilities (prebriefing)*: Any member who is skilled and exhibits leadership qualities can be a team leader. The team leader should possess good communication skills and facilitate all team members to participate in the resuscitation process.
- *Counseling of the parents*: A senior team member must preferably do antenatal counseling in extreme preterm gestation (≤28 weeks' gestation) or identify high-risk factors. It is essential to provide important information on outcomes, discuss options, and informed decision-making.
- *Prepare equipment*: One must assemble all equipment per the checklist and check their optimal functionality (**Table 2** and **Figs. 1A to D**).
- *Postresuscitation team debriefing*: To help to identify areas for improvement

Equipment Check

The radiant warmer needs to be preheated in manual mode with 100% heater output before delivery. The functioning of a wall-mounted suction device, self-inflating bag, laryngoscopes, and "T" piece resuscitator must be performed ahead of the neonate's delivery (**Figs. 1A to D**). It is recommended to use a checklist to ensure the timely availability of all equipment.

Asepsis and Precautions

All members of the team must perform hand washing, wear sterile gloves, and an apron. Use masks, goggles, face shields, and impervious aprons in high-risk cases [maternal hepatitis B or C, human immunodeficiency virus (HIV) or severe acute respiratory syndrome coronavirus 2 (SARS-CoV-2 infection)]. **Flowchart 1** summarizes the steps of neonatal resuscitation as per the ILCOR 2015.

ASSESSMENT AT BIRTH

Questions to be Asked at Birth

Newly born infants requiring resuscitation can be generally identified by rapidly assessing the answers to the question:
- Is the baby breathing or crying? A baby who is not breathing well or is gasping requires intervention.
- Is the baby born term?
- Does the baby have a good muscle tone?
  If the answer to the questions is "yes," the newly born infant may stay with the mother for routine care. Observation of breathing, activity, and color must continue.
  If the answer to any of the questions is "No," the infant should proceed to initial steps on the radiant warmer and receive one or more of the following actions in sequence:

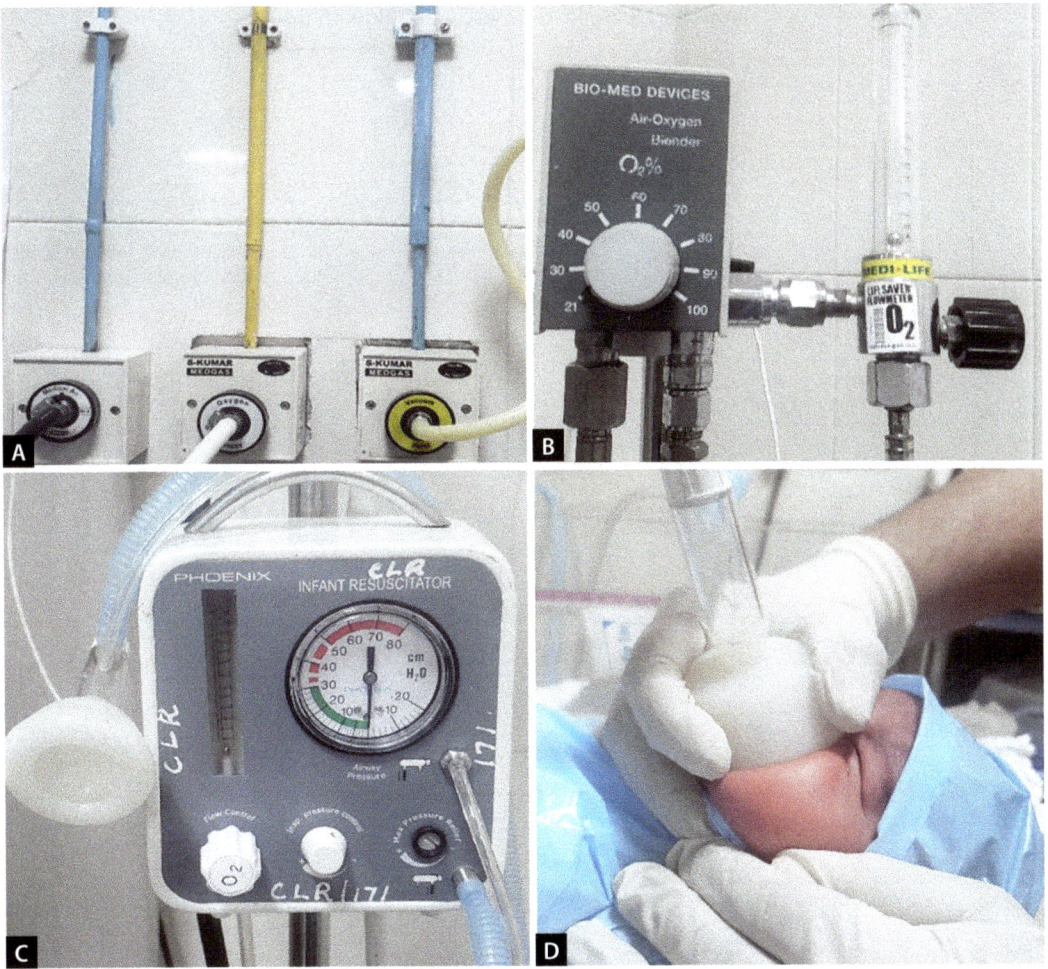

Figs. 1A to D: Equipment preparation before resuscitation. (A) Air, oxygen, and suction ports; (B) Blender and flow meter; (C) T-piece resuscitator; (D) Neonate receiving delivery room continuous positive airway pressure (CPAP) using T-piece device.

- Initial steps in stabilization (warm and maintain normal temperature, position, clear secretions only if copious and or obstructing the airway, dry, stimulate).
- Ventilate and oxygenate
- Initiate chest compressions
- Administer epinephrine and volume

ROUTINE CARE

If the answer to all three above rapid evaluation questions is "Yes" (term neonate, breathing at birth, and good muscle tone), the baby can remain with the mother and have routine care performed on the mother's chest or abdomen. Warmth is maintained by direct skin-to-skin contact and covering the baby with warm linen. If necessary, secretions in the upper airway can be cleared by wiping the baby's mouth and nose with a cloth. Gentle suction with a bulb syringe should be reserved for babies that have meconium-stained fluid, secretions that are obstructing breathing, and those that are having difficulty clearing their secretions. After these steps, continue monitoring the newborn's breathing, tone, activity, color, and temperature every 15 minutes in the first 1 hour.

PLACENTAL TRANSFUSION AND DELAYED CORD CLAMPING

Placental transfusion in the form of delayed cord clamping has innumerable benefits to the neonate. It is recommended to delay the cord clamping for at least 30–60 seconds in all neonates who do not require resuscitation. Cord milking should not be done in neonates <28 weeks. Resuscitation with intact cord using mobile resuscitation trolleys in depressed neonates is under evaluation.

INITIAL STEPS

If the answer to any of the three questions is "No" (preterm, not breathing, or poor tone), one must proceed to "initial steps." The initial steps and the subsequent assessment should be *completed within 60 seconds of birth* **(Fig. 2)**.

- *Provide warmth*: Place the neonate under a radiant warmer. Ensure that the neonate's body temperature is maintained between 36.5 and 37.5°C. Attach the temperature sensor to the baby's skin and switch the warmer to servo-controlled mode.

SECTION 6 | Delivery Room Management

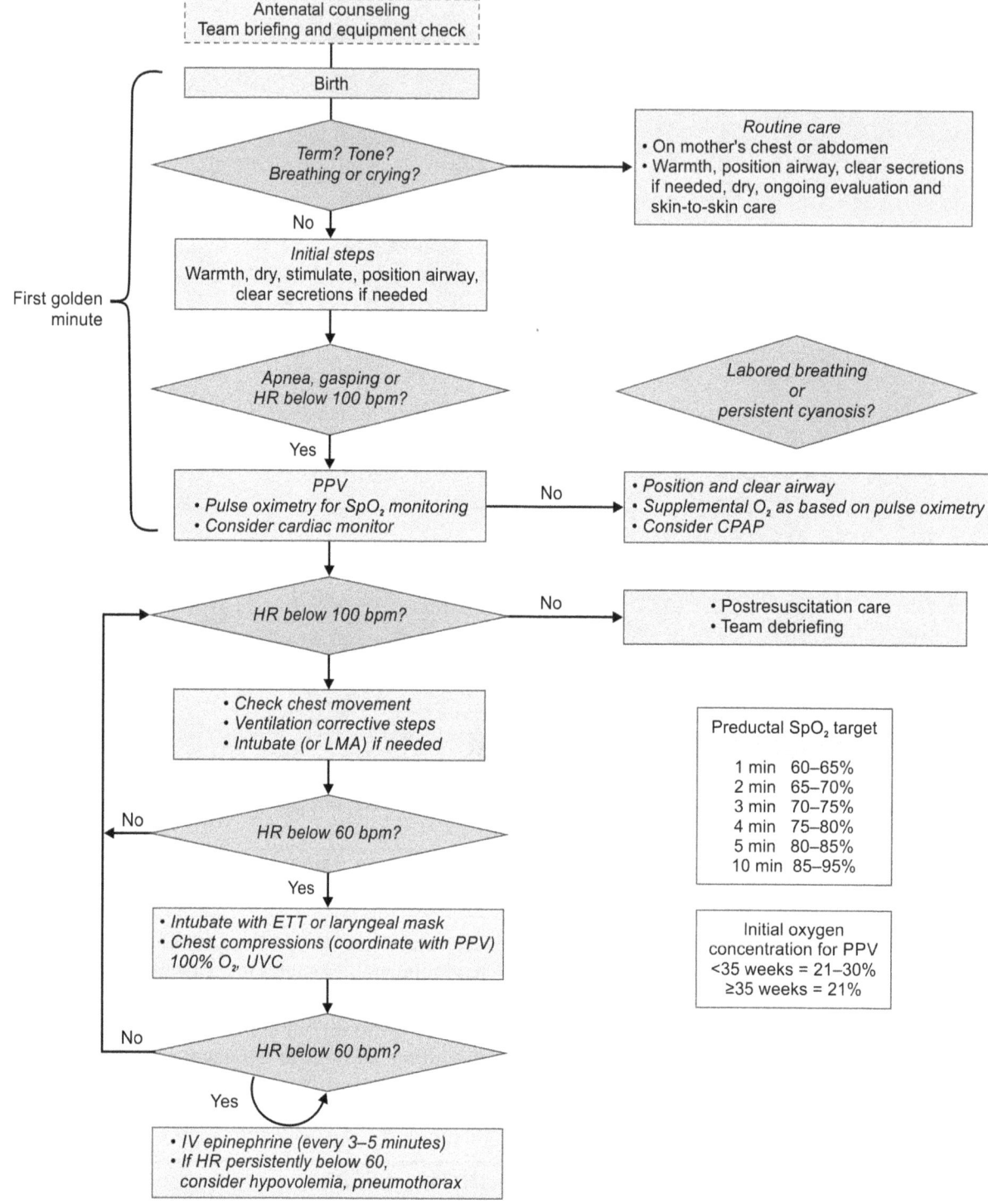

Flowchart 1: Neonatal resuscitation algorithm.

(bpm: beats/min; CPAP: continuous positive airway pressure; ETT: endotracheal tube; HR: heart rate; ILCOR: International Liaison Committee on Resuscitation; IV: intravenous; LMA: laryngeal mask airway; PPV: positive pressure ventilation; UVC: umbilical venous catheter)
Source: Adapted from ILCOR 2021

- *Dry the neonate* using dry, warm linen. Remove the wet linen immediately. For babies, <32 weeks' gestation, cover immediately in a plastic sheet before drying.
- *Tactile stimulation* may be provided by gentle rubbing of the back.
- *Position* the head and neck *to open the airway* in neutral or slightly extended in the sniffing position.
- *Clear secretions (only if necessary):* Gently suction the *mouth followed by the nose* using a 12–14 F suction catheter connected to 80–100 mm Hg negative pressure if the baby is not breathing, if secretions are obstructing

the airway, if there is meconium-stained fluid or before starting PPV.

Thermal care

- The admission temperature of newly born infants is a strong predictor of mortality. Hypothermia is also associated with morbidities such as the increased risk of intraventricular hemorrhage, respiratory distress, hypoglycemia, and late-onset sepsis.
- It is recommended that the temperature be maintained between 36.5 and 37.5°C after birth. The use of radiant warmers and plastic wrap with a cap in combination with other strategies, including increased room temperature, thermal mattresses, and the use of warmed humidified resuscitation gases, may be reasonable to prevent hypothermia in infants born at <32 weeks of gestation (**Fig. 3**). Delivery room temperature must be >25°C.

MANAGEMENT OF NEONATES BORN THROUGH MECONIUM-STAINED AMNIOTIC FLUID

If the infant is vigorous, with good muscle tone and respiratory efforts, routine care can be given as in the previous section. If an infant presents with poor muscle tone and inadequate breathing efforts or heart rate < 100/min (nonvigorous), the initial steps of resuscitation should be completed as in the previous section under a radiant warmer. PPV should be initiated if the infant is apneic or the heart rate is <100/min after the initial steps are completed.

In a recent Cochrane meta-analysis comparing routine tracheal suction versus no suction in nonvigorous neonates born through meconium-stained amniotic fluid, there was no difference in the incidence of mortality or meconium aspiration syndrome (MAS). Hence, tracheal suctioning is not indicated in nonvigorous infants born through meconium-stained amniotic fluid unless there is evidence of tracheal obstruction while providing PPV. However, a team skilled in intubation should still be present in the delivery room.

ASSESSMENT OF NEONATE AFTER INITIAL STEPS

After the performance of the initial steps, we must assess
- *Breathing*: Whether the neonate has regular breathing efforts
- *Heart rate*: Auscultation of the precordium is the preferred physical examination method for the initial assessment of the heart rate. To estimate heart rate, listen with a stethoscope for 6 seconds, and multiply the number of heartbeats by 10, e.g., if 10 beats are counted in 6 seconds, the heart rate is 100 bpm. Heart rate should be above 100 bpm.

It is recommended to use a pulse oximeter for monitoring if the neonate requires beyond the initial steps (although this is more simplified in the Indian guideline (NSSK: Navjaat Shishu Suraksha Karyakram). An electrocardiogram is recommended wherever feasible.

Further steps are as follows:
- If the baby is not breathing or the heart rate is <100 bpm, initiate PPV

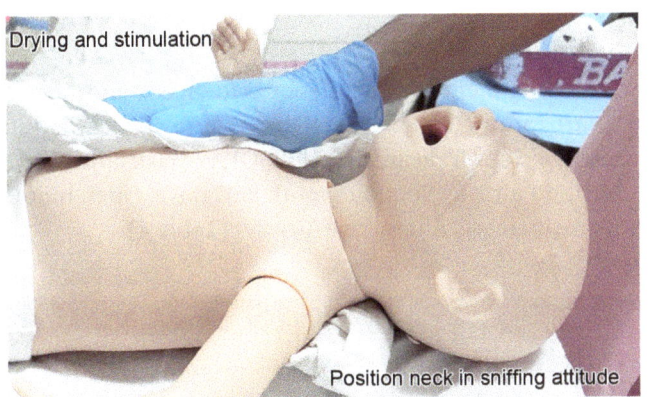

Fig. 2: Initial steps under a radiant warmer. Suction only if needed. Remove wet linen.

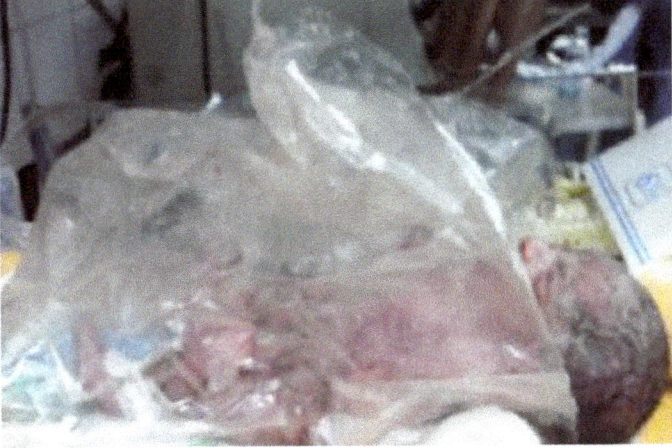
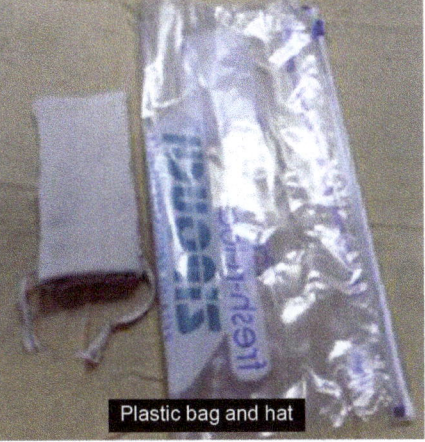

Fig. 3: Thermoregulation in preterm neonates. Preterm neonates are received in a plastic bag without drying. The plastic bag or wrap is removed in the NICU after thermal stabilization.

- If the baby is breathing and the heart rate is >100 bpm but has labored breathing, start continuous positive airway pressure (CPAP) using a T-piece resuscitator with a tight seal over the nose and mouth.
- If the baby is breathing normally with a heart rate > 100 bpm, but the SpO_2 is below the target range, free-flow oxygen can be administered targeting the minute specific oxygen saturation levels in **Figures 1A to D** using:
  - Oxygen tubing or oxygen mask held close to the baby's nose and mouth
  - T-piece resuscitator held loosely
  - Flow inflated bag and mask

POSITIVE PRESSURE VENTILATION

Indications

Neonates who do not breathe (apnea or gasping) within the first 30 seconds after birth or are persistently bradycardic (heart rate < 100/min) despite appropriate initial actions (including tactile stimulation) may receive PPV at a rate of 40–60/min. The concept of "FIRST GOLDEN MINUTE" is the time needed to ensure ventilation of the lungs. Ventilation of the lungs is the KEY step of resuscitation.

Initial Fractional Inspired Oxygen Concentration (FiO_2) to be Used

- Initially use 21% oxygen (room air) for term infants and 21–30% for preterm infants <35 weeks' gestation (increase to 100% if chest compressions are started).
- This may be done by using a blender connected to the inlet of the PPV device.

Devices for Providing Positive Pressure Ventilation

There are three devices to provide PPV: Self-inflating bag, flow inflating bag (anesthesia bag), and T-piece resuscitator.

The relative advantages and disadvantages are summarized in **Table 3**.

Assessing the Effectiveness of Positive Pressure Ventilation

- The best indicator of successful PPV is a rising heart rate.
- After initiating PPV, check the heart rate after 15 seconds (**Flowchart 2**).
- If heart rate is increasing, continue PPV and do a second assessment after another 15 seconds.
- If the heart rate is not increasing, then assess if the chest is moving.
- If the chest IS moving, continue PPV for another 15 seconds and assess the heart rate. If the chest is NOT moving, then take corrective ventilation steps immediately.
- After ventilation corrective steps are done, do a second assessment of the baby's heart rate after 30 seconds of PPV that moves the chest.

Ventilation Corrective Steps

When there is ineffective ventilation evidenced by no increase in heart rate or absent chest rise, perform ventilation-corrective steps indicated by MR SOPA (Mask adjustment, Reposition airway, Suction mouth and nose, Open mouth, Pressure increase, Alternative Airway) (**Table 4**).

TABLE 3: Positive-pressure ventilation devices.

Self-inflating bag	Flow inflating bag	T-piece resuscitator
Does not need a gas source	Needs a gas source	Needs a gas source
Cannot provide PEEP unless PEEP valve is added	Can provide PEEP and CPAP	Can provide PEEP
Cannot provide free-flow oxygen	Can provide free-flow oxygen	Can provide free-flow oxygen
PIP cannot be controlled (depends on the depth of compression of the bag)	PIP cannot be controlled	Controlled delivery of PIP

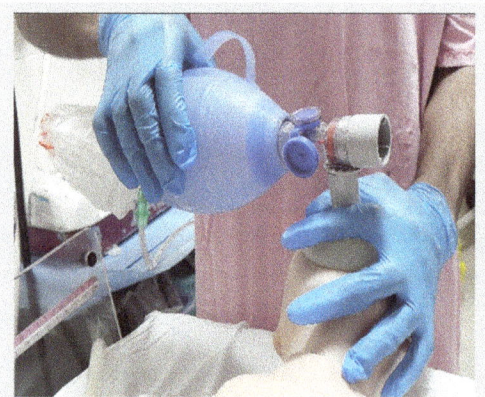
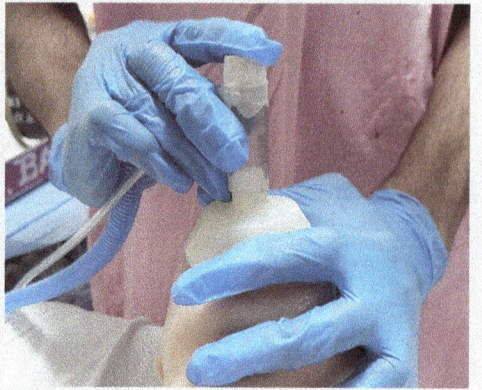

(CPAP: continuous positive airway pressure; PEEP: positive end-expiratory pressure; PIP: peak inspiratory pressure)

Endotracheal Intubation

- The indications of intubation are prolonged or ineffective bag mask ventilation while initiating chest compressions and special circumstances such as congenital diaphragmatic hernia or direct tracheal suction if thick secretions obstruct the airway.
- Use the nasotragal length (NTL) method for calculating the depth of insertion.
- Measure the distance (cm) from the baby's nasal septum to the ear tragus. Depth of insertion of ET tube can be calculated using NTL +1 cm.
- ET tubes of sizes 2.5, 3.0, and 3.5 are used in neonates. Choose the appropriate size based on weight or gestational age and birth weight.

Flowchart 2: Steps after initiating positive pressure ventilation (PPV).

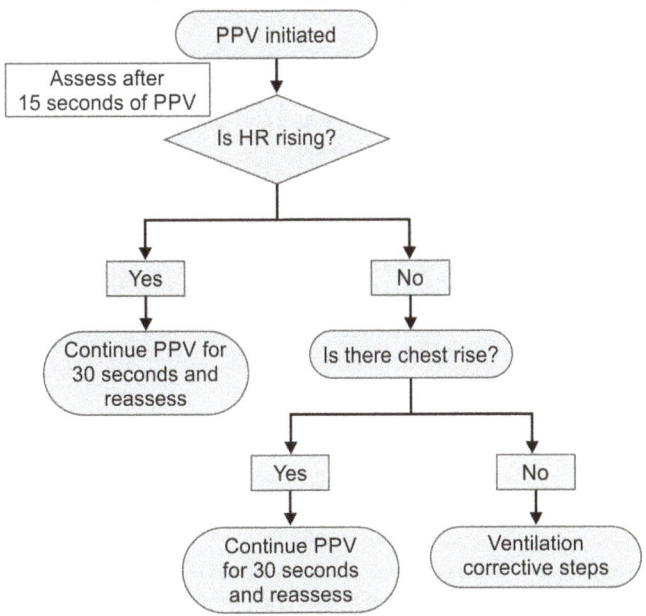

(HR: heart rate)

CHEST COMPRESSIONS

Indication

Chest compressions must be initiated when the heart rate is <60/min, despite adequate ventilation (30 seconds of PPV that moves the chest).

Technique

- Compressions are given on the lower third of the sternum to a depth of one-third of the anterior-posterior diameter of the chest. To provide this correctly, place the thumbs on the sternum below an imaginary line connecting the baby's nipples **(Fig. 4)**.
- The two-thumb technique is better than the two-finger technique, based on higher blood pressure and coronary perfusion pressure with the former with less rescuer fatigue. Importantly encircle the chest, providing support to the baby's back.
- The ratio should be 3:1 of compressions to ventilation, with 90 compressions and 30 breaths to achieve 120 events per minute. Use the phrase "One-and-Two-and-Three and-Breathe-and" while doing this to provide

	Corrective steps	Actions
TABLE 4: Ventilation-corrective measures ("MR SOPA").		
M	Mask adjustment	Reapply the mask. Consider the 2-hand technique
R	Reposition airway	Place head neutral or slightly extended
Provide five breaths PPV and reassess chest movement		
S	Suction mouth and nose	Use a bulb syringe or suction catheter
O	Open mouth	Open the mouth and lift the jaw forward
Provide 5 breaths PPV and reassess chest movement		
P	Pressure increase	Increase peak inspiratory pressure (PIP) in 5–10 cm H$_2$O increments, max. 40 cm
Provide 5 breaths PPV and reassess chest movement		
A	Alternative airway	Place an endotracheal tube or laryngeal mask
Try PPV and assess chest movement and breath sounds		

(PPV: positive pressure ventilation)

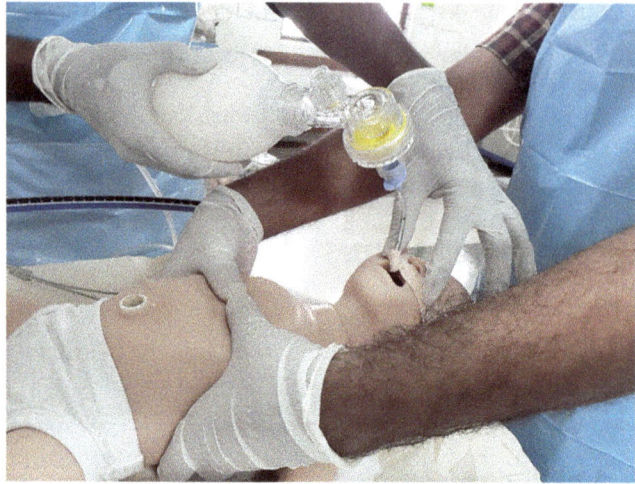

Fig. 4: Coordinated positive-pressure ventilation and chest compressions.

chest compressions when counting 1, 2, and 3 followed by release. During the "breathe" phase-deliver PPV.
- It is recommended to intubate the neonate and connect to 100% oxygen before initiating chest compressions.
- It is suggested to call for help before starting chest compression, anticipating the need for vascular access, and medications after this step.
- After 60 seconds of coordinated PPV and chest compressions, reassess the heart rate. Stop compressions if the heart rate is 60/min or higher. Otherwise, go to the next step.

MEDICATIONS

Epinephrine and normal saline are the two medications used in neonatal resuscitation.

Indications for Drugs
- If the heart rate remains <60/min despite adequate ventilation and chest compressions, administration of epinephrine is indicated.
- The recommended route of epinephrine is intravenous through the umbilical vein. However, one dose of intratracheal adrenaline may be considered in time for securing venous access.
- Volume expansion with normal saline is indicated in shock from acute blood loss (e.g., bleeding vasa previa, fetal trauma, cord accidents, fetomaternal hemorrhage) associated with persistent bradycardia and evidence of poor perfusion (like prolonged capillary fill) **(Table 5)**.

SPECIAL SITUATIONS

The critical considerations for resuscitation in special situations are summarized in **Table 6.**

TABLE 5: Drugs for neonatal resuscitation.

Drug	Epinephrine	Volume expander
Concentration	1:10,000 epinephrine (0.1 mg/mL). Do not use 1:1,000 concentration	Normal saline (0.9% NaCl) or type-O Rh-negative blood
Route	• Intravenous through the umbilical vein (preferred) • Endotracheal only while intravenous access is being obtained	Intravenous or intraosseous
Preparation	• Dilute 1:1,000 ten times: Take 1 mL of 1:1,000 solution in a 10 mL syringe and add 9 mL of Normal saline • Load this in a 1-mL syringe should be labeled "Epinephrine-IV" • 3- to 5-mL syringe should be labeled "Epinephrine-ET only"	Volume is drawn into a 30- to 60-mL syringe (labeled)
Dose	• Intravenous = 0.2 mL/kg • Endotracheal = 1 mL/kg	10 mL/kg
Administration	• Administer as quickly as possible • *Intravenous*: Flush with 0.5–1 mL normal saline • *Endotracheal*: PPV breaths to distribute into lungs	Over 5–10 minutes
Frequency	Repeat every 3–5 minutes if the heart rate remains <60 bpm	—
	Note that intraosseous administration is an alternative to the intravenous route	

POSTRESUSCITATION CARE

Neonates receiving PPV need to be monitored in a facility with a neonatal intensive care unit (NICU) for postresuscitation care. For those who are 36 weeks and more, with evidence of moderate-to-severe encephalopathy resulting from asphyxia, therapeutic hypothermia needs to be considered.

DISCONTINUATION/NONINITIATION OF RESUSCITATION

- Resuscitation may be discontinued if there are no signs of life for 20 minutes, despite all resuscitative measures and the absence of correctable causes. It is imperative to discuss the details with the team members and family before discontinuation.
- If the neonate shows any signs of life, further care and appropriate treatment need to be initiated, and continuation of care may be decided in discussion with the family.
- Resuscitation may be withheld in established conditions such as anencephaly, trisomy 13 and 18, and extreme prematurity (<24 weeks).

CHAPTER 42 | Neonatal Resuscitation

TABLE 6: Resuscitation in special situations.

COVID-19 positive mother	• Needs a separate delivery area • Use full PPE (overalls, caps, gowns, shoe covers, N95 mask, face shield) • Delayed cord clamping and skin-to-skin contact can be done as routine
Congenital diaphragmatic hernia	• Avoid bag and mask ventilation • Elective endotracheal intubation • Feeding tube and decompress the bowel • Gentle ventilation • Role of EXIT to be discussed
Hydrops fetalis	• A team of four members may be necessary • In addition to initial steps and intubation, consider pleural and ascitic tap • Saline bolus for hypovolemia
Pierre Robin sequence	• Prone position • Nasopharyngeal airway • Anticipate difficult intubation
Pneumothorax	• It can be diagnosed by auscultation with a clinical exam, transillumination, lung ultrasound, or X-ray • Needle aspiration is the emergency treatment modality
Bradycardia, despite adequate ventilation and good perfusion	Congenital heart block needs to be evaluated
Resuscitation out-of-hospital facility	• Use the same principles of resuscitation • Use plastic bags for temperature maintenance • Mouth-to-mouth needs to be considered
Extremely preterm	• Remember to have a polythene wrap, a thermal mattress, T-piece resuscitator, blender, 00 laryngoscope blades, 2.5 mm-size endotracheal tube • Wrap the baby in polythene wrap before drying • Use T-piece resuscitator to provide PPV • Blender to give 21–30% oxygen for PPV • Consider surfactant if neonate requires intubation

(PPE: personal protective equipment; PPV: positive pressure ventilation)

CHAPTER AT A GLANCE

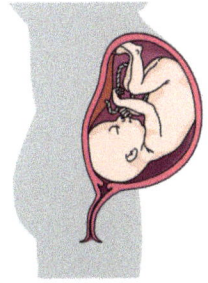

1 Four pre-birth questions
- Gestational age?
- Amniotic fluid clear?
- Additional risk factors?
- Umbilical cord management plan?

4 Dose of epinephrine
- Intravenous 0.2 mL/kg
- Endotracheal 1 mL/kg
- Dilution: 1:10,000
- Flush with 3 mL saline

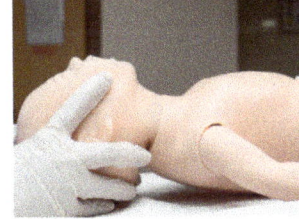

2 Initial steps
- Warm, dry, stimulate
- Position airway
- Clear secretions if necessary

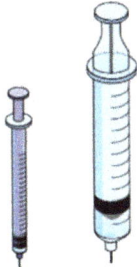

- Intravenous 0.2 ml/kg epinephrine
- Saline flush important

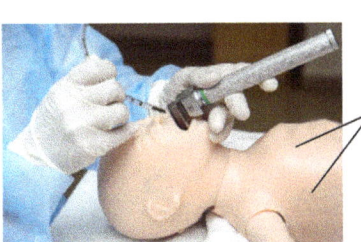

3 Cardiac monitor
When an alternate airway becomes necessary, a cardiac monitor is recommended for accurate heart rate assessment

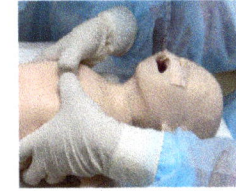

5 Cessation of resuscitation
In the confirmed absence of heart rate after complete resuscitative efforts for 20 minutes, cessation of resuscitation effort can be considered (individualized based on patient and contextual factors)

Pertinent updates in the neonatal resuscitation guidelines. Adapted from 8th edition of NRP.

KEY POINTS

- Anticipation and preparation for every birth are essential.
- Delayed cord clamping and skin-to-skin contact are essential components of routine care.
- Ventilation is the most critical step for ensuring effective ventilation.
- For preterm newborns <35 weeks of gestation, resuscitation should be initiated with 21–30% oxygen, and the oxygen concentration should be titrated to achieve target preductal saturation.
- Thermal care during resuscitation is an essential component in preterm neonates.
- For nonvigorous neonates born through meconium-stained fluid, the initial steps should be completed, followed by PPV if the infant is not breathing or the heart rate is <100 bpm. Routine endotracheal intubation is not recommended.

SUGGESTED READING

1. Aziz K, Lee HC, Escobedo MB, Hoover AV, Kamath-Rayne BD, Kapadia VS, et al. Part 5: Neonatal Resuscitation: 2020 American Heart Association Guidelines for cardiopulmonary resuscitation and emergency cardiovascular care. Circulation. 2020;142(16_suppl_2):S524-50.
2. Weiner G, Zaichkin J (Eds). Textbook of Neonatal Resuscitation, 8th edition. Dallas, TX: American Academy of Pediatrics and American Heart Association; 2021.

CHAPTER 43

Umbilical Cord Management

Sindhu Sivanandan, Yavana Suriya Venkatesh

INTRODUCTION

The placenta is the gas exchange organ of the fetus. The lungs take up this function at birth, and the alveoli hitherto filled with fluid is replaced by air. The pulmonary vascular resistance falls, and the blood flow through the lung increases. When the umbilical cord is clamped and cut at birth, the neonate is separated from the low-resistance placenta. The systemic vascular resistance increases and the entire cardiac output depends on oxygenated blood from the lungs. The smooth transition to extrauterine life can be severely impacted by cord clamping and abrupt removal of placental circulation. A delay in cord clamping facilitates placental transfusion, whereby a significant amount of blood is transferred to the neonate in the first few minutes after birth. This volume is to the tune of 80–100 mL of blood for term infants, approximately one third of total neonatal blood volume.

OBJECTIVES

- Know the physiology of placental transfusion at birth
- Understand the benefits of delayed cord clamping in term and preterm neonates
- Discuss the role of umbilical cord milking and intact cord resuscitation
- Understand cord management strategies in specific situations

PHYSIOLOGY OF PLACENTAL TRANSFUSION

Physiological Changes after Immediate Cord Clamping

The umbilical vein provides oxygenated blood from the placenta and contributes to the right ventricular (RV) filling. Following immediate umbilical cord clamping (defined as clamping the cord shortly after birth, usually within the first 15–20 seconds), the RV output falls by about 50%, significantly affecting the left ventricular (LV) output. This state of low cardiac output exists until the lungs become aerated and pulmonary blood flow increases. Studies in lambs have demonstrated that clamping the umbilical cord before ventilation is established leads to a hemodynamic imbalance with decreased systemic blood pressure, heart rate, and fluctuation in cerebral blood flow. A smooth extrauterine transition can be ensured when umbilical cord clamping is delayed (**Fig. 1**). Delayed umbilical cord clamping is defined as cord clamping at least 30–60 seconds after birth.

Factors Affecting Placental Transfusion

- *Timing of cord clamping*: At birth, the proportion of blood distributed between the infant and the placental circuits is 67% and 33%, respectively. This proportion increases to 80:20 by 1 minute (i.e., almost half of the blood is transferred by 1 minute). Thus, placental transfusion is proportional to the time cord clamping is delayed. Which further changes to 87:13 by 3–5 minutes.
- *Infant's position relative to the placenta*: The position of the baby compared to the level of the placenta (at the perineum or on the mother's chest or abdomen) does not seem to impact the volume of placental transfusion

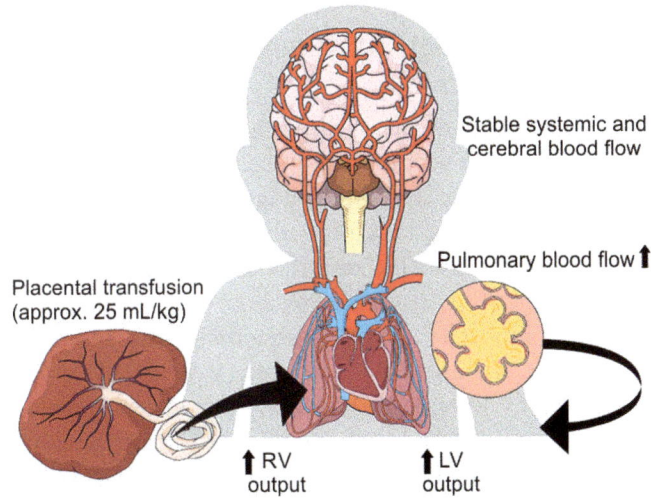

Fig. 1: Changes in transitional circulation during delayed cord clamping.
(LV: left ventricle; RV: right ventricle)

among term vaginally delivered infants if the provider waits for at least 2 minutes.
- *Infant's respiratory effort*: Sheep experiments had shown that during inspiration, the umbilical venous blood flow reduces, possibly due to an increase in intrathoracic pressure, irrespective of the mode of breathing (spontaneous or mechanical ventilation).
- *Uterine contraction*: Uterine contractions facilitate placental transfusion. The uterine contraction that delivers the fetus contributes to one third of the placental transfusion. Subsequent uterine contractions during the third stage of labor facilitate the process. Oxytocin is given at the onset of the third stage of labor accelerates placental transfusion.

CORD MANAGEMENT STRATEGIES

Delayed Cord Clamping

Given the benefits of delayed cord clamping (DCC), it is prudent to wait for at least 30–60 seconds after birth in vigorous term and preterm neonates.

Benefits of Delayed Cord Clamping in Term Neonates

The blood volume of term infants following DCC is approximately 90 mL/kg compared to 70 mL/kg following immediate cord clamping (ICC). This additional blood provides 40–50 mg/kg of extra iron. The Cochrane systematic review showed that the term infants subjected to DCC had higher birth weight (100 g higher) and hemoglobin concentration (2 g/dL) at birth. Even though the increase in hemoglobin did not persist at later assessments, the infants had higher iron stores (serum iron, total body iron, ferritin, and transferrin saturation) at 3 and 6 months. The increment in iron stores translates to 75 mg of iron or more than 3 months' requirement in a 6-month-old infant. Some studies showed that there may be a small risk of jaundice in DCC infants **(Table 1)**.

Benefits of Delayed Cord Clamping in Preterm Neonates

The Cochrane review on DCC in preterm infants showed that DCC is associated with lower in-hospital mortality, reduced risk of intraventricular hemorrhage (IVH) of all grades, stable blood pressure, and lesser need for blood transfusion **(Table 1)**. DCC did not increase the risk of jaundice requiring phototherapy. The Australian Placental Transfusion Study, the largest study enrolling 1,566 preterm infants, compared immediate clamping (≤10 seconds after delivery) to delayed clamping (≥60 seconds after delivery). The investigators did not note any difference in the composite primary outcome of death or major morbidity (severe brain injury, severe

TABLE 1: Benefits of delayed cord clamping in term and preterm infants.

Term infants	Preterm infants
Physiological: Spontaneously breathing infants have better oxygen saturation (10% higher) up to 10 minutes after birth, lower heart rates, and early establishment of regular breathing	*Physiological*: • Hemodynamic stability • Reduced need for inotropes and fluid boluses in the first 24 hours of life • Increased superior vena cava blood flow • Better left ventricular output • Higher cerebral oxygenation index
Clinical outcomes: • Higher weight at birth (higher by 100 g) • Higher hemoglobin at 24–48 hours (higher by 2 g/dL) • Higher iron stores at 4–6 months' age	*Clinical outcomes*: • Reduces in-hospital mortality by 30% (95% CI 2–50%) • Lesser risk of any intraventricular hemorrhage (no difference in rates of severe IVH). The Australian trial did not show any difference in IVH • Less need for packed cell transfusion • Better motor scores on Bayley assessment at 18 months corrected age

(CI: confidence interval; IVH: intraventricular hemorrhage)

retinopathy of prematurity, necrotizing enterocolitis, or late-onset sepsis) by 36 weeks of postmenstrual age.

Delayed Cord Clamping and Early Neurodevelopmental Outcomes

A follow-up study of a randomized trial of 400 low-risk term infants noted no difference in neurodevelopment outcome between DCC and ICC groups at 4 years of age but better fine motor functions among boys in subgroup analysis. In another study, preterm infants randomized to the DCC arm showed better motor function at 18 months corrected age than ICC infants. These effects could be related to the decreased incidence of iron-deficiency anemia, and iron plays a critical role in normal brain development and function.

Umbilical Cord Milking

Umbilical cord milking (UCM) is proposed as an alternative to DCC when neonates require immediate resuscitation at birth. UCM consists of gently milking a long segment (20 cm) of the umbilical cord toward the baby. The cord is then allowed to refill, and the process is repeated two to four times before clamping the cord. UCM can be performed when the infant is still attached to the placenta (intact UCM) or after clamping and cutting a long umbilical cord segment (cut UCM).

Umbilical cord milking was comparable to DCC in term and late-preterm infants in improving hemoglobin levels at birth and 6-8 weeks of life. In preterm infants, UCM was noted to be associated with a higher risk of IVH. The premature infants receiving cord milking or DCC (PREMOD 2) trial comparing UCM and DCC among preterm infants <32 weeks' gestation was stopped before completion when the first interim analysis revealed a significantly increased risk of severe IVH with cord milking. Due to the higher risk of IVH, the recent Neonatal Resuscitation Program (NRP) recommends against cord milking among infants <28 weeks' gestation.

Physiological Based Cord Clamping

Physiological based cord clamping (PBCC) refers to the approach wherein the infant's physiological status determines cord clamping than a fixed time-based approach. Studies in lambs had shown that establishing lung aeration when the newborn is still attached to the placenta results in better hemodynamic transition. In most trials, nonvigorous infants were excluded. However, this population might benefit when respiratory support [positive-pressure ventilation or continuous positive airway pressure (CPAP)] is provided with an intact cord.

Custom-made resuscitation tables have been used to facilitate PBCC or intact cord resuscitation. These tables can be taken closer to the maternal side, and care providers receive the infant onto this table and proceed with resuscitation while the cord is still intact. In one study, the umbilical cord was clamped after the neonate was stable as indicated by heart rate > 100 bpm, spontaneous breathing on CPAP with tidal volumes > 4 mL/kg, and acceptable oxygen saturation. The challenges in performing PBCC include the need for real-time monitoring of vital parameters during resuscitation, prevention of hypothermia, difficulty in performing extensive resuscitation when additional staff is needed, and neonates with short umbilical cords.

Researchers from Nepal randomized vaginally delivered late preterm and term infants who do not breathe spontaneously after initial steps to intact cord resuscitation or early cord clamping. The intact cord group received positive-pressure ventilation at the mother's bed without advanced equipment except for a pulse oximeter, and the cord was clamped at 3 minutes of age. In the intact cord group, infants established regular breathing earlier and had higher oxygen saturation and a higher Apgar score at 1, 5, and 10 minutes, and no adverse effects. This study showed the feasibility of intact cord resuscitation in low-resource settings.

Maternal Effects of Delayed Cord Clamping

Delayed umbilical cord clamping does not lead to adverse outcomes in the mother, such as lower hemoglobin level, postpartum hemorrhage, or the need for blood transfusion.

SPECIAL SITUATIONS

Neonates Needing Immediate Resuscitation

There is currently insufficient evidence to recommend delayed versus early cord clamping for neonates who need resuscitation at birth. Until more evidence is available, it is reasonable to clamp the cord immediately and proceed with resuscitation.

Conditions where Immediate Cord Clamping are Indicated

Early cord clamping is recommended in the following situations due to the risk of maternal hemorrhage or the need for immediate neonatal resuscitation.
- Severe maternal hemorrhage, hypotension, or hemodynamic instability
- Abnormal placentation (previa/abruption)
- Cord prolapse, rupture, or avulsion

Multiple Pregnancies and Intrauterine Growth Restriction

Twin and triplet pregnancies pose unique challenges. There are concerns about twin-to-twin transfusion in monochorionic placentation, the well-being of the second fetus, and maternal risk of postpartum hemorrhage. In a retrospective study, the authors demonstrated the feasibility of implementing DCC in preterm monochorionic and dichorionic multiple pregnancies with comparable clinical outcomes to singletons undergoing DCC.

In fetuses with intrauterine growth restriction (IUGR) or abnormal doppler, the uteroplacental perfusion may be compromised, and resuscitation at birth may be anticipated. In a randomized trial comparing DCC versus ICC, neonates with antenatally diagnosed IUGR (a majority had normal Doppler) receiving DCC showed better superior vena caval and systemic blood flows. They had higher serum ferritin levels at 3 months without adverse effects.

In twin pregnancies and IUGR fetuses, there is limited data to make recommendations about DCC.

The neonatal and obstetric teams should weigh the relative risks and benefits of immediate or DCC in such situations.

Rh Incompatibility

Infants with suspected Rh incompatibility were generally excluded from DCC due to fears of increasing the risk of jaundice and anemia. A randomized study showed that DCC performed in Rh-alloimmunized infants (Rh-negative mothers with positive indirect Coomb's test) improves hematocrit at 2 hours of life without increasing the need for double-volume exchange transfusion or duration of phototherapy. If the fetus is born with hydrops or requires immediate resuscitation, early cord clamping may be reasonable.

HIV-positive Mothers

The World Health Organization (WHO) recommends DCC in HIV-positive pregnant women as DCC's benefits far outweigh the theoretical risk of mother-to-child transmission of the virus. On the other hand the National AIDS Control Organization, India recommends ICC to prevent mother-to-child transmission. In a retrospective study, the authors compared ICC and DCC during cesarean section among HIV-positive mothers. The neonates who received DCC had higher hemoglobin at 1 month of age, and all the infants tested negative for HIV-PCR up to 18 months of life. The additional risk of mother-to-child transmission of HIV posed by DCC in women with high viral load or those not on antiretroviral therapy are unknown.

Delayed Cord Clamping in the Context of Cord Blood Banking

The yield of cord blood and the total nucleated cell content (a threshold greater than 1.5 million nucleated cells) are decreased when cord clamping is delayed for 60 seconds and further decreased when clamping is delayed for 2 minutes. The benefits of DCC to the baby far outweigh the possibility that the banked cord blood might be put to later use in a public bank. Families who wish to bank umbilical cord blood need to be counseled about the cost-to-benefit of the procedure and the risk of denying the benefits of DCC to their infant.

IMPLEMENTING DELAYED CORD CLAMPING

Planning and Communication

Despite the established benefits and the various organizations, including the WHO, NRP, and the American College of Obstetrics and Gynecology (ACOG), recommending ≥30–60 seconds of DCC, cord clamping practices vary across institutions. Routine implementation requires reaffirmation and communication between the obstetric and neonatal care providers before all deliveries. Team communication helps to weigh the relative risks and benefits of immediate or delayed umbilical cord clamping in particular situations.

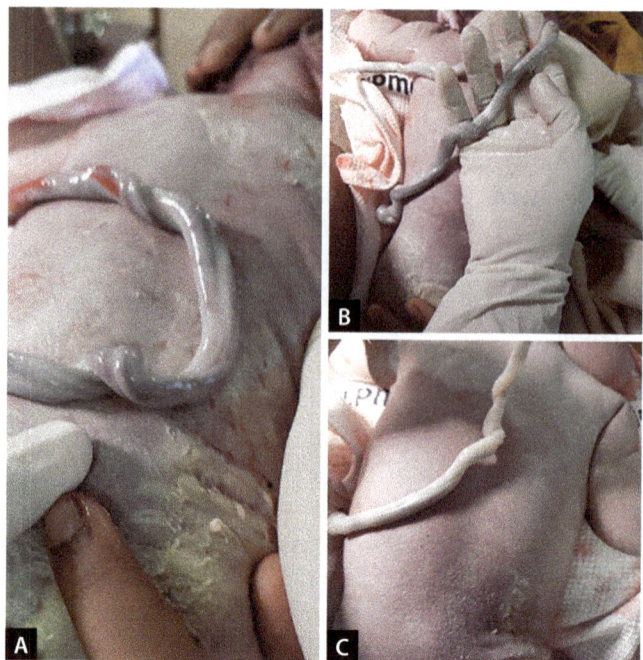

Figs. 2A to C: Delayed cord clamping during routine care. Note the change in the appearance of the cord from turgid at 30 seconds (A) still filled at 1 minute (B), pale and constricted at 2 minutes (C).

Care of the Neonate during Delayed Cord Clamping

The labor room quality improvement initiative (LaQshya) of the Government of India recommends DCC for 1–3 minutes. In neonates requiring routine care, the baby is received on the mother's abdomen, dried, and stimulated to breathe while awaiting umbilical cord clamping **(Figs. 2A to C)**. In cesarean delivery, the newborn can be placed on the maternal abdomen or held by the surgeon or assistant until the umbilical cord is clamped. The team managing the mother or the baby can demand early cord clamping if maternal hemodynamic instability or the need for immediate neonatal resuscitation is noted.

Active Management of the Third Stage of Labor during Delayed Cord Clamping

Delayed cord clamping does not alter the active management of the third stage of labor (AMTSL), including oxytocin which should be administered immediately after the birth of the baby. If the placental circulation is not intact (placenta previa, abruption, or umbilical cord avulsion), ICC is appropriate.

CHAPTER 43 | Umbilical Cord Management

CHAPTER AT A GLANCE

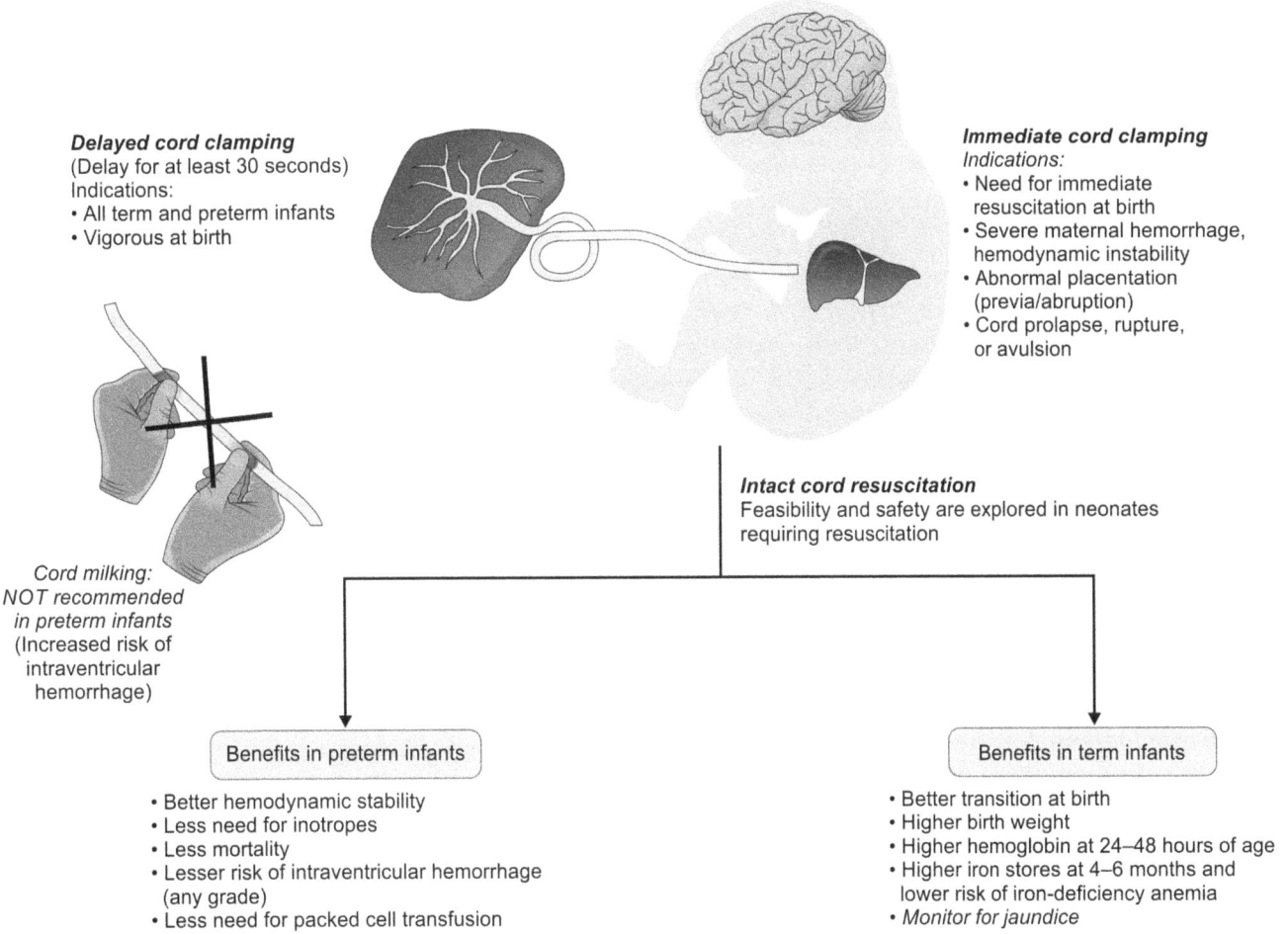

Delayed cord clamping
(Delay for at least 30 seconds)
Indications:
- All term and preterm infants
- Vigorous at birth

Cord milking:
NOT recommended in preterm infants (Increased risk of intraventricular hemorrhage)

Immediate cord clamping
Indications:
- Need for immediate resuscitation at birth
- Severe maternal hemorrhage, hemodynamic instability
- Abnormal placentation (previa/abruption)
- Cord prolapse, rupture, or avulsion

Intact cord resuscitation
Feasibility and safety are explored in neonates requiring resuscitation

Benefits in preterm infants
- Better hemodynamic stability
- Less need for inotropes
- Less mortality
- Lesser risk of intraventricular hemorrhage (any grade)
- Less need for packed cell transfusion

Benefits in term infants
- Better transition at birth
- Higher birth weight
- Higher hemoglobin at 24–48 hours of age
- Higher iron stores at 4–6 months and lower risk of iron-deficiency anemia
- *Monitor for jaundice*

KEY POINTS

- Health providers should delay umbilical cord clamping by 1–3 minutes in all vigorous term and preterm neonates irrespective of the mode of delivery.
- In term infants, DCC increases hemoglobin levels at birth and improves iron stores at 4–6 months of life. Term infants receiving DCC need monitoring for jaundice.
- In preterm infants, DCC is associated with lower mortality, improved hemodynamic stability, and lower incidence of IVH.
- Cord milking is not recommended in preterm infants born before 28 weeks due to a higher risk of IVH.
- In situations where uteroplacental perfusion or umbilical cord flow may be compromised, neonatal and obstetric teams must assess the risks and benefits in deciding about the optimal cord management strategy.

SUGGESTED READING

1. Balasubramanian H, Ananthan A, Jain V, Rao SC, Kabra N. Umbilical cord milking in preterm infants: a systematic review and meta-analysis. Arch Dis Child Fetal Neonatal Ed. 2020;105(6):572-80.
2. Delayed umbilical cord clamping after birth: ACOG committee opinion Summary, Number 814. Obstet Gynecol. 2020;136(6):1238-9.
3. Niermeyer S. A physiologic approach to cord clamping: clinical issues. Maternal Health Neonatol Perinatol. 2015;1(1):21.
4. Rabe H, Gyte GM, Diaz-Rossello JL, Duley L. Effect of timing of umbilical cord clamping and other strategies to influence placental transfusion at preterm birth on maternal and infant outcomes. Cochrane Database Syst Rev. 2019;9:CD003248.
5. UshaDevi R, Mangalabharathi S, Prakash V, Thanigainathan S, Shobha S. Delivery room care and neonatal resuscitation while on intact placental circulation: an open-label, single-arm study. J Perinatol. 2021;41(7):1558-65.

44

Perinatal Asphyxia

Rajendra Prasad Anne, Avantika Gupta

INTRODUCTION

The transition from intrauterine life to extrauterine life is challenging to both the mother and the fetus. Any impairment of this process can disrupt blood and oxygen supply to the fetus, resulting in perinatal asphyxia, which accounts for a quarter of four million neonatal deaths and 3.2 million stillbirths globally each year. Survivors are at risk of neurodevelopmental impairment, including cerebral palsy and learning disabilities.

OBJECTIVES

- To review the risk factors for perinatal asphyxia
- Assessment of antepartum and intrapartum of fetal well-being
- Management of a mother with fetal distress
- Management of a neonate with perinatal asphyxia
- Prognostication of neonates with perinatal asphyxia
- Counseling parents appropriately

RISK FACTORS FOR PERINATAL ASPHYXIA

The various antepartum and intrapartum risk factors for perinatal asphyxia are listed in **Table 1**. The pregnancies with these risk factors, usually labeled as high-risk pregnancies, need close antenatal monitoring and timely intervention to avoid perinatal asphyxia.

TABLE 1: Antepartum and intrapartum risk factors for perinatal asphyxia.

Antepartum risk factors	Intrapartum high-risk factors
- Age > 40 years - Fetal growth restriction - Hypertensive disorder in pregnancy - Oligohydramnios - Multiple pregnancy - Antepartum hemorrhage - Prolonged rupture of membranes (>18 hours) - Chorioamnionitis - Complicated diabetes mellitus	- Antepartum hemorrhage - Meconium-stained liquor - Fever > 38°C - Prolonged first/second stage of labor - Uterine hyperstimulation (prostaglandin/oxytocin use) - Cord prolapse - Rupture uterus - Difficult instrumental delivery - Shoulder dystocia

ANTEPARTUM AND INTRAPARTUM ASSESSMENT OF FETAL WELL-BEING

Commonly used methods for monitoring fetal well-being include fetal movement count by the mother, nonstress test (NST) or cardiotocograph (CTG), and ultrasound biophysical profile (BPP). These antepartum fetal surveillance programs are primarily focused at reducing stillbirths. There is insufficient data to say whether they reduce neonatal encephalopathy or cerebral palsy.

Fetal movement count: The "count-to-10" method recommends the pregnant woman to count fetal movements at the same time each day. Healthcare providers should be contacted if less than ten movements are perceived in a 2–3-hour period. This surveillance is started around 28 weeks' gestation and continued throughout pregnancy. Recurrent episodes of reduced fetal movement can be associated with poor fetal outcomes and may indicate early delivery. While studies do not show a decrease in the incidence of stillbirths, this is an inexpensive self-monitored tool with out the need of technology.

Non-stress test: This a noninvasive method using a CTG machine to identify fetuses at risk of intrauterine death and is done from 28 to 32 weeks of gestation. In a normal fetus, fetal heart rate (FHR) accelerates in response to fetal movement (cardiovascular reflex response to neurological activity). While interpreting the NST, a systematic approach need to be followed: Assessment of the baseline FHR, heart rate variability, presence of accelerations, decelerations, and contractions. The NST is labeled as reactive if at least two accelerations of 15 bpm lasting at least 15 seconds, with normal variability and baseline, are detected in a 20-minute interval.

Interpretation based on the Royal College of Obstetricians and Gynaecologists (RCOG) or the International Federation of Gynecology and Obstetrics (FIGO) guidelines can be used to identify fetuses who are at distress. A reactive (normal) NST is predictive of fetal well-being, and a nonreactive (abnormal) trace warrants further evaluation. The most common cause of nonreactive NST is fetal sleep.

The CTG changes predictive of perinatal asphyxia are reduced variability associated with tachycardia or recurrent variable decelerations, recurrent late decelerations, atypical variable decelerations, prolonged deceleration >3 minutes, bradycardia, and sinusoidal pattern. In the presence of meconium or abruption, even a suspicious trace may indicate fetal distress. An early passage of large or thick meconium increases the risk of hypoxic-ischemic encephalopathy (HIE).

Ultrasound biophysical profile (BPP): BPP comprising fetal movements, fetal tone, and fetal breathing and liquor volume using ultrasound with or without FHR assessment is another commonly used technique.

All the above tests need to be interpreted based on fetal condition and maternal risk factors. Fetuses with growth restriction are at higher risk of asphyxia. The use of Doppler velocimetry of uterine artery, fetal umbilical, middle cerebral artery, and the ductus venosus pulsatility indices may guide monitoring and planning delivery.

Intrapartum fetal well-being monitoring: Intermittent auscultation and continuous CTG are used for monitoring during labor. While intermittent auscultation is acceptable for low-risk pregnancies, electronic FHR monitoring is recommended for high-risk pregnancies. While CTG has been shown to decrease neonatal seizures, no impact on cerebral palsy is reported. Its widespread use has resulted in the increase in cesarean section rates. One has to keep in mind that the studies which form the basis of these results were not powered for these outcomes and done in an era (1970-1990) when CTG equipment, interpretation, and clinical experience were evolving.

Fetal scalp pH monitoring is a useful adjunctive test which can also assess intrapartum fetal well-being and reduce the interventions resulting from CTG monitoring. The presence of FHR acceleration in response to digital stimulation in labor correlates well with a fetal pH > 7.20. In some centers in India, fetal scalp lactate is used instead of scalp pH, as it requires <0.5 mL of blood and results can be obtained quickly. Other parameters such as fetal pulse oximetry, fetal electroencephalogram (EEG), and near-infrared spectroscopy have also been used for intrapartum assessment.

Some essential points to be remembered while monitoring fetal well-being:

Consider the complete clinical scenario (gestational age, high-risk factors, history of drug intake, stage, and rate of progress of labor) and not just the result of any test, while making clinical decisions

Try to look for the cause of an abnormal test result, and if reversible, intervene timely to avoid adverse fetal outcome.

Always compare the results of the fetal well-being test with the previous results to see the progression of abnormality.

Obstetricians should be trained in the interpretation of the results.

TIMING OF PERINATAL ASPHYXIA

About 80% of events resulting in perinatal asphyxia occur intrapartum, while the remaining antepartum and postpartum. Acute sentinel events include placental abruption, cord accidents (cord prolapse, cord avulsion, or bleeding vasa previa), rupture uterus, maternal cardiac arrest, all necessitating emergency delivery, and sudden out-of-hospital births without healthcare personnel in attendance. Such sentinel birth events may be noted in only 10-20% of neonates with perinatal asphyxia. In most others, a combination of maternal events, cord blood gas acidemia, and need for resuscitation points toward perinatal asphyxia.

MANAGEMENT OF A MOTHER WITH FETAL DISTRESS

If the CTG is suspicious or pathological, the following steps may be considered for intrauterine resuscitation and further measures based on the clinical scenario **(Fig. 1)**:

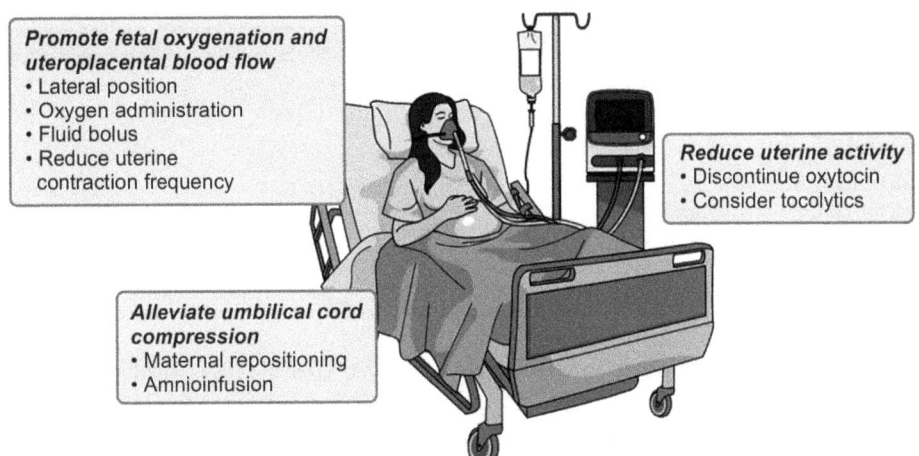

Fig. 1: Various intrauterine resuscitative measures to promote oxygen delivery to the fetus when fetal heart rate patterns suggest fetal hypoxemia.

- Change maternal position to lateral (left or right) position.
- Correct hypotension and dehydration by giving intravenous fluid bolus of nonglucose-containing fluid such as Ringer's lactate.
- Treat uterine hyperstimulation by reducing or stopping oxytocin if it is being used or by offering a tocolytic drug (subcutaneous terbutaline 0.25 mg).
- Oxygen may be administered to the mother; however, the evidence for its benefit is limited.
- Amnioinfusion may be considered in variable decelerations following cord compression, especially when facilities for emergency cesarean section are unavailable or there is undue delay in performing it.
- Response to fetal scalp stimulation can be reassuring and can be done before doing fetal scalp pH test to avoid unnecessary sampling.
- Per vaginal examination should be done to rule out cord prolapse and to see color of liquor.
- Start preparing the patient for urgent delivery simultaneously when there is prolonged deceleration or bradycardia depending on the stage of labor.

CORD BLOOD GAS ANALYSIS

Cord blood gases can reflect fetal hypoxia. Umbilical arterial sample are preferred to venous samples, as they represent fetal metabolic status and also correlate well with neonatal outcomes. Indications for umbilical cord gas analysis are:
- Neonatal asphyxia (need for resuscitation at birth)
- Nonreassuring FHR patterns
- Difficult vaginal delivery
- Cesarean section for fetal indications
- Preterm delivery, small for gestational age fetus

Paired cord blood gases are preferred but umbilical artery sample is the single best specimen. **Figure 2** shows the method to obtain cord gas after delivery of the neonate. The normal umbilical arterial blood parameters and interpretation are given in **Box 1**.

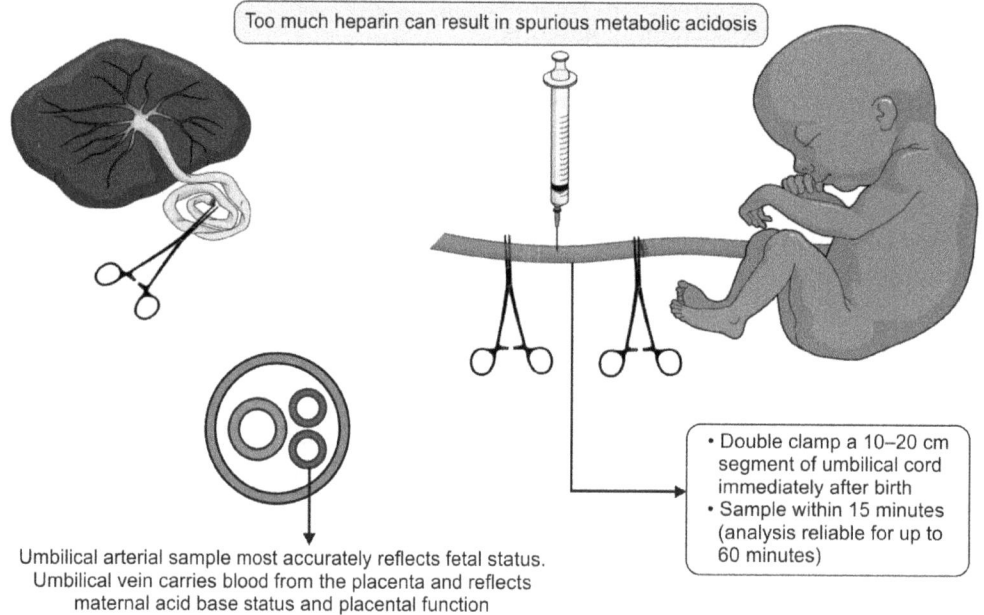

Fig. 2: Procedure to obtain umbilical arterial cord gas after birth.

BOX 1: Umbilical cord arterial gas parameters and interpretation of fetal acidosis.

Normal umbilical arterial blood parameters (5th and 95th centiles):
- pH   7.12–7.35
- pO_2 6.2–27.6 mm Hg
- pCO_2 41.9–73.5 mm Hg
- Base deficit –9.3 ± 1.5 mmol/L
- Bicarbonate 18.8–28.2 mmol/L

Interpretation:
- Umbilical artery pH < 7.0, or base deficit ≥12 mmol/L indicates that an intrapartum event could have contributed to hypoxic component
- If the cord arterial gas pH is >7.20, it is unlikely that intrapartum hypoxia played a role in causing neonatal encephalopathy

Points to note:
- The presence of metabolic acidosis does not exclude other causes of asphyxia or encephalopathy (such as prematurity, birth trauma, infection, meconium aspiration, structural brain malformations, antenatal insult)
- Absence of metabolic acidosis at birth does not exclude hypoxia or acidosis during pregnancy

POSTNATAL MANAGEMENT OF A NEONATE WITH PERINATAL ASPHYXIA

Neonatal Resuscitation
Two trained personnel should attend all pregnancies with risk factors and one should be skilled in extensive resuscitation. Follow neonatal resuscitation protocol. All neonates requiring resuscitation must be shifted to a neonatal intensive care unit (NICU) for observation and early identification and management of HIE.

Supportive Care
Perinatal asphyxia leads to multiorgan dysfunction (Table 2), and management includes prevention and management of the neonate from ongoing injury.

Examination
Objective assessment of neurological status must be performed with Thompson or Modified Sarnat score (Table 3). These can help in timely initiation of neuroprotective measures. Any neonate with a suspicion of HIE should be examined by two experienced neonatologists before a decision on providing therapeutic hypothermia (TH) is taken (Figs. 3A and B). An amplitude-integrated EEG (aEEG), when available, is a useful adjunct to clinical examination.

Supportive Management
- *Thermoregulation*: Maintain normothermia till a decision on TH is taken.
- *Fluids and electrolytes*: Provide maintenance intravenous fluids. Minimal enteral nutrition can be started in stable neonates even when undergoing TH.
- *Respiratory care*: Respiratory failure may need mechanical ventilation. Monitor oxygenation.
- *Hemodynamic support*: Myocardial dysfunction can lead to poor perfusion (delayed capillary refill), bradycardia, hypotension, and shock. Fluid bolus may be detrimental in the presence of myocardial dysfunction. Inotropic support and echocardiographic assessment are needed.
- Identification and management of sepsis

TABLE 2: Multisystem involvement in hypoxic ischemia encephalopathy.

Organ system	Complications
Central nervous system (72%)	• Encephalopathy • Seizures, hemorrhage
Cardiovascular system (29%)	• Myocardial injury • Cardiogenic shock • Arrhythmias
Respiratory system (26%)	• Persistent pulmonary hypertension • Respiratory failure • Pulmonary edema
Renal (42%)	• Acute kidney injury • Syndrome of inappropriate antidiuretic hormone secretion
Gastrointestinal (29%)	• Necrotizing enterocolitis, hemorrhage, hepatic injury, cholestasis,
Hematological and metabolic	• Thrombocytopenia, polycythemia, hypoglycemia, lactic acidosis

TABLE 3: The modified Sarnat staging for neonatal encephalopathy.

Parameter	Normal	Mild encephalopathy	Moderate encephalopathy	Severe encephalopathy
Level of consciousness	Alert, responsive to external stimuli	Hyperalert, stare, jitteriness, high-pitched cry, exaggerated response	Lethargic	Stupor/coma
Spontaneous activity	Changes position when awake	Normal /decreased	Decreased	No activity
Posture	Predominantly flexed	Mild flexion of distal joints	Moderate flexion	Decerebrate
Tone	Strong flexor tone	Normal/slight increase	Hypotonia	Flaccid/rigid
Primitive reflex: • Suck • Moro	• Strong, easily illicit • Complete	• Weak, poor • Partial response	• Weak but has a bite • Incomplete	• Absent • Absent
Autonomic system: • Pupils • Heart rate • Respiration	• In dark: 2.5–4.5 mm • Light: 1.5–2.5 mm • 100–160 bpm • Regular	• Mydriasis • Tachycardia >160 • Hyperventilation >60	• Constricted • Bradycardia<100 • Periodic breathing	• Deviation/dilated/NR • Variable • Apnea/requires ventilation
Seizure	None	None	Common; focal or multifocal	Uncommon (excluding decerebration)

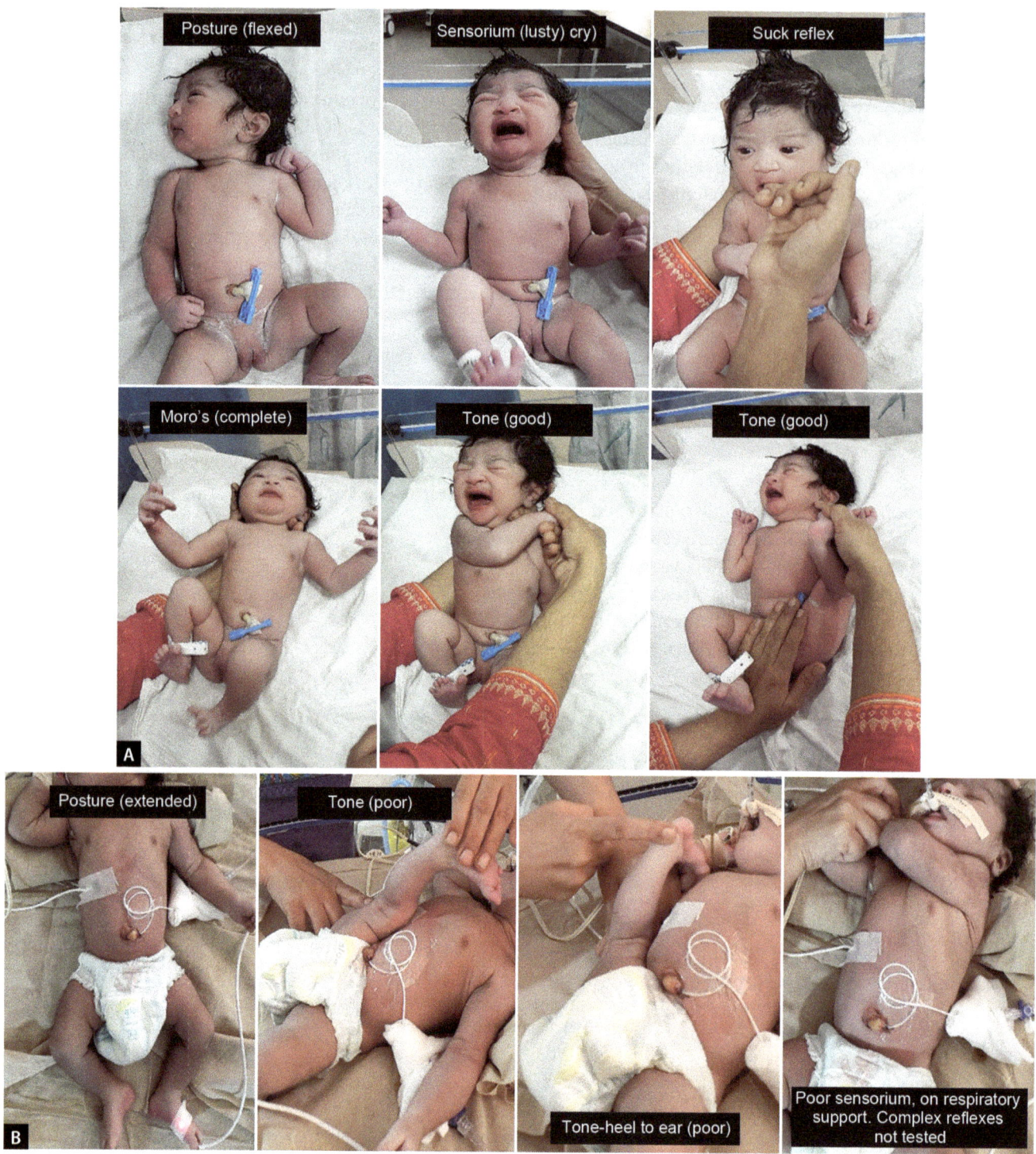

Figs. 3A and B: (A) Neurological examination of a neonate at 1 hour of age. The neonate required positive pressure ventilation for 1 minute. The Apgar scores were 5 and 8 at 1 and 5 minutes of age. Umbilical arterial gas showed a pH of 7.1 and base deficit of 14 mEq/L. Neurological examination is normal. Neonate requires continued monitoring; (B) The neonate required intubation and positive-pressure ventilation. The Apgar scores were 3 and 6 at 1 and 5 minutes of age. Umbilical arterial gas showed a pH of 7.0 and base deficit of 18 mEq/L. Neurological examination shows severe encephalopathy. Neonate satisfies cooling criteria.

- *Seizure management*: More than half of the neonates who develop seizures due to HIE have them in first 6–12 hours. In neonates with HIE, the seizures are frequently subtle (orolingual and ocular) or electrographic only. Thus, relying only on clinical evaluation can result in underdiagnosis of seizures. Seizures increase cerebral metabolic rate in a tissue with already compromised perfusion, and result in further excitotoxicity. All clinical and electrographic seizures warrant treatment with antiepileptics. Phenobarbital is the drug of choice but several recent reports suggest levetiracetam as an effective alternate drug.

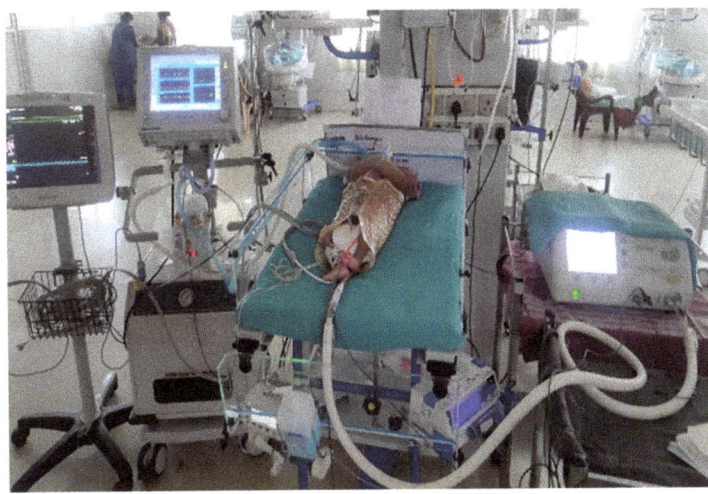

Place — Level-3 NICU

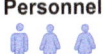
Personnel — Trained personnel; 24x7 monitoring

Paraphernalia
- Cooling device
- Multipara monitors
- Mechanical ventilation
- Supportive care

Protocol and policy
- Timely identification of eligible neonates
- Evidence based protocolized care
- Neurodevelopmental follow-up

Fig. 4: Prerequisites for initiating therapeutic hypothermia in a unit. The figure shows a neonate receiving therapeutic hypothermia. Servocontrolled hypothermia device, mechanical ventilator, and equipment for core temperature and hemodynamic monitoring are seen.

- *Ongoing monitoring*: Evaluate for end-organ injury (hemogram, renal function tests, liver function tests, coagulation profile, troponin, creatine kinase—muscle brain, electrocardiogram, and echocardiography). Continuous monitoring of vital parameters, blood sugar, urine output, electrolytes, and neurological status are of utmost importance.

Neuroprotective Strategies

After stabilizing the hemodynamics, the priority will be to initiate neuroprotective strategies. The neonate should preferably be transferred to a tertiary care center with TH facilities. The prerequisites for initiating TH include **(Fig. 4)** an appropriate *place* (at least a well-established level II/level III NICU is preferred), *personnel* [trained pediatrician and nursing staff; round the clock monitoring), *paraphernalia* (radiant warmer; cooling device; rectal and surface probes for temperature monitoring; multiparametric monitors that can measure temperature, heart rate, respiratory rate, noninvasive blood pressure and SpO2; arterial blood gas (ABG) machine; mechanical ventilator; glucometer; desirable to have amplitude integrated EEG and MRI facilities], and protocols (timely identification of HIE; ensuring TH for eligible infants within 6 hours of birth; evidence-based standard *protocol* for providing and monitoring TH; standardized neurodevelopmental follow-up, and continuing staff education).

Mechanism of Therapeutic Hypothermia

Therapeutic hypothermia helps limit brain injury by decreasing energy consumption, extracellular glutamate accumulation, free radical generation, inflammation, and apoptosis. It is more effective when initiated within the initial 6 hours (window period) before secondary energy failure ensues.

Any neonate with severe metabolic acidosis in cord blood gas (pH < 7.0 or base deficit > 16) and moderate or severe

TABLE 4: Criteria for initiating therapeutic hypothermia.

Eligibility criteria (all)	• Gestational age > 35 weeks AND • Birth weight > 1,800 grams AND • No major congenital anomaly (chromosomal, or life-threatening malformation) AND • Age < 6 hours
Essential criteria (at least one of these)	• pH < 7.0 (cord blood or arterial blood in <1 hour age) OR • Base deficit > 16 mmol/L (cord blood or arterial blood in <1 hour age) OR • Need for positive pressure ventilation at 10 minutes age OR • Apgar scores less than 5 at 10 minutes of age
Neurological criteria	Moderate-to-severe encephalopathy according to modified Sarnat staging

encephalopathy based on an objective examination qualifies for TH if gestational age is greater than 35 weeks and infant is less than 6 hours of age. The examination guiding the decision on TH should be preferably performed in the first hour. It is important to start TH as soon as indicated for the best neuroprotective results. The criteria used for initiating TH are provided in **Table 4**.

Devices

Therapeutic hypothermia can be administered using servo-controlled devices or phase change materials (PCM). Although servo-controlled devices are preferred, in resource-limited settings, PCM have been successfully used to administer TH. The phases of TH include an initial rapid cooling to a rectal temperature of 33.5°C, continuation for 72 hours, and rewarming at 0.5°C per hour. There is no added benefit with longer duration or deeper cooling

Monitoring

The infant needs meticulous monitoring of hemodynamics, organ dysfunction status, and neurological assessment while on TH. It is preferable to establish central venous and arterial access, give minimal oral feeds, provide analgesia with opioids, and evaluate hematological and biochemical parameters 12–24 hourly. Electrolytes and acid–base status may need more frequent monitoring.

Benefits

Randomized clinical trials have showed that therapeutic hypothermia for neonatal HIE results in reduction in death or major neurodevelopmental impairment at 18 months of age. Follow-up of these infants show that the benefit persists in childhood. In a recent randomized cooling trial from low-middle income countries, the benefits of therapeutic hypothermia was not observed. This is contrary to the findings from high income settings. The majority of enrolled infants were born at a peripheral center and later referred to the cooling units. Both antenatal and intrapartum care are essential pillars to prevent perinatal asphyxia and postnatal management alone is unlikely to benefit where care at birth is poor. The readers are referred to the position statement and guidelines for the use of therapeutic hypothermia to treat HIE in India by the National Neonatology Forum of India.

Transport of Asphyxiated Neonate to a Tertiary Center for Cooling

Hospitals with limited facility for cooling should transport eligible neonates within 6 hours to another referral unit. During transport, maintain normothermia. Passive cooling strategies (removal of external heat sources to the newborn) can lead to body temperature fluctuations and severe hypothermia that is more harmful. Hence, when facilities for TH are not available and the neonate cannot be safely transferred to a referral center within 6 hours of life (unstable neonate, poor transportation facilities, or long travel time), the neonate should be continued with normothermia and supportive measures in the birthing unit.

Alternative Neuroprotective Strategies

Several other modalities have been tried as adjuncts to TH to provide additional neuroprotective benefits. Erythropoietin, allopurinol, and melatonin were noted to have some additional benefits when used along with TH. Although xenon was found to be safe, no additional benefits were observed.

PROGNOSIS OF PERINATAL ASPHYXIA

The common adverse outcomes related to HIE are cerebral palsy and intellectual impairment. Apgar scores and extended Apgar scores do not correlate well with long-term neurological outcomes as they are subjective and other factors also influence them. The poor prognostic factors for long-term neurodevelopmental impairment are:

- Need for chest compressions for more than 1 minute during resuscitation, onset of respiration beyond 10 minutes, and base deficit greater than 16 in cord blood gas. In a retrospective study, Shah et al. observed that each variable increased the risk of adverse outcome (death or neurodevelopmental delay) from the baseline by 15%
- *Grade of encephalopathy*: Death or severe adverse outcome has been observed in 75% of infants with severe encephalopathy, 25–50% with moderate encephalopathy, and <1% with mild encephalopathy.
- Presence of seizures increases the risk of neurological sequelae by 40-fold.
- Electroencephalographic patterns of burst suppression, prolonged interburst intervals (>20 seconds), and isoelectric tracing are associated with poor outcomes. Amplitude-integrated EEG patterns of continuous low-voltage, burst suppression, and flat tracings indicate a poor prognosis.
- On cranial ultrasound, the features of basal ganglia abnormalities, focal parenchymal abnormalities and featureless appearance predict poor outcomes.
- Magnetic resonance imaging is the best neuroimaging modality to establish the timing and pattern of insult, and to predict prognosis. In presence of a normal MRI, the neonate is unlikely to develop neurodevelopmental abnormalities. Specifically, neonates with moderate-to-severe lesions in basal ganglia and thalamus have poor motor and cognitive outcomes. Abnormal signal in posterior limb of internal capsule (PLIC) indicates poor motor outcomes. Predominant involvement of parasagittal watershed regions and predominant white mater injury result in more prominent cognitive defects than motor defects.
- On MR spectroscopy, the parameters of lactate-to-N-acetyl aspartate ratio (Lac/NAA) and N-acetyl aspartate-to-creatine ratio (NAA/Cr) offer valuable prognostic information.

PARENTAL COUNSELING

Parental counseling of a neonate with perinatal asphyxia is challenging to neonatologists and obstetricians, because of medicolegal implications. Often the cause of litigation is inadequate or incorrect communication among the staff and with the parents.

- Whenever a situation of fetal distress arises, discuss with the parents, taking into consideration the clinical scenario including the assessment of the stage of labor, about the options of termination of pregnancy and the mode of delivery.

- Explain the possible need for resuscitation at birth and NICU admission, in cases where delivery is planned following assessment suggesting fetal distress.
- When TH is deemed necessary, the parents should be made to understand the benefit of the intervention based on available facts.
- Medical records should be accurate, complete, and objective to reflect the events during labor and birth and also the plan and management of healthcare providers.
- Parental support should be provided during entire hospitalization and follow-up period with detailed neurological assessments during each of these visits.
- A root-cause analysis should be performed for any sentinel event, adverse events and near miss events. Problem-solving and corrective action should be undertaken.

CHAPTER AT A GLANCE

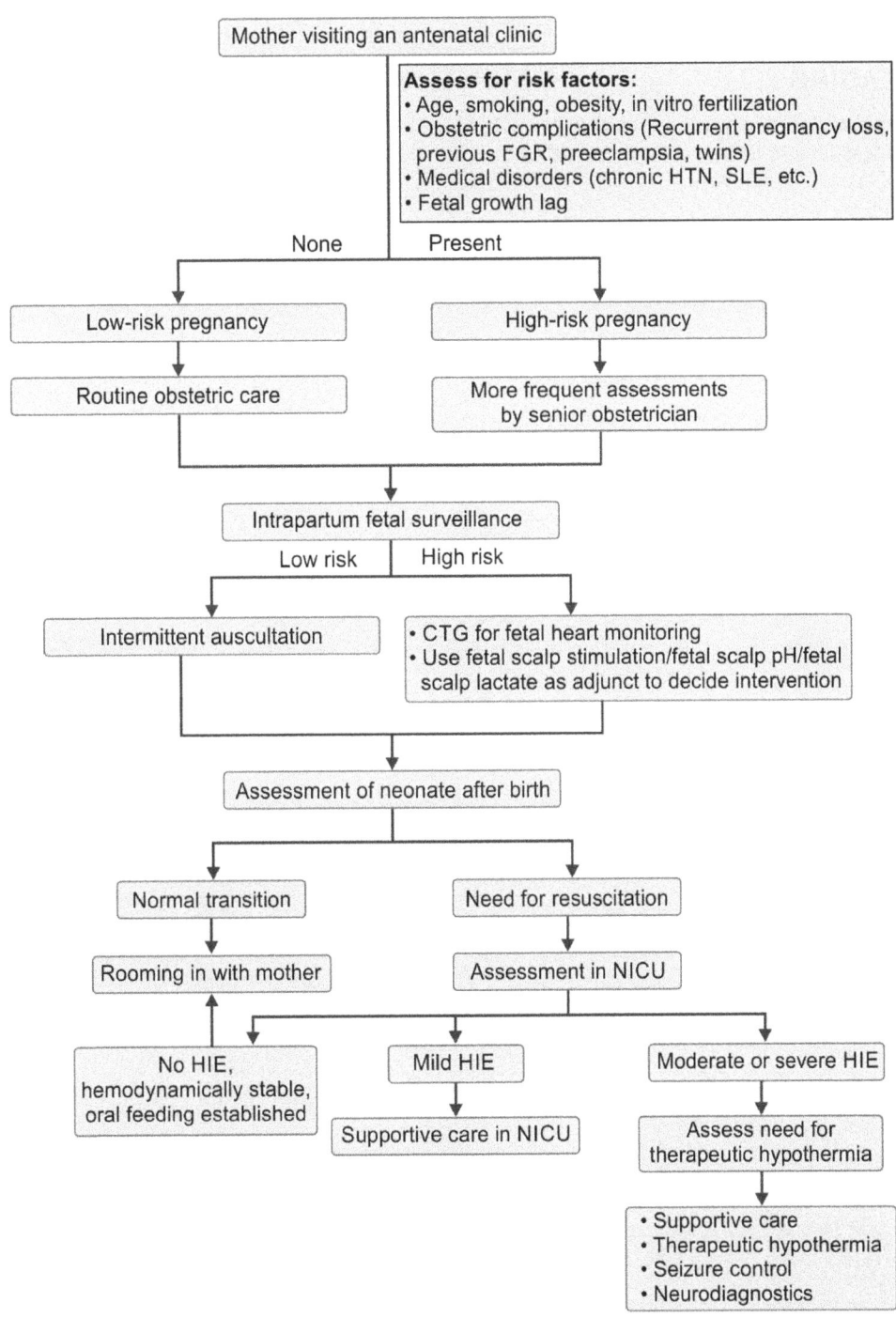

(CTG: cardiotocograph; FGR: fetal growth restriction; HIE: hypoxic-ischemic encephalopathy; HTN: hypertension; NICU: neonatal intensive care unit; SLE: systemic lupus erythematosus)

KEY POINTS

- It is essential to identify pregnancies based on antenatal risk factors for perinatal asphyxia.
- Intrapartum assessment of fetal well-being can guide early identification of fetal hypoxia and the obstetric management (intrauterine resuscitation, timing, and mode of delivery).
- All neonates requiring resuscitation should be offered postresuscitation care and evaluated systematically for neurological status and end organ injury.
- When HIE is detected, neuroprotective measures should follow hemodynamic stabilization of the neonate.
- Prognostication of the neonates relies primarily on neurological syndrome, seizures, electroencephalography, and neuroimaging.

SUGGESTED READING

1. Arulkumaran SS. Best Practice in Labour and Delivery, 2nd edition. Cambridge: Cambridge University Press; 2016.
2. Ayres-de-Campos D, Spong CY, Edwin Chandraharan, for the FIGO Intrapartum Fetal Monitoring Expert Consensus Panel. FIGO consensus guidelines on intrapartum fetal monitoring: Cardiotocography. Int J Gynecol Obstet. 2015
3. Jacobs SE, Berg M, Hunt R, Tarnow-Mordi WO, Inder TE, Davis PG. Cooling for newborns with hypoxic ischaemic encephalopathy. Cochrane Database Syst Rev. 2013;2013(1):CD003311.
4. National Neonatology Forum, India. Position Statement and Guidelines For Use of Therapeutic Hypothermia to treat Neonatal Hypoxic Ischemic Encephalopathy In India, October 2021. Available from http://nnfi.org/assests/pdf/NNF_Position_statement_and_Guidelines_for_TH%20_Final_(10112021)-converted.pdf.
5. NICE guidelines. Intrapartum care for healthy women and babies. Clinical Guideline 190. London: National Institute for Health and Care Excellence (UK); 2014.
6. Volpe JJ (Ed). Volpe's Neurology of the Newborn, 6th edition. Philadelphia, PA: Elsevier; 2018.

CHAPTER 45

Care at Birth

Manikumar S, Thenmozhi G

INTRODUCTION

Each year 2.8 million neonates die. Three-quarters of neonatal deaths occur in the first 7 days of life, particularly within 24 hours of age. Prematurity, birth asphyxia, and sepsis are the leading causes of neonatal mortality. Essential newborn care (ENC) practices and care during the golden hour after birth can significantly decrease neonatal morbidity and mortality. Neonatal resuscitation and delayed cord clamping are dealt with separately. This chapter will focus on care at birth and particular aspects of preterm care.

OBJECTIVES

- Know the components of essential newborn care
- Know the unique aspects in managing a preterm and low birth weight neonate at birth.

ESSENTIAL NEWBORN CARE

Essential newborn care refers to key practices in the care of the newborn at the time of birth and in the immediate postnatal period, regardless of the place of delivery. The components of ENC as recommended by the World Health Organization (WHO) include:
- Initiating skin-to-skin contact
- Early initiation of breastfeeding
- Thermal care of the newborn
- Prevention of infection (dry cord care, eye care, hand hygiene).

Skin-to-skin Contact at Birth

The first hour after birth is a unique period where a mother-infant dyad can establish a symbiotic relationship. At birth, when neonate requires only routine care, the baby is delivered onto the mother's abdomen, dried with a dry cloth, and delayed cord clamping is done. Then the neonate is nursed over the mother's chest with the face turned to one side and covered with a warm towel (**Fig. 1**). Once settled in the skin-to-skin position with the mother, temperature,

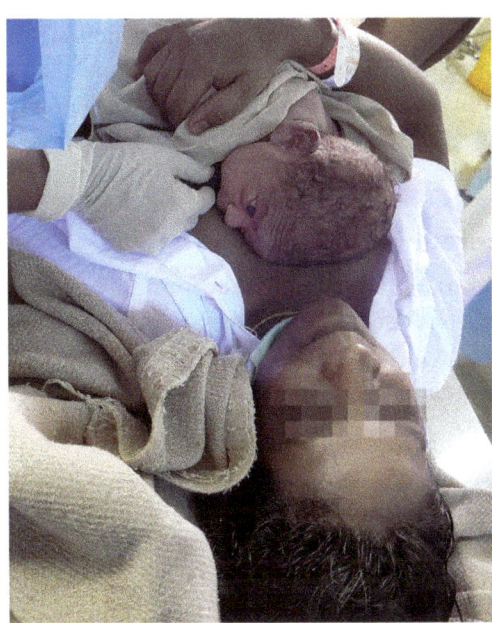

Fig. 1: Skin-to-skin contact at birth.

color, and respiratory efforts should be monitored every 15 minutes for the first hour of life. During cesarean section, the newborn infant may be positioned horizontally above the sterile drape. The advantages of skin-to-skin care are provided in **Table 1**. Mother-infant dyad should be continuously monitored during this period to assist if either of them needs help.

Early Initiation of Breastfeeding

Early initiation (within 1 hour of birth) of breastfeeding and exclusive breastfeeding through the first 6 months of age are both low cost interventions that decrease neonatal mortality. Exclusive breastfeeding is defined as providing only breast milk and no other liquids or solids, not even water except vitamins, minerals, or medicines such as oral rehydration solution or antibiotics. According to the recent National Family Health Survey (NFHS) data, <50% of neonates are breastfed within the first hour of life, and only 60–70% are exclusively breastfed until 6 months of life.

TABLE 1: Advantages of skin-to-skin care

Maternal benefits	Neonatal benefits
• The release of oxytocin helps in earlier expulsion of the placenta and reduced postpartum hemorrhage • Less stress • Better mother-infant bonding • Early establishment of breastfeeding	• Better thermoregulation • Reduced crying • Effective breastfeeding • Higher exclusive breastfeeding rates until 6 months after birth • Higher blood glucose levels

In resource-limited settings, nulliparity, cesarean delivery, lack of skin-to-skin care at birth, multiple births, low birth weight (LBW), and need for resuscitation at birth are associated with delayed breastfeeding initiation. The World Health Organization (WHO) recommends that mothers receive physical assistance to initiate breastfeeding and not just counseling alone. The other recommendations for early initiation of breastfeeding are listed in **Box 1**.

Thermoregulation

Hypothermia is associated with mortality, higher risk of infections, and metabolic derangements. The *"warm chain"* is a set of ten interlinked procedures carried out at birth and in the postnatal period to prevent hypothermia. These are listed next.

BOX 1: Supporting breastfeeding initiation at birth.

Support at birth
- Assistance in initiating skin-to-skin contact immediately after birth
- Support mothers to initiate breastfeeding as soon as possible after birth
- Provide practical support to establish breastfeeding and manage common breastfeeding difficulties
- Teach mothers how to express breast milk and feed infants in case of temporary separation
- Encourage responsive feeding and support mothers to identify infant's early feeding cues
- Health facilities should ensure zero separation of mother-infant dyads except when either of them needs specialized medical care

Additional support
- Discourage prelacteal feeds and other drinks to the baby
- Preterm infants need additional support, including nonnutritive sucking and oral stimulation until breastfeeding is established
- If expressed breast milk is indicated, paladai, Katori-spoon, or cup feeding is preferable to bottle-feeding

Provision of enabling environment
- Have a written breastfeeding policy that is communicated to staff and parents
- Healthcare providers need to be trained to offer breastfeeding support
- Pregnant women and their families should receive counseling in the antenatal period about the benefits of breastfeeding
- Provide ongoing support for breastfeeding mothers even after discharge from the hospital

The steps of warm chain are:
- Warm delivery room (25°C), with no draughts of air
- Immediate drying
- Initiate skin-to-skin care at birth
- Provide warm clothing
- Early and exclusive breastfeeding
- Postpone bathing for the first 24 hours
- Keep the mother and baby together
- Kangaroo care for stable LBW babies
- Warm transport
- Educate care providers on hypothermia prevention, recognition, and management of hypothermia.

Asepsis at Birth

All neonates should be handled with strict asepsis after birth. Handwashing is the essential step in maintaining asepsis. Birth attendant and maternal hand washing significantly reduces neonatal mortality by 40%. The five cleans at birth are:
1. Clean hands—handwashing
2. Clean place
3. Clean cloth for wrapping the baby
4. Clean cord cut with a clean blade
5. Clean cord clamp (or a clean thread).

Adherence to the five cleans can lead to a 27% reduction in sepsis-related deaths in a health facility. Use a clean, sterile cloth for cleaning and wrapping the baby at birth. It has to be gentle enough not to remove the vernix caseosa. The newborn who requires antibiotics because of suspected sepsis should be given the first dose of antibiotic as per the unit policy after obtaining blood culture. Also, ensure proper biomedical waste management practices in the delivery room.

Care of the Umbilical Cord

The cord must be cut 2-3 finger breadths away from the insertion site at the umbilicus. If it is long, there is a risk of contamination with urine and feces. If too short, there is a small risk of clamping the bowel because of a small omphalocele, which may be missed easily. Use a sterile blade/scissor to cut the cord. A cord clamp is usually preferred. Caution is exercised when using a tie, as it may get loosened when the cord dries up. A normal umbilicus has two arteries and a single vein. A single umbilical artery may be associated with renal anomalies, intrauterine growth restriction, or prematurity. However, routine ultrasound for renal anomalies is not warranted as the prevalence of renal malformations is low.

World Health Organization recommends dry cord care, which implies keeping the cord clean and dry, exposed to air, or covered by a clean cloth. If soiled, the cord can be cleaned with soap and water. The application of 4% chlorhexidine for cord care reduces the risk of neonatal mortality and omphalitis when births occur in community settings in regions with high neonatal mortality. In hospital births with strict adherence to asepsis, dry cord care is recommended.

The risk factors for umbilical sepsis or omphalitis include home births, poor asepsis at birth, LBW, prolonged rupture of membranes, umbilical catheterization, and chorioamnionitis. The common organisms causing omphalitis are *Staphylococcus aureus*, followed by *Streptococci* and Gram-negative bacilli. Rarely, anaerobic and polymicrobial infections may occur. Prompt management of omphalitis with broad-spectrum antibiotics (combination of antistaphylococcal penicillin and aminoglycoside) may prevent complications like intra-abdominal abscesses, portal venous thrombosis, peritonitis, and abdominal wall cellulitis. Bloodstream infection and meningitis must be ruled out in neonates presenting with systemic signs.

Umbilical cord granuloma is a common problem in neonates that presents as a soft, moist, pink lesion at the base of the cord. This results from the excess tissue that is left behind after cord separation. The lesion can be treated with a simple application of a pinch of cooking salt over the granuloma twice a day for a few days. The granuloma shrinks and dries in due course.

Cord Gas Examination

Umbilical cord gases provide information about fetal acid-base status. Low cord pH is substantially associated with neonatal mortality and morbidity and cerebral palsy in childhood. Fetal acidosis is diagnosed when cord arterial pH is <7 or cord base deficit is >12 mmol/L. Neonatal complications occur can occur in 10% of neonates who have fetal acidemia and the rate of complications can increase to 40% in neonates with severe acidosis (base deficit greater than 16 mmol/L at birth). The indications for cord gas estimation as per ACOG include:
- Cesarean delivery for fetal compromise
- Need for resuscitation at birth (low 5-minute Apgar score)
- Severe growth restriction
- Fetal distress on cardiotocography
- Meconium-stained liquor
- *Others*: Maternal thyroid disease, intrapartum fever, or multifetal gestation.

When cord blood sampling is anticipated, the cord should be double clamped and from this isolated segment, the sample can be obtained within 60 minutes after birth.

Eye Care

Eye care is given with two separate swabs for either eye with a single gentle swipe from the medial to lateral end. Antibiotic prophylaxis with 1% silver nitrate eye drops or 0.5% erythromycin eye ointment is provided in certain countries to decrease the incidence of ophthalmia neonatorum due to *Neisseria gonorrhoeae*. With a decrease in gonococcal infections and improvement in hygienic practices at birth, the role of antibiotic eye prophylaxis is questioned.

If a neonate presents with signs of conjunctivitis within the first 4 weeks of birth, a conjunctival swab should be sent for Gram stain and culture. If Gram-negative diplococci are isolated, treatment with parenteral cephalosporins should begin immediately. Infants with chlamydial infection can be treated with oral antibiotics. Most other bacterial conjunctivitis can be treated locally except *Pseudomonas* infection.

Baby Identification

The baby identification tag (tied both to mother and baby) must have at least the following details—name, hospital number, sex, birth weight, and date and time of birth. Always double-check as a routine, especially in high delivery load institutes. Radiofrequency identity tags are also used. Recording the footprint of the baby in the delivery case record is still being practiced in many institutes. However, it has to be remembered that its sensitivity in resolving disputes is poor (20%).

Recording Anthropometry

The electronic weighing machines with a preferred accuracy of at least 5 g have primarily replaced the previously popular salter-type weighing scales with an accuracy of 50 g. The scale should be placed on a level flat surface. Ensure to educate the delivery team on zero, tare, and the freeze value function. Use a sterile cloth/single-use sterile cover over the weighing tray and use the TARE function to account for the weight of these. The weighing machine needs to be calibrated weekly once.

Head circumference should be measured using a nonstretchable tape above the eyebrows in the front and the maximum protuberance of the skull at the back (**Fig. 2**). Head circumference <3 SD below mean on sex-specific growth charts indicates microcephaly.

Standards of Birth Weight

Birth weight after delayed cord clamping is 20–30 g/kg higher than with early cord clamping. If delayed cord clamping becomes the standard practice, the mean-term birth weight will be approximately 100 g higher. From an epidemiological point of view, this is a dramatic shift. The baby is weighed preferably after the initial cardiorespiratory stabilization. The weight decreases linearly during the first 24 hours with a median decrease of 20 g/kg for a full-term baby 12 hours after a vaginal delivery. For term infants, plot the weight on Multicenter Growth Reference Study (WHO-MGRS) growth chart. For preterm infants, INTERGROWTH-21 or Fenton's charts can be used. Neonates whose birth weight is <10th centile on the growth charts are labeled as small for gestational age (SGA).

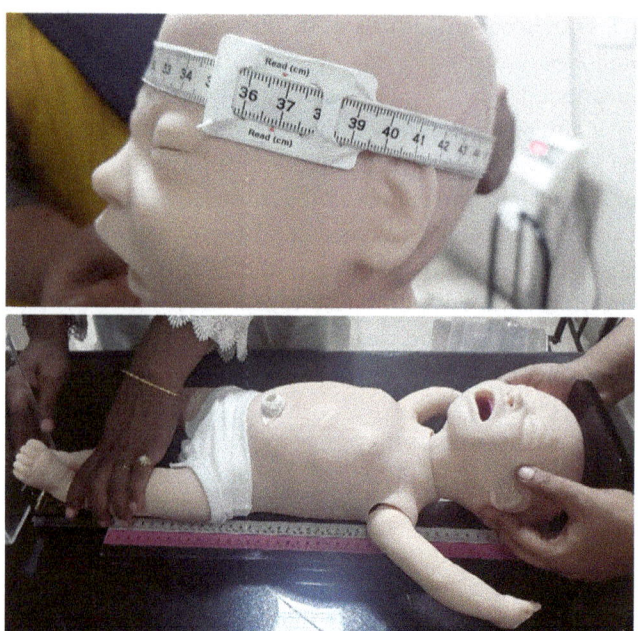

Fig. 2: Measuring head circumference and length.

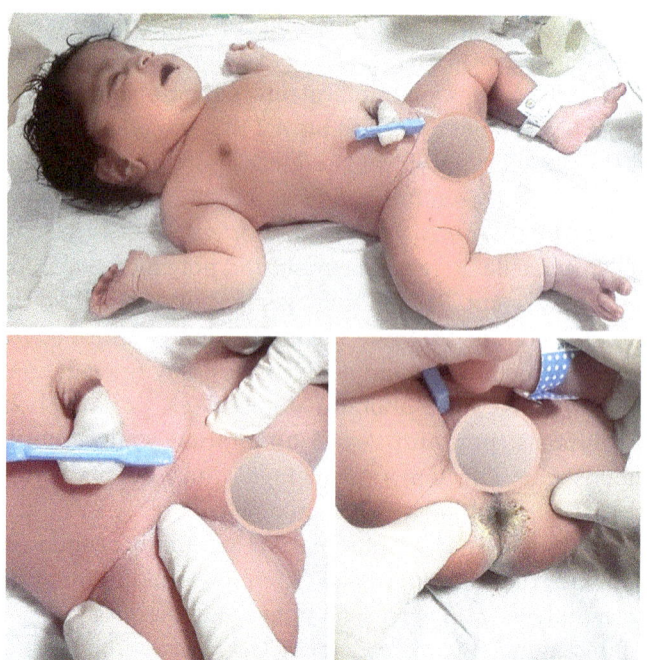

Fig. 3: Systematic examination at birth to rule out major malformations. Check the femoral pulses and ensure patency of the anus.

Neonates who have experienced fetal growth restriction can be identified at birth based on specific parameters. A consensus-based definition of growth restriction is:
- Birth weight less than the third percentile on population-based or customized growth charts.
- *OR at least 3 out of 5 of the following*: Birth weight <10th centile, head circumference <10th centile, length <10th centile, prenatal diagnosis of fetal growth restriction, and maternal pregnancy information (e.g., hypertension or preeclampsia).

The significance of identifying SGA and growth-restricted neonates is that they are at higher risk of complications both in the short and long term.

Administration of Vitamin K

All neonates delivered in any health facility must receive vitamin K at birth. The preferred formulation is vitamin K1 (phytonadione) which is available as a 1 mg vial for a single baby. The dose of vitamin K is 1 mg for neonates > 1.5 kg and 0.5 mg for neonates <1.5 kg birth weight. It is given intramuscularly in the anterolateral thigh using a 26-gauge needle attached to a 1 mL syringe. Even if a baby has to be referred, always give it before referral. Vitamin K administration has important implications for ensuring quality—the number of vials indented in the delivery room versus the number of babies delivered, is an easy indicator to ensure administration. Missed doses at birth can result in a higher risk of vitamin K deficiency bleeding, where the most typical presentation is intracranial hemorrhage.

Delivery Point Screening

As part of the Rashtriya Bal Suraksha Karyakram (RBSK) government program, delivery point screening for congenital disabilities is essential. **Figure 3** demonstrates the systematic examination at birth to rule out malformations. Salient examinations are discussed below:
- *Eye:* The eyes should be examined using an ophthalmoscope, with the lens power set at 0 and the examiner standing approximately 18 inches away. Project the light simultaneously onto both eyes. The presence of symmetrical red reflex in both eyes is normal. The presence of opacity (leukocoria) or asymmetry of the red reflex may indicate cataract, chorioretinitis, retinoblastoma, or other etiologies
- *Femoral pulse and cardiac examination*: Palpate the femoral pulses. A good volume pulse does not rule out coarctation of the aorta, as the ductus maybe patent to supply the descending aorta. Screening for congenital cyanotic heart disease using pulse oximetry is recommended before discharge and after 24 hours of life.
- *Genital examination:* Patency of the anus should be confirmed. Determination of the sex of the neonate is an essential part of the birth examination. The presence of clitoromegaly or fused labia, bilateral undescended testes, micropenis, or bifid scrotum (**Fig. 4**) indicates disorders of sexual differentiation. In such cases the sex of the baby should not be assigned until investigations are done. Parents need to be shown the abnormality and counseled. Endocrinology and genetic opinion should be obtained.
- *Spine examination:* Sacral dimple is commonly noted. The presence of hair, lipoma, or pigmentation may indicate spina bifida occulta. A simple sacral dimple is <0.5 cm in diameter, located within 2.5 cm of the anal verge, and not associated with cutaneous markers. In the

absence of these criteria, a spinal ultrasound should be done to look for spina bifida.

- *Hip examination:* With the infant supine and hips flexed to 90°, stabilize the pelvis. Each hip should be examined separately. The Barlow and the Ortolani maneuvers should be performed sequentially on each hip. The Barlow maneuver involves adducting the hip while pushing the thigh posteriorly to see if the hip can be dislocated, while the Ortolani maneuver involves abducting the hips while pushing the thigh anteriorly and relocates reducible hips (**Figs. 5A and B**). In either test, a click or a clunk is felt when the femoral head dislocates/relocates into the acetabulum. A follow-up hip examination within 2 weeks followed by a hip ultrasound is recommended if the test is positive. Female infants born by breech delivery and those with a family history of developmental hip dysplasia should undergo an ultrasound of the hip.

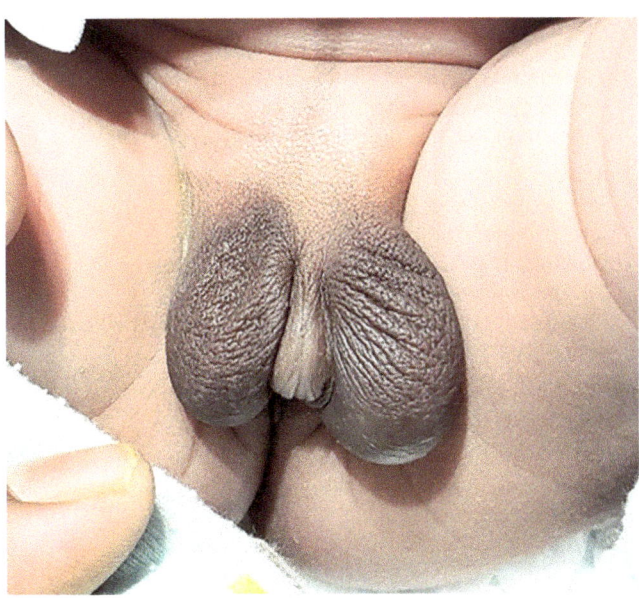

Fig. 4: Ambiguous genitalia. Bifid scrotum with palpable gonads, micropenis, and perineal hypospadias.

Communication

Communicate with the parents and relatives at the time of birth, sex of the baby, birth weight, and the condition at birth. Show the baby and the identity tag. Counseling for preterm birth ideally should happen before the baby is born.

Respectful Maternity Care

Respectful maternity care is an approach which is women-centerd and friendly care based on the principle of ethics and respecting the human rights. It aims to provide quality care and improve women's and newborns' experiences during childbirth. The Labor room Quality improvement initiative (LaQshya) by the government aims to reduce preventable maternal and neonatal mortality, morbidity, and stillbirths. The mother should be encouraged to move around freely and let the mother choose her comfortable birth position. A birth companion provides personal and emotional support to the mother. They can help in early initiation of breastfeeding. Stress during delivery can be reduced by planning timely travel to health facility and respectful care by staff. The normal progress of labor should be respected and unnecessary induction or augmentation of labor or operative deliveries should be avoided. Provide a stimulating environment for the mother-baby dyad in the delivery room. Health facilities preferably should implement the Labor-Delivery-Recovery (LDR) concept, where the whole process of labor, delivery, and 4 hours postpartum happen in the same cot. These will serve as a primer to improve the standards and practices in the delivery room. The components of respectful maternity care that improves the overall experience of women at childbirth and promotes neonates' cognitive development are highlighted in **Figure 6**.

GOLDEN HOUR MANAGEMENT OF THE PRETERM INFANT

The golden hour care for preterm infants helps standardize care practices to improve clinical outcomes such as survival,

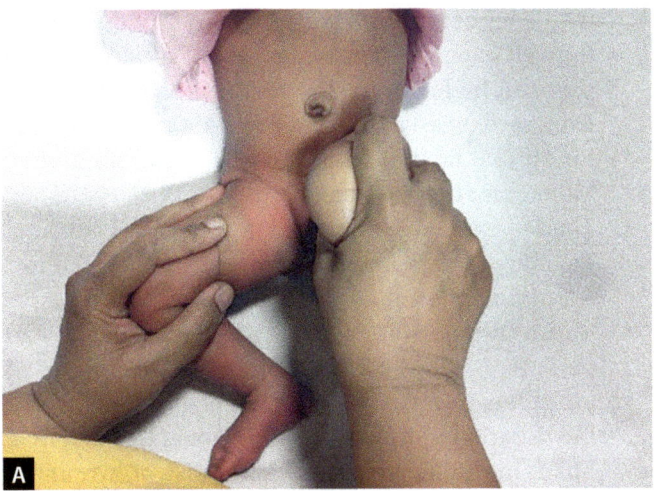
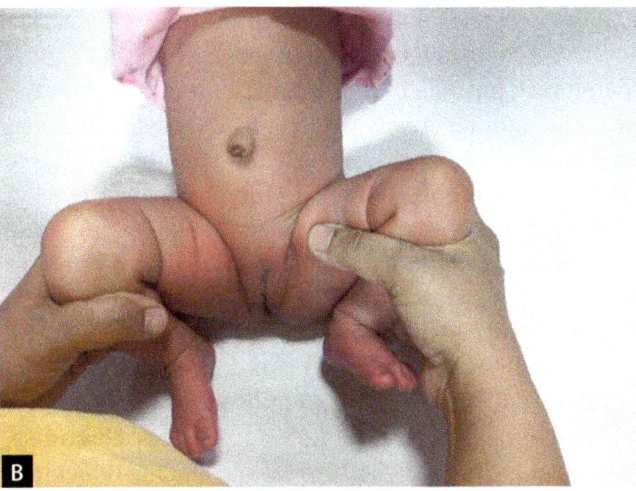

Figs. 5A and B: Hip examination for developmental dysplasia of hip. (A) Barlow's maneuver (adducting the hip while pushing the thigh posteriorly dislocates an unstable hip); (B) Ortolani maneuver (abducting the hips while pushing the thigh anteriorly relocates reducible hips).

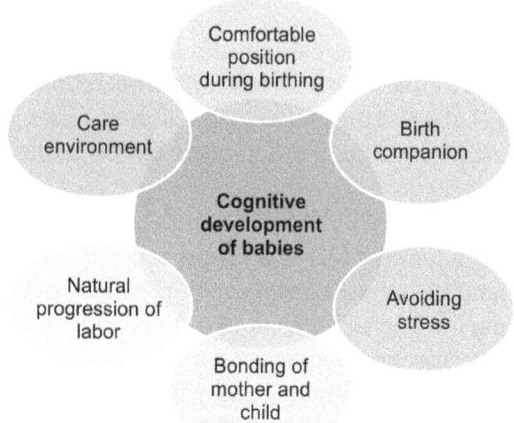

Fig. 6: Components of respectful maternity care as per the national "LaQshya" inititative for promoting cognitive development of babies.

intraventricular hemorrhage, chronic lung disease, and retinopathy of prematurity and neurodevelopment. The golden hour care encompasses care in the delivery room, thermoregulation, ventilation and oxygenation, nutritional support, and infection prevention. These are summarized in **Box 2**. Coordinated management during the golden hour requires teamwork, communication, and organization.

CARE OF LOW BIRTH WEIGHT INFANT

Neonates weighing <2,500 g at birth are called LBW infants. LBW may be due to prematurity or growth restriction. These infants have special needs and are at higher risk of morbidity and mortality compared to term appropriate for gestational age neonates.

Neonates with fetal growth restriction, particularly those where insult is in the latter half of have characteristic features are shown in **Figure 7A**. They have a relatively large head with an undergrown trunk and extremities and a scaphoid-appearing abdomen. The anterior fontanel may be large from decreased membranous bone formation. The skin is dry and loose with folds due to the paucity of subcutaneous fat. They have a characteristic old wizened man look and appear hyperalert. A passage of meconium in utero can stain the cord, skin, and fingernails yellow-green. Growth-restricted neonates are at higher risk of morbidity, including asphyxia, meconium aspiration, persistent pulmonary hypertension of the newborn, hypoglycemia, polycythemia, temperature instability, and long-term complications like poor catch-up growth and neurodevelopmental impairment.

Late preterm infants are neonates born between 34 and 36 weeks of gestational age and comprise three-fourths of all preterm infants. They are often overlooked because of their size but are at risk of respiratory distress, jaundice, apnea, hypoglycemia, hypothermia, and feeding difficulties at birth. These neonates are at risk of neurodevelopmental impairment and need follow-up (**Fig. 7B**).

BOX 2: Golden hour management of preterm infants.

Delivery room care:
- Antenatal counseling
- Delivery room temperature 25–28°C
- Follow NRP guidelines
- Supplies for thermoregulation (plastic wrap, hat) in addition to radiant warmer and transport incubator
- T-piece resuscitator, blended oxygen, and pulse-oximeter are essential to provide gentle ventilation and adherence to target oxygen saturation

Thermoregulation:
- Continue to monitor the temperature. Admission temperature is monitored as a quality indicator of good resuscitation in the delivery room
- Early initiation of Kangaroo mother care

Ventilation and oxygenation:
- Early initiation of CPAP
- Early rescue surfactant
- Monitor oxygen saturation and titrate FiO_2 based on pulse oximetry
- Early initiation of caffeine therapy when indicated

Cardiovascular support:
- Early intravenous access
- Judicious use of fluid resuscitation and vasopressors

Nutrition:
- Secure central lines when indicated
- Total parenteral nutrition whenever indicated
- Monitor blood sugars
- Early enteral feeding
- Exclusive use of human milk (Mother's milk or pasteurized donor milk)

Prevention of infection:
- Hand hygiene
- Investigate and treat sepsis

(CPAP: continuous positive airway pressure; NRP: neonatal resuscitation program)

Management

- *Feeding*: Breastfeeding efficacy may take time. The frequency of feeding should be every 2 hours, including through the night. If neonates cannot suckle adequately, they can be fed *expressed* breast milk using a paladai. Expressed breast milk can be stored at room temperature for up to 6 hours and in the refrigerator for 24 hours. Monitor for hypoglycemia.
- *Thermoregulation*: Skin-to-skin contact at birth should be followed by Kangaroo Mother Care (KMC). Provide warm clothing, mittens, and hat. Delay bathing.
- *Kangaroo mother care*: All LBW babies should be started on KMC as soon as they are stable. *The benefits of* KMC are numerous; it increases breastfeeding rates as well as the duration of breastfeeding. Neonatal mortality and infant mortality are reduced. The risk of hypothermia and infection is reduced. There is better mother infant bonding, better weight gain, and helps in early discharge.

CHAPTER 45 | Care at Birth

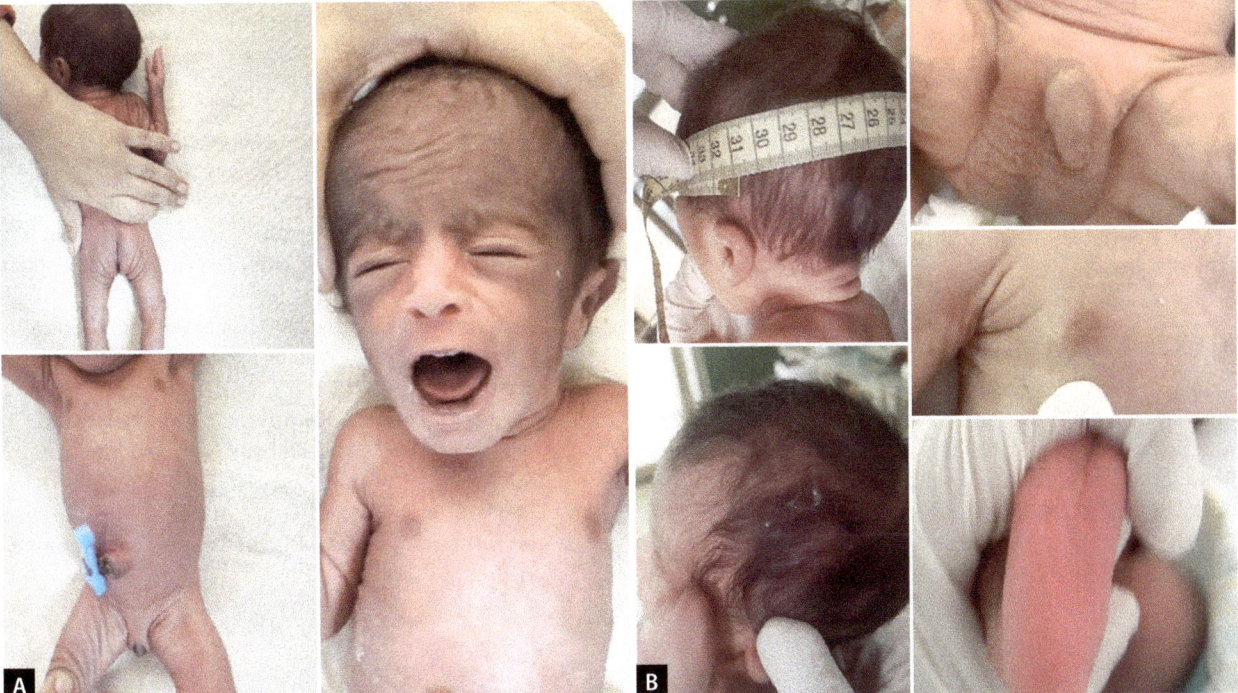

Figs. 7A and B: (A) Features of a neonate with intrauterine growth restriction. Loose skin folds, paucity of subcutaneous fat, and triangular facies; (B) Late preterm 34 weeks neonate—note the wooly hair, paucity of scrotal rugae, descended testes, smaller breast bud, and creases only in the **anterior** part of the sole. The head size is appropriate for gestation.

Chapter at a Glance

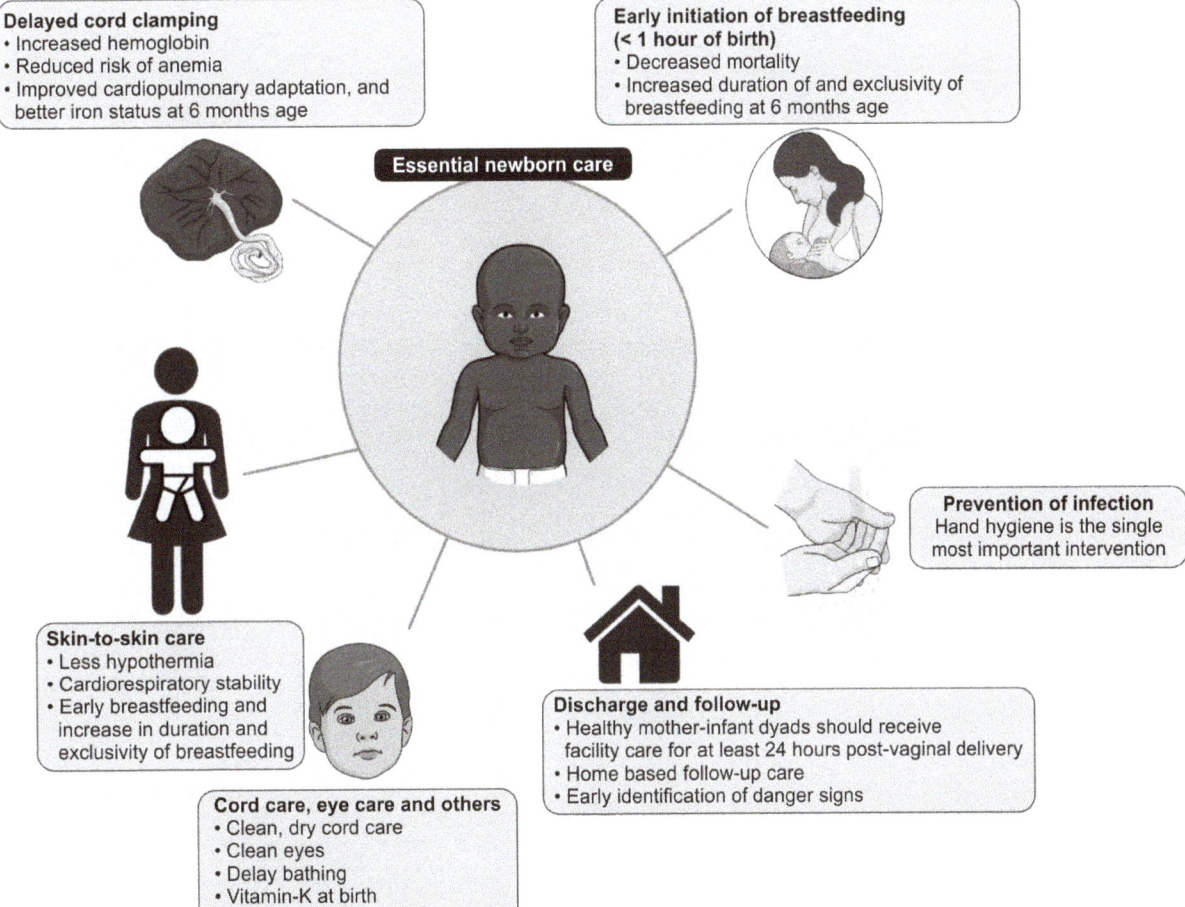

Delayed cord clamping
- Increased hemoglobin
- Reduced risk of anemia
- Improved cardiopulmonary adaptation, and better iron status at 6 months age

Early initiation of breastfeeding (< 1 hour of birth)
- Decreased mortality
- Increased duration of and exclusivity of breastfeeding at 6 months age

Essential newborn care

Prevention of infection
Hand hygiene is the single most important intervention

Skin-to-skin care
- Less hypothermia
- Cardiorespiratory stability
- Early breastfeeding and increase in duration and exclusivity of breastfeeding

Cord care, eye care and others
- Clean, dry cord care
- Clean eyes
- Delay bathing
- Vitamin-K at birth
- Birth vaccination

Discharge and follow-up
- Healthy mother-infant dyads should receive facility care for at least 24 hours post-vaginal delivery
- Home based follow-up care
- Early identification of danger signs

KEY POINTS

- Care at birth influences short- and long-term outcomes in the neonate.
- Skin-to-skin care at birth among stable neonates promotes early initiation of breastfeeding.
- Respectful maternity care during childbirth is a fundamental right that has a positive impact on mother-infant dyad.
- Preterm neonates need additional efforts to maintain thermoregulation.

SUGGESTED READING

1. Aziz K, Lee HC, Escobedo MB, Hoover AV, Kamath-Rayne BD, Kapadia VS, et al. Part 5: Neonatal Resuscitation: 2020 American Heart Association Guidelines for Cardiopulmonary Resuscitation and Emergency Cardiovascular Care. Circulation. 2020;142(16_suppl_2):S524-50.
2. LaQshya guidelines. [online] Available from http://nhm.gov.in/New_Updates_2018/NHM_Components/RMNCH_MH_Guidelines/LaQshya-Guidelines.pdf[Last" http://nhm.gov.in/New_Updates_2018/NHM_Components/RMNCH_MH_Guidelines/LaQshya-Guidelines.pdf[Last accessed November 2021].
3. Marshall S, Lang AM, Perez M, Saugstad OD. Delivery room handling of the newborn. J Perinat Med. 2019;48(1):1-10.
4. Martherus T, Oberthuer A, Dekker J, Hooper SB, McGillick EV, Kribs A, et al. Supporting breathing of preterm infants at birth: a narrative review. Arch Dis Child Fetal Neonatal Ed. 2019;104(1):F102-7.
5. Nosherwan A, Cheung PY, Schmölzer GM. Management of extremely low birth weight infants in delivery room. Clin Perinatol. 2017;44(2):361-75.
6. Sharma D. Golden 60 minutes of newborn's life: Part 1: preterm neonate. J Matern Fetal Neonatal Med. 2017;30(22):2716-27.
7. Trevisanuto D, Testoni D, de Almeida MFB. Maintaining normothermia: why and how? Semin Fetal Neonatal Med. 2018;23(5):333-9.

CHAPTER 46

Postnatal Care and Discharge Planning

Tanushree Sahoo, Abhishek S Aradhya, Monica Gupta

INTRODUCTION

The "First 1000 Days" period extends between the pregnancy and the child's second birthday. Comprehensive care during this period of rapid physical growth and brain development ensures survival and optimal neurodevelopment. The postnatal period begins immediately after delivery and lasts for the first 6 weeks. According to the recent estimate, nearly 40% of stillbirths and two thirds of neonatal deaths happen during birth and within 48 hours. The first week of life itself, accounts for nearly three-fourths of all neonatal deaths. Most deaths can be prevented by comprehensive postnatal care, including early initiation and maintenance of breastfeeding, provision of warmth, maintaining asepsis, early detection of common birth defects, and prompt treatment initiation.

OBJECTIVES

- Discuss the care of the neonate in the postnatal period
- Screen the neonate for common disorders
- Identify common postnatal issues of the mother-infant dyad
- Plan discharge from the hospital

CARE IN THE POSTNATAL PERIOD

Detailed Examination

Apart from the examination at birth, a thorough repeat head-to-toe examination should be done within the first 24 hours of life to pick up congenital anomalies and birth trauma. It should include auscultation of the heart and lungs and gestational age assessment. Particular attention should be paid to checking the patency of the anal orifice, occult midline defects, femoral pulses, and hips. A cardiac murmur may be normal immediately after birth but may indicate abnormality on the second or third day after birth.

The first stool is passed by 24 hours of life in 99% of healthy, full-term neonates. Delayed passage of meconium by 48 hours of life in a term neonate warrants evaluation by physical examination and abdominal radiograph. Causes include lower intestinal tract obstruction such as Hirschsprung disease, intestinal atresia, imperforate anus, meconium ileus, or meconium plug syndrome, maternal drugs during delivery (magnesium sulfate, opiates), or hypothyroidism. Preterm neonates exhibit a delay in the passage of first stool due to decreased gut motility.

Most neonates, irrespective of gestation, pass urine by 24 hours, 92% by 24 hours, and 99% by 48 hours. A neonate who has not voided by 24 hours needs evaluation. Review maternal history for oligohydramnios, asphyxia, antenatal ultrasound for renal anomalies, and drugs given to mothers.

Term babies may lose up to 10% of weight after birth and usually regain their birth weight by day 10–14. Weight loss up to 3% per day is considered normal. The risk factors for excessive weight loss include primigravida mother, cesarean delivery, late preterm. Excessive weight loss should be evaluated by feeding assessment, ongoing lactation support, and may also require serum sodium monitoring.

Warm Environment

The babies should be kept in the euthermic range in the postnatal ward by adequate clothing (at least two-layer clothing with caps, socks, and mittens) and frequent breastfeeding. Low birth weight babies (especially < 2 kg birth weight) should be offered kangaroo mother care at least 8–10 hours/day. The benefits of kangaroo care are:
- Decreased hypothermia
- Higher exclusive breastfeeding rate
- Fewer episodes of apnea or bradycardia
- Better weight gain
- Early discharge
- Decreased neonatal mortality
- Less nosocomial infection
- Lesser readmission rates

Rooming-in and Supine Sleeping

The mother and baby should be kept in the same room and preferably in the same bed. The neonate should be nursed on a hard surface with a supine position (sleep on their back) to avoid the risk of sudden infant death syndrome. Infants need protected sleep, and care should be taken to avoid loud noise and painful stimuli. Breast milk, sucrose, or facilitated tucking should be considered for any painful procedures like sampling in the postnatal ward.

Immunization

All neonates should receive a birth dose of oral polio, intradermal BCG, and hepatitis B vaccine after birth, preferably before discharge. The birth dose of hepatitis B should preferably be given within 24 hours of life. In preterm babies with a birth weight of < 2 kg, the birth dose hepatitis B vaccine may be less immunogenic, and hence three doses should be administered later.

Bathing

Since vernix caseosa protects the skin, vigorous rubbing to wipe it away at birth should be discouraged. Bathing should be postponed during the hospital stay and till the cord falls off. However, wiping or sponging a baby in lukewarm water over frequently soiled areas (around neck, anus, and genitalia) can be considered during the hospital stay. In premature babies, bathing can be postponed, and sponging should be considered for an initial couple of days till the baby gains adequate weight (2.5 kg). Soap for bathing should ideally match the neonates' body pH (slightly acidic) and be odorless.

OIL MASSAGE

Oil massage is a low-cost traditional practice that has shown multiple benefits for preterm neonates in low-middle income country (LMIC) settings. It is known to improve skin circulation, maintain better skin integrity, improve weight gain and reduce sepsis. A gentle massage using any commonly available vegetable oils (e.g., coconut, sunflower, and olive) can be done for neonates. One must not instill oil into the ear or cord.

PREDISCHARGE SCREENING AND CHECKS

All newborn infants should undergo screening for the following disorders before discharge from the hospital, depending on availability. A detailed neurological examination including state-to-state variability, neuromuscular maturity, or any stigmata of the neurocutaneous syndrome to be done.

Hearing

Out of every 1,000 live births, 1–3 can have a moderate or severe hearing impairment. The risk is tenfold higher in neonates with risk factors. Hence, universal hearing screen is recommended for all neonates before discharge **(Fig. 1)**. The Indian Academy of Pediatrics recommends a two-stage

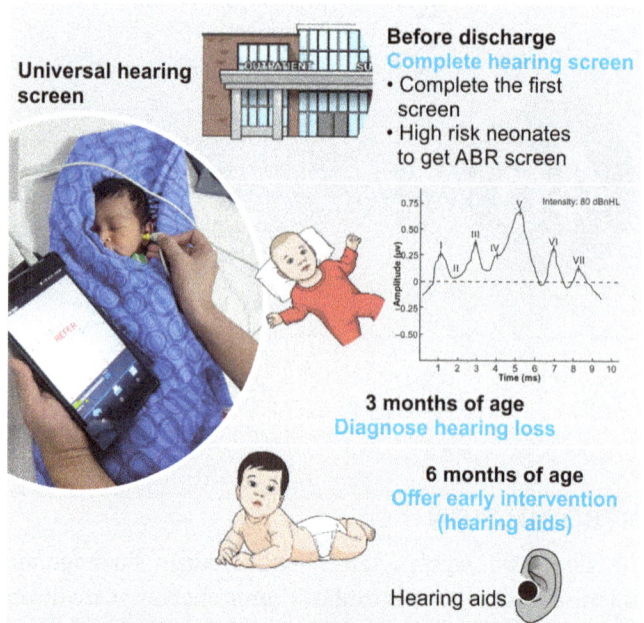

Fig. 1: Screening for neonatal hearing loss. Figure inset shows otoacoustic emission (OAE) screen being performed. According to the Early Hearing Detection and Intervention (EHDI) Program 1-3-6 rule, hearing screening no later than 1 month of age, a diagnosis no later than 3 months of age and early intervention services no later than 6 months age.
(ABR: auditory brainstem response)

screening protocol with otoacoustic emissions (OAE) as the first screen, and auditory brainstem response (ABR) as the second step. If the first OAE is "refer", it should be repeated at 6 weeks during the immunization visit. If again abnormal, it has to be confirmed with ABR and a complete audiological evaluation should be undertaken before 3 months of age and hearing aids should be offered by 6 months of age. Neonates with risk factors for hearing loss and NICU graduates should preferably undergo ABR as the first step as OAE can fail to detect sensorineural hearing loss.

Vision

All neonates at birth should be inspected for any gross eye anomalies like white cornea, congenital cataracts. Red reflex should be tested using a hand held ophthalmoscope within the first 48 hours of life. Normal red reflexes are bilaterally symmetrical red or orange, while the absence of it or black shadows or flecks mandates urgent ophthalmological referral **(Fig. 2)**.

Common Metabolic and Genetic Disorders

Newborn screening for congenital metabolic conditions is recommended. In India's Expanded Newborn Screening study on 18,000 neonates, the common disorders identified were congenital hypothyroidism, congenital adrenal hyperplasia (CAH), and glucose-6-phosphate dehydrogenase (G6PD) deficiency followed by aminoacidopathies. The sample for metabolic screening consists of heel prick blood

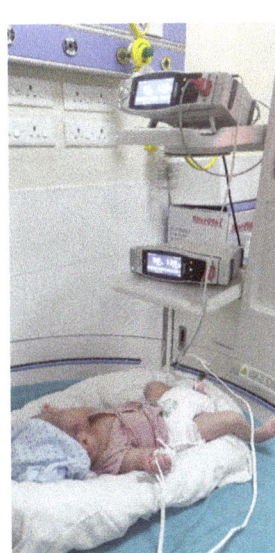
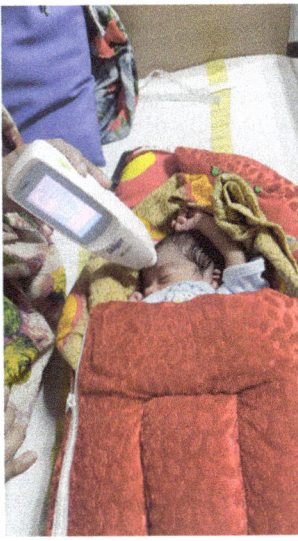
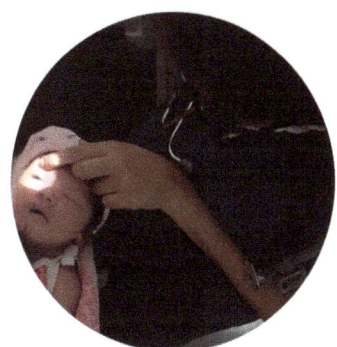
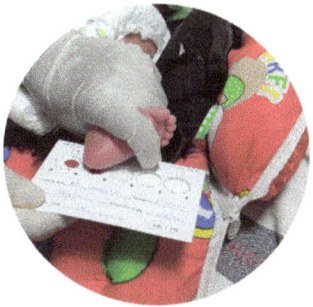

Pulse oximeter screen for critical congenital heart disease | Predischarge screening for jaundice | Screening for red reflex | Inborn error of metabolism screen

Fig. 2: Components of predischarge newborn screening include pulse oximetry screen for congenital cyanotic heart disease, jaundice screen, red reflex, and common inborn errors of metabolism.

impregnated into special filter paper (dried blood spot) taken between 72 hours and 7 days of life. The samples are transported to a central laboratory for testing. In centers with high birth rates and early discharge policy, the sample can be taken after 24 hours of age after adequate breastfeeding is established. Once the screening for common disorders is implemented in a unit, it can be expanded to various other disorders in a phased manner.

Developmental Dysplasia of the Hip

A hip examination should be performed before discharge and documented. Hip instability (positive Ortolani or Barlow's tests) should be confirmed by ultrasonography of the hip. Selective ultrasonography of the hip can be considered at 6 weeks, if there are signs of hip instability clinically, breech presentation in the third trimester, or positive family history. The hip examination needs to be continued in each visit during follow-up until the baby attains walking.

Critical Congenital Heart Disease Screening

All newborns should undergo pulse oximetry testing after 24 hours of life to rule out critical congenital heart defects. A newborn is said to have "passed the test" if the saturation values are more than 95% in both right hands and lower limb with less than 3% difference. Saturation values of less than 90% in both the right upper and lower limbs are labeled as failed screening. All intermediate values are subjected to rescreening once or twice at an hourly interval. Infants who fail screening or have intermediate results should undergo a detailed cardiological evaluation, including echocardiography.

Neonatal Jaundice

A visual assessment of jaundice followed by transcutaneous evaluation of jaundice (wherever available) is a must before discharge. The measured value should be plotted on the Bhutani's pre-discharge bilirubin nomogram. Any neonate with bilirubin values in high risk or high intermediate zone should not be discharged, while neonates with bilirubin in the low intermediate zone should be followed up after 24–48 hours of discharge. Infants born before 37 weeks of gestation, ABO or Rh incompatibility setting, family history of jaundice, sepsis, or asphyxia are at risk for jaundice. Neonates need early follow-up for jaundice if discharged before 48 hours of life.

COMMON POSTNATAL ISSUES OF MOTHER AND INFANT DYAD

Common postnatal problems encountered by the mother and infant are discussed in **Table 1**.

HARMFUL POSTNATAL PRACTICES

Common harmful postpartum practices that are practiced by lay health workers based on traditional beliefs are given

TABLE 1: Common postnatal problems and their management.

Problem	Management
Flat nipple or retracted nipple	Ideally identified antenatally and management initiated before birth. Postnatally use syringing technique followed by proper attachment and latching
Cracked nipple	Usually, a consequence of improper attachment and positioning. Address proper breastfeeding technique. Apply hindmilk and continue milk expression. Avoid soap to wash breast. Commercial lubricants do not offer any advantages
Engorged breasts	The breasts are swollen, hard, and painful. Typically occurs after 48 hours when milk let down has been established. Hot fomentation followed by frequent feeding or expression of milk. If not treated correctly, it may lead to breast abscess occasionally
Fever in the neonate (temperature > 37.5°C)	Common causes of hyperthermia are dehydration, environmental conditions (high ambient temperature or over clothing), and sepsis. Rule out dehydration due to excessive weight loss and sepsis
Hypothermia (temperature <36.5°C)	Prevent using appropriate clothing and Kangaroo care. Other causes are hypoglycemia and sepsis, which need to be ruled out, if hypothermia persists
Regurgitation	Small amounts of regurgitation are normal and can be conservatively managed, if weight gain is adequate
Constipation or loose stools	Stool frequency can vary from 3 to 5 times a day (due to the small volume of the stomach and gastro-colic reflex) to once in 3 days. Unless there are signs of diarrhea (features of dehydration inform of decreased urine output, tachycardia) or constipation (in the form of abdominal distension or vomiting), the frequency of stool passage should not be a matter of concern
Urine frequency	Neonates pass urine less frequently in the first few days of life (1–3 times a day) that increases later. Assessment of urine frequency can be challenging if the baby passes urine each time with the stool and is on absorbent diapers
Diaper rash	Manifests with redness and excoriation in the perianal area (typically at the region of contact with diaper). The absence of involvement of creases and satellite lesions typically distinguishes these lesions from candidiasis. These lesions can often be treated by simple measures like cotton nappies, keeping the area dry, and applying lubricants like petrolatum/zinc oxide

below. To improve maternal and neonatal health, these practices must be addressed before discharge.
- Pre-lacteal feeds (honey, sugar water) and discarding colostrum resulting in delayed initiation of breastfeeding.
- Restriction of certain foods to the mother in the belief of better wound healing and to prevent harmful effects in the newborn.
- *Poor self-hygiene, cord, and eye care practices*: Applying turmeric, ghee to the cord, early bathing of the neonate, and poor maternal hygiene.

DISCHARGE PLANNING

When to Discharge

Discharge can be planned after all the following criteria are satisfied:
- A normal physical examination and no abnormality detected during the hospital stay.
- Vitals are normal and stable for at least 12 hours before discharge.
- Completed at least two successful breastfeedings and mother is confident about latching, swallowing, and infant satiety.
- Mother is confident of taking care of baby, well aware of danger signs, and follow up visits.
- Baby has passed urine and meconium
- The baby has received the birth dose of immunization
- Risk assessment for jaundice has been done and screening tests as per hospital policy is done.

Generally, most of the term neonates are fit for discharge after 24–48 hours in vaginal delivery and by 72 hours in LSCS, if all of the above criteria are satisfied. A preterm neonate may take a much longer duration for discharge.

Discharge Preparedness

At the time of discharge, the mother should be handed over the mother-child protection (MCP) card and encouraged to go through the card while emphasizing early child development, including age-appropriate development milestone tracking by parents, positive parenting practices, and early identification of danger signs. The danger signs are:
- Presence of fever (axillary temperature >37.7°C) or hypothermia (axillary temperature < 36.5°C)
- Fast breathing (Respiration rate more than > 60/min)
- Severe chest indrawing
- Poor feeding/letharg
- Abdominal distension and vomiting
- Bleeding from any site
- Convulsion
- Yellow discoloration of palm and sole

With the appearance of any of the above danger signs, the parents should immediately seek medical care.

Emergency contact numbers for teleconsultation (preferably available 24 × 7) should be mentioned in the discharge paper. Usually, babies need to be called after 48 hours and no later than 72 hours after discharge to assess general health, feeding adequacy, mother-infant interaction, and jaundice. Studies have identified jaundice, dehydration, and feeding difficulties as the most common reasons for readmission.

Discharge Medications

Vitamin D needs to be started at 400 IU/day and continued till 1 year of age. Regular multivitamins are not needed in term exclusively breastfed infants, but oral iron is recommended from 6 months of age. Preterm very low-birth infants need additional calcium, phosphorus, and iron supplements.

POSTPARTUM CARE AND ADVICE FOR MOTHER'S HEALTH

Mothers face the challenge to adapt to multiple physical, social, and psychological changes after delivery. Recovery from the changes in the childbirth and the associated hormonal changes, transition to parenthood and learning to feed and care of the newborn present considerable challenges for women. Optimum postpartum care provides an opportunity to promote the overall health and well-being of women as well to aid in her transition to being a mother.

Care after Birth (Within First 24 Hours)

- All postpartum women should have regular assessment of vaginal bleeding, uterine contraction, fundal height, temperature, and heart rate (pulse) during the first 24 hours starting from the first hour after birth. Blood pressure should be measured immediately after birth and they should be encouraged to void within 6 hours after birth. These assessments will aid in the early identification of complications such as hypo or hypertension, development of sepsis, urinary retention, and postpartum hemorrhage, which needs interventions to reduce the maternal morbidity.
- Mothers who deliver vaginally should be taught pelvic floor exercises before discharge. Perineal wound care for vaginally delivered women and abdominal wound care for women who underwent cesarean section should be taught before discharge. They should be advised follow up consultation, if signs of infection like fever, foul-smelling vaginal discharge, wound discharge, excessive bleeding, painful breast engorgement, or any bladder or bowel problems.
- At the time of discharge, written recommendation for follow to ensure well-being as well for any ongoing medical issues should be documented in the records and should be given to the patient and communicated to appropriate family members to ensure continuation of care during the postpartum. They also should be provided with the information of whom to contact, in cases of emergency.

Postpartum Care after 24 Hours

- In the subsequent visits/contact all mothers should be enquired about general well-being and symptoms or signs suggestive of any postpartum complications. Special care should be taken to assess the emotional well-being of the mothers as well to address any concerns regarding the breastfeeding.
- All mothers should be counseled about the physiological process of recovery after birth, and advised to consult health care professional incase of any problem. They should be counseled about hygiene, especially about hand washing.
- Mother should be advised to consume healthy food, refrain from smoking and alcohol, take plenty of water and other liquids, and adequate rest for optimum milk output. She should be encouraged to continue night feeding also. All breastfeeding mothers should also be advised iron, calcium, and vitamin D supplementation for the initial 3 months following birth. Advantages of early ambulation and plenty of fluids to prevent venous thrombosis in high-risk mothers should be emphasized.
- Mothers should be counseled on birth spacing and family planning. Contraceptive options should be discussed, and contraceptive options, which could be used safely while breastfeeding such as copper T, low dose progesterone pill (Mini Pill), or depot medroxy-progesterone acetate should be provided.
- The emotional well-being of all postpartum females should be assessed, and proper psychological support should be provided before discharge. A mother who has lost her baby should receive additional supportive care and if needed should receive counseling from perinatal mental health team. At each subsequent postnatal contact, mothers should be enquired about their emotional well-being, and the supports they are receiving from family and others as well as their coping strategies for dealing with day-to-day matters. They should be encouraged to talk about or to report back to the hospital in cases of any changes in mood, emotional state, and behavior.
- *Long-term issues on health*: Mothers with medical conditions such as hypertension, obesity, heart disease, thyroid disorders, renal disorders, etc., should be counseled regarding the importance of timely follow-up with the obstetric team or their primary treating team. Medications such as anti-epileptics, psychotropic medications should be reviewed to ensure adjustment of dosage after delivery.

CHAPTER AT A GLANCE

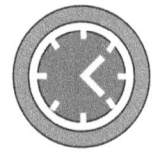

First 24 hours

Neonate

Birth-1 hour
- Assess breathing
- Delayed cord clamping
- Skin-to-skin care
- Early initiation of breastfeeding

1–24 hours
- Weight, eye, and cord care
- Complete clinical examination
- Vitamin-K prophylaxis
- Birth vaccination

Mother

Maternal
- Assess for vaginal bleeding, uterine contraction, fundal height
- Monitor vital signs (Temperature, heart rate, and blood pressure) Document passage of urine within 6 hours

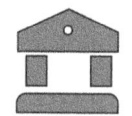

Beyond 24 hours

- Thermoregulation
- Rooming-in
- Detailed clinical examination
- Exclusive breastfeeding
- Identify preterm and low-birth weight neonates who require additional care
- Predischarge screening
- Discharge preparedness

- Assess urination and urinary continence, bowel movements, healing of perineal wound and lochia
- Ask for symptoms; headache, fatigue, back pain, perineal pain and perineal hygiene, breast pain, and uterine tenderness

Care at home

Postnatal visits
Mother-baby dyad should be provided a total of four postnatal visits by midwives or community health workers
- First day (24 hours in case of home delivery)
- Day 3 (48–72 hours)
- Between days 7 and 14
- 6 weeks

Assess physical and emotional well-being of mother, breastfeeding and neonatal danger signs
- Maternal iron and folic acid should be continued for 3 months postpartum

---

KEY POINTS

- The postnatal period is a vulnerable transitional period for mother-infant dyad associated with higher maternal and neonatal mortality.
- Comprehensive care, including exclusive breastfeeding, thermal care, cord care, hand hygiene, and kangaroo care, can decrease neonatal deaths.
- Mothers need active support with breastfeeding.
- Risk assessment for jaundice is necessary before discharge, with follow-up plans.
- Active involvement of both family members and health care workers are needed for a smooth transition of postnatal care from health care facility to home.

SUGGESTED READING

1. American Academy of Pediatrics Subcommittee on Hyperbilirubinemia. Management of hyperbilirubinemia in the newborn infant 35 or more weeks of gestation. Pediatrics. 2004;114(1):297-316.
2. Martin GR, Ewer AK, Gaviglio A, Hom LA, Saarinen A, Sontag M, et al. Updated strategies for pulse oximetry screening for critical congenital heart disease. Pediatrics. 2020;146(1): e20191650.
3. Ministry of Health & Family Welfare, Government of India (2014). India Newborn Action Plan (INAP): National Health Mission [online]. Available from https://www.newbornwhocc.org/INAP_Final.pdf. [Last accessed November, 2021].
4. National Rural Health Mission (2013). Operational guideline: Rashtriya Bal Swasthya Karyakram (RBSK): Child Health Screening and Early Intervention Services under NRHM [online]. Available from http://cghealth.nic.in/nhmcg/Informations/RMNCH/7Rastriya_Bal_Swaasthya_karyakaram.pdf. [Last accessed November, 2021]
5. Young Infants Clinical Signs Study Group. Clinical signs that predict severe illness in children under age 2 months: a multicentre study. Lancet. 2008;371(9607):135-42.

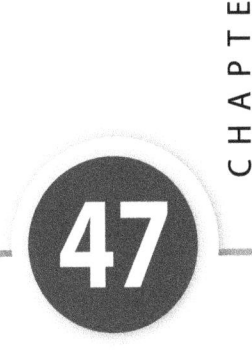

47. Surgical Conditions Presenting at Birth

Srishti Goel, Vikram Khanna

INTRODUCTION

Surgical conditions (both congenital and acquired) are common neonatal emergencies constituting 4–12% of the total neonatal intensive care unit admissions. Timely diagnosis and appropriate management have greatly improved the outcomes and survival of neonates with surgical problems. This chapter provides an overview of clinical presentation and approach to diagnosing and managing common newborn surgical emergencies.

OBJECTIVES

- Understand the spectrum and clinical presentation of surgical conditions presenting at birth.
- Understand the approach to diagnosis and management of surgical emergencies.

SPECTRUM OF SURGICAL CONDITIONS

The conditions requiring surgery can be both congenital (around 85–90% of all cases) and acquired. Gastrointestinal (GIT) anomalies are the leading causes of neonatal surgical emergencies, followed by respiratory and central nervous system problems **(Table 1)**. Among GIT causes, esophageal atresia with or without trachea esophageal fistula, intestinal atresia, and anorectal malformation (ARM) are common.

ANTENATAL DIAGNOSIS AND MANAGEMENT

Antenatal Diagnosis

When surgical conditions that require multidisciplinary care are diagnosed in the antenatal period, the following are recommended:
- In-utero transfer and planned delivery in a well-equipped center with optimal obstetric, neonatal, and surgical facilities.
- Prenatal counseling regarding prognosis and likely outcome.
- Fetal surgical intervention based on existing facilities.
- Planning delivery and postnatal care to optimize neonatal outcomes.

Fetal Therapy

Fetal surgical interventions are available in certain centers for some congenital malformations **(Table 2)**. Fetal access is gained either through maternal laparotomy and open hysterotomy or via minimally invasive percutaneous fetoscopic surgery. Ex-utero intrapartum therapy (EXIT), usually done for large fetal neck masses and complex airway malformations, involves stabilizing airway and fetal intervention immediately after delivery while maintaining uteroplacental circulation (i.e., the umbilical cord is intact). Due to associated obstetric risks such as preterm labor, premature rupture of membranes, and chorioamnionitis, fetal surgery should be reserved for conditions wherein the fetus is at risk of intrauterine or early fetal demise with suboptimal and inadequate postnatal therapy. Other prerequisites include the availability of accurate prenatal diagnosis, the absence of life-threatening associated anomalies or chromosomal syndromes, and facilities for multidisciplinary team management with comprehensive prenatal counseling.

APPROACH TO DIAGNOSIS AND MANAGEMENT

Clinical Presentation

Most surgical conditions present with the following features:
- Respiratory distress at or soon after birth
- Vomiting (bilious or non-bilious) or abdominal distension
- Delayed passage of meconium or absent anal opening
- Defect in abdominal wall
- Hydronephrosis
- Masses (Renal, inguinal, scrotal, or lumbosacral)

This section gives a simple algorithm-based approach to the diagnosis and management of common neonatal surgical conditions based on clinical presentation **(Flowcharts 1 and 2)**.

Always rule out medical causes that present with similar symptoms such as surfactant deficiency, pneumonia, meconium aspiration syndrome, sepsis, necrotizing

TABLE 1: Surgical conditions presenting in the newborn.

Congenital causes	Most common (85–90%)
Malformations of the central nervous system (15–20%)	• Neural tube defects (NTD; meningomyelocele) • Hydrocephalus • Arnold Chiari malformation • Dandy-walker malformation
Malformations of laryngo-tracheobronchial tree (10–15%)	• Choanal atresia • Laryngotracheal clefts, laryngeal webs • Tracheal agenesis • Congenital high-airway obstruction syndrome (CHAOS) • Congenital lobar emphysema (CLE) • Cystic congenital-pulmonary airway malformation (CPAM) • Pulmonary sequestration • Congenital diaphragmatic hernia (CDH) • Diaphragmatic eventration
Congenital heart disease (5–10%)	Duct-dependent systemic or pulmonary circulation
Gastrointestinal malformations (GI) (35–60%)	• Esophageal atresia (EA) with or without tracheoesophageal fistula (TEF) • Hypertrophic pyloric stenosis • Intestinal atresia, web, stenosis (Duodenal, jejunal and ileal and colonic) • Annular pancreas • Meconium ileus, meconium peritonitis, meconium plug syndrome • Malrotation and midgut volvulus • Hirschsprung's disease • Anorectal malformations (ARM) • Mesenteric cysts • Incarcerated inguinal hernia • Abdominal wall defects (Omphalocele, gastroschisis)
Malformations of genitourinary tract (3–5%)	• Obstructive and non-obstructive hydronephrosis (HDN) • Posterior urethral valve/bladder outlet obstruction (PUV/BOO) • Exstrophy of bladder • Cloacal exstrophy • Testicular torsion • Hypospadias • Epispadias
Acquired conditions (10–15%)	Necrotizing enterocolitis, perforation of the gut, peritoneal adhesions

TABLE 2: Conditions amenable to in-utero fetal intervention.

Condition	Type of fetal surgery
Congenital diaphragmatic hernia	Fetal endoscopic tracheal occlusion (FETO) using balloon at 26–29 weeks followed by removal at 34–36 weeks or ex-utero intrapartum therapy (EXIT) procedure
Congenital pulmonary airway malformation (CPAM)	*Macrocystic CPAM at < 32 weeks*: In utero drainage via thoraco amniotic shunt (TAS)
Fetal hydrothorax secondary to lymphatic malformations of the thoracic duct	Percutaneous thoracocentesis or thoraco-amniotic shunt
Sacrococcygeal teratoma	Debulking, ablation, or devascularization using radiofrequency or laser sources. Surgical resection in the neonatal period
Fetal neck masses (Cystic hygroma, teratoma)	• Open fetal resection • EXIT-to-airway procedure and EXIT-to-resection procedure to permit the safe establishment of airway before delivery
Meningomyelocele	Open repair via maternal laparotomy and open hysterotomy at 19–26 weeks
Lower urinary tract obstruction (posterior urethral valve, bladder outlet obstruction)	• *Percutaneous vesico-amniotic shunt*: Most common • Fetoscopic cystoscopy guided valve ablation • Open fetal vesicostomy

CHAPTER 47 | Surgical Conditions Presenting at Birth

Flowchart 1: Approach to surgical conditions presenting with respiratory distress at or soon after birth.

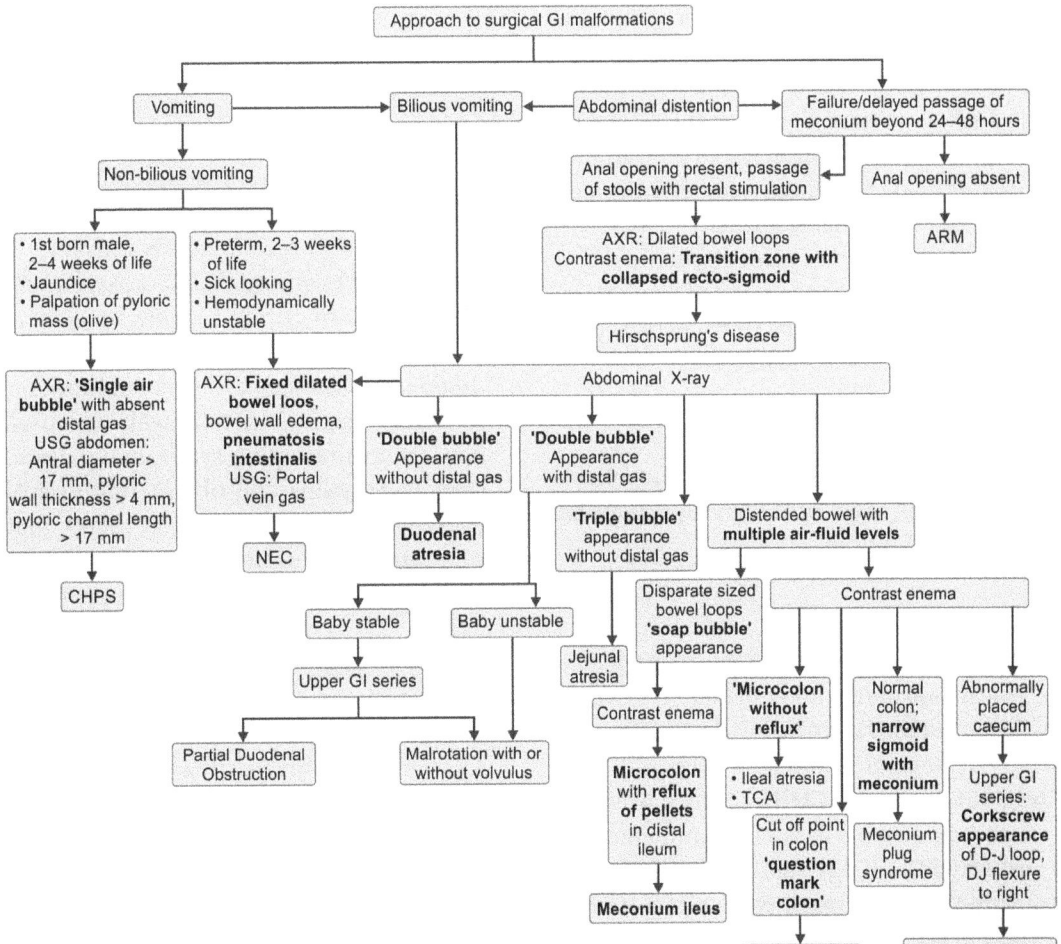

(BMV: bag and mask ventilation; CDH: congenital diaphragmatic hernia; GIT: gastrointestinal tract; PPHN: persistent pulmonary hypertension; USG: ultrasound; NG: nasogastric)

Flowchart 2: Approach to diagnosis of common neonatal gastrointestinal surgical conditions.

(ARM: anorectal malformation; AXR: abdominal X-ray; CHPS: congenital hypertrophic pyloric stenosis; NEC: necrotizing enterocolitis; TCA: total colonic aganglionosis; GIT: gastrointestinal tract; USG: ultrasound)

enterocolitis (NEC), and feed intolerance due to prematurity, infection, or metabolic abnormalities.

Examine the neonate for associated system anomalies [e.g., vertebral, anorectal, cardiac, trachea-esophageal, radial, renal, and limb (VACTERL) defects] and syndromes (Trisomies and aneuploidies). Workup for associated anomalies includes echocardiography, ultrasonogram of brain and kidney, and X-rays of the spine and vertebral defects.

Respiratory Conditions

Causes

Congenital diaphragmatic hernia (CDH) and diaphragmatic eventration, esophageal atresia (EA) with or without tracheoesophageal fistula (TEF), bilateral choanal atresia, congenital pulmonary airway malformation (CPAM), congenital lobar emphysema (CLE), and malformations of the laryngo-tracheobronchial tree. Underlying mechanisms include airway obstruction, pulmonary compression, collapse or displacement, and parenchymal disease or insufficiency.

Clinical Manifestations

Suspect surgical disorders when respiratory distress is associated with any one of the following signs or symptoms **(Flowchart 1)**:
- Drooling of saliva with attacks of choking or cyanosis postfeeding and failure to pass a nasogastric (NG) tube in stomach—EA with or without TEF.
- Cyclical cyanosis with failure to pass a catheter through bilateral nostrils—bilateral choanal atresia.
- Scaphoid abdomen with evidence of mediastinal shift on clinical examination—CDH or eventration of diaphragm.
- Bulging hemithorax with mediastinal shift, decreased air entry, and hyper-resonance—CPAM or CLE.

Investigations

Chest X-ray (CXR) **(Fig. 1)**, ultrasound of the chest, computerized tomography, and bronchoscopy may be needed.

Management

Preoperative management should focus on the maintenance of temperature, airway, breathing, and circulation (TABC), and minimizing the risk of aspiration by head-end elevation (15–30°), insertion of Replogle tube (in cases with EA/TEF), and NG tube (in cases with CDH). Positive pressure ventilation through bag and mask is contraindicated in neonates with suspected CDH, and immediate intubation should be performed in those with severe respiratory distress.

Surgical therapy involves definitive repair after immediate stabilization. The timing of surgery depends on the type and severity of the disorder, the presence of associated anomalies, and the baby's general condition. It is advisable to delay primary repair in cases with extreme prematurity, hemodynamic instability, and pulmonary hypertension. Mild cases of CLE and CPAM are managed conservatively, with surgery being reserved for severe cases.

Gastrointestinal Conditions

Surgical malformations of the GIT tract commonly present with vomiting (bilious or non-bilious), abdominal distention, and failure or delayed passage of meconium beyond 24–48 hours **(Flowchart 2)**. Proximal GI obstructions are predominantly present with vomiting and minimal abdominal distention, usually limited to the upper abdomen, while distal GI obstruction presents with early and diffuse abdominal distention with or without bilious vomiting and delayed passage of meconium. Obstructions distal to the ampulla of vater presents with bile-stained vomiting.

Bilious vomiting represents a life-threatening emergency and should be considered "malrotation" unless proven otherwise. Rule out nonsurgical causes such as septic ileus, paralytic, ileus, and immaturity of GIT in preterm neonates.

Causes

- *Bilious vomiting*: Malrotation with or without midgut volvulus, intestinal atresia, web, stenosis (duodenal, jejunal, ileal, and colonic), annular pancreas, obstructing peritoneal bands, persistent omphalomesenteric duct, Hirschsprung's disease, and vascular anomalies (aberrant superior mesenteric artery, portal vein). Acquired causes include sepsis and NEC.
- *Non-bilious vomiting includes congenital hypertrophic pyloric stenosis (CHPS), upper duodenal stenosis/web (above ampulla of Vater) and NEC.*
- *Abdominal distention*: Congenital intestinal obstruction (due to intestinal atresia, web, stenosis, meconium ileus, meconium plug syndrome, malrotation with or without volvulus and obstructing peritoneal bands), Hirschsprung's disease, anorectal malformations, pneumoperitoneum, NEC and septic ileus, and peritoneal adhesions and strictures (post GI surgery/NEC).
- *Failure or delayed passage of meconium*: Nonpassage or delayed passage of meconium beyond 24–48 hours of life should be taken as Hirschsprung's disease or ARM unless proved otherwise. Always inspect for the presence of an anal opening. The absence of anal opening indicates ARM, and presence should alert for Hirschsprung's disease. A perineal fistula or an abnormal connection with the genitourinary tract (rectovaginal, rectovesical, and rectourethral fistula) may be present in around 80% of males and more than 95% of female babies with ARM.

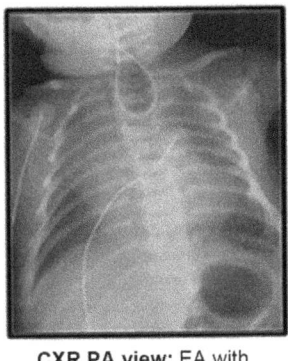
CXR PA view: EA with TEF (Curled up NG tube in upper esophagus with stomach bubble)

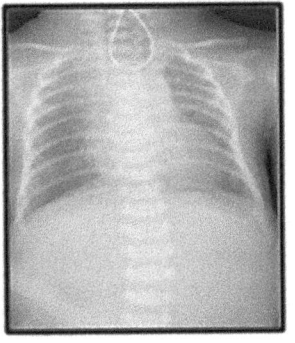
CXR PA view: EA without TEF (Curled up NG tube in upper esophagus with absence of stomach bubble)

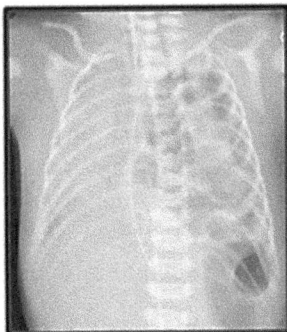
CXR PA view: CDH (Bowel loops in hemithorax with mediastinal shift)

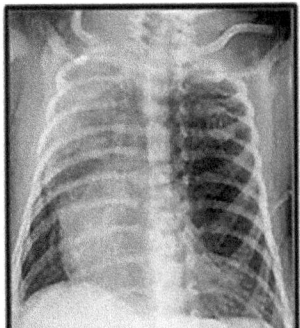
CXR PA view: CLE (Hyperlucent area in lung herniating to opposite side with mediastinal shift)

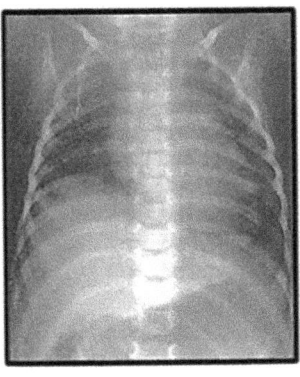
CXR PA view: Diaphragmatic eventration (Elevation of diaphragm with smooth unbroken outline)

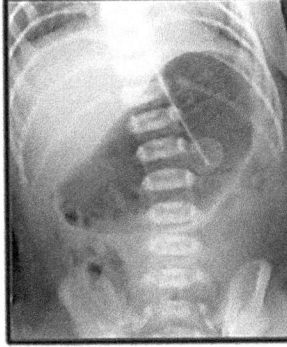
AXR supine view: CHPS (single air bubble)

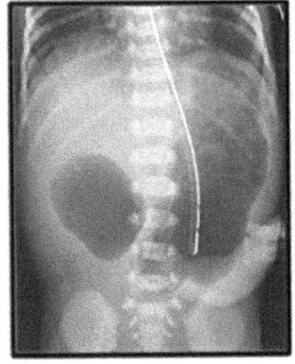
AXR supine view: DA (Double bubble appearance)

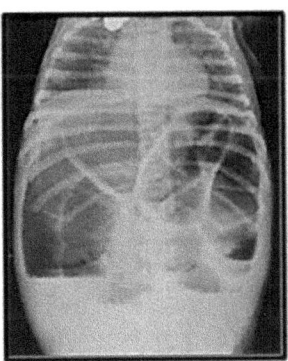
AXR: Ileal atresia (Distended bowel with multiple air-fluid levels)

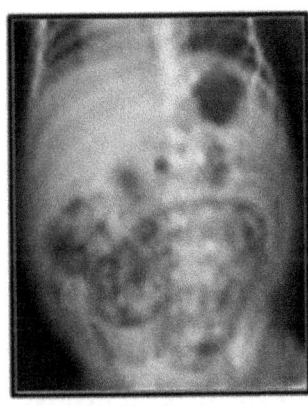
AXR supine view: NEC (Fixed dilated bowel loops, pneumatosis intestinalis)

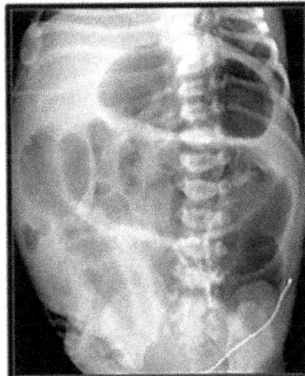
AXR meconium ileus (Disparate bowel loops)

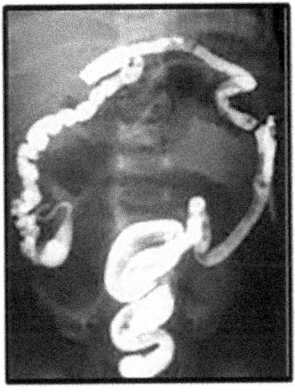
Contrast enema: TCA (Microcolon without reflux)

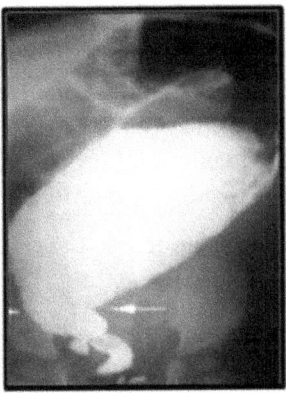
Contrast enema: Hirchsprung's disease (Transition zone)

Fig. 1: Appearance of common surgical conditions on diagnostic imaging.
(AXR: abdominal X-ray; CDH: congenital diaphragmatic hernia; CHPS: congenital hypertrophic pyloric stenosis; CLE: congenital lobar emphysema; CXR: chest X-ray; DA: duodenal atresia; EA/TEF: esophageal atresia/tracheo-esophageal fistula; NEC: necrotizing enterocolitis; TCA: total colonic aganglionosis)

Investigation

Plain radiographs of the abdomen (anteroposterior, left lateral decubitus, and cross-table lateral views) are the single most important investigation for neonatal GI malformations. Contrast studies with nonionic water-soluble contrast (upper GI series and contrast enema) help to diagnose a proximal and distal bowel obstruction. **Figure 1** outlines the radiological appearance of common GI malformations presenting in the neonatal period.

Other investigations include an ultrasound abdomen with a Doppler to evaluate the relationship of superior mesenteric artery and vein (normally artery lies to the left of a vein; reversed in cases with malrotation). The presence of hyper-myelinated axons with the absence of ganglion cells in myenteric plexus on rectal biopsy confirms the diagnosis of Hirschsprung's disease.

Management

Supportive treatment forms the mainstay of therapy initially. Preoperative management should focus on maintaining TABC, fluid and electrolyte balance, and decompression of the GIT using continuous NG tube suction and close monitoring of vitals and urine output.

Definitive surgery usually involves resection followed by end-to-end anastomosis. "Malrotation with or without volvulus" should be managed on an urgent basis to prevent devascularization of the gut and subsequent gangrene. The gut is de-rotated, the base of the mesentery is widened, and Ladd's bands are divided. Contrast enema is not only diagnostic but is also therapeutic in cases with meconium ileus and meconium plug syndrome. The presence of fistula and its type play an important role in deciding the treatment plan in babies with ARM. While the management commonly involves slow dilatation with Hegar's dilators followed by delayed repair in cases with perineal fistula, babies without fistula or those with high ARM require colostomy with the definitive repair of the defect at the later stages.

Hydronephrosis

Antenatal hydronephrosis (HDN) refers to the anteroposterior diameter (APD) of renal pelvis ≥4 mm and ≥7 mm in the second and third trimester, respectively. Half to two-thirds of cases of antenatal HDN are transient and resolved by the third trimester. Babies with postnatal HDN are at increased risk of developing renal damage, urinary tract infections (UTI), and vesicoureteric reflux (VUR) and hence require long-term follow-up with or without surgery.

Causes: Include pelvi-ureteric junction (PUJ) obstruction, vesicoureteric junction (VUJ) obstruction, VUR, posterior urethral valve or bladder outlet obstruction (PUV/BOO), ureterocele, megaureter, and multicystic dysplastic kidney.

Investigation: Pregnant women with antenatally diagnosed HDN in their fetus should undergo periodic follow-up USG scans based on the severity to assess disease progression. It is advisable to rule out lower urinary tract obstruction (LUTO), oligohydramnios, renal dysplasia, and other extrarenal structural and chromosomal anomalies, the presence of which indicates a poor prognosis and requires referral to higher centers with facilities for prenatal testing and counseling.

All cases with antenatal HDN should undergo postnatal USG KUB within the 3rd-7th day of life (preferably before hospital discharge) except those with suspected LUTO or PUV/BOO, where the postnatal USG is performed earlier within the first 24-48 hours of life (**Flowchart 3**).

Neonatal HDN is defined as APD ≥ 7 mm. The subsequent evaluation depends on the severity of HDN as assessed by the society of fetal urology (SFU) classification or APD of the renal pelvis.

- *Normal USG KUB in the first week of life*: Repeat USG at 4-6 weeks.
- *Mild unilateral/bilateral HDN (APD < 10 mm or SFU grade 1-2)*: Sequential ultrasound after 1-2 months and 3-6 monthly until resolution.
- *Unilateral/bilateral hydronephrosis (APD > 10 mm, SFU grade 3-4 or ureteric dilatation)*: Perform micturating cystourethrogram (MCU) to rule out LUTO or VUR.

Indication of MCU

- *Babies with suspected LUTO*: Perform MCU within 24-72 hours of life.
- *Moderate-to-severe HDN (SFU 3-4; renal APD > 10 mm) or presence of dilated ureter*: Perform MCU at 4-6 weeks of age.

Indication of Diuretic Renography

Diuretic renography is performed at 6-8 weeks of life in babies with moderate-severe unilateral or bilateral HDN and normal MCU evaluation.

Management: Neonates with LUTO or PUV/BOO should undergo PUV fulguration and those with obstructed HDN, and/or reduced/worsening differential renal function should undergo Pyeloplasty. Provide antibiotic prophylaxis (Cephalexin, cotrimoxazole or nitrofurantoin) in cases with VUR though the first year of life and those with moderate or severe HDN (SFU 3-4; renal APD > 10 mm) or dilated ureter while awaiting evaluation (**Flowchart 3**). It is important to screen all babies with HDN for UTI and renal damage by periodic evaluation of blood pressures, urinalysis, and estimation of renal function tests.

COMMON NEWBORN SURGICAL EMERGENCIES

This section provides a brief description and management of the common neonatal surgical emergencies.

Congenital Diaphragmatic Hernia

- *Incidence*: 1 in 3,000-4,000
- Left-sided CDH is common (80%). Etiology-failure of closure of pleuroperitoneal folds resulting in herniation of intestinal contents. Associated with pulmonary hypoplasia.
- *Antenatal markers*: Polyhydramnios, intestinal loops in fetal hemithorax
- *Postnatal diagnosis*: Bowel loops in Hemithorax with mediastinal shift

Flowchart 3: Approach to neonatal conditions presenting with antenatal and postnatal hydronephrosis (HDN).

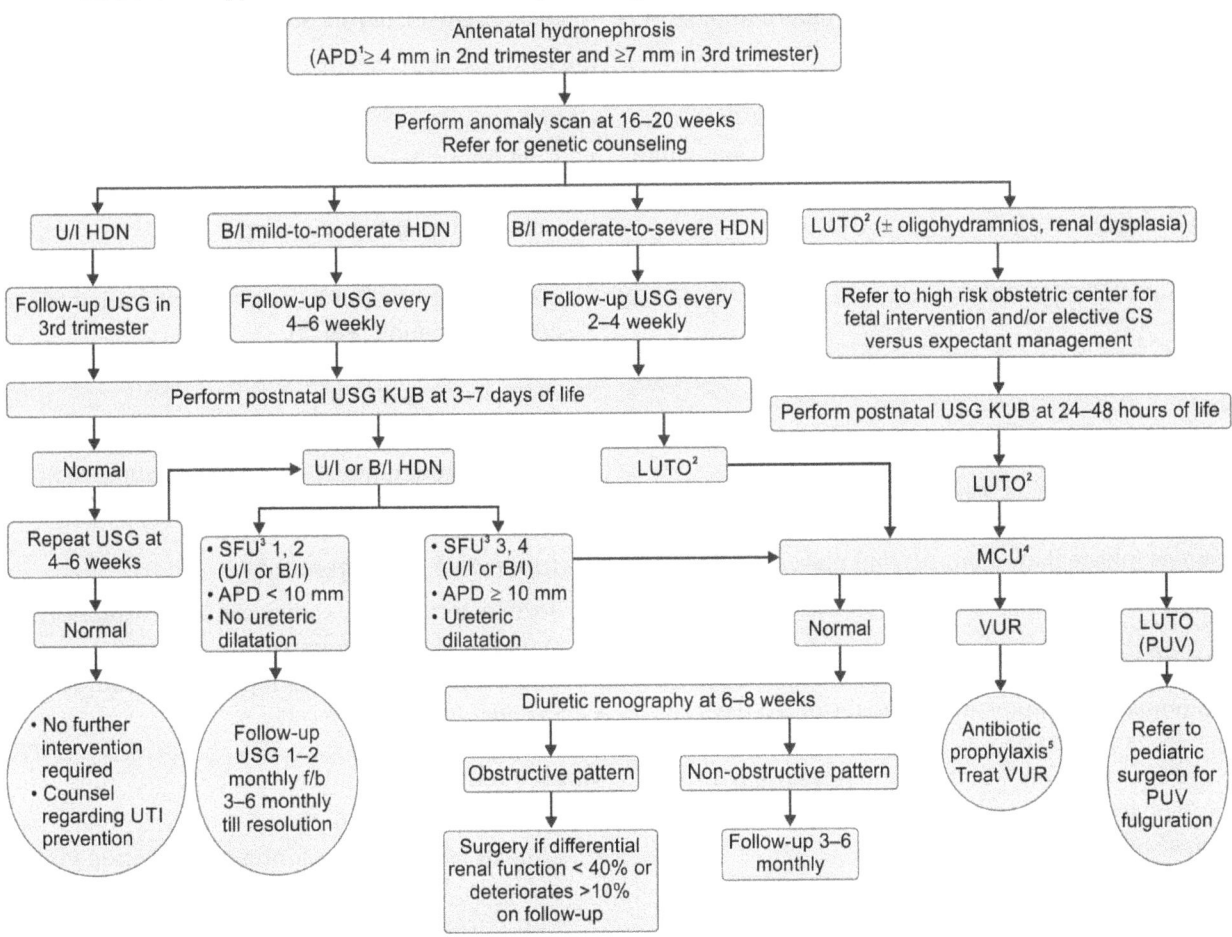

(APD: anteroposterior diameter of the renal pelvis; LUTO: lower urinary tract obstruction; MCU: micturating cystourethrogram; SFU: staging proposed by society of fetal urology; USG KUB: ultrasound of kidney, ureter, and bladder; UTI: urinary tract infection; VUR: vesicoureteric reflux PUV: posterior urethral valve).
Severity of HDN is graded based on the classification proposed by SFU or APD of renal pelvis.
[1]APD of renal pelvis is measured in transverse axial plane at level of renal hilum. Neonatal HDN is defined as APD ≥ 7 mm (Mild: 7–9 mm, moderate: 10–15 mm, severe: > 15 mm).
[2]Lower urinary tract obstruction is suggested by bilateral hydroureteronephrosis along with dilated bladder and posterior urethra and bladder wall thickening.
[3]SFU classification: Grade 0: Normal, no splitting of renal pelvis, grade 1: Slight separation of central renal echo complex. Grade 2: Dilated renal pelvis with visualization of single or few calyces, grade 3: SFU grade 2 with enlarged fluid filled calyces throughout the kidney and normal parenchyma thickness. Grade 4: SFU grade 3 with thinned out renal parenchyma. (Mild-HDN: SFU grade 1–2, moderate-to-severe HDN: SFU grade 3–4).
[4]Perform MCU within 24–72 hours of life in babies with suspected LUTO and at 4–6 weeks of age in other cases with moderate-to-severe HDN (SFU 3–4; renal APD > 10 mm) or dilated ureter.
[5]Provide antibiotic prophylaxis (Cephalexin, cotrimoxazole or nitrofurantoin) in all cases with VUR through the first year of life and those with moderate or severe hydronephrosis (SFU 3–4; renal APD > 10 mm) or dilated ureter while awaiting evaluation.

Preoperative Management

- Decompress gut with orogastric tube
- Avoid bag and mask ventilation
- Optimize oxygenation, gentle ventilation, and permissive hypercapnia
- Treat persistent pulmonary hypertension of the newborn

Surgical Management

- *Severe antenatally diagnosed cases*: Delivery by EXIT.
- *Timing of surgery*: Delayed for 48–72 hours for stabilization. Surgical placement of herniated abdominal contents back into abdomen using a thoracic or abdominal approach).

Postoperative Care

- Optimization of oxygenation and gentle ventilation
- Begin enteral feeds as soon as the NG aspirates decrease
- *Survival*: 30–70%

Esophageal Atresia with/without Tracheaesophageal Fistula

- Incidence: 1 in 3,000–4,500

- *Clinical features*: Respiratory distress, frothing, or excessive salivation from mouth and failure to pass NG tube
- *Associated anomalies*: VATER or VACTERAL (25%), single umbilical artery, trisomy 13, 18, 21
- *Antenatal markers*: Polyhydramnios, absent/small stomach bubble
- *Postnatal diagnosis*: Pouch sign on CXR

Preoperative Management

- NPO
- Continuous proximal pouch decompression (Replogle tube)
- Head end elevation

Surgery: Operate soon as baby is clinically stable. Surgery involves division of TEF and primary esophageal repair with esophago-esophageal anastomosis and placement of chest drain.

Postoperative Care

- Anastomosis under pressure: ventilate for 3–5 days
- Begin feeds as soon baby is stable
- Contrast swallow on 7–10th day; remove drain and NG tube, if no leak
- *Survival*: 85–90%

Duodenal Atresia

- *Incidence*: 1 in 5,000
- *Clinical features*: Bilious vomiting (80%; obstruction distal to ampulla of Vater), abdominal distention (limited to upper abdomen).
- *Associated anomalies*: Down's syndrome (25%), VATER or VACTERAL (25%), cardiac anomalies.
- *Antenatal markers*: Polyhydramnios, "double-bubble appearance" of the distended stomach and proximal duodenum on prenatal imaging.
- *Postnatal diagnosis*: "Double bubble" sign along with the absence of distal gas on AXR.
- *Preoperative management*: NPO and continuous NG suction
- *Surgery*: Kimura's duodenoduodenostomy (open or laparoscopic)
- *Postoperative care*: Nutrition support (parenteral nutrition with the initiation of enteral feeds) and observe for recurrent strictures, constipation.
- *Survival*: > 95%

Omphalocele

- *Incidence*: 1 in 5,500
- *Clinical features*: Gut contents herniating via anterior abdominal defect (2–15 cm) covered with transparent membrane and umbilical cord attached on top.
- *Associated anomalies (50–80%)*: Cardiac, congenital diaphragmatic hernia, trisomy.

Preoperative Management

- Nurse supine
- Continuous NG suction
- Encase intestinal contents in bowel bag/cover with warm saline gauze and plastic wrap.
- Large defects can be painted with silver nitrate or mercurochrome (0.5%) or povidone-iodine to promote eschar formation (**Fig. 2**).

Surgical Management

Surgery is usually delayed for 6 months after birth but is performed immediately, if the sac is ruptured. Primary closure of the defect is done.

Postoperative Management

- Begin enteral feeds as soon as the NG aspirates decrease
- Manage associated anomalies
- Observe for abdominal compartment syndrome
- *Survival*: 70–80%

Gastroschisis

- *Incidence*: 1 in 14,000–15,000
- *Clinical features*: Gut contents herniating via anterior abdominal defect (3–6 cm), usually right to cord base with normal umbilical cord insertion. There is no sac (**Fig. 3**).
- *Associated anomalies (10–15%)*: Intestinal atresia. Always associated with intestinal malrotation.
- *Antenatal markers*: Ventral wall defect containing GI contents
- Preoperative care:
  - Nurse supine
  - Nil oral, continuous NG suction

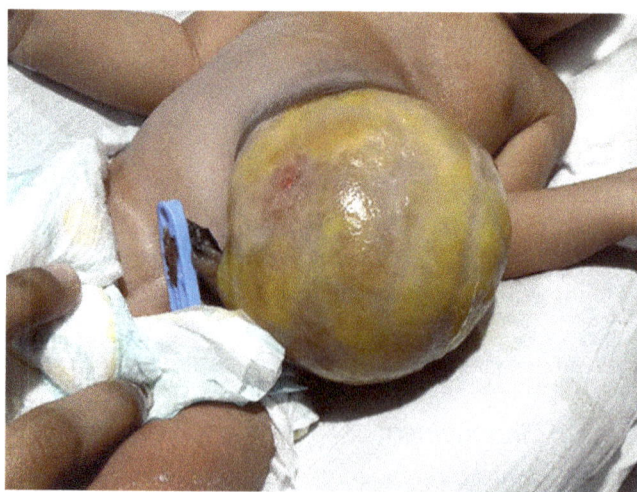

Fig. 2: Neonate with giant omphalocele painted with silver sulfadiazine.

- Encase intestinal contents in a bowel bag or cover with warm saline gauze and plastic wrap.
- *Surgery*: Small defects can be repaired immediately after birth. Silo (sealed plastic device) suspension with daily compression is usually required in larger defects.
- *Postoperative*: Nutrition support (Prolonged TPN with early initiation of enteral feeds). Observe for abdominal compartment syndrome, small bowel syndrome.
- *Survival*: 90–95%

Hirschsprung's Disease

- *Incidence*: 1 in 5,000 births
- The condition is due to the absence of ganglion cells in the distal colon or rectum due to the arrest of caudal migration of neural crest cells. The aganglionic segment of the bowel fails to relax, causing obstruction.

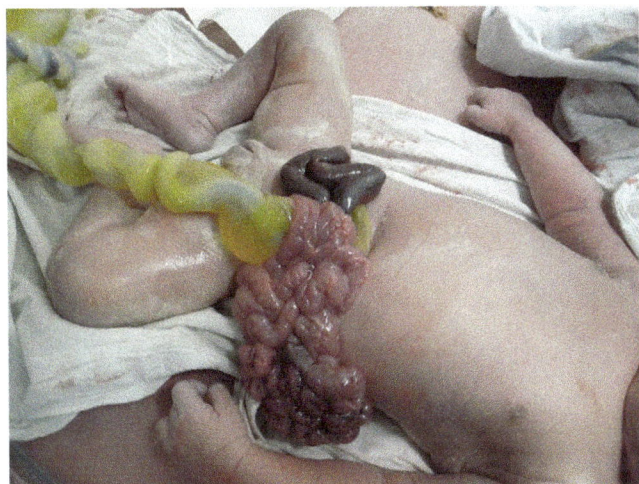

Fig. 3: Gastroschisis-intestines herniating through a defect to the right of the umbilical cord base and the absence of a sac.

- *Clinical features*: Failure to pass stools within 48 hours, Abdominal distention, bilious vomiting (rare).
- *Associated anomalies*: Down syndrome (8–16%)
- *Investigations*: Dilated bowel loops on abdominal X-ray. Characteristic "transition zone" on contrast enema. Rectal biopsy confirms the diagnosis (hyper-myelinated axons, absence of ganglion cells in myenteric plexus).
- *Management*: In mild cases, rectal washes with saline (twice/thrice daily) can be started, and oral feeds continued. A colostomy is performed, if the bowel is not decompressed with saline washes. Definite surgical treatment is planned (rectal pull-through procedure) by 6–8 weeks. (Swenson's, Soave, Duhamel's)
- *Postoperative*: Nutrition support (parenteral nutrition with early initiation of enteral feeds). Observe for constipation, enterocolitis (diarrhea, abdominal pain, and distention).
- *Survival*: 80–95%

Malrotation with Midgut Volvulus

- *Incidence*: 1 in 6,000
- *CF*: Bilious vomiting, rapid clinical deterioration and hemodynamic instability (in cases with associated volvulus) on day 3–5 of life. **Bilious vomiting = Malrotation unless proved otherwise**.
- *Investigations*: Dilated bowel loops, paucity of gas or non-specific.
- Upper GIT contrast study—shows duodenojejunal flexure (DJ) to right, cork-screw appearance of DJ junction **(Fig. 4)**.
- *Surgical management*: Emergency procedure. Ladd's Procedure (De-rotation of volvulus, broadening of the mesentery, division of bands, incidental appendectomy).

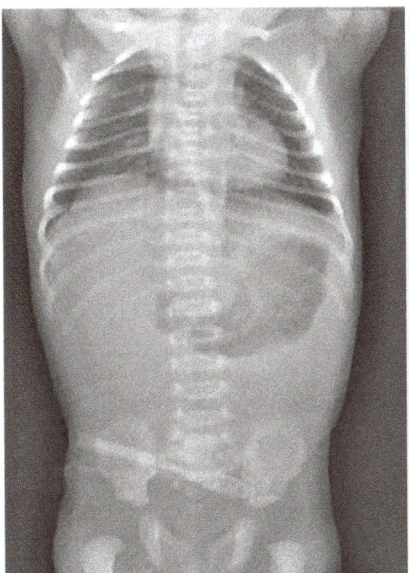 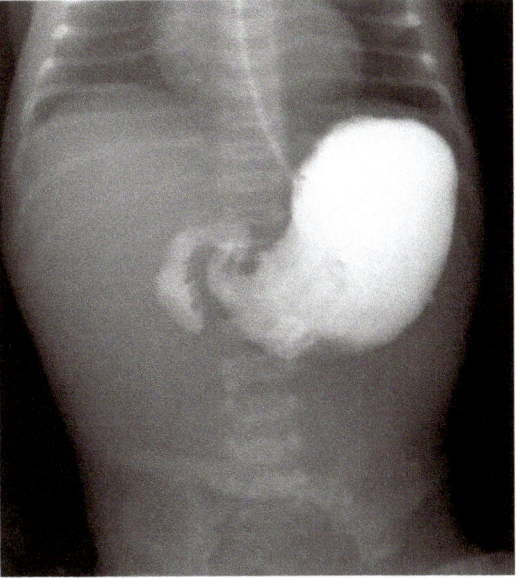

Fig. 4: Malrotation. Plain X-ray shows a paucity of bowel gas. In contrast study, the duodenojejunal flexure is to the right of the vertebra.

- *Postoperative care*: Nutrition support (parenteral nutrition with the initiation of enteral feeds). Observe for recurrent volvulus, strictures, constipation.
- *Survival*: > 95%

Anorectal Malformation

- *Incidence*: 1 in 4,000–5,000
- Fistula present in 85% males (recto-bulbar fistula) and 95% females (ano-vestibular)
- *Clinical features*: Non-passage of meconium, abdominal distention, absent anal opening, flat perineum
- *Associated anomalies (50–70%)*: VATER/VACTERL/CHARGE, genitourinary, cardiac, GIT, spinal, trisomy 21
- *Investigations*: Dilated bowel loops in an X-ray. Absence of rectal gas in cross-table lateral X-ray.
- *Management*: Depends on the presence of perineal fistula (obvious after 24 hours). If a perineal fistula is present **(Fig. 5)**, anoplasty is done. If no fistula, then colostomy.
- Definitive surgery is posterior sagittal anorectoplasty at 6–8 weeks.

Postoperative Care

- Begin feeds as soon as the baby passes stool
- Anal opening dilatation with Hager's dilators till 6–12 months
- Observe for constipation/fecal incontinence
- *Survival*: 95% or more

Meningomyelocele

- *Incidence*: 1 in 2,000
- Meningomyelocele is due to failure of closure of the neural tube
- *Clinical features*: Red, raw neural structure at thoracolumbar-spinal region without overlying skin or dura with CSF leakage **(Fig. 6)**.
- *Associated anomalies*: The majority have Arnold Chiari type 2 malformation and hydrocephalus.
- *Antenatal markers*: Raised maternal serum alpha-fetoprotein, lemon, and banana sign in antenatal ultrasound.

Preoperative Care

- Nurse in prone/left lateral position
- Cover defect with saline-soaked gauze
- Avoid latex gloves
- Evaluate for neurological deficits, hydrocephalus, limb defects, palpable bladder, and anal patency
- *Timing of surgery*: Primary closure is done immediately in cases with open neural tube defect
- *Postoperative*: Multidisciplinary team approach (urology, orthopedics, pediatrics, neurosurgeon, geneticist)
- *Survival*: 60–80%

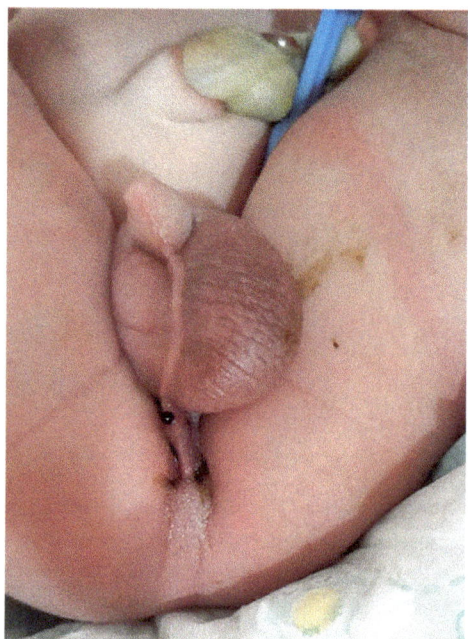

Fig. 5: Absent anal opening. Note the meconium pearls along the median raphe.

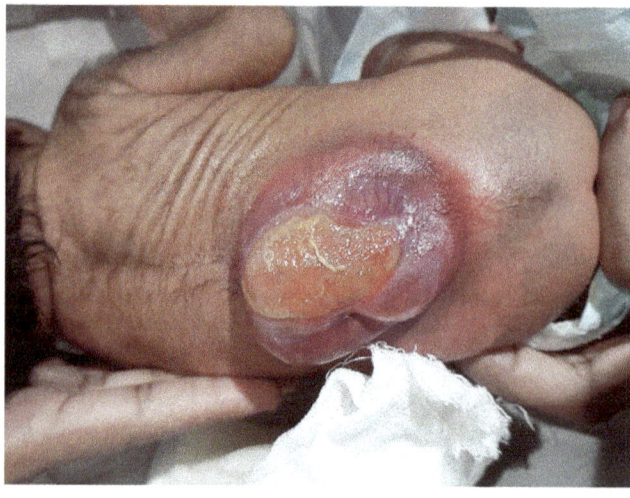

Fig. 6: Open neural tube defect.

CHAPTER 47 | Surgical Conditions Presenting at Birth

CHAPTER AT A GLANCE

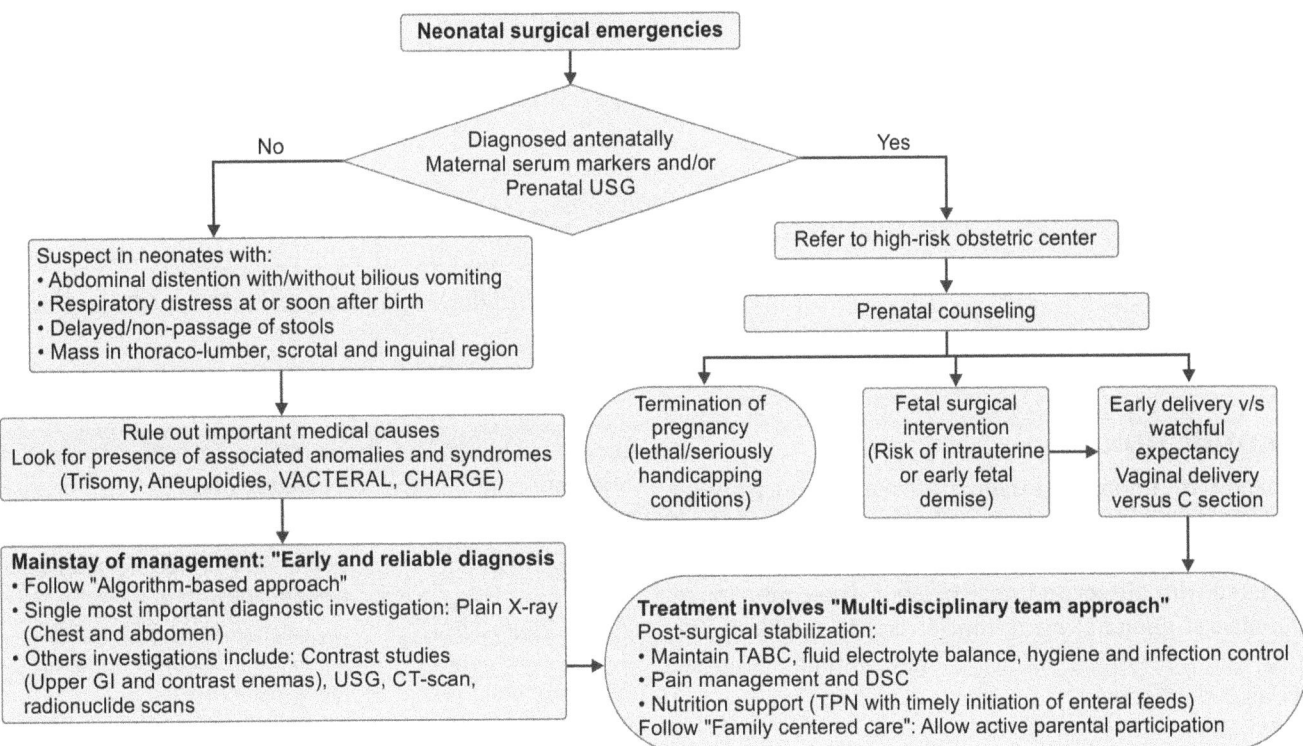

(CHARGE: coloboma, heart defect, choanal atresia, growth restriction, genital hypoplasia and ear anomalies; DSC: definite surgical care; TPN: total parenteral nutrition; TABC: temperature, airway, breathing, and circulation; VACTERAL: vertebral, anorectal, cardiac, trachea-esophageal, radial, renal, and limb

KEY POINTS

- Fetuses with major anomalies require in-utero transfer to a tertiary care center with optimal obstetric, surgical, and neonatal care.
- Bilious vomiting in a neonate is malrotation of gut unless proved otherwise.
- Management of congenital diaphragmatic hernia is medical, with surgery planned after physiological stabilization.

SUGGESTED READING

1. Chandrasekharan PK, Rawat M, Madappa R, Rothstein DH, Lakshminrusimha S. Congenital Diaphragmatic hernia - a review. Matern Health Neonatol Perinatol. 2017;3:6.
2. Lockridge T, Caldwell AD, Jason P. Neonatal surgical emergencies: stabilization and management. J Obstet Gynecol Neonatal Nurs. 2002;31(3):328-39.
3. Pani N, Panda CK. Anesthetic consideration for neonatal surgical emergencies. Indian J Anaesth. 2012;56(5):463-9.
4. Puligandla PS, Skarsgard ED, Offringa M, Adatia I, Baird R, Bailey M, et al. Diagnosis and management of congenital diaphragmatic hernia: a clinical practice guideline. CMAJ. 2018;190(4):E103-12.
5. Sinha A, Bagga A, Krishna A, Bajpai M, Srinivas M, Uppal R, et al. Revised guidelines on the management of antenatal hydronephrosis. Indian J Nephrol. 2013;23(2):83-97.

Birth Trauma

Chanchal Kumar, S Thanigainathan, Charu Sharma

INTRODUCTION

Neonatal birth trauma is a traumatic event or injury during the process of birth leading to structural damage or functional impairment of a neonate. These injuries are primarily associated with the second stage of labor. The approximate incidence of neonatal birth injuries is 0.06–0.08% of live births. Life-threatening injuries are rare, and most injuries have a good prognosis.

OBJECTIVES

- Discuss various risk factors associated with birth trauma.
- Describe common birth injuries, their evaluation, management, and prognosis.

RISK FACTORS

Risk Factors for Birth Trauma

The risk factors for birth trauma are listed below and the related injuries are provided in **Table 1**:

- Fetal factors:
  - Macrosomia (birth weight > 4,000 g)
  - Prematurity
  - Abnormal fetal presentation
- Mode of delivery:
  - Forceps delivery
  - Vacuum extraction
  - Breech delivery
  - Precipitous delivery
  - Cesarean section
- Maternal factors:
  - Maternal age less than 16 years or more than 35 years
  - Primigravida
  - Obesity
  - Cephalopelvic disproportion
  - Short stature
  - Pelvic abnormalities

TABLE 1: Risk factors and related injuries.

Risk factor	Related injuries
Forceps delivery	Facial nerve injuries
Vacuum extraction	Depressed skull fracture, subgaleal hemorrhage
Instrumental vaginal delivery (forceps or vacuum or both)	Cephalohematoma, intracranial hemorrhage, shoulder dystocia, retinal hemorrhages
Breech presentation	Brachial plexus palsy, intracranial hemorrhage, gluteal lacerations, long bone fractures
Macrosomia	Shoulder dystocia, clavicle fracture, rib fracture, cephalohematoma, caput succedaneum
Abnormal presentation (face, brow, transverse, compound)	Excessive bruising, retinal hemorrhage, lacerations
Prematurity	Bruising, intracranial, and extracranial hemorrhage
Precipitous delivery	Bruising, intracranial, and extracranial hemorrhage, retinal hemorrhage

Source: Adapted from Akangire G, Carter B. Birth injuries in neonates. Pediatr Rev. 2016;37(11):451-62.

HEAD AND NECK INJURIES

Extracranial Injuries (Fig. 1)

Skull Fracture

Skull fracture may occur during instrumental vaginal delivery and can be associated with intracranial or extracranial injury. A skull radiograph should be performed in case of suspicion of fracture on clinical assessment or abnormal neurological signs. There are three commonly described fracture patterns-linear, depressed and occipital osteodiastasis.

1. *Linear fracture* is nondepressed and usually needs only close monitoring.
2. *Depressed fractures* greater than 1 cm in depth increases the possibility of intracranial hemorrhage such as subdural or subarachnoid hemorrhage.

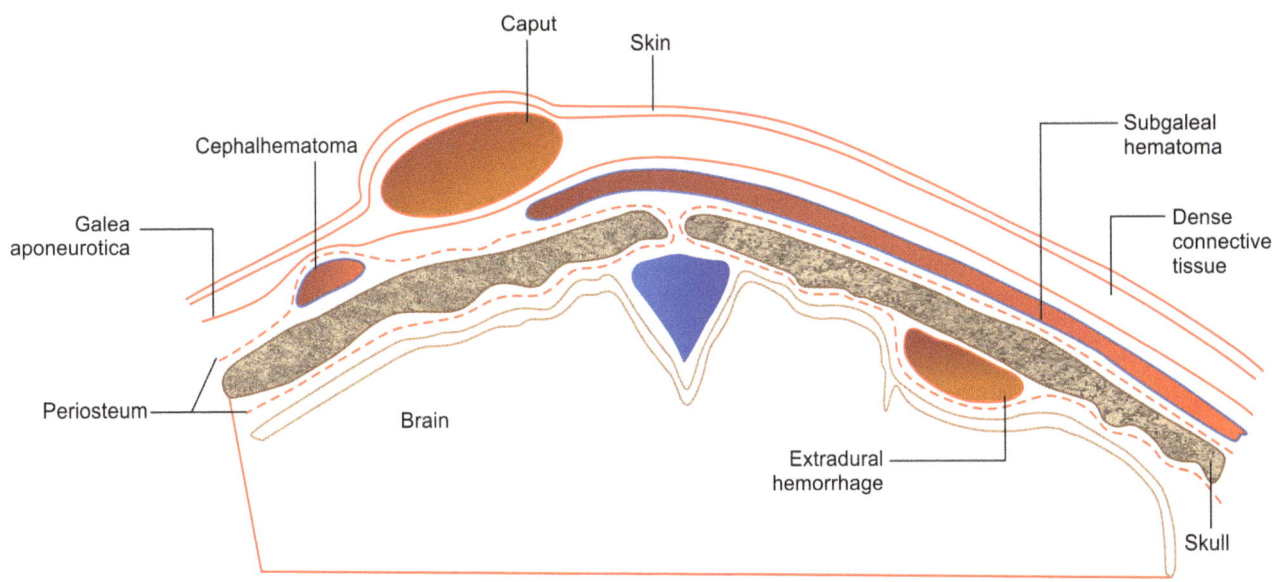

Fig. 1: Types of extracranial hemorrhages.

3. *Occipital osteodiastasis*, mainly seen in breech presentation, is the separation of the squamous and lateral portion of the occipital bone and may be associated with cerebellar contusion and hemorrhage. A dural tear may lead to leptomeningeal cyst formation later.

Investigations: Computed tomogram (CT) with multiplanar and 3D reconstruction is an excellent tool for diagnosis. Magnetic resonance imaging (MRI) can be considered, if CT does not offer sufficient information.

Management: Neurosurgical consultation is indicated for those with evidence of bone fragments in the cerebrum, localizing signs, raised intracranial pressure, cerebrospinal fluid (CSF) accumulation below galea, depressed fracture greater than 1 cm, and nonimprovement to conservative management.

Cephalohematoma

Cephalohematoma is a subperiosteal collection of blood due to rupture of superficial veins between the skull and periosteum during instrumental vaginal delivery. The swelling is well-demarcated, without any overlying skin findings, and confined by the suture lines. It is not present at birth and usually evolves over 24 hours or more. The lesion is usually unilateral but may be bilateral. Skull fracture may be observed with it 5% of cases. A CT scan needs to be performed if a skull fracture is suspected or neurologic signs are present. Anemia is usually not significant; however, there can be significant hyperbilirubinemia. It usually resolves within 8 weeks; however, a palpable nodule can be present until 3–4 months, if calcified. Incision and drainage are contraindicated unless associated with secondary infection. Osteomyelitis and subdural empyema are rare complications.

Subgaleal Hemorrhage

The blood collection under aponeurosis of the scalp is due to rupture of emissary veins. Even though it is reported following spontaneous birth, it is more commonly associated with instrumental vaginal deliveries. The lesion is ill-defined, not confined by suture lines, and can extend up to the supraorbital ridge anteriorly, temporal fascia laterally, and nape of the neck posteriorly. It can accommodate up to 40% of total blood volume, and every 1 cm increase in occipitofrontal circumference (OFC) may indicate 40 mL of blood loss. The clinical presentation varies from being asymptomatic at birth to rapidly progressive shock. Coagulopathy is a significant risk factor for subgaleal bleed in noninstrumental deliveries.

Caput succedaneum: This is an important differential for subgaleal hemorrhage (**Table 2**). It is subcutaneous edema that usually presents over the presenting part of the scalp at birth. The lesion is ill-defined and not confined by suture lines. The management is conservative, and it usually resolves spontaneously within 4–6 days. Encephalocele is to be considered in case of a large caput if it increases in size beyond 24 hours after birth or does not diminish by 48–72 hours, especially if associated with neurological deficit or hemodynamic instability.

Management of subgaleal hemorrhage:
- Monitor vitals, head circumference, fluid intake, and urine output. Serial hematocrit can help in monitoring. In cases where the size is increasing, rule out coagulopathy by assessing platelet count, prothrombin time (PT), activated partial thromboplastin time (aPTT), and international normalized ratio (INR).
- Aggressive volume replacement (10–20 mL/kg) with packed red blood cells or whole blood is warranted in shock or anemia.
- Transfuse fresh frozen plasma or platelets as needed.

TABLE 2: Differentiation of the types of scalp injury.

	Caput succedaneum	Cephalohematoma	Subgaleal hemorrhage
Site of fluid/blood collection	Subcutaneous tissue	Sub-periosteal	Under aponeurosis
Presentation	At birth	After 24 hours	Evolves over few hours
Reason	Pressure at presenting part	Rupture of bridging veins	Rupture of emissary veins
Clinical manifestation	Swelling at presenting part. Ill-defined, not confined by suture lines	Usually well-demarcated, unilateral, confined by suture lines, hyperbilirubinemia	Ill-defined swelling over the scalp, not confined by suture lines, extending up to the orbital ridge, temporal fascia, and nape of the neck, hypovolemia, hyperbilirubinemia
Hemodynamic instability	Uncommon	Uncommon	High risk if extensive hemorrhage
Management	Conservative	Conservative	Volume resuscitation with correction of associated coagulopathy
Resolution	Within 4–6 days	Within 6–8 weeks	Resolves gradually

- Appropriate management of hyperbilirubinemia
- Surgical evacuation of hematoma is rarely needed
- Prognosis depends on the severity of the hemorrhage, and a full recovery can occur, if its recognized early and aggressive correction of hypovolemia is done.

Facial Injury

Fracture of the mandible, maxilla, lacrimal bones, and nasal bone, dislocation, and hematoma are the expected facial injuries due to malpresentation at birth. Improper application of forceps may also lead to these injuries. Facial injury may manifest with ecchymosis, edema, respiratory distress, and feeding difficulty. Without treatment, it can lead to deformity. CT scan is needed in case of temporal and cribriform plate injury. Expert consultation should be obtained promptly. The hematoma of the pinna needs drainage to prevent the development of cauliflower ear. Full-thickness laceration of the scalp, face, cheek, and ear can occur in cesarean section and requires suturing.

Sternocleidomastoid Injury

Sternocleidomastoid (SCM) injury can be caused by either muscle compartment syndrome or rupture and hematoma formation during birth. Manifestations include torticollis, palpable mass in SCM, and head tilt to the side of the injury. Initial management is conservative with stretching exercises. Surgery is indicated if the torticollis is present beyond 6 months of age.

Clavicle Fracture

The clavicle is the most common bone injured during the birth process. Shoulder dystocia, breech presentation, and macrosomia are the risk factors. There are two forms: (1) incomplete fracture, which may not be symptomatic at birth and usually, presents with callus formation at 7–10 days; (2) complete fracture presents with crepitus, pain, bony irregularity, and pseudoparalysis. Chest X-ray is confirmatory. Management is conservative with a sling application or pinning the sleeve with the shirt to limit the movement. Healing is generally complete.

Intracranial Injuries (Fig. 2)

When to Suspect Intracranial Hemorrhage

- Acute deterioration-altered sensorium, irritability, bradycardia, absent doll's eye movements, unequal pupils, Opisthotonos, tonic posturing, hypotonia, abnormal respiration, and acute deterioration on the ventilator.
- Seizures
- Apnea
- Raised fontanel, loss of pulsatility of the fontanel
- Bloody CSF tap in intraventricular hemorrhage (IVH) or subarachnoid hemorrhage.

Subdural hemorrhage (SDH): Bleeding between the dura mater and the arachnoid layer of the brain due to rupture of the bridging veins. It is noted in deliveries following abnormal labor or difficult delivery. It is the most common intracranial hemorrhage in term infants and occurs mainly in interhemispheric or tentorial locations. Posterior fossa SDH can lead to brainstem compression and hydrocephalus. A CT scan is indicated when SDH is suspected. Most of the neonates with SDH are managed with supportive care and treatment of seizures. An urgent neurosurgical consultation is needed for progressive brainstem dysfunction, tense bulging fontanelle, or opisthotonos. Resolution usually occurs without any long-term sequel in the majority of the cases.

Extradural hemorrhage (EDH): Tight adherence between the skull and dura, especially at the level of the sutures in neonates, is considered to be protective from EDH. Collection of blood outside dura due to rupture of the middle meningeal artery may occur following forceps delivery or in those predisposed to coagulopathy. Cephalhematoma and skull fracture are common associations. The presentation may vary from being asymptomatic or with seizures, and rarely it can lead to death. A small EDH (asymptomatic, <1 cm lesions) does not require surgical management. However, neonates with large EDH with hemodynamic

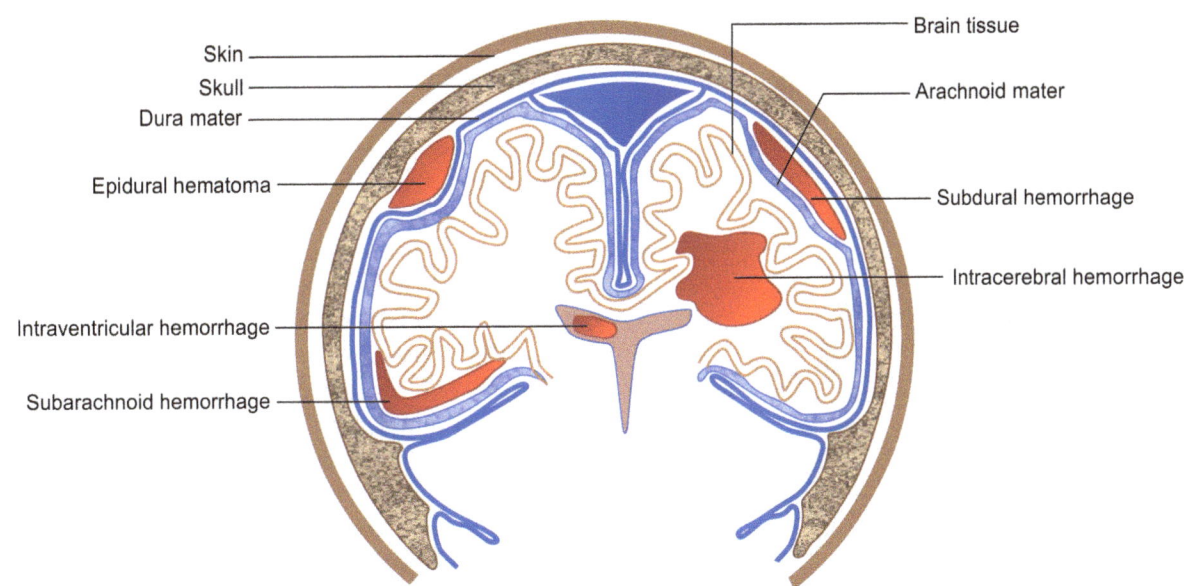

Fig. 2: Types of intracranial hemorrhage.

changes and neurological impairment may warrant early surgical evacuation with craniotomy.

Subarachnoid hemorrhage: Collection of blood under the arachnoid layer of the brain due to rupture of bridging veins. Conservative management is followed as most cases resolve spontaneously. Surgical evacuation is considered in case of herniation. Hydrocephalus is a rare complication. Serial monitoring of OFC can aid in early diagnosis.

Intraventricular hemorrhage: Usually associated with preterm birth, IVH is related to birth injury in term infants. Instrumental delivery is the major risk factor. Treatment is supportive with the maintenance of blood pressure, volume status, and correction of coagulopathy. Packed cell transfusion is needed in case of large IVH.

Retinal hemorrhage: Usually associated with instrumental deliveries due to increased venous congestion and pressure during delivery. It may be associated with ocular or periorbital injury, including hyphema, vitreous hemorrhage, laceration, or orbital fracture. It usually resolves spontaneously in 1–2 weeks. Associated optic nerve injury increases the risk of visual impairment. Prompt diagnosis and treatment are necessary for other ocular injuries.

NERVE INJURIES

Facial Nerve Injury

Usually facial nerve injury results from the compression of the peripheral branch of the facial nerve by incorrect application of forceps. Loss of nasolabial fold, partial closing of the eye (ptosis), and drooping mouth with a deviation of mouth to the unaffected side are common features. It usually resolves in 2–3 weeks. This is to be differentiated from the congenital absence of depressor anguli oris muscle where eye and forehead muscles are unaffected, and the nasolabial fold will be intact. Improvement following traumatic facial nerve injury can be observed within days, and complete recovery may take weeks to months. In cases where spontaneous recovery does not occur, surgical intervention may be needed to avoid permanent disfigurement.

Brachial Plexus Injury

Brachial plexus injury involves the paresis of upper arm muscles due to injury of spinal roots C5-T1. It commonly occurs with lateral traction of the infant's neck during a difficult delivery in shoulder dystocia. Injury can vary from edema or hemorrhage to tearing of the nerve roots from the spinal cord completely. Brachial plexus palsy can present as:

- Erb-Duchenne palsy **(Fig. 3)**:
  - Injury to C5-6, the most common form of brachial plexus palsy.
  - It leads to weakness of the shoulder and arm, with hand muscles remaining intact.
  - The arm retains a position of adduction and internal rotation, fully extended at the elbow, with pronation of the forearm and flexion of the wrist.
  - Absent biceps reflex, asymmetric Moro's reflex, and intact grasp reflex.
  - Phrenic nerve injury may be associated.
- Klumpke palsy:
  - Injury to C8-T1, rare form of brachial plexus injury.
  - The upper arm and shoulder movements are intact, but with weakness of the wrist and hand.
  - Biceps reflex intact, asymmetric Moro's reflex, and loss of grasp reflex.
- *If all nerve roots are involved*: Total arm paresis with associated sensory loss.
- *Horner syndrome*: Ipsilateral miosis, ptosis, and enophthalmos; damage to sympathetic outflow via nerve root T1.

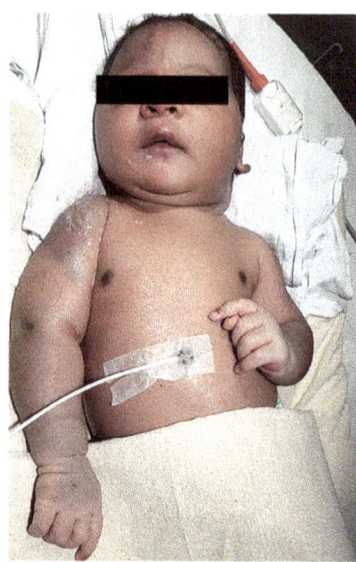

Fig. 3: Clinical photograph of a neonate with Erb's palsy. Note the internally rotated arm, extended elbow, and pronated forearm. (Printed with permission).

Complete plexus palsy and Klumpke palsy have guarded outcomes.

Diagnosis is clinical. A chest X-ray is needed to rule out clavicle or humerus fracture.

Management

Physiotherapy with passive range of motion exercise at shoulder, elbow, and wrist is the mainstay of treatment and started within the first week. The affected arm should not be immobilized during the first few days unless there is an associated bone fracture. The prognosis is good if anti-gravity movement in biceps and shoulder abduction appears by 3 months of age. Surgical exploration is needed in pan-plexopathy, pre-ganglionic nerve root lesion, neurotmesis lesion, and incomplete functional recovery by 3–6 months of age. CT myelography or MRI is indicated before surgery.

Phrenic Nerve Injury

Phrenic nerve injury is caused by lateral hyperextension of the neck during birth, exerting excessive stretch to the cervical nerve roots. It is associated with brachial plexus palsy in 75% of cases. The neonate presents with respiratory distress, cyanosis, and asymmetrical chest movement due to weakness of the diaphragm on the affected side. Chest X-ray may show an elevated diaphragm dome on the affected side, and ultrasonography/fluoroscopy shows paradoxical movement during inspiration. The neonate is managed with supportive care with continuous positive airway pressure or mechanical ventilation as needed and airway care. Most neonates improve within 1–3 months without permanent sequelae. Diaphragmatic plication may be needed in refractory cases and in those with recurrent pneumonia or atelectasis.

Spinal Cord Injury

Spinal cord injury can be caused by hyperextension of the neck, breech delivery, or severe shoulder dystocia. Incomplete mineralization of the vertebrae and laxity of the ligaments predispose to spinal injuries in the neonate. The upper cervical cord is commonly involved in shoulder dystocia and cephalic presentation, whereas lower cervical and upper thoracic involvement occurs in complicated breech deliveries. The clinical manifestation depends on the site of injury. High cervical or brainstem injury is associated with respiratory failure and shock with poor survival outcomes. Lower cord injury may present with extremity paralysis, absence deep tendon reflex, urinary retention, constipation, bilateral brachial plexus injury, and contractures. Careful resuscitation, including immobilization of the head, neck, and spine, prevents further damage. Neurology and neurosurgery consultation should be obtained promptly. Radiographs, CT, and MRI help make the diagnosis. The prognosis depends upon the site and severity of the injury.

LONG BONE INJURIES

Humerus and femur are commonly injured long bones. There are two forms: (1) incomplete or greenstick fracture may not be noticed until swelling, pain, and callus formation occurs by 7–10 days; (2) complete fracture presents with bony deformity. Chest X-ray is needed for confirmation. It usually heals with splinting for 2 weeks. Pavlik harness can be used for splinting femur even in unilateral condition. A displaced fracture requires closed reduction and casting. Radial nerve injury may be seen in displaced humerus fractures. Complete healing without limb shortening is expected. Epiphyseal separation presents with pain and tenderness and can lead to growth abnormality, if severe. USG is the investigation of choice, as epiphysis is not ossified. Immobilization by splinting is needed for 2 weeks.

SOFT-TISSUE AND VISCERAL INJURIES

Soft-tissue Injuries

Petechiae and ecchymosis can develop due to a sudden increase in venous pressure because of tight nuchal cord, breech presentation, or precipitous delivery. Scalp electrode or scalpel use during cesaran and lead to abrasion and laceration. Treatment is supportive except for suturing needed for deep wounds.

Subcutaneous fat necrosis is not usually present at birth and is caused by focal pressure on adipose tissue. It presents as a well-demarcated, irregular, firm, non-pitting swelling within 2 weeks after birth. The common sites involved are the face, extremity, trunk, and buttock. No treatment is required, although the infant is followed for the development of hypercalcemia. It usually resolves within several weeks or months.

Intra-abdominal Injuries

Hepatic Injury

The liver is the most common solid organ to get injured. Macrosomia, breech presentation, and hepatomegaly are major risk factors. Subcapsular hematoma may be initially asymptomatic at birth. Later manifestations of blood loss such as tachycardia, tachypnea, jaundice, or shock occur. Abdominal wall discoloration may be noted due to rupture of hematoma. Management includes volume restoration, correction of coagulopathy, and probably surgical exploration.

Splenic Injury

Splenic injury is an uncommon traumatic injury as the newborn's spleen is well protected due to its anatomical position. Clinical manifestations due to blood loss can occur along with a palpable mass on the left side. Management of blood loss and correction of coagulopathy is recommended. Surgical exploration is warranted in cases where bleeding is uncontrolled or if the infant's condition is unstable and should aim at salvaging the spleen.

Adrenal Hemorrhage

Macrosomia and breech presentation are the major risk factors. Adrenal hemorrhage is usually unilateral, and the right side is commonly involved. Clinical manifestations include fever, flank mass, pallor, abdominal wall discoloration, and signs of adrenal insufficiency like poor feeding, vomiting, irritability, listlessness, and shock. USG abdomen is the investigation of choice. The management includes volume restoration, coagulopathy, steroid therapy, and surgical exploration in severe bleeding.

CLINICAL AND MEDICOLEGAL IMPLICATIONS

Neonates born after instrumental vaginal delivery or difficult second stage should be clinically examined for trauma. Clinicians must document the injury in detail in case records and communicate with family members. Neonates with trauma should be assessed for pain and offered pain relief.

While maternal, fetal, and obstetric risk factors play a role in birth trauma, some cases (e.g., brachial plexus palsy, intracranial hemorrhages) can occur without risk factors. These cases are attributed to endogenous factors that antedate or occur during normal labor. Cesarean section decreases the risk but does not eliminate birth trauma. Thus, cesarean section is not the solution to prevent birth trauma, as it would lead to unacceptably high rates of operative delivery without benefits. Adequate training and experience in the conduct of instrumental delivery are essential.

CHAPTER AT A GLANCE

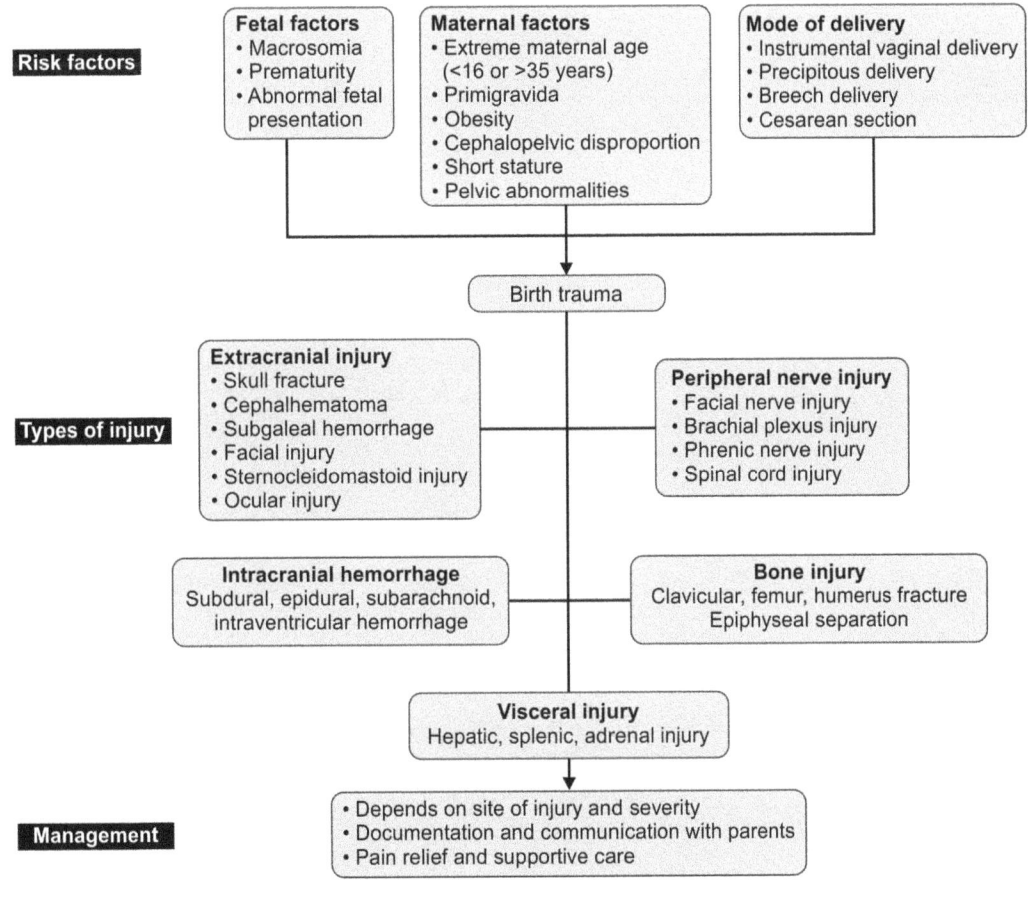

KEY POINTS

- Macrosomia, difficult delivery, breech extraction, and instrumental vaginal delivery are the major risk factors for birth trauma.
- Subgaleal hemorrhage should be closely monitored and may require aggressive fluid resuscitation.
- Erb's palsy is the most common brachial plexus injury, and shoulder dystocia is a significant risk factor. It should be managed by close follow-up and physical therapy until 3–4 months of age.
- Intracranial hemorrhage, spinal injury, diaphragmatic palsy, and visceral injuries are life-threatening.
- Careful documentation of birth injuries and efficient communication with parents is essential.

SUGGESTED READING

1. Akangire G, Carter B. Birth injuries in neonates. Pediatr Rev. 2016;37(11):451-62.
2. McKee-Garrett T. Delivery room emergencies due to birth injuries. Semin Fetal Neonatal Med. 2019;24(6):101047.
3. Parker LA. Part 1: early recognition and treatment of birth trauma: injuries to the head and face. Adv Neonatal Care. 2005;5(6):288-97.
4. Parker LA. Part 2: Birth trauma: injuries to the intraabdominal organs, peripheral nerves, and skeletal system. Adv Neonatal Care. 2006;6(1):7-14.
5. Rosenberg AA. Traumatic birth injury. Neoreviews. 2003;4(10):e270-6.
6. Smith BW, Daunter AK, Yang LJ-S, Wilson TJ. An update on the management of neonatal brachial plexus palsy-replacing old paradigms: A review. JAMA Pediatr. 2018;172(6):585-91.

CHAPTER 49

Ethical and Medicolegal Issues in the Perinatal Period

Niharika Allu, Femitha Pournami

INTRODUCTION

During our daily practice, we face many ethical, moral, and legal dilemmas. Some examples include a decision on initiating or withholding resuscitation for a periviable birth, aggressive management or surgical care of a neonate with life-threatening anomalies, or the end-of-life care of a severely asphyxiated neonate on a ventilator. These dilemmas stem from considerations for the quality of life of the neonate, acting in the neonates' best interest, respecting parental wishes and cultural preferences, and the law of the land.

OBJECTIVES

- Understand the rights of the mother and newborn
- Learn management of ethical dilemmas using case examples
- Learn about medicolegal problems in perinatal practice and how to prevent them

RIGHTS OF THE MOTHER AND NEWBORN

In 1948, the United Nations adopted the Universal Declaration of Human Rights—a milestone in history that said, "all human beings are born free and equal in dignity and rights". In 1989, the International Convention on the Child's Rights recognized that children need special safeguards and care due to their physical and mental immaturity. In 2001, at the World Congress of Perinatal Medicine at Barcelona, the rights of the mother and newborn were laid down called the "Declaration of Barcelona". In 2011, the Parma Charter provided a detailed list of the rights of the newborn (**Box 1**).

The Respectful Maternity Care Charter in 2019 articulates the rights of both mothers and newborns, especially in the context of receiving maternity care in a health facility. The well-being of the mother and newborn during childbirth are interconnected and healthcare providers should protect the basic human rights of both individuals (mother and baby). Both have the right to respect, dignity, highest standard of health, and freedom from discrimination. The mother has

BOX 1: The Parma charter of the rights of the newborn.

- Every newborn is entitled to life and the best levels of health regardless of racial, geographic, religious, sociocultural, or gender discrimination
- Every live newborn is entitled to appropriate assistance during delivery that should be guaranteed regardless of gestational age, weight, sex, the presence of malformations, and other factors
- Every newborn, healthy or ill, is entitled to the best care, social protection, and safety
- Every newborn has the right to be born in the most suitable place based on risk factors or needs
- The newborn must be guaranteed vicinity to its parents (Rooming-in and family-centered care must be guaranteed)
- When the neonate's health is at stake due to abuse or other circumstances, appropriate legal and organizational measures should be undertaken
- No medical procedure, including those for research purposes, may be performed on the newborn without the informed parental consent *except during emergencies in the newborn's best interests*
- To promote psychological and physical development, every newborn is entitled to be breastfed (or alternate means when mother's milk is unavailable)
- Every neonate is entitled to appropriate treatment, and palliative care, and pain control in the event of severe illness (extreme prematurity, malformations, or life-threatening conditions)
- Every newborn is entitled to be registered after birth, given a name, and acquiring nationality. Any disowned newborn is entitled to be adopted with optimum guarantees, considering that the child's interests must prevail at all times
- The newborn is a very special "citizen" who has rights but no duties and who, for the recognition of his/her rights, depends totally on the attention and commitment of others

right to confidentiality, information, and informed consent. The charter also recognizes the newborn as an individual with autonomous rights, and every decision made by the mother or caregiver must consider the baby's best interest. Physicians and health systems have an essential role in ensuring the mother-infant dyad's health, safety, and dignity by protecting their fundamental human rights.

BIRTH AT PERIVIABLE GESTATION

Case Scenario

A neonatologist is called to attend the delivery of a neonate with a gestational age of 24 weeks based on the last menstrual period (LMP) and an estimated fetal weight of 450 g. What antenatal counseling should be provided, and how should the neonatal team proceed during resuscitation?

Outcomes at Periviable Gestations

At periviable gestations (22–24 weeks), the risk of neonatal mortality and long-term neurodevelopmental impairment is high. Neonatal care practices and outcomes vary across nations. Among infants born at 22–25 weeks in Australia and New Zealand, 40% died and 10% had severe neurodevelopmental impairment between 2 and 3 years of age. In a population-based cohort of US-born infants, the survival at 1 year was 31%, 42%, and 64%, respectively, for neonates at 22, 23, and 24 weeks when active resuscitation was provided. At 25 weeks, survival was 80%. In an Indian cohort of extremely low-birth-weight infants (mean gestational age 28 weeks), survival to discharge was 60%. Therefore, it is essential to involve parents in decision-making at periviable gestations, and the goals are family-centered. This also needs to be individualized based on the institute/hospital perinatal birth statistics. Most organizations recommend offering comfort care to infants born at less than 22 weeks of gestation and full resuscitation from 25 weeks onward. The period between 22 and 24 weeks is considered a gray zone.

Antenatal Counseling at Periviable Gestation

The components of antenatal counseling at periviable gestation are:
- Assessment of risk to neonate based on the best available information
- Communication of risks to parents
- Encourage shared decision making and offer family-centered care
- Offer ongoing support

Risk Assessment

- *Gestational age*: Gestational age is the most critical determinant of outcome. However, the assessment is inaccurate. An individual woman's ovulatory cycles have a wide variation, and the ultrasound has an accuracy of around ±5 days in the first trimester and ± 2 weeks in the second trimester.
- *Other determinants*: Estimated birth weight, female gender, administration of antenatal corticosteroids, singleton birth, are associated with improved outcomes.

Parents are under stress when delivery is anticipated at early gestations, and the time available for counseling is often limited. The physician should be sensitive to the parents' religious, social, and cultural backgrounds. The language should be simple. Whenever possible, the obstetricians and neonatologists should meet the prospective parents together. When meeting with parents, the physicians should provide the following information, which facilitate their decision making:

- Expected outcomes (survival and neurodevelopment); preferably institution-specific data should be provided.
- Discuss treatment options (comfort care vs. full resuscitation and management). Active management includes interventions such as surfactant therapy, mechanical ventilation, and parenteral nutrition. If a decision is made not to resuscitate, provide comfort care and encourage family bonding.
- Options for redirection of care during resuscitation and early neonatal period. Each neonate is unique; thus, decision-making should be individualized and modified in light of new information/clinical situations.

Communication between obstetric and neonatal team members improves optimal decision-making. Institutions should develop policies and procedures for counseling and management at periviable gestations. The use of visual aids providing institution specific survival and morbidity of preterm infants helps parents understand better (**Figs. 1 and 2**). Shared decision-making with the family and the parent's wishes for their unborn child is important. Additional counseling sessions regardless of parental decisions and consultation from hospital social workers and palliative care units should be provided.

Decision Making in the Delivery Room

During resuscitation of a periviable neonate, providers offer care based on the shared decision-making and the hospital's policies. However, the neonates' condition at birth also has a strong bearing on further care (**Flowchart 1**). If a comfort care decision had been taken but the neonate is noted to be vigorous at birth, the providers can redirect care and provide appropriate respiratory support. The neonate should be transferred to intensive care unit and further management provided. Similarly, if the neonate responds poorly to resuscitation in a case where parents opted for full care, the care pathways need to be reconsidered. The decision for full care versus comfort care should be individualized based on continued assessment. Palliative care, pain relief and family support should be offered when a decision to withdraw or withhold care is made.

Case Progression

In the case provided, a shared decision making was done and parents opted for comfort care. The neonate had poor tone but had some respiratory efforts that improved after initial steps. The neonate was transferred to intensive care unit on continuous positive airway pressure (CPAP). A senior physician assessed the neonate and felt appropriate

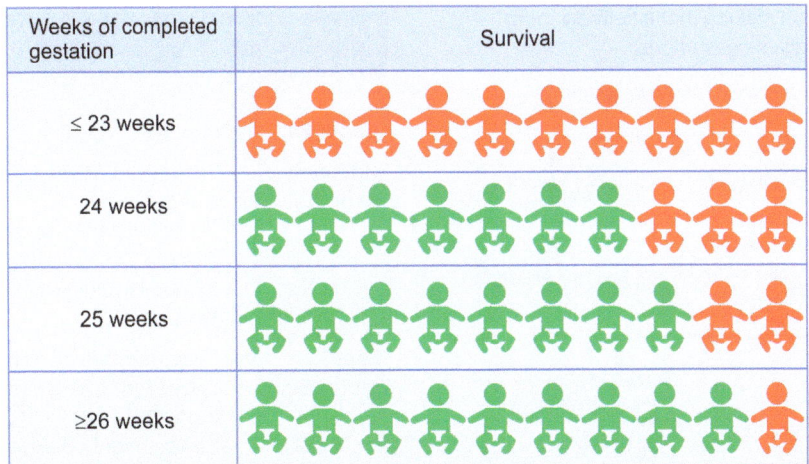

Fig. 1: Example of visual aid depicting survival (*green icon = proportion of survivors at discharge out of every 10 live born neonates*) at extremely low gestations. If gestational age estimation is inaccurate, estimated weight can be used as a surrogate.
Source: Adapted from author's unit at KIMS Health, Trivandrum, India.

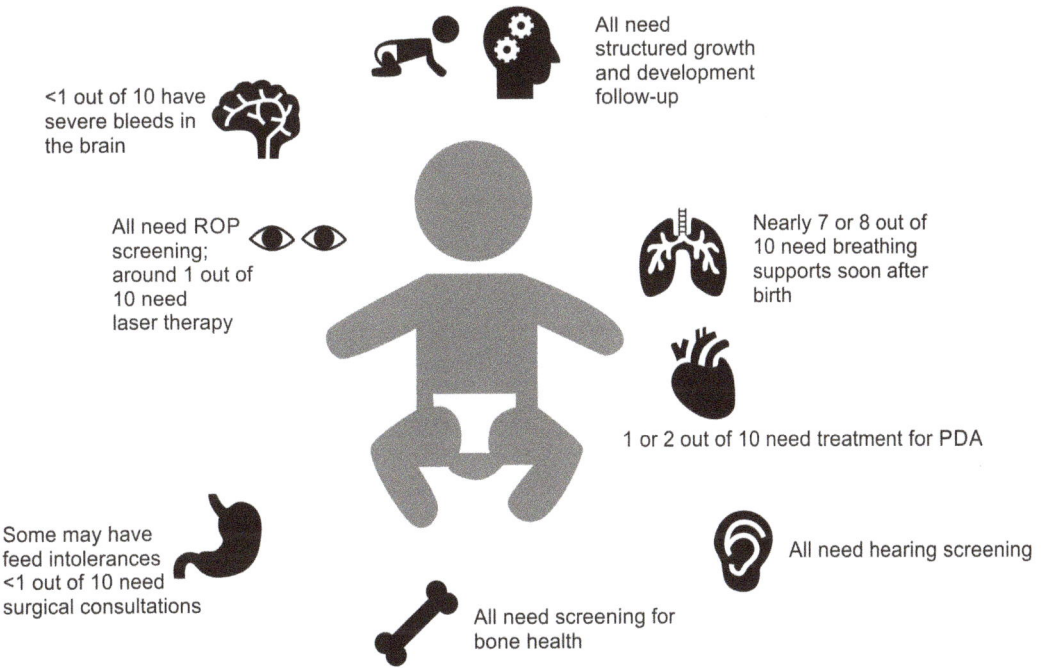

Fig. 2: Example of visual aid depicting expected morbidity and follow up needs in neonates <32 weeks gestation. These tools assist physicians in conveying complex information to patients.
(PDA: patent ductus arteriosus; ROP: retinopathy of prematurity)
Source: Adapted from author's unit at KIMS Health, Trivandrum, India.

to provide further respiratory support. Parents were consulted and the team proceeded with intubation and surfactant. However, on day 2 of life a large intraventricular hemorrhage and clinical worsening was noted. Care plans were redesignated to comfort care.

MAJOR MALFORMATIONS DIAGNOSED IN FETUS/NEWBORN

Case Scenario-2

In an antenatal ultrasound scan, a fetus is detected to have massive hydrocephalus. The fetus has additional malformations, including an open neural tube defect, omphalocele, and short limbs. The pregnancy is already at 26 weeks gestation, and termination is not an option. What are the ethical issues in this case, and how can management be offered?

Antenatal Counseling

Perinatal or fetal palliative care is an active approach that encompasses physical, emotional, and social components to improve the quality of life (QOL) for the unborn baby or neonate and supports the family. Management addresses the distressing symptoms, providing comfort care and bereavement support.

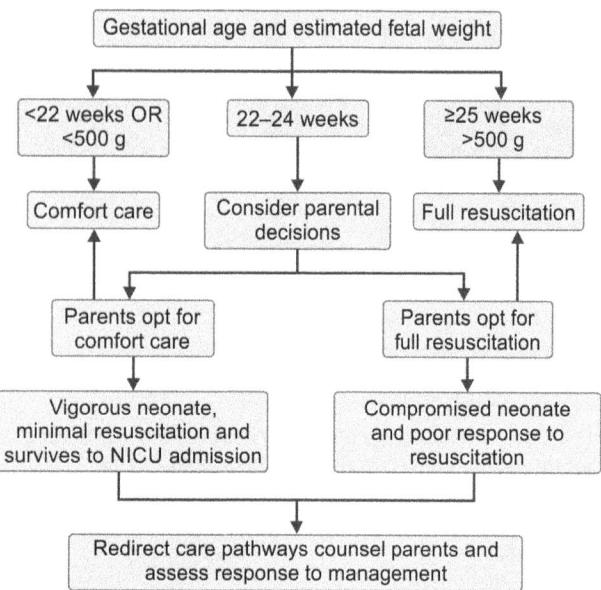

Flowchart 1: Decision making in the delivery room at periviable gestations.

(NICU: neonatal intensive care unit)

The following should be considered when counseling parents with malformed fetuses:
- How certain is the diagnosis of malformation or genetic abnormality (check if amniocentesis, karyotyping, or a detailed ultrasound was performed)?
- How well can one make a judgment about prognosis during pregnancy or after birth?

Based on the best available information of the diagnosis and prognosis of the condition, the physicians and parents should engage in open discussion and act in the unborn child's best interest (**Table 1**).

A palliative care plan (**Table 2**) should be planned that fully respects the life of the unborn child with options such as:
- Offering comfort care in the delivery room or NICU
- Planning of discharge from the hospital when it is likely that the baby may live longer
- Detailed investigations and a trial of management where the prognosis is uncertain.

The same considerations can be applied if major malformations are diagnosed in the postnatal period.

MEDICOLEGAL ISSUES IN PERINATAL PERIOD

Medicolegal issues are gaining importance in India. Medical negligence refers to breach (by a physician or a hospital) in the legal duty to care. A patient can file a litigation in court of law when a breach in standard of care, diagnosis or a therapeutic intervention is noted leading to harm. In an analysis of the judgments obtained from all the District Consumer Courts of South India, the common causes of obstetric litigations were birth asphyxia and traumatic injury to new born. The reasons for alleging negligence were inadequate documentation and improper consent taking processes on the part of the doctors.

TABLE 1: Examples of fetal conditions and management options based on prognosis.

Condition	Examples	Management options
Uniformly poor	• Trisomy 13, 15, or 18 • Anencephaly • Large encephaloceles • Acardia • Bilateral multicystic dysplastic kidneys	Palliative care at resuscitation and later
Poor prognosis	• Thanatophoric dwarfism • Lethal forms of osteogenesis imperfecta • Severe oligohydramnios with suspected pulmonary hypoplasia • Severe hydrocephalus with minimal brain growth	Parental choice, individualize goals of care when recognizing uncertainty
Prognosis is uncertain or variable	• Severe oligo or anhydramnios • Complex or severe cases of meningomyelocele • Hypoplastic left heart syndrome • Pentalogy of Cantrell (ectopia cordis) • Giant omphalocele • Idiopathic nonimmune hydrops • Multiple severe anomalies	Offer assessment and trial of treatment

TABLE 2: Palliative care options for the neonate born with major life-threatening malformation.

Resuscitation status	Comfort measures	Family-centered care
Options: • Do not intubate • No assisted mechanical ventilation • No chest compressions	• Dry, stimulate • Provide warmth • Allow parents to see the neonate and hold her Interventions in NICU (based on need): • Nasal cannula or oxygen hood • Pain relief (Morphine, 0.05 mg/kg IV q15 minutes for obvious signs of pain/distress) • Oro gastric feeds or intravenous fluids • Comfort measures (swaddling, kangaroo care)	• Allow rooming-in • Ensure privacy, if possible, in a separate area or room • Allow parents to hold or huddle with the infant • Offer emotional support to the family • Religious practices within safety norms of the unit in the presence of clergy/religious leaders, if the family opts • Explanations on what to expect before death (e.g., gasping, visible cardiac pulsations during severe bradycardia) • Reduce distressing alarms

(NICU: neonatal intensive care unit)

Medicolegal issues are important for families and have significant cost implications for organizations.

Case Study

A 24-year-old primigravida was admitted in labor following an uncomplicated antenatal period. The obstetric resident noted that liquor was meconium stained when the membranes ruptured. Cardiotocogram was applied but there was difficulty in obtaining the trace. The resident noted decelerations at several occasions but was not sure of interpretation. Observing that the cervix was 8 cm dilated, oxytocin infusion was started to augment labor. The consultant arrived and noted late decelerations. The oxytocin drip was stopped and an emergency cesarean was planned. A male infant 3.2 kg was delivered. The Apgar scores at 1 and 5 minutes were 2 and 6. The cord arterial gas analysis showed a pH was 7.2 and base deficit was 10. The neonate was transferred to neonatal unit for postresuscitation care. There was mild encephalopathy that improved after 24 hours. The baby was transferred to postnatal ward on day 2 of life and discharged home on breastfeeding by day 4 of life. At 6 months of age, the neonate was noted to have poor head control and had not attained social smile and at 12 months the child was diagnosed to have cerebral palsy. The parents sought legal opinion with allegations that poor intrapartum care and delay in performing cesarean section led to cerebral palsy.

In medicolegal cases, it is important to establish that there was indeed a definite breach of duty AND that the injury was directly caused by breach of duty. Often the medicolegal claim might be sought years after the alleged event. The following are considered in such claims:
- The neurological deficit in the child
- Whether the deficit was due to birth asphyxia?
- Are there alternate etiologies?
- Whether there was any breach of duty during delivery and postnatal care?

The American Academy of Pediatrics and the American College of Obstetricians and Gynecologists have developed a checklist to establish if there is a reasonable causal link between birth asphyxia and later cerebral palsy. The four criteria that must be met are:
1. Fetal acidosis as evidenced by umbilical cord arterial pH less than 7 and base deficit of 12 mmol/L or more.
2. Early onset moderate or severe encephalopathy in infants ≥34 weeks gestation
3. Cerebral palsy of the spastic quadriplegic or dyskinetic type
4. Exclusion of other etiologies that can explain the neurological injury such as trauma, coagulopathy, infectious, or genetic disorders.

In this case, the court agreed that there was delay in recognition of fetal distress, but the physicians had taken appropriate action and had documented events correctly. They also recognized that the cerebral palsy is not causally related to perinatal depression.

A breach of duty or medical negligence can be related to incorrect diagnosis (failure to recognize fetal distress, imminent uterine rupture, or interpret cardiotocography), negligence related to poor patient counseling (not informing the risk of shoulder dystocia in a pregnant diabetic woman with a large fetus, or the risk of neonatal problems in periviable gestations) or negligence related to poor standard of care (administering wrong medication, not properly skilled in instrumental delivery, or cesarean section leading to trauma to mother or baby).

Prevention of Medicolegal Claims

The best way to handle any medicolegal litigation is to prevent them. **Box 2** lists preventive measures related to obstetric practice. Since negligence claims may be made many years later it is important to preserve documents such as antenatal register, birth register, case records (along with partograms, cardiotocography, and ultrasound reports), and the Preconception and Prenatal Diagnostic Technique (PCPNDT) registers. It is recommended to preserve obstetric records for 21 years.

MEDICAL LEGAL ISSUES IN ASSISTED REPRODUCTIVE TECHNIQUES (ART) OR SURROGACY

With advances in medicine couples with infertility can achieve the dream of becoming parent with the assistance of new technologies called as ART such as in vitro fertilization, intracytoplasmic sperm injection (ICSI), etc. Recently, the option to have a child with help of a surrogate mother (who carries and deliver the child) in cases, where it is physically or medically impossible and/or is not desirous to carry a child, has opened opportunities but with many legal challenges. However, the introduction of the recent Assisted Reproductive Technology (Regulation) Bill, 2020 has attempted to regulate the issues and standardize the protocols for ART and surrogacy.

The rights of child born through ART is guided by the clause 31 of the act which states "The child born shall be deemed to be a biological child of the commissioning couple and the said child shall be entitled to all the rights and privileges available to a natural child only from the commissioning couple under any law for the time being in force. A donor shall relinquish all parental rights over the child or children, which may be born from his or her gamete".

In cases of surrogacy the following shall be followed:
- Surrogate mother should not use or register in the name of the commissioning couple for whom she is acting as surrogate as this would pose legal issues, particularly in the untoward event of maternal death.

> **BOX 2:** Prevention of medicolegal claims in obstetric practice.
>
> *Maternal care:*
> - Obtain adequate obstetrical history to identify risk factors
> - Anticipate for shoulder dystocia and cephalo pelvic disproportion, especially in patients with risk factors such as big baby, short stature
> - Document cardiotocograph findings based on recommended classification and act appropriately
> - Judicious use of oxytocin to induce or augment labor
> - Early recognition of delayed labor, malpresentation or cord prolapse, lack of progress in labor
> - Once a decision to carry out cesarean section or instrumental delivery is made, avoid undue delays
> - Provide the highest standards of care
>
> *Neonatal care:*
> - The pediatrician or neonatal care provider should be available in-house (24 × 7)
> - Equipment for resuscitation should be available and functional
> - Resuscitation should be according to recommended guidelines
> - Neonates sustaining perinatal asphyxia or birth injury should be observed in a suitable facility
> - Monitor the neonate for encephalopathy and seizures
> - Timely initiation of therapeutic hypothermia
> - Refer the baby timely to a higher facility, if the center does not have skilled personnel or facility
> - Identification tag should be placed on the neonate as well as the mother. It may contain the name of the mother +/- father, sex, time of birth, birth weight and date of birth and the hospital number, based on the unit policy
>
> *Documentation and communication:*
> - Discussions among obstetric, neonatal teams, and parents prior to delivery
> - Accurate and honest documentation of examination findings, reports, and interpretation
> - Legible notes, with signature, printed name with date and time
> - The patient details should be noted in all pages
> - In case of emergency or verbal orders, a retrospective note should be made as soon as possible and the timing of the entry noted
> - Appropriate parental counseling and shared decision making

- The birth certificate shall be in the name of the commissioning parents. The ART clinic should also provide a certificate to the commissioning parents giving the name and address of the surrogate mother.
- All the expenses of surrogate mother during the period of pregnancy and postnatal care relating to pregnancy should be borne by the commissioning couple.
- The surrogate mother would also be entitled a monetary compensation from the commissioning couple for agreeing to act as a surrogate.
- Surrogate mother shall relinquish all parental rights related with the offspring in writing.

CHAPTER AT A GLANCE

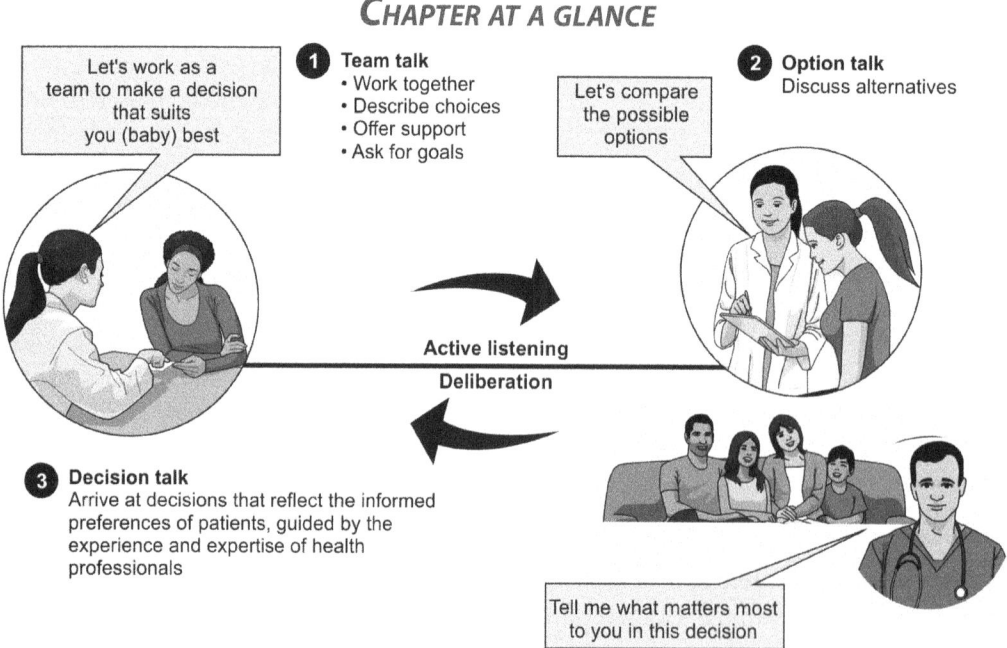

The crux of the chapter is good communication between the health professionals and the parents. The three-talk model can be used for shared decision-making. The figure depicts conversational steps starting with providing support, followed by providing options, helping parents to compare and discuss the risks and benefits of alternate options, finally helping with informed preferences. (Adapted from, A three-talk model for shared decision making: multistage consultation process. BMJ 2017)

KEY POINTS

- Individual hospital and unit policies must be drawn up and approved by concerned stakeholders for anticipated ethically difficult situations.
- The rights of both mothers and newborns (including the right to respect, dignity, highest standard of health, and freedom from discrimination) must be protected.
- Ethical dilemmas may arise at various situations in obstetric care including management at periviable gestation, fetuses or neonates with major malformations, termination of pregnancy, and artificial reproductive technologies.
- Parental counseling with accurate information and shared decision making is important.
- Comfort care or palliative care decisions should be made in consultation with parents and all providers should act in the best interest of the unborn fetus or neonate.
- The best means of handling medicolegal litigations is preventing them.
- Careful, accurate, and honest record keeping is important. Incomplete/unclear records are a poor defense; no records at all is no defense.

SUGGESTED READING

1. Bevilacqua G, Corradi M, Donzelli GP, Fanos V, Gianotti D, Magnani C, et al. The Parma Charter of the Rights of the Newborn. J Matern Fetal Neonatal Med. 2011;24(1):171.
2. Carrera JM, Cabero L, de Gruyter W. Declaration of Barcelona on the Rights of Mother and Newborn. Barcelona: Proceedings of the 5th World Congress of Perinatal Medicine; 2001.
3. Mishra S, Mukhopadhyay K, Tiwari S, Bangal R, Yadav BS, Sachdeva A, et al. End-of-Life care: Consensus statement by Indian Academy of Pediatrics. Indian Pediatr. 2017;54:851-9.
4. The American College of Obstetricians and Gynecologists and the Society for Maternal-Fetal Medicine. Obstetric care consensus: *Interim update. Periviable birth*. Obstet Gynecol. 2017;130(4):e187-99.
5. Tiwari S, Kuthe A. Care at the edge of viability: legal and ethical issues. NIJP. 2016;5.2:76-80.

SECTION 7

Miscellaneous

Arjit Mohapatra, Sindhu Sivanandan, Anish Keepanasseril

- **Stillbirth**
  Priyadarshini V, Anish Keepanasseril
- **Placental Examination**
  Saubhagya Kumar Jena, Tapas Som

CHAPTER 50

Stillbirth

Priyadarshini V, Anish Keepanasseril

INTRODUCTION

Perinatal mortality rate, which includes stillbirth and early neonatal mortality, is a key quality-of-care indicator of pregnancy and childbirth care. With improvement in health care, neonatal mortality has declined over the years, but the stillbirth rates (SBR) have remained steady. India accounts for 0.34 million of the 1.9 million stillbirths globally in 2019, making it the highest contributor. The perinatal mortality rate in India in 2017 was 23 per 1,000 live births, with stillbirths alone contributing to 5 per 1,000 live births. To reduce perinatal mortality, there is a need to implement an integrated systematic approach during pregnancy, labor, and newborn care. The Indian New-born Action Plan, launched in 2014, aims to achieve single-digit SBR by 2030 with an annual reduction in SBR or 4.4%. The progress in preventing stillbirths is slow compared with reductions in neonatal mortality rate. We need tremendous effort and investment in ending preventable stillbirths.

OBJECTIVES

- To understand the definition of stillbirth
- To identify the risk factors associated with stillbirth
- To learn the optimal investigation algorithm for stillbirths
- To adopt strategies during pre-pregnancy, antenatal, and intrapartum periods to bring down stillbirths.

DEFINITION OF STILLBIRTH

Stillbirth refers to a baby born with no signs of life after the period of viability. Viability is generally assessed based on gestational age (generally 20 weeks or 28 weeks depending on the setting) **(Table 1)**, where gestational age is not available, birth weight or length at birth is used as surrogates. The International Classification of Diseases (ICD) definition of late fetal deaths is used for international comparisons of stillbirths. ICD (10th and 11th revisions) defines late fetal death as the in-utero death of a fetus with a birth weight of

TABLE 1: Definitions of stillbirth.

International Classification of Diseases 10th revision (ICD 10) definitions (birth weight is given priority over gestational age)	• Late fetal death 1,000 g or more or 28 weeks or more or 35 cm or more • Early fetal death 500 g, or more or 22 weeks or more or 25 cm or more
WHO definition (refers to ICD definitions of late fetal deaths	• For international comparison, stillbirth is defined as a fetus who dies after 28 weeks of pregnancy but before or during birth • For reporting, stillbirth is defined as fetal death ≥22 weeks of gestation, or with a birth weight of ≥500 g or body length of ≥25 cm, before or during labor and birth
India (Health Management Information system), Ministry of Health Government of India	• Stillbirth has been defined as complete expulsion or extraction of a baby from its mother where the fetus does not breathe or show any evidence of life, such as the beating of the heart or a cry or movement of the limbs • For sentinel surveillance in the country, the following definitions will be used • *Early fetal deaths*: Death of a fetus weighing at least 500 g or after 20 completed weeks gestation, or with a crown-heel length of 25 cm or more • *Late fetal deaths*: Fetal death weighing at least 1,000 g or a gestational age of 28 years completed weeks or a crown-heel length of 35 cm or more

≥1,000 g or a gestational age of ≥28 weeks (if birthweight is not available) a body length of ≥35 cm (if gestational age is not available). The Core Stillbirth Estimation Group (CSEG) recommends using gestational age rather than birthweight and omitting the length criterion as gestational age is a better predictor of maturity and viability.

Note:
- The varying definitions of stillbirths is generally due to variation in the viability thresholds adopted by different nations.
- The SBR calculated based on gestational age and birth weight thresholds do not give similar results. Hence, the definition should be based on only one parameter, and gestational age threshold is the most appropriate.
- Despite being important, stillbirths were not included in the millennium development goals (MDGs) and are not tracked by the United Nations or the Global Burden of Disease. They are now included in the Early Newborn Action Plan.

Based on the timing of occurrence of fetal death, stillbirth can be classified as antepartum (*macerated stillbirth*; fetal death before labor) or intrapartum (*fresh stillbirth*; fetal death during labor or birth process) **(Table 2)**.

Stillbirth Rate

Stillbirth rate is the number of stillbirths at 28 weeks gestation or more per 1,000 total births (live births plus stillbirths). In 2015, India ranked first in the global burden of stillbirths, with 22 per 1,000 total births. A survey of nine Indian states between 2010 and 2013 reported a stillbirth of 10 per 1,000 total births, with variation between 4.2 and 14.8. The current annual reduction rate (ARR) of stillbirth is 2.4%. According to the Indian Newborn Action Plan, the plan is to reduce stillbirths to <10 per 1,000 births by 2030. This requires intensified efforts and an ARR of stillbirths by 4.2%.

Causes of Stillbirth

The most common risk factors for stillbirth in the developing world include advanced maternal age, prematurity, lack of adequate care in the antepartum and intrapartum period, multiple gestation, and maternal morbidity. The risk factors for stillbirth are listed in **Box 1**.

Classification of Stillbirth

Various classification systems are reported in the literature, mainly based on the presumed cause of death or associated pregnancy-related complications. A systematic uniform way of recording the cause of death and the factors leading to it will help understand the causes and aid in formulating strategies leading to reducing the stillbirth rates. Different classification systems include Causes of Death and Associated Conditions (CODAC), Wigglesworth, Aberdeen, Perinatal Society of Australia and New Zealand-Perinatal Death Classification (PSANZ-PDC), Relevant Condition at Death (ReCoDe), and Tulip system. Among the various classification systems, CODAC retains most of the information related to the factors contributing to the stillbirth, whereas others, such as the PSANZ-PDC and ReCoDe, are user-friendly and easier to implement. Currently, ReCoDe **(Box 2)** is the only system dedicated to the classification of stillbirths causes. It is preferable in low to middle-income settings such as ours to use a classification system based on clinical features.

INVESTIGATION OF STILLBIRTH

Currently, evaluation following stillbirth is mainly influenced by the availability of the relevant investigation, the family's financial constraints, and also guided by personal or cultural beliefs. Stillbirths from unknown causes account for 25–60% in various reports. A systematic evaluation comprises reviewing relevant history, laboratory investigation, placental histopathology, and fetal autopsy, which are needed to detect a contributory factor leading to stillbirth. Adopting such a uniformly agreed protocol in the evaluation will help to reduce the proportion of unclassified stillbirths.

Maternal History

Obtain a thorough maternal history to get information about general conditions or symptoms associated with risk

TABLE 2: Comparison between antepartum and intrapartum stillbirth.	
Antepartum stillbirth	*Intrapartum stillbirth*
Fetal death before labor (generally before 12 hours of labor)	During the labor or birth process
The skin shows discoloration or darkening, redness, peeling, and breakdown. Therefore, called a macerated stillbirth. Signs of skin maceration begin at 6–12 hours after fetal death	Fetal heart rate is present at the onset of labor. In settings where fetal heart rate monitoring is not available, the fetus's skin is frequently used to estimate the timing of the stillbirth. The skin is intact, therefore called a fresh stillbirth
Generally due to antenatal risk factors, including congenital malformations. Prevention should focus on quality antenatal care and family planning	Prevention should focus on quality care during labor and childbirth
Overall, 55% of stillbirths occur in the antenatal period	The proportion of intrapartum stillbirth varies from 10% in developed countries to 60% in South Asia

> **BOX 1:** Risk factors for stillbirth.
>
> *Maternal factors*
> *Demographic/social risk factors:*
> - Advanced maternal age (also teenage pregnancy)
> - Nulliparity
> - Smoking and illicit drug use during pregnancy
> - Obesity
> - Inadequate prenatal care
> - Lower socioeconomic status
>
> *Maternal medical conditions and infections:*
> - Diabetes mellitus
> - Hypertensive disorders
> - Thrombophilia and thromboembolic disorders
> - Autoimmune disease
> - Epilepsy
> - Severe anemia
> - Cyanotic heart disease
> - Infections (HIV, malaria, syphilis—an important preventable cause in developing countries)
>
> *Family/previous obstetric history:*
> - Consanguinity history
> - Familial disorders/inherited conditions—recurrent spontaneous abortions, venous/pulmonary thromboembolism
> - The previous child born with structural or chromosomal anomaly/syndrome documented developmental delay
>
> *Fetal factor:*
> - Congenital anomaly or infection
> - Fetal growth restriction
> - Previous fetal demise
> - Multiple gestations
> - Pregnancy lasting 42 weeks or more
>
> *Cord/placental factors:*
> - Abnormalities of structure, length, or insertion of the umbilical cord
> - Umbilical cord prolapse
> - True knot of the umbilical cord
> - Large or small placenta
> - Abruption
> - Placental tumors

> **BOX 2:** Classification of stillbirth by Relevant Condition at Death.
>
> *Fetus:*
> - Lethal congenital anomaly
> - Infection
> - Chronic
> - Acute
> - Nonimmune hydrops
> - Iso-immunization
> - Feto-maternal hemorrhage
> - Twin-twin transfusion
> - Fetal growth restriction
> - Other
>
> *Umbilical cord:*
> - Prolapse
> - Constricting loop or knot
> - Velamentous insertion
> - Other
>
> *Placenta:*
> - Abruptio
> - Previa
> - Vasa previa
> - Placental insufficiency/infarction
> - Others
>
> *Amniotic fluid:*
> - Chorioamnionitis
> - Oligohydramnios
> - Polyhydramnios
> - Others
>
> *Uterus*
> - Rupture
> - Other

factors. Maternal medical illness, obstetric history, exposure to medications, infections during pregnancy, family history (including consanguinity) with a three-generation pedigree including stillborn infants should be obtained. Recurrent pregnancy losses (RPL) or previous babies with developmental delay or malformations may point to single-gene disorders. History of arrhythmias and sudden death in the previous sibling may point to long QT syndrome. Review maternal records to obtain the accurate gestational age, antenatal visits and examinations, laboratory investigations, and ultrasound details.

Investigations

The maternal investigations that are considered for stillbirth are given in **Box 3**.

Fetal and Placental Examination

In addition to examining the fetus, stillbirth evaluation should include gross and histologic examination of the placenta, umbilical cord, membranes, genetic evaluation, and partial or complete fetal autopsy **(Box 4)**.

Placental examination by a pathologist is the single most crucial aspect. It can reveal abruption, umbilical cord thrombosis, velamentous cord insertion, and vasa previa. It can also give clues to infection, genetic abnormalities, and anemia. In twin gestations, chorionicity should be established, and vascular anastomoses identified.

Autopsy

"Perinatal autopsy" is the postmortem examination of the fetus to establish and confirm the cause of stillbirth. It is the most useful diagnostic test in determining the cause of stillbirth. The yield is more significant when dysmorphic features, inconsistent growth measurements, anomalies, hydrops, or growth restriction. If families do not consent for a complete autopsy, partial autopsy, minimal tissue sampling, ultrasonography, and magnetic resonance imaging can be offered but are less informative than a complete autopsy.

The family's cultural and religious beliefs must be respected, and attempts to persuade them to choose postmortem must be avoided. Written consent is a must for

> **BOX 3:** Maternal investigations in stillbirth.

Maternal/family history—to assess the presence of risk/contributing factors in the previous and current pregnancy is the key in guiding further evaluation

Maternal blood tests:

- Hematology and biochemistry

  Complete blood count
  Renal and liver function test } Preecclampsia, organ failure in sepsis, obstetric cholestasis
  C-reactive protein

- *Blood glucose, hemoglobin A1C, thyroid profile:* Diabetes, hypothyroid
- *Coagulation profile:* Disseminated intravascular coagulation
- *Kleihauer–Betke (KB) or acid elution test:* To diagnose lethal feto-maternal hemorrhage, a significant cause of late fetal death. Also, to decide the level of requirement of anti-RhD gammaglobulin. KB test should be recommended for all women, not simply those who are RhD-negative, and sample must be obtained before birth as red cells might clear quickly from maternal circulation
- Serology for cytomegalovirus, toxoplasma, parvovirus B19, rubella and syphilis
- Maternal thrombophilia screen—indicated if evidence of fetal growth screen restriction or placental disease. The association between inherited thrombophilias and stillbirth is weak, and the results do not guide management in a future pregnancy
- Maternal antibody testing:
  - Maternal red cell antibody (immune hemolytic disease)
  - Maternal Ro and La antibodies (maternal autoimmune disease)—if fetal hydrops found
  - Maternal alloimmune platelet antibody (alloimmune thrombocytopenia)—if fetal intracranial hemorrhage found on postmortem

Maternal toxicology—to rule out toxins or substance abuse such as cocaine–guided by the history or clinical features, if indicated

- *Maternal microbiology* (culture of urine, high vaginal swabs, and blood) in cases with maternal fever, reduced liquor volume of a history suggestive of prolonged rupture of membranes
- In cases when the contributory factor cannot be assigned

> **BOX 4:** Examination of the fetus, placenta, and membranes in stillbirth.

Examination of the fetus:

- Preferably done by a perinatal pathologist or neonatologist to identify malformation and syndromic features
- Weight, length, and head circumference
- Photographs of the fetus and placenta
- Frontal and profile photographs of the whole body

Sex determination: In macerated and hydropic fetuses, the determination of sex may be difficult. Two experienced healthcare practitioners (midwives, obstetricians, neonatologists, or pathologists) should inspect the baby. If there is any difficulty, rapid karyotyping using quantitative fluorescent polymerase chain reaction (QF-PCR) or fluorescence in situ hybridization (FISH) should be offered.

Ultrasound (and Amniocentesis where indicated):

- Rule out fetal abnormalities
- Measure fetal biometry
- Assessment of amniotic fluid volume
- Amniocentesis for cytogenetic analysis/microbiological assessment

Postmortem radiological imaging will aid in detecting the skeletal anomalies which may be missed on an external inspection (**Figs. 1A and B**).

Placental examination:

- Gross appearance of the cord, membranes, and placenta
- Detailed microscopic assessment of the placenta and cord
- Bacterial culture of the swabs taken between the amnion and chorion
- Karyotyping/Microarray of amnion and placental tissue

any invasive procedure or tissues taken for genetic analysis. The process of the autopsy must be explained, including the likely appearance of the baby afterward. The baby must be treated with dignity.

Labor and Birth

The timing and the mode of delivery are based on an informed discussion with the mother and her family. It should consider the family's wishes, maternal condition, and the safety of the method used for the termination. The discussion should also include how the expectant management and waiting for the spontaneous onset of delivery may affect the findings at the autopsy of the fetus, as many features might be distorted once the maceration of the baby sets in. Vaginal birth is the preferred mode of delivery after a stillbirth. The development of complications such as DIC is reported to

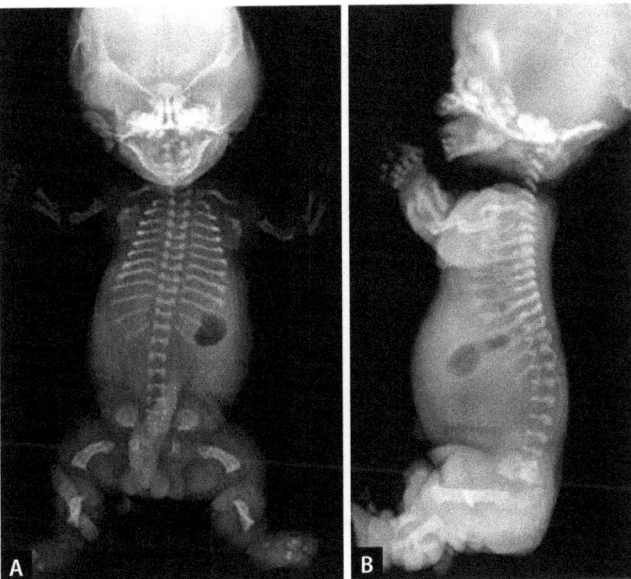

Figs. 1A and B: Radiograph of the fetus (Infantogram). (A) *Anteroposterior view:* Large skull, narrow thorax, short thick bowed tubular bones of extremities; (B) *Lateral view:* Severe flattening of vertebral bodies (platyspondyly), short ribs (Thanatophoric skeletal dysplasia).

occur after 3–4 weeks of stillbirth. However, most mothers have spontaneous onset of labor within that time frame, so the counseling aiming to reduce the anxiety and ensuring support to the family remains the critical factor in cases of expectant management when opted.

FOLLOW-UP AND GRIEF MANAGEMENT

After investigations are completed, the results of the autopsy, placental examination, and other tests should be communicated to the family promptly. Records should document the events and contributory factors of stillbirth. However, despite an exhaustive review, the cause may remain elusion in about one-quarter of stillbirths. Healthcare providers should offer emotional support and bereavement counseling to the parents based on the family's personal, social, and religious backgrounds.

SPECIAL SITUATIONS

Rhesus D-negative Women with Fetal Loss

Major feto-maternal hemorrhage can result in stillbirth, and a KB test is recommended to aid in the diagnosis. In most cases, the sensitizing event would have occurred much before the time frame for administering anti-D. However, given the advantage it offers, all women with Rh-negative blood group with stillbirth should be offered anti-D unless the baby's blood group is ascertained from cord blood or typed with maternal cell-free DNA (cfDNA). The dose of anti-D can be guided by quantification of the fetal blood cells using the KB test.

Women with Recurrent Fetal Loss

Recurrent pregnancy loss is defined as two or more fetal losses, known to affect 1% of fertile couples. Risk factors associated with recurrent loss include unbalanced translocations in the parents, inherited thrombophilia (Factor V Leiden, prothrombin gene mutation, protein S deficiency), and antiphospholipid antibodies (lupus anticoagulant or anticardiolipin antibody). The role of endocrine factors (Luteal phase deficiency) and anatomic factors (uterine anomalies, cervical insufficiency) is not entirely understood. Even though TORCH infection has been attributed to causing stillbirth, it has not been associated with recurrent fetal loss. The risk of recurrence of stillbirth is 2–10 times higher in a subsequent pregnancy. The goal of managing recurrent loss is to identify the appropriate cause by systematic evaluation and offer specific treatment.

STRATEGIES FOR PREVENTION OF STILLBIRTH

Higher national coverage of antenatal care is strongly associated with lower antepartum stillbirths. Strategies to prevent intrapartum stillbirths involve timely, high-quality care around the time of birth **(Fig. 2)**. Fetuses with low birth weight and gestational age and those with fetal growth restriction are at the highest risk of stillbirth. Early identification of high-risk pregnancies and optimum management is essential. The three delays model is relevant for stillbirths, too—these include delays in recognizing danger signs, delay in care-seeking due to social or economic barriers, or distance and lack of transport, and delay in receiving high-quality health facility care. The preventive strategies should include the spectrum of care covering prepregnancy, antenatal, and intrapartum care. Interventions are best packaged and provided through linked service delivery methods tailored to suit existing healthcare systems. Services are best integrated to provide a continuum of care from before pregnancy through to postnatal care. Interventions should be delivered as a package through the health system, with skilled care at birth and emergency obstetric caretaking priority. More complex interventions could be added as mortality declines and the capacity of the health system increases.

In LMICs, which account for 92% of the worldwide burden of stillbirth, universal coverage of care (99%) with intervention packages can prevent one million (45%) third-trimester stillbirths, 50% of maternal deaths, and 1.4 million (43%) neonatal deaths. This comes at a meager additional cost of US$ 2–3 per person.

Janani Suraksha Yojana

India's Janani Suraksha Yojanass (JSY) program is an example of government-initiated activity linked to

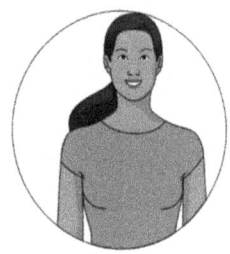

Reproductive health
- Elective abortion where legal
- Emergency reproductive and gynecological care
- Family planning

Preventive care
- Periconceptional folate
- Prevent obesity
- Smoking cessation
- Reduction of exposure to indoor pollution

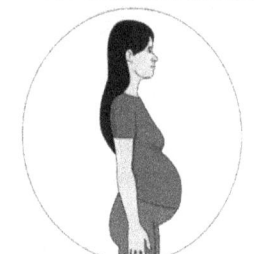

Basic antenatal care
- Birth preparedness
- Malaria prevention
- Detection and management of syphilis
- Tetanus toxoid immunization
- Prevention of mother-infant transmission of HIV

Advanced antenatal care
- Detection and management of hypertensive disorder or pregnancy
- Detection and management of diabetes

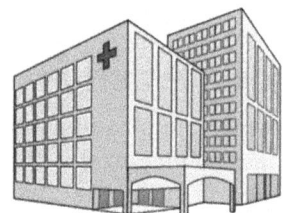

Emergency obstetric and newborn care (EmONC)
Basic
- Parenteral antibiotics to prevent puerperal infection
- Anticonvulsants for treatment of eclampsia and preeclampsia
- Uterotonic drugs for postpartum hemorrhage
- Manual removal of the placenta
- Assisted vaginal delivery (vacuum extractions)
- Removal of retained products of conception
- Neonatal resuscitation

Comprehensive
All above + cesarean section and blood transfusion

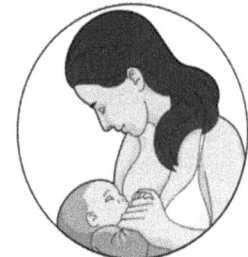

Immediate newborn care
- Delayed cord clamping
- Thermoregulation
- Immediate breastfeeding
- Infection prevention

Fig. 2: Strategies to prevent stillbirths covering prepregnancy, antenatal, and intrapartum periods.

Overall target is to decrease maternal mortality ratio and infant mortality rate, and to increase institutional deliveries

- Registration
- Early identification of complicated cases
- Providing at least three antenatal visits
- Postdelivery visits
- Immunization
- Organizing appropriate referral and provide referral transport mother

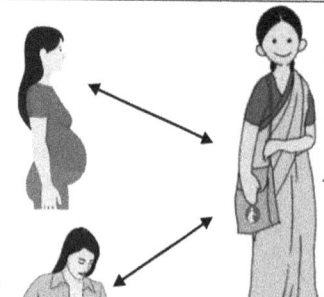
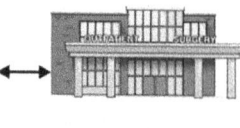
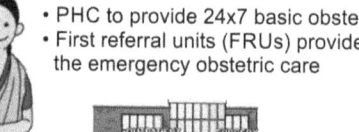

- PHC to provide 24x7 basic obstetric care
- First referral units (FRUs) provide the emergency obstetric care

- Field level health worker coordinates
- Cash assistance to mother and ASHA worker for institutional deliveries

Fig. 3: India's Janani Suraksha Yojana, a conditional cash transfer program to increase births in health facilities.

the health system to decrease maternal and neonatal mortality rates **(Fig. 3)**. Started in 2005, the JSY program is the world's largest conditional cash transfer scheme that provides incentives to women of low socioeconomic status giving birth in a health facility. The community health workers identify pregnant women and help them to get to the health facility. They also facilitate women to receive at least three antenatal care visits, immunization for the neonate, a postnatal examination, and early referral to a health facility. Studies have shown that the JSY program had increased the coverage of three antenatal visits by 15–20% and institutional deliveries by about 30%. Although perinatal and neonatal deaths were reduced by about 10%, the change in maternal mortality was not significant. Reasons speculated were poor quality of care at health facilities and most public hospitals in rural areas lacking adequate skilled staff and supplies, equipment, and infrastructure and effective systems of communication and referral. Therefore, it is mandatory to improve both coverage and quality of care.

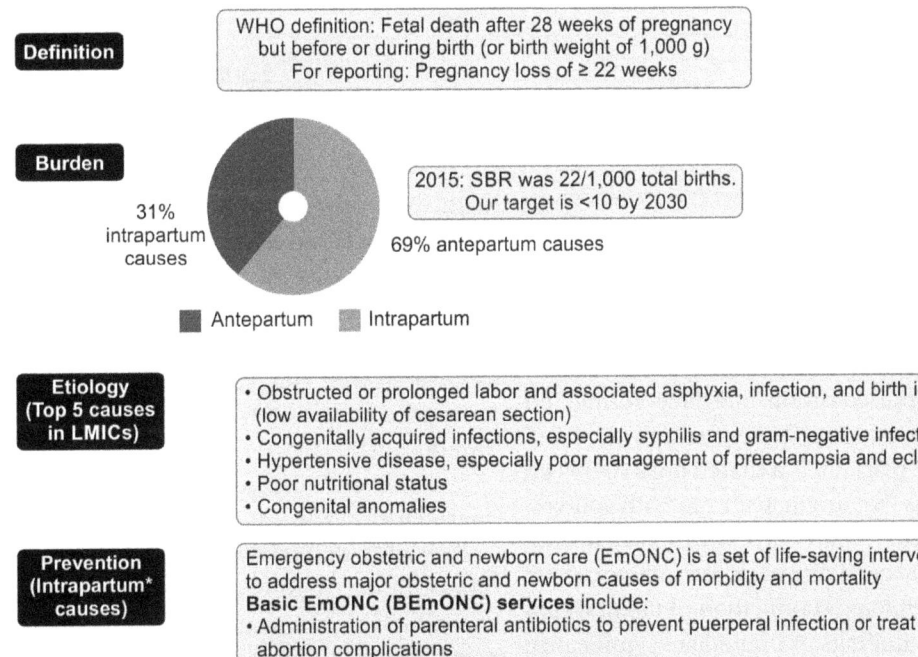

KEY POINTS

- The stillbirth rate is a key indicator of the quality of care during pregnancy and childbirth.
- India's Newborn Action Plan aims to end preventable stillbirths to achieve a "Single Digit stillbirth rate" by 2030.
- Detailed systematic approach aids in detecting the cause of stillbirth; placental examination and fetal autopsy are essential parts of the investigation.
- The most common risk factors for stillbirth in the developing world include advanced maternal age, prematurity, lack of adequate care in the antepartum and intrapartum period, multiple gestation, and maternal morbidity.
- Prevention of stillbirths should extend throughout the continuum of care from the prepregnancy, antenatal and intrapartum period.
- Can prevent 1.1 million stillbirths and 1.4 million neonatal deaths each year with universal coverage and good quality care, and a meager additional cost of US$ 2–3 per person.

SUGGESTED READING

1. de Bernis L, Kinney MV, Stones W, Ten Hoope-Bender P, Vivio D, Leisher SH, et al.; Lancet Ending Preventable Stillbirths Series study group; Lancet Ending Preventable Stillbirths Series Advisory Group. Stillbirths: ending preventable deaths by 2030. Lancet. 2016;387(10019):703-16.
2. Lawn JE, Blencowe H, Waiswa P, Amouzou A, Mathers C, Hogan D, et al.; Lancet Ending Preventable Stillbirths Series study group; Lancet Stillbirth Epidemiology investigator group. Stillbirths: rates, risk factors, and acceleration towards 2030. Lancet. 2016;387(10018):587-603.
3. Lim SS, Dandona L, Hoisington JA, James SL, Hogan MC, Gakidou E. India's Janani Suraksha Yojana, a conditional cash transfer programme to increase births in health facilities: an impact evaluation. Lancet. 2010;375(9730):2009-23.
4. Management of Stillbirth: Obstetric Care Consensus No, 10. Obstet Gynecol. 2020;135(3):e110-32.
5. Miller ES, Minturn L, Linn R, Weese-Mayer DE, Ernst LM. Stillbirth evaluation: a stepwise assessment of placental pathology and autopsy. Am J Obstet Gynecol. 2016;214(1):115.e1-6.

51

Placental Examination

Saubhagya Kumar Jena, Tapas Som

INTRODUCTION

Viviparity is a reproductive mode where the embryo develops inside the mother's womb, and the mother gives birth to a live young. In placental viviparity, zygotes and embryos get physiological support from the placenta, the maternal-fetal contact zone, or the common interface connected through the umbilical cord to supply oxygen, nutrition, and excretion of wastes. The placenta is a shared organ between the mother and the fetus that originated from both sources. Maternal or fetal disorders may have an impact on the placenta. Conversely, placental disorders can influence fetal or maternal health. Therefore, examination of the placenta may provide additional findings of immediate significance for further management, and the findings may be related to the prognosis of the neonate or future pregnancies. The histopathological examination (HPE) is indicated in fetal or neonatal death cases where etiology is unknown.

OBJECTIVES

- To review the development of the placenta.
- To discuss the clinical significance of abnormal development, the position of the placenta.
- To discuss the specific indications for placental examination.
- To discuss the assessment of placental function before birth.
- To discuss the examination of the placenta after birth.

DEVELOPMENT OF PLACENTA

The placenta is formed from two sources, namely from trophoblasts of fetal origin and decidua basalis of maternal origin. Trophoblastic cells differentiate to form cytotrophoblast and syncytiotrophoblast. The syncytiotrophoblast invades the endometrium at the beginning of the second week. Vacuoles appear within the syncytium, and gradually these vacuoles fuse to form lacunae. Lacunar spaces enlarge to create intercommunicating networks with each other. Trophoblastic cells continue to invade the endometrium and erode the endothelial lining of the maternal capillaries. Lacunar spaces become continuous with the sinusoids.

At the end of the second week, the blastocyst all around is covered with villi. However, the villi only on the embryonic pole grow to develop the future placenta (chorionic frondosum).

At the end of the third week, the extraembryonic mesoderm invades into the structure of the villi. Mesodermal cells further differentiate into blood vessels inside the villi. These blood vessels later communicate with the blood vessels of the connecting stalk through the chorionic plate (extraembryonic mesoderm). The cells of the cytotrophoblast gradually proliferate and penetrate the syncytiotrophoblast as columns. The cells penetrate the tip of the villi to reach the endometrium where the cells proliferate and establish connection between similar extensions to form a shell-like structure called outer cytotrophoblast shell. On the maternal side, the adjoining part of decidua basalis, the decidual plate is intimately connected to the cytotrophoblastic shell. A few villi extend from the chorionic plate to the decidua basalis, known as anchoring villi, from which the free villi hang that help in the exchange of nutrients and others. Maternal blood vessels or sinusoids penetrate the roof of the cytotrophoblast shell to establish uteroplacental circulation.

Later, several septa arise from the decidual plate (basalis) toward the lacunar spaces during the fourth month, dividing the placenta into several cotyledons. These septa do not touch the chorionic plate, and the core is constituted of maternal tissue. However, the surface is formed by syncytiotrophoblast. The umbilical cord developed from the connecting stalk forms the connection between the embryo with the placenta. Placental size increases with the expansion of the uterus. At term, it covers approximately 15–30% of the internal uterine surface, discoid in shape, contains about 150 mL of maternal blood in the intervillous space, covered internally by amnion and externally by decidua basalis.

FUNCTION

- *Exchange of gases:* The exchange of oxygen and carbon dioxide takes place by simple diffusion against the concentration gradient. Gaseous exchange depends upon the placental blood flow.
- *Exchange of nutrients and electrolytes:* It allows water, electrolytes, and nutrients including glucose, amino acids, fatty acids, and vitamins to pass from maternal to fetal blood. It eliminates urea and other waste products into the maternal blood.
- *Transmission of maternal antibodies:* Maternal antibodies pass through the placenta to protect the fetus from infection (diphtheria, tetanus, measles, rubella). Passage of IgG antibodies against fetal Rh or ABO blood group antigens may lead to isoimmunization.
- *Hormone production:* Placenta also synthesizes many hormones that are extremely important for the continuation of pregnancy and growth of the fetus. Human chorionic gonadotropin (hCG) is produced by the placenta, the activity of which is similar to LH before pregnancy.
- *Immunological defense:* The placenta functions as a shield against infection of the fetus. As the developing fetus's innate and adaptive immune defenses are poorly equipped to fight infections, the placenta acts as an immunological barrier and protects the fetus.

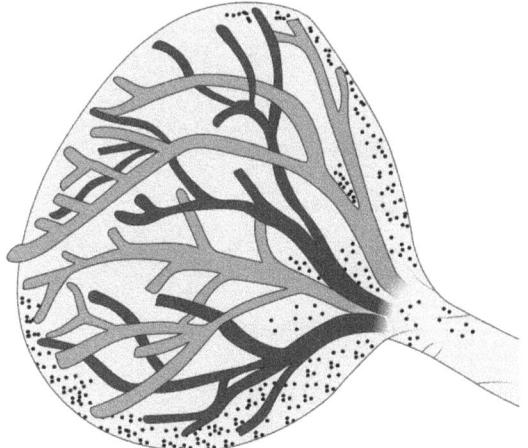

Fig. 1: Marginal insertion of cord.

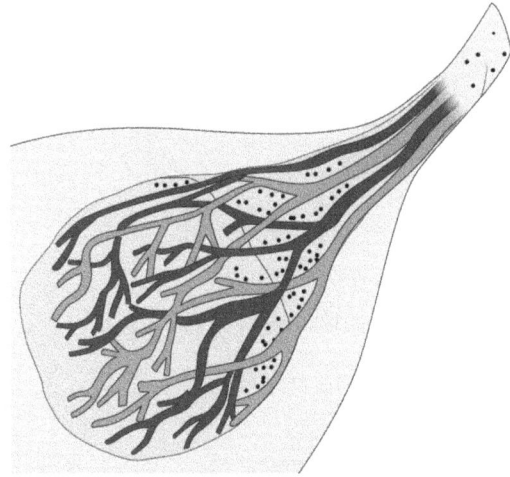

Fig. 2: Velamentous insertion of cord.

ABERRATION IN IMPLANTATION

Attachment of placenta depends on the site of implantation. Implantation occurs typically in the upper part of the body of the uterus. However, abnormal implantation can lead to compromise in fetal growth and endanger the life of the mother. Abnormal placentation may occur in the following sites:
- *Lower uterine segment*: Placenta previa (marginal or complete type is usually associated with antepartum and postpartum hemorrhages).
- *Tubal*: Interstitial, ampulla, and isthmus of the uterine tube (ectopic pregnancy)
- Abdominal in relation to the mesentery
- *Ovarian*: It leads to teratoma formation

ABNORMALITIES ACCORDING TO THE INSERTION OF THE UMBILICAL CORD (GENERALLY AT OR NEAR THE CENTER)

- Paracentral insertion
- *Marginal or battledore placenta* **(Fig. 1)**: The cord is attached at the margin of the placenta (7%).
- *Velamentous insertion* **(Fig. 2)**: The umbilical cord is attached with the fetal membranes close to the peripheral margin of placenta (1%). Chance of fetal blood loss increases with the velamentous/membranous insertion of the cord.

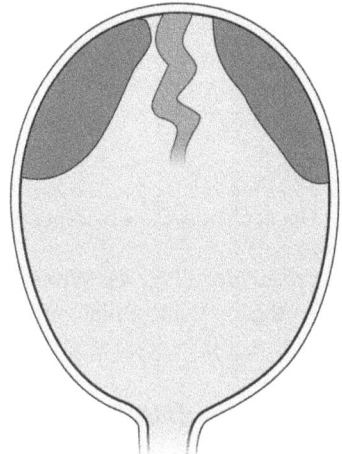

Fig. 3: Bilobed placenta.

ABNORMALITIES BASED ON THE STRUCTURE OF LOBULATIONS

- *Lobed placenta* **(Fig. 3)**: When associated with velamentous or membranous vessels, increases the risk of fetal bleeding.

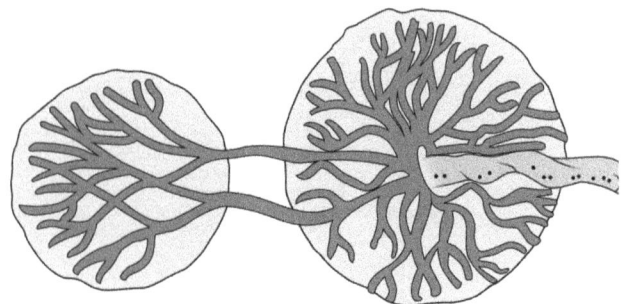

Fig. 4: Placenta succenturiata.

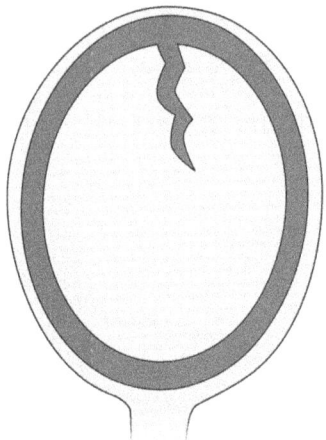

Fig. 5: Placenta membranacea.

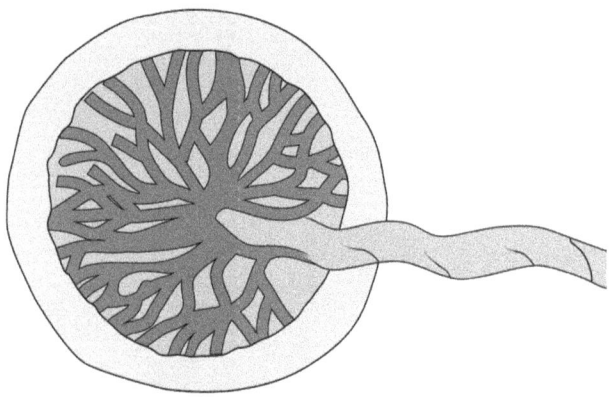

Fig. 6: Circumvallate placenta.

- *Placenta succenturiata* (**Fig. 4**): Where a small part is separated from the rest of the placenta. Small part may be retained in utero increases the risk of postpartum hemorrhage.
- *Placenta membranacea* (**Fig. 5**): Where chorionic villi are persisting all around the blastocyst. Mothers usually present with early bleeding and placenta previa. Often affected pregnancies terminate in preterm deliveries.
- *Circumvallate placenta* (**Fig. 6**): Where the margins of the placenta are covered by decidua, is often associated with acute or chronic maternal hemorrhages.

INDICATIONS FOR PLACENTAL EXAMINATION

All placentas should be examined grossly after delivery in the labor room by the personnel conducting the labor/

TABLE 1: Indications of placental examination.

Fetal/Neonatal	Placental	Maternal
• Stillbirth/perinatal death • Hydrops • Multiple pregnancies • Prematurity/postmaturity • Major malformations • IUGR • Infections • Seizures • Required NICU admissions • Perinatal asphyxia	• Abnormal fetal/placental weight • Extensive infarction • Meconium staining • Retroplacental hemorrhage • Infections • Excessive fibrin deposition • Chorangioma • Villous atrophy	• Bad obstetric history • Maternal disorders (PET, SLE, drug abuse) • Infections/fever • Abruptio • Polyhydramnios • Oligohydramnios • Repetitive bleeding

(IUGR: intrauterine growth restriction; NICU: neonatal intensive care unit; PET: preeclampsia; SLE: systemic lupus erythematosus)

delivery. However, pathologists may be asked for gross and microscopic examination in certain specific conditions. Some of those are mentioned in **Table 1**.

EXAMINATION OF PLACENTA

In the first trimester, with confirmation of gestational sac, implantation of placenta is also confirmed. Ultrasonographic studies assess placental function, and sometimes magnetic resonance imaging (MRI) may be required to confirm the abnormality in detail before intervention.

Examination of the Placenta before Birth

Ultrasonographic Assessment

A methodical sonographic evaluation of the placenta should include location, visual estimation of the size (and, if appearing abnormal, measurement of thickness and or volume), implantation, morphology, anatomy, as well as a search for anomalies, such as additional lobes and tumors (**Fig. 7**). Further assessment for multiple gestations consists of examining the intervening membranes (if present).

Doppler Assessment of Umbilical Artery

Doppler investigation of the fetal–placental circulation (umbilical artery, intraplacental circulation), as well as the uterine arteries, is performed to assess placental function. The assessment of umbilical blood flow provides information on blood perfusion of the fetal–placental unit (**Fig. 8**). The diastolic blood flow velocity component in the umbilical artery increases with advancing gestation. In pregnancies complicated by placental dysfunction, there may be a reduction in the number of functional villi and/or small blood vessels with, as a result, increased

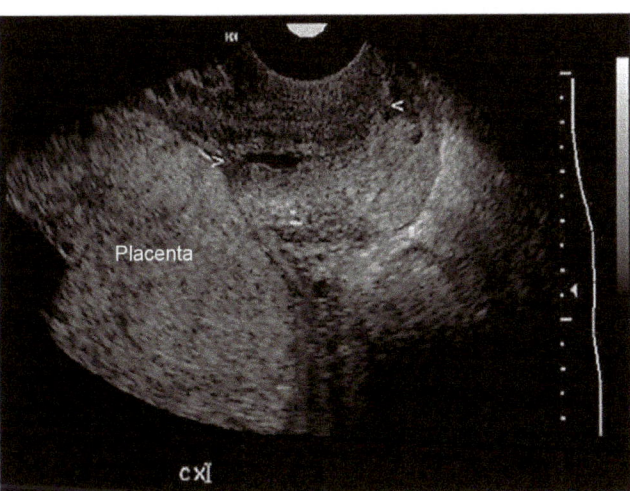

Fig. 7: Complete placenta previa in TV-USG.

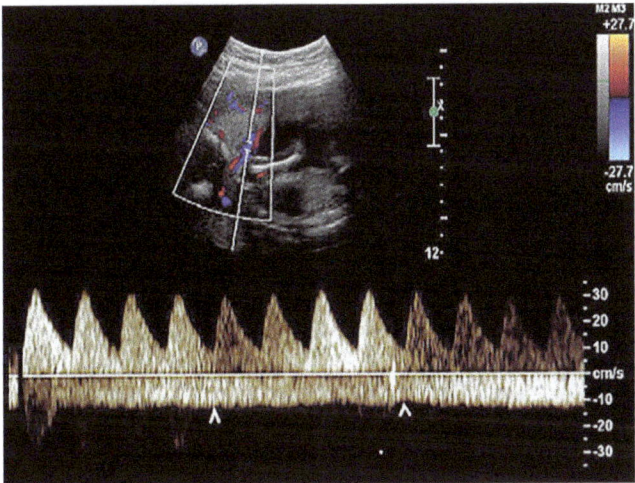

Fig. 8: Normal Doppler in the umbilical artery.

impedance, reflected, mainly, by a decrease in end-diastolic velocity. When the resistance increases even more, the forward flow may be negligible or absent (absent end-diastolic velocity).

Further increase in the resistance causes reversed end-diastolic velocity, which is considered a late step in the cascade of events leading to intrauterine fetal demise. Doppler assessment of the umbilical arteries was found to improve the outcome of high-risk pregnancies and reduce hospital admissions. On the contrary, routine Doppler ultrasound in low-risk or unselected populations does not seem to benefit a mother or newborn.

Magnetic Resonance Imaging

Magnetic resonance imaging is indicated in the diagnostic workup when ultrasound evaluation is equivocal or for patients with high clinical risk factors for placenta accreta. In cases where ultrasound has already made a definitive diagnosis, MRI is often used to plan the cesarean section delivery and peripartum hysterectomy.

Chorionic Villous Sampling

Chorionic villus sampling, sometimes called "chorionic villous biopsy" is a form of prenatal diagnosis to determine chromosomal or genetic disorders in the fetus. It entails sampling of the chorionic villus and testing it for chromosomal abnormalities.

Examination of Placenta after Birth

Macroscopic Examination

Photography: Photographic records are essential, and the caregiver can accomplish these quickly before storing the placenta at 4°C or fixation in 10% formalin (1:10 dilution of 40% formalin).

Gross examination: The following features are routinely looked for the singleton pregnancies:

- *Weight:* A healthy term fresh placenta weighs about 500–600 g. The usual ratio between fetal and placental weight is 6/7:1. The heavy placenta is noted in hydrops, GDM, whereas the light-weight placenta is seen in intrauterine growth restriction (IUGR)/placental insufficiency.
- *Diameter of the placenta and shape:* It is often round to oval in shape, can be elliptical. The diameter is 20–25 cm when round in shape with 2–2.5 cm thickness. However, all measurements can vary depending on the weight of the baby, diseases of the fetus and mother.
- *Umbilical cord:*
  - The usual length in term healthy neonates is approximately 50–55 cm with a diameter of 2–2.5 cm. The cord has the same length as the baby (Leonardo da Vinci). Short cord (<32 cm at term) is often noted in osteogenesis imperfecta, thanatophoric dysplasia, abdominal wall defects, and fetal akinesia syndrome. Long cord (>100 cm at term) may lead to increased perinatal complications like knots, entanglements, prolapse that may cause fetal distress or demise.
  - It is also spirally twisted (counterclockwise if seen from the fetal end 7:1) to protect the umbilical vessels. No or less coiling or twisting 2–2.5/10 cm (coiling index < 0.19/cm) is associated with adverse perinatal outcomes, whereas excessive coiling sometimes is associated with increased frequency of preterm labor.
  - The cord is usually attached to the center. Sometimes attachment is eccentric or marginal. Knots (false and true), cysts, thrombi (protein C deficiency), hemorrhages, varicosities, aneurysms, tumors (angioma and teratoma), and odor (fetid smell in *E. coli* infection, sweet smell in *L. monocytogenes*) are also looked for along with its attachment **(Fig. 9)**.
- *Membranes:* The membrane consists of two layers—amnion and chorion. The amnion should be separated

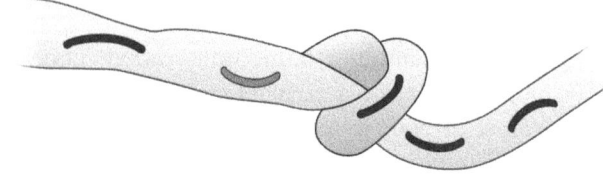

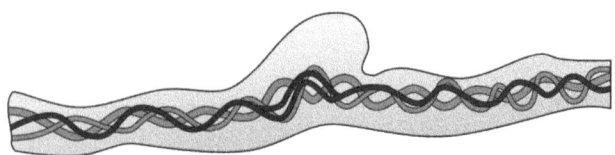

Fig. 9: Cord with false (top), true (bottom) knots.

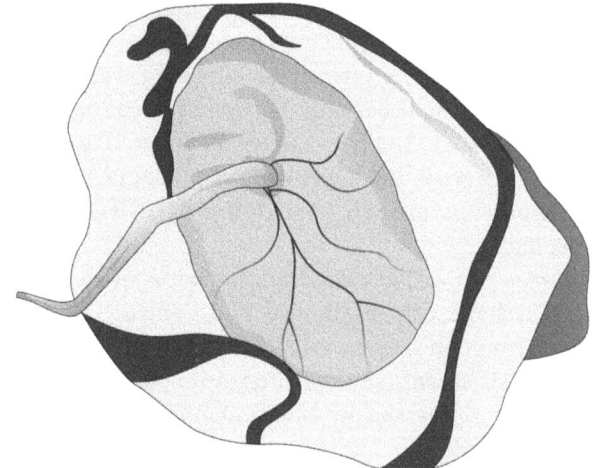

Fig. 10: Opaque fetal surface – infection.

from the chorion at the base of the cord by pulling the amnion back to ensure the presence of two layers. Completeness of the membranes should be observed.
- *Fetal surface:* This surface usually looks shiny, with visible veins crossing underneath the arteries. It looks dull and opaque in chorioamnionitis, greenish in meconium-stained amniotic fluid (MSAF). Amnion nodosum is a finely granular and dull amniotic surface often noted with oligohydramnios **(Fig. 10)**.
- *Maternal surface:*
  - It is divided into 15-20 cotyledons by septa, and the usual color is deep maroon. This surface should also be looked for retroplacental clot/hematoma (signs of abruptions—old/recent, size of clots), calcifications (pale white), missing cotyledons (no cotyledonary divisions in maternal floor infarction).
  - *Infarction:* Fresh infarcts are dark red, whereas old infarcts are yellow to white. Maternal hypertension, preeclampsia, eclampsia, IUGR, and maternal systemic lupus erythematosus are associated with placental infarcts. Clinical associations fairly correlate with the extent of involvement, especially when >15% of the placenta is involved.

- *Cut section:* While cutting the placenta, infarction (yellow to white), thrombi inside the intervillous space, and solid tumor (chorioangioma), if any, should be looked at.

In addition, the features that are additionally looked for the multiple pregnancies include the membranes that divide the sac (two vs. four), and vascular anastomoses. Generally, the dividing membranes of dichorionic diamniotic placentas (DADC) are four-layered, opaque due to interposition of old blood vessels or decidua, and form a ridge over the placenta where they meet between each other.

Microscopic Examination

Placental tissues sent for HPE are collected from the following six sites: membranes (amnion and chorion), normal-appearing tissues (two), margin (one), tissue appearing abnormal (one), and cord/cord insertion (one). Usually, H&E stain is used for routine HPE. However, other special stains can be used for specific purposes.

Placental tissue for viral/cytogenetic/metabolic studies/DNA studies: Villous tissue is usually taken from the mid-portion of the placenta or subamniotic chorionic plate. Chromosomal analysis can also be done, especially in situations where the fetus is macerated. A small chorion with bit of fetal vessels is cut and transferred to tissue culture media for this purpose. For the metabolic study, villous tissue (10-20 g) should be frozen quickly in liquid nitrogen within 10 minutes after thorough washing in buffered saline. Then the tissue can be stored at –80°C for subsequent examinations. For electron microscopy, minced villous tissue should be placed in glutaraldehyde.

Lesions suggestive of histologic chorioamnionitis:
- On gross examination, the fetal surface appears dull and opaque.
- Presence of diffuse maternal infiltration of chorion or subchorionic fibrin by neutrophils originating in the intervillous space or decidual postcapillary venules. It can also be accompanied with fetal neutrophilic response within the walls of large veins and arteries of the cord or chorionic plate. Adverse outcomes associated with chorioamnionitis include spontaneous prematurity, neonatal sepsis, and fetal central nervous system (CNS) injury.

Lesions consistent with maternal malperfusion (MMP):
- Retroplacental hemorrhages
- Vascular changes include acute atherosis, chronic perivasculitis, mural hypertrophy, fibrinoid necrosis, absence of spiral artery remodeling, arterial thrombosis, and persistence of intramural endovascular trophoblast in the third trimester (decidual arteriopathy).
- Villous changes include increased syncytial knots, villous agglutination, increased intervillous fibrin deposition, distal villous hypoplasia, and villous infarcts.

- Severe MMP is an important cause of fetal growth restriction (FGR), preterm birth, intrauterine fetal death (IUFD), and fetal CNS injury. Milder MMP can be associated with late spontaneous preterm birth.

Lesions consistent with fetal thrombotic vasculopathy (FTV):
- Thrombosis of the chorionic plate and stem villous vessels, avascular villi, intramural fibrin deposition, villous stromal-vascular karyorrhexis, stem vessel obliteration, and vascular ectasia.
- FTV has been associated with FGR, IUFD, fetal CNS injury, and fetal vascular disruptions, including stroke, porencephaly, intestinal atresia, and limb deficiencies.

Underlying maternal conditions that can increase the risk of FTV in subsequent pregnancies include diabetes, antiphospholipid syndrome, thrombophilic mutations, and antiplatelet antibodies.

Villitis of unknown etiology (VUE): Villitis of unknown etiology is defined by maternal lymphohistiocytic infiltration of the fetal stroma of terminal villi, but often extending to the small vessels of upstream villi. High grade is defined as the presence of multiple foci, on more than one section, at least one of which shows inflammation affecting more than ten contiguous villi is associated with FGR. Diffuse VUE, often associated with perivillous fibrin deposition, can cause IUFD.

Placental Examination Report

Name of the patient: _____

History: _____

Photography

Taken - Yes/No, B&W/Color

Macroscopic examination

Weight: _____ gm

Size: _____ x _____ x _____ cm

Cord: _____ Insertion site: Central _____ Eccentric _____ cm from the margin

Type of insertion: Marginal _____ Velamentous _____ Vasa previa _____

Vessels - 3 or 2, Thrombosis - Yes/No, Knots - Yes/No, Twist - Yes/No

Membranes: _____ Color: Normal/opaque/green

Point of rupture from margin _____ cm

Marginal _____ Circumvallate _____

Amnion nodosum _____

Fetal surface: _____ Vessels _____

Maternal surface: _____ Color: Normal/pale _____

Intact - Yes/No, Calcification - Marked/normal No

Abruptio - Yes/No, Recent/Old, Size _____ cm

Cut surface: _____ Infarct _____ % of total, Old/Recent

Tumors _____ Others _____

Microscopic examination _____

Diagnosis _____

CHAPTER AT A GLANCE

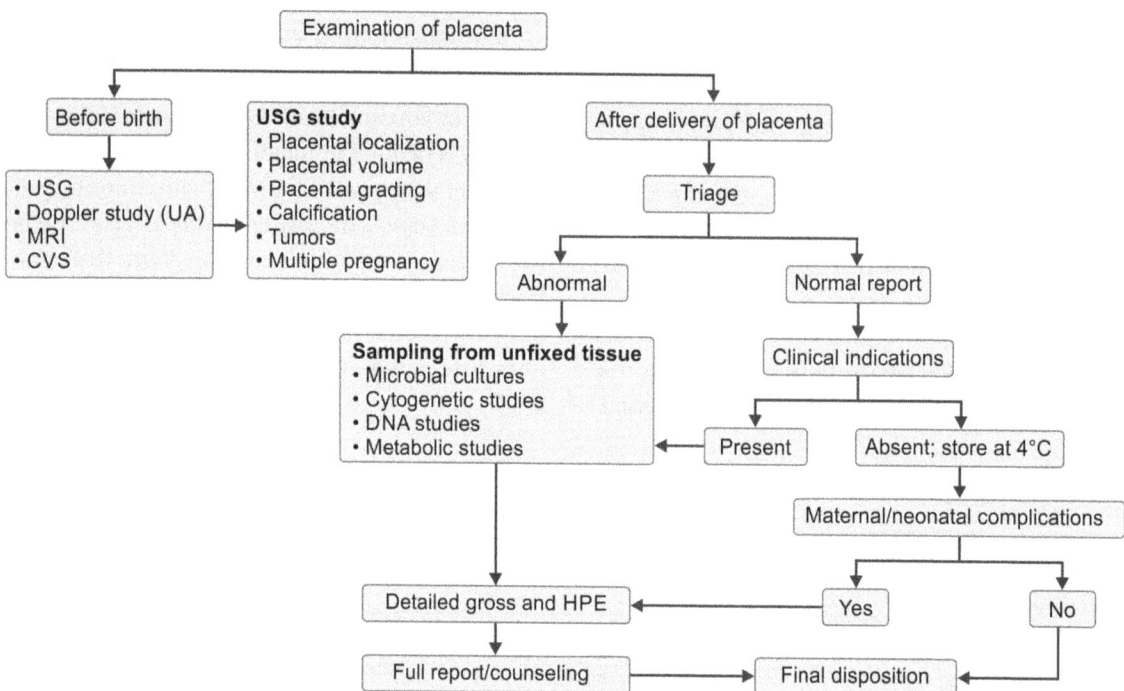

(HPE: histopathological examination; CVS: chorionic villus sampling; MRI: magnetic resonance imaging; USG: ultrasonography)

KEY POINTS

- All placentas should be examined by healthcare professional conducting deliveries. However, triaging must be done based on the clinical conditions and availability of the facilities for gross and microscopic examination by the pathologists.
- Many abnormalities can be detected before birth accurately by USG. Functional assessment can also be performed using Doppler velocimetry studies.
- Placental tissue must be preserved appropriately based on the type and methods of examination required (Culture, Karyotyping, DNA studies, HPE).
- Additional information obtained after placental evaluation can assist in the immediate management of mother or infant, improved management of subsequent pregnancies for the conditions that have recurrence risks, the institution of early intervention to improve long-term outcomes.

SUGGESTED READING

1. Benirschke K, Burton GJ, Baergen RN. Pathology of the Human Placenta. 6th edition. Berlin: Springer Science & Business Media; c2012.
2. Devi VS. Inderbir Singh's Human Embryology. 11th edition. New Delhi, India: Jaypee Brothers Medical Publishers; 2018.
3. Kaplan CG. Examination of placenta. Lab Med. 2007;38(10): 624-8.
4. Langston C, Kaplan C, MacPherson T, Manci E, Peevy K, Clark B, et al. Practice guideline for examination of the placenta: Developed by the Placental Pathology Practice Guideline Development Task Force of the College of American Pathologists. Arch Pathol Lab Med. 1997;121(5):449-76.
5. Schuett GW. Biology of the Vipers. Eagle Mountain, Utah: Eagle Mountain Pub; c2002.
6. Yetter III JF. Examination of the placenta. Am Fam Physician. 1998;57(5):1045-54.

Index

Page numbers followed by *b* refer to box, *f* refer to figure, *fc* refer to flowchart, and *t* refer to table

A

Abdomen 38, 309
Abdominal circumference 87, 93
　thoracic to 201
Abdominal wall defects, fetal anterior 81*t*
Abortions 211
　risk of 261
Abruptio placenta 279
Abruption 312
　placenta 184*t*
Absolute neutrophil count 120
Acardiac twin, size of 208
Accelerations 18
Achondroplasia 70
Acid-fast bacillus 274, 278
Acromegaly 124
Activated partial thromboplastin time 138, 142
Acute respiratory distress syndrome 142, 266, 289, 292
Acyclovir 263
　intravenous 253, 263
　prodrug of 247
Adenomatoid malformation, congenital pulmonary 25
Adenovirus 228
Adrenocorticotropic hormone 124
Aedes
　aegypti 265, 266
　albopictus 265, 266
Agyria 44
Aicardi syndrome 44
Alanine aminotransferase 189
Alcohol 153
Allopurinol 320
Alpha-fetoprotein 5, 41, 86
Alpha-thalassemia 26
Aminoglycoside 325
Amniocentesis 6
Amniotic fluid 84*f*, 198, 199, 200*f*, 202, 218, 220, 271
　abnormalities 200
　embolism 134
　functions of 199*f*
　index 14, 142, 189, 192, 199
　levels 206
　measurement 198
　　methods of 198
　meconium-stained 303
　methods of 199
　part of 198
　production, pathways of 199*f*
　regulation 198
　role of 199*f*
　testing 220, 232
　viral polymerase chain reaction 103
　volume 11, 202
　　abnormalities of 199

Ampicillin 165, 221
Ampulla 373
Anal
　atresia 106
　opening, absent 346*f*
Anemia 127, 129, 189, 235, 257
　causes of 127
　consequences of 128
　hemolytic 128
　physiologic 127
　prevention of 25
　risk of 311
　treatment of 25, 130*t*
Anencephaly 40, 41*f*
Anesthesia 196
　general 195, 196
　regional 196
Aneuploidy 3
　screening for 3, 103, 107
Aneurysms 40
Angiotensin receptor blockers 121, 150, 151
Angiotensin-converting enzyme 56, 150, 151
　inhibitors 36, 121, 151, 195
Anorectal malformations 80, 81, 337, 339, 346
Antenatal care 120, 195
　visits 370
Antenatal corticosteroids 166*t*, 170, 172, 173, 175, 180, 220
　benefits of 171, 172
　courses of 172
　dosing regimens of 171
　mechanism of action of 170, 171*f*
　rescue course of 172
　safety of 220
　trial 180
　use of 173, 174
Antenatal hydronephrosis 67, 342, 343*fc*
　evaluation of 67*fc*
　management of 67*fc*
Antenatal hydrops fetalis, diagnostic criteria for 95*t*
Antenatal management 80, 82, 96
Antenatal monitoring 96, 206
Antenatal steroids 165, 170, 191
Antenatal ultrasound scan 357
Antepartum fetal surveillance 12*t*, 14
　tests for 11
Antepartum hemorrhage 164, 183, 183*fc*, 186
　management of 186
　pathophysiology of 184*fc*
Antepartum stillbirth 366
Anterior abdominal wall defects 81
Antibiotic 151, 220, 323
　prophylaxis 325
　role of 180
　therapy 220
　treatment 246
Antibody 287
　test 252

Anticardiolipin antibody 369
Anti-citrullinated protein antibody 143
Anticoagulant 151
Antiepileptics 36, 151, 335
　drugs 157, 159
　effect of 157*t*
Antigen detection 253
Antihypertensive 190*t*
　medication 151
Antimicrobial therapy 165
Antineoplastic agents 149
Antinuclear antibody 138
Antioxidant strategies 181
Antiphospholipid antibody syndrome 7, 134, 138, 140-142, 189, 193, 212, 213, 369
　effect of 142
　pathogenesis of 141
Antipsychotic drugs, effects of 158*t*
Antiretroviral therapy 280*t*, 283
Antistaphylococcal penicillin 325
Antithyroid peroxidase antibodies 138
Anti-tubercular therapy 277
Antivirals 248
　role of 247
　use of 249
Anxiety 153
Aortic arch, interrupted 55
Aortic isthmus Doppler 89
Aortic stenosis 57
Aortopulmonary collateral arteries, major 60
Apgar scores 318*f*, 320
Aplasia 51
Apnea 273, 304, 328
Aqueduct stenosis 40
Aqueous penicillin G 257
Arterial perfusion, reversed 208
Arthralgia 265, 268
Asepsis 300, 324
Aspartate aminotransferase 134, 189
Asphyxia, timing of 315
Aspirin 193
　prophylaxis, risk factors for 193*t*
　use of 6
Assisted reproductive techniques 204, 359
Atresia, intestinal 337
Atrial septal defect 55, 57, 60, 151
Atrium, right 57
Attention deficit hyperactivity disorder 122, 153, 155
Atypical hemolytic uremic syndrome 134
Auditory brainstem response 250
Autoimmune 213
　disease 7
　　hormone-controlled T-cell responses influence progression of 137*f*
　disorders 137, 141*t*
　hemolytic anemia 128
　thyroid diseases 138

Index

Automated auditory brainstem response 98
Autopsy 114, 367
  conventional 38
Autosomal dominant 110, 113
  polycystic kidney disease 62, 63
Autosomal recessive 110, 113
  polycystic kidney disease 62, 63
Auxiliary nurse midwives 174
Azathioprine 140
Azithromycin 165, 257

B

Bacille calmette-guérin 278, 282
  vaccination 283
Bacteriuria, asymptomatic 163
Bag and mask ventilation 339
Ballantyne syndrome 98
Balloon atrial septostomy 59
Barlow's maneuver 327f
Barlow's test 333
Basalis 372
Benzathine penicillin 257
Benzodiazepines 151
Beta-blockers 138
Beta-human chorionic gonadotropin 3, 5, 9, 86
Betamethasone 166
Beta-thalassemia 3, 129
Bifid scrotum 327f
Bilious vomiting 340, 345
Bilirubin-induced neurological dysfunction 98, 99
Biophysical profile 13t, 14, 26, 101, 189, 192
Biophysical tests 12t
Biparietal diameter 82
Birth
  asphyxia 358
  defects 35, 36t
    major 35
    minor 35
    prevention of 25
    types of 35
  management at 90
  trauma 348
    risk factors for 348
  weight, standards of 325
Biventricular repair 60
Bladder
  anomalies of 64
  exstrophy of 81
  outlet obstruction 27, 338
Blake's pouch cyst 40
Blalock-Taussig shunt 60
Bleeding vasa previa 306, 315
Blindness 252
Blood
  components
    choice of 97
    proportion of 97
  flow 4
  indices 129t
  outside, collection of 350
  pressure 134, 186, 188, 190t, 192, 310
  sugar level 8
  tests 220
  transfusion 249
  urea nitrogen 189
  volume 97
Blue-berry muffin rash 245
Bochdalek hernia 48
Body mass index 125, 163, 189
Bone
  and mineral metabolism, disorders of 123t
  disorders of 122
  marrow biopsy 135
Brachial plexus injury 351
Bradycardia 317
Brain 188, 247
  malformations 43t
Brainstem evoked response audiometry 98, 269
Breastfeeding 209, 277, 293
  early initiation of 323
  exclusive 277, 282
Breastmilk 277
  use of 249
Breasts, engorged 334
Breathing 303
Breech delivery 348
Bronchial atresia 52
Bronchoalveolar lavage 232
Bronchopulmonary dysplasia 92, 209
  development of 222
Bronchopulmonary sequestration 48, 50, 50f
  diagnosis of 50f
Brownie nose pigmentation 267, 267f

C

Caffeine 154
Calcinosis 142
Calcium supplementation, high-dose 193
Cantrell variant, pentalogy of 81
Caput succedaneum 349
Carbamazepine 151
Carbimazole 122, 138
Carcinoma, hepatocellular 286
Cardiac arrhythmia, treatment of 25
Cardiac defect 59, 60
Cardiac malfromations 54
Cardiac septal defects 240
Cardiomyopathy 21, 156, 159
Cardiotocography 12, 321
  categorization 19
  continuous 209
  trace 18f
Cardiovascular disease 196
Cardiovascular reflex 314
Cataract 232, 240, 252, 326
Cebocephaly 42f
Central nervous system 16, 45, 106, 108, 134, 148, 150, 154, 250, 252-254, 292
  anomalies 202
  development 40
  disease 252
  dysfunction 11
  malformations 40
    clinical classifications of 40
Centrofacial pigmentation 267f
Cephalohematoma 349
Cerebellar hypoplasia 247
Cerebral
  hemorrhage 195
  palsy 177
Cerebroplacental ratio 87, 93
Cerebrospinal fluid 44, 230, 232, 253-255, 259, 269, 275
Cerebrovascular accident 142
Cervical
  cerclage 164
  insufficiency 215
  length measurements 164
  lymphadenopathy 233
  weakness 212
Cervicovaginal secretions 244
Cervix, ripening of 219
Cesarean section 122, 139, 209, 348
  lower segment 21
  rates 315
Chest 38
  compressions 305, 306f
  X-ray 341
Chikungunya 227, 228, 230, 261, 266, 267
  infection 267
  virus 261, 266
Choanal atresia 347
  bilateral 340
Choledochal cysts 83
Chorioamnionitis 164, 165, 218, 219, 222, 279
  clinical 164
  diagnosis of 220
  pathophysiology of 218
Chorioangiomas 201
Chorionic villus
  biopsy 375
  sampling 6, 8, 75, 100, 109, 110, 113, 378
Chorionicity 204, 205, 205f
Chorioretinitis 252, 326
Chromosomal abnormality
  frequency of 36t
  percentage of 36
Chromosomal defects, markers of 5
Chromosomal disorders 110
Chromosomal microarray 6, 36, 100
Chronicity 205
Circumvallate placenta 374, 374f
Cisterna magna, large 247
Citrate phosphate dextrose 99
Clavicle fracture 350
Cobblestone lissencephaly 44
Cocaine 149
Coloboma 347
Colonic atresia 81
  anorectal malformations of 80
Comparative genomic hybridization 110
Complete blood count 135, 138, 189, 192, 220, 250, 253
Computed tomography 38
Congenital cystic adenoid malformation 36
Congenital pulmonary airway malformation 48, 49, 49f, 51t, 338, 340
Conjoined twins 208
Conjunctivitis 268
Consanguinity 367
Constipation 334
Continuous positive airway pressure 79, 301f, 302, 304, 311, 328, 356
Contraction stress test 14
Convulsion 334
Coomb's test
  direct 105, 106
  indirect 97, 100, 105, 106, 311
Cord
  accidents 306, 315
  avulsion 315
  blood

banking 312
 gas analysis 316
 platelet count 139
 clamping 309, 309f, 311, 312
  delayed 301
  maternal effects of delayed 311
  physiological based 311
  timing of 309
 gas examination 325
 management strategies 310
 marginal insertion of 373f
 prolapse 315
 velamentous insertion of 373f
Coronavirus disease 230
Corpus callosum 40
 dysgenesis of 43
Cortical atrophy 262
Cortical development, disorders of 44
Cortical malformation 36
Corticosteroids 166, 293
 long-term risks of 174
 use of 291
Cotrimoxazole prophylaxis 281, 281t
Counseling
 antenatal 75, 76, 103, 300, 356, 357
 genetic 42, 43
COVID-19 230, 289, 290
 care centers 290
 hospitals 290
 management of 290, 291, 293, 293t
 pregnancies 290
 severity, classification of 292t
 signs of 292
 status 290
 symptoms of 292
C-reactive protein 143, 165, 222, 253
Creatine kinase 319
Critical congenital heart disease
 delivery room management of 58
 screening 333
Crown-rump length 3
Cryptorchidism 65, 65f
 congenital 65
Cushing's syndrome 124
Cyanosis 273
Cyanotic heart disease, congenital 333f
Cyclophosphamide 140
Cysts
 bronchogenic 48, 51
 hepatic 83
Cytomegalovirus 26, 78, 90, 100, 101, 108, 148, 150, 151, 227, 228, 230, 244, 250
 abnormalities in 247t
 congenital 78, 247,
 diagnosis of 246
 infection 44, 244-247
 interpretation of 246t
 laboratory diagnosis of 248
 vaccine 249

D

Daily fetal movement count 192
Dandy-Ealker malformation 44
Day care setting, prevention in 249
Death, causes of 366
Decidua 218
 basalis 372
Decidual arteriopathy 376

Deep tendon reflex, loss of 194
Deep vein thrombosis 142
Defensins 249
Delayed cord clamping 310-312
 benefits of 310
Delivery 167, 258
 intent for 164
 management of 139
 mode of 90, 135, 144, 208, 220, 290, 348
 options 129
 plan 208
 point screening 326
 room
  care 328
  management 66, 82, 297
  placental examination in 90
 timing of 89, 90, 121, 195, 290
Dengue 227, 228, 266
 viral infection 265
 virus 230, 261, 265
Deoxyguanosine triphosphate 263
Depressed fractures 348
Depression 153
Dexamethasone 140, 166
Diabetes insipidus 119, 123
Diabetes mellitus 103, 149, 151
 gestational 3, 8, 14, 105, 119, 120, 125, 173, 175, 207, 290
 insulin-dependent 124
 maternal 104, 104t, 201
 type 1 119
 type 2 119
Diamniotic dichorionic twins 206, 209
Diamniotic-monochorionic twins 209
 diagnosis of 206f
Diaper rash 334
Diaphragm, development of 48
Diaphragmatic plication 352
Diastolic blood
 flow velocity 374
 pressure 190
Diastrophic dwarfism 70
Dichorionic-diamniotic 205
 pregnancy 205
 twins, diagnosis of 206f
Dichorionic-monoamniotic twins 205
Diethylene-triamine-pentaacetate 68
Diphtheria 373
Direct fluorescent antibody 258
Direct-acting antiviral agents, development of 287
Disability adjusted life years 127
Disproportionate intrauterine growth intervention trial 89
Disseminated intravascular coagulation 136, 142
Distal bowel obstruction 341
Diuretic renography, indication of 342
Dizygotic twins 205, 208
Doppler velocimetry 13
Double bubble sign 344
Double volume exchange transfusion 97, 99
Double-outlet right ventricle 55, 60
Down's syndrome 113fc, 245, 344
Drugs 143
Ductus arteriosus 59, 60
Ductus venosus 4
 Doppler 88, 89f
 flow 4
 waveforms 88

Duodenal atresia 79, 341, 344
Duodenojejunal flexure 345f
Dural fistula 40
Dusky-bowel appearance 82
Dye dilution technique 198
Dyspnea 202
Dysuria 252

E

Eagle-Barrett syndrome 66
Ear anomalies 347
Ebolavirus 228
Ebstein's anomaly 57f, 148, 151
Ecchymosis 350
Echocardiography 98, 156, 319
Echoviruses 228
Ecidual plate 372
Eclampsia 187, 193, 290
 complications of 194
 prevention of 6
Ectopia 63
Edema 350
Efavirenz 280
Electrocardiogram 98, 101, 319
Electroencephalogram 253
Electrolytes 317
 exchange of 373
Elevated liver enzymes 128, 195
Embryos 372
Encephalitis 252, 263, 267
Encephalocele 40
Encephalopathy
 grade of 320
 mild 320
End-diastolic flow 29
 absent 190, 207
 reversal of 207
Endocrine function 119
Endotracheal intubation 305
Endotracheal tube 302
Epilepsy, pregnancy with 157
Epinephrine 306
Epithelial cells, lymphocytic infiltration of 142
Epstein-Barr virus 228
Erb-Duchenne palsy 351, 352f
Ergotamine 149
Erythrocyte sedimentation rate 143, 274
Erythromycin 165, 257, 320
Erythropoietin 99
Escherichia coli 219
Esophageal anomalies 78
Esophageal atresia 78, 340, 341, 343
Estimated fetal weight 81, 87, 93
Ethambutol 276-278
Ethylenediaminetetraacetic acid 75
Ex utero intrapartum treatment 25
Exomphalos 81
Expected delivery date 205
Extracellular glutamate accumulation 319
Extracorporeal membrane oxygenation 49, 58, 59, 61
Eye 254, 326
 abnormalities 38
 care 325

F

Face 38
Facial nerve injury 350, 351

Fanconi anemia 26
Fast breathing 334
Fatty liver, acute 134, 157, 159
Femoglobin 127t
Femoral pulse 326
Ferric carboxymaltose 130
Ferritin 310
Fetal
   abdomen, transverse section of 84f
   abnormalities, minor 5
   acidosis, interpretation of 316b
   actocardiograph 13
   akinesia syndrome 74
   alcohol
      spectrum 153
      syndrome 149
   anemia 25, 27f, 202
   anomaly, targeted imaging for 214
   arrhythmias 24, 26t
   autopsy 38
   birth defect 36, 37
   bleeding disorders, risk of 21
   blood sampling 21, 21t
   bradyarrhythmia, management of 25
   brain
      cellular architecture of 177
      coronal view of 84f
   cardiac balloon valvuloplasty 25
   cardiovascular
      malformations 54
      system, development of 54
   complications 206, 207, 222
   compromise, pathophysiology of 11
   congenital heart disease 56b
   death 4
   demise 154
   disorders 33
   distress 196
   echocardiographic parameters 58, 59
   echocardiography 26, 56, 56f
   effects 119, 196
   electroencephalogram 315
   endoscopic tracheal occlusion 49
   examination 367
   fibronectin 164
   gastrointestinal
      disorders, antenatal diagnosis of 84
      sonographic examination 78
   genetic testing 36
   genital differentiation 62
   goiter 25, 26f
   growth restriction 14, 16, 21, 86, 90, 104, 105, 173, 175, 190, 192, 321
      prediction of 87
      prevention of 87
      risk factors for 86t
      selective 28, 29
   growth scans 190
   heart
      development of 54
      rate 11, 12, 16, 17, 21, 26, 191, 192, 315f
   hydrothorax 28
   hypothyroidism 138
   hypoxemia 315f
   infections 103, 107, 246
      risk of 240fc
   interventions 57
   intra-abdominal cyst 83
   kidney 62
   loss 138, 369
      recurrent 369
   lung
      development, stages of 47
      fluid 198
      malformations 47
      maturity 291
   magnetic resonance imaging 36, 48
   magnetoencephalography 13
   malformation 240
      development of 47t
   membranes 218
   monitoring 193
      intrapartum 16, 20
      maternal and fetal indications for 10t
   morbidity 142
   movement count 314
   neck
      coronal section of 26f
      masses 338
   neurodevelopment, impaired 138
   nutrition 198
   oxygenation 18
   pulse oximetry 315
   reduction, selective 29
   scalp stimulation 21
   screening 74
   sepsis 21
   single-gene disorders 113fc
   skin 198
   structural anomalies 110
   surface 376
   surgery 25
   surveillance 206
      emerging methods of 13
   tachyarrhythmia, management of 25
   therapy 24, 25b, 337
      ethics of 24
      types of 24
   thoracic malformations 47
   thorax, transverse section of 56f
   toxoplasma infection, diagnosis of 234
   trauma 306
   treatment 24
      failure, risk of 258
      team 24
   ultrasonography 36, 63
   varicella, diagnosis of 263
   venous circulation 13
   ventriculomegaly 41
   well-being
      antepartum assessment of 314
      assessment of 10, 190
      intrapartum assessment of 314
      monitoring, intrapartum 315
Fetoscopic
   endoluminal tracheal occlusion 28, 30
   laser photocoagulation 28
   selective laser photocoagulation 29f
   surgical therapy 24
Fetus 198, 218
   examination of 368b
   malformations diagnosed in 357
   normal 314
   radiograph of 369f
Fever 148, 245, 262, 268
   high-grade 265
   low-grade 220
   presence of 334
Fibrosis, cystic 78
Figure-of-eight appearance 44f
First-line anti-tubercular treatment 277
First-trimester
   combined test 6fc
   screening 3f
Fissure, interhemispheric 42f
Fluids 317
Fluorescence in situ hybridization technique 6, 45, 110
Folate deficiency 127
   anemia 127
Folic acid 105
   antagonist 149
   concentrations 129
   deficiency 149
Folinic acid 237
Forceps delivery 348
Forebrain, midline malformations of 42
Free beta-human chorionic gonadotropin 109
Free thyroxine 122

G

Ganciclovir 248, 253
   therapy 248
Gardnerella vaginalis 219
Gases, exchange of 373
Gastrointestinal
   anomalies 83, 202, 337
   malformations 78
   tract 129, 154, 199, 252, 339
Gastroschisis 79, 81-83, 344, 345f
Genetic
   disorders 70, 103, 110, 332
      counseling guidance on 112t
   factors 163, 213
   screening 71
   testing 112t
Genital anomalies 65
Genital hypoplasia 347
Genitalia, ambiguous 327f
Genitourinary system malformation 62
Gentamicin 221
Germinal matrix-intraventricular hemorrhage 177
Gestation neonates, small for 91f
Gestational age 14, 356
   estimation of 205
   small for 86, 93, 184
Gestational diabetes mellitus 3, 8, 14, 105, 119, 120, 125, 173, 175, 207, 290
   complications of 138
   prevalence of 104
   screening for 120fc
Gestational sacs 205
Gestosis 187
   classification of 188t
   scoring system 7, 187, 189t
Glasgow coma scale 186
Glomerular filtration rate 187
Glucocorticoids 140
Glucose-6-phosphate dehydrogenase 332
Graft versus host disease 249
Gram-negative
   bacilli 325
   diplococci 325
Granulocyte cerebrospinal fluid 250
Granuloma, hepatic 272
Graves' disease 137, 138, 149
   management of 138

Index

Great artery
  congenitally corrected transposition of 25
  transposition of 55, 60
Growth
  charts 90
  discordance 206
  restriction 245, 347
    fetal 87t, 328
    intervention trial 89
  retardation 128

H

H1N1 influenza
  infection 263, 264, 265fc
  virus 261
Haemophilus influenzae 245, 282
Hair, presence of 326
Hashimoto's thyroiditis 138
Head and neck injuries 348
Headache 264
  acute onset of 188
Health
  care workers 174
  information 279
  long-term issues on 335
Hearing 332
  assessment 277
  loss, sensorineural 244
Heart
  block, congenital 140
  defect 347
  development 54f
    stages of 55
  disease 156
    acquired 156
    adult congenital 156, 159
    congenital 54, 55t, 57, 58, 61, 76
    ischemic 196
    pregnancy with 156
  failure 139
    congestive 59, 208
  rate 56, 302, 303, 305
    baseline 17
    fetal 314
Heavy alcohol consumption 153
Hemagglutinin 263
  antigen 263
Hemangioma 148
Hematocrit 97
Hematological disorder 133
Hematological tests 189
Hematology 187
Hematoma 40
Hemoglobin 129, 130, 131
  C disease 128
  electrophoresis 8
  glycated 103
  S-beta-thalassemia 128
Hemogram 319
Hemolysis, elevated liver enzymes, low platelet count syndrome 123, 133, 134, 157, 175, 187, 195, 209, 234
Hemolytic-uremic syndrome 134, 135
Hemophilia 21
Hemorrhage 40
  adrenal 353
  antepartum 154, 183, 184
  extracranial 349f, 350

fetal 184
fetomaternal 95, 95f, 306
intracranial 36, 139, 188, 245, 348, 350, 351f
intraventricular 171, 175, 303, 310, 351
postpartum 134, 193, 202, 222, 266, 335
retinal 351
risk factors of antepartum 183
subarachnoid 351
subdural 350
subgaleal 349
vitreous 351
Hemorrhagic disease 159
Hepatic calcification 83, 84f
Hepatitis 245, 248
  A 228, 284
    vaccine 282, 284
    virus 284, 288
  B 21, 228, 282, 285
    immune globulin 285, 288
    infection 285b, 286fc
    monovalent vaccine 285
    surface antibody 285, 286
    surface antigen 285, 286
    vaccination 285, 286, 286b
    virus 138, 230
  C 21, 228, 286
    virus 138, 286-288
  D 287
    virus 287
  E 287
    virus 287, 288
  fulminant 252
  severe 263
  viruses 284
Hepatomegaly 235
Hernia
  congenital diaphragmatic 28, 30, 48, 48f, 305, 307, 338-342
  isolated congenital diaphragmatic 28
Herpes simplex virus 227, 228, 230, 251-253, 254, 255
  diagnosis of neonatal 253t
  infections 251
    clinical features of 252t
    treatment, maternal 253t
  prevalence of 251
  transmission of 251
Herpesvirus 228
Heterotopia 40
High airway obstruction, congenital 25, 101
High pulsatility index 193
Higher order multiple-gestation triplets 208
High-frequency oscillatory ventilation 49
High-peak systolic velocity 27f
High-performance liquid chromatography 8, 100
Hip
  developmental dysplasia of 327f, 333
  examination 327, 327f
  instability 333
Hirschsprung's disease 80, 345
Holoprosencephaly 43
  classification of 42
  diagnosis of 43
  etiology of 43
Hormonal therapy 25
Hormone production 373
Horner syndrome 351
Human chorionic gonadotropin 125, 373
Human enterovirus 228, 230

Human immunodeficiency
  infection 282, 282t
  syndrome 138
  transmission 279
  virus 21, 128, 133, 228, 230, 279, 281-283, 300
Human parechovirus 232
Human platelet antigen 135
Hybrid lesions 47
Hydroceles 148
Hydronephrosis 66f, 342
  antenatal 66
Hydropic neonates 97
Hydrops fetalis 95, 97fc, 202, 307
Hydroxychloroquine 140, 293
Hygienic food 284
Hygroma, cystic 338
Hyperbilirubinemia 246, 349
Hypercalcemia
  development of 352
  familial hypocalciuric 123
Hyperechoic lung lesion 50f
Hyperglycemia 119
  incidence of 119t
Hyperimmune globulin 247
  role of 247
Hyperparathyroidism 122
Hyperplasia, congenital adrenal 332
Hyperprolactinemia 123
Hypertension 65, 105, 187, 321, 335
  chronic 195
  gestational 104, 191, 192fc
  management of 196
  pharmacological management of 190
Hypertensive disorders 103, 104, 187
Hypertensive emergency,
  management of 191, 191fc
Hyperthermia 148, 195
Hyperthyroid 122
Hyperthyroidism 122, 149
  management 119
  subclinical 121
Hyphema 351
Hypogammaglobulinemia 282
Hypoglycemia 92, 303, 328
Hypoparathyroidism 123
Hypoplasia 268
Hypoplastic
  adrenal cortex 151
  left heart syndrome 55, 57, 59, 61
  right heart syndrome 55
Hypospadias 65
Hypotension 19, 82, 317
Hypothalamo-pituitary thyroid 121
Hypothermia 235, 319f, 328, 334
Hypothyroidism 121, 122
  congenital 195, 332
Hypotonia 128
Hypotonic fetal urine 198
Hypoventilation 143
Hypoxemia-ischemia, prevention of 181
Hypoxia 18
  chronic 11
Hypoxic ischemia encephalopathy 317t, 321

I

Immune hydrops 99fc
  fetalis 95
    postnatal management of 98fc
  management of 96
  pathophysiology of 95, 96fc

Immune thrombocytopenia 133, 134, 135b, 136
   purpura 138
      therapeutic options for 139t
      without bleeding 139t
Immunization 264, 282, 332
   active 263, 285
Immunoglobulin 249
   G 253
   intravenous 97, 130, 135, 136, 139, 264
   M antibody 284
Immunological defense 373
Imperforate anus 80f
Implantation, abnormal 373
In utero fetal intervention 338t
In vitro fertilization 6, 109, 189, 213, 216, 359
Induction 40
Infarction 376
Infection 163, 227, 252, 367
   active 276
   asymptomatic 235, 237
   bacterial 219
   chronic 128
   congenital 227, 229f, 230t, 231b, 273, 225
   first-episode 253
   intra-amniotic 218, 221t
   intrauterine 164
   mechanism of 218
   pathogenesis of 229f
   postpartum 246
   prevention of 25, 328
   puerperal 143
   subclinical 235
   treatment of 25
Inflammation 319
   acute chronic 129
   prevention of 181
Influenza 228, 263
   vaccine, inactivated 264, 282
   virus 263
   virus, type A 263
Inherited thrombophilic defects 212
Injuries
   extracranial 348
   hepatic 353
   intra-abdominal 353
   intracranial 350
Intellectual disability 262
Internal capsule, posterior limb of 320
Interventricular septum 57
Intestinal duplication cyst 83, 84f
Intracytoplasmic sperm injection 7, 189, 359
Intrapartum cardiotocography interpretation 19
Intrapartum
   management 280
   risk factors 299
   stillbirth 366
Intraplacental circulation 374
Intrauterine fetal
   blood transfusion 25
   death 122
   demise 193, 208, 209
Intrauterine growth
   restriction 76, 87t, 106, 122, 150, 158, 159, 184, 196, 200, 206, 257f, 311, 329f, 374
      risk of 138
      severe 78
   retardation 267, 269
Intrauterine transfusion 27, 96, 97, 99, 105, 106
Invasive testing 6
   role of 246

Iodides 138
Ionizing radiation 107, 148
Iron
   deficiency anemia 127
      consequences of 128b
      evolution of 128f
   intravenous 130t
   supplementation 131
Isoimmunization 103, 373
   etiology of 95
   mechanism of 95
Isoimmunized pregnancy 105
   counseling in 106fc
Isolated fever, classification of 219t
Isolation 258, 263
Isoniazid 275, 276, 278
Ivermectin 293

J

Janani Suraksha Yojana 369, 370f
Jaundice 235, 245, 273, 328, 333f
   evaluation of 333
   neonatal 333
   risk of 311
Jejunal atresia 79
   diagnosis of 79f
Jejunoileal atresia 79

K

Kangaroo mother care 328
Karyotype 113
Ketoacidosis, diabetic 125
Kidney 111, 187
   anomalies of 62
   congenital anomalies of 62
   disease
      chronic 128, 139, 158, 159
      cystic 62
   disease, end-stage 63
   injury, acute 266
   nonvisualization of 201
   ureter, and bladder, ultrasound of 343
Kimura's duodenoduodenostomy 344
Klebsiella 221
Klumpke palsy 351

L

Labor
   active management of third stage of 312
   and birth 368
   and delivery, stress of 143
   premature 154
   stage of 316
Labor-delivery-recovery concept 327
Laceration 351
Lactate dehydrogenase 192
Lactoferrin 249
Lacunae 372
Large intestine, disorders of 80
Laryngeal mask airway 302
Last menstrual period 167
Late deceleration 18, 18f
Late preterm 170
   delivery 258
Late syphilis, treatment of 257
Latent tuberculosis infection 274
Lead 148

Leucodepletion decreases 249
Left atrium 54, 56, 57
Left ventricle 54-57, 309
   outflow tract 56
Leptomeningeal cyst 349
Lesion
   consistent 376
   hybrid 48
   mixed 48
Leukocoria 326
Leukocytes 249
Leukocytosis, maternal 165
Leukoencephalopathy syndrome, posterior reversible 188
Leukomalacia, periventricular 177, 221
Limb
   abnormalities 111, 150
   buds 69
   short 357
Linear fracture 348
Lipoma, presence of 326
Lissencephaly 40, 44
Listeria monocytogenes 221
   infection 219
Lithium 36, 148
Liver 187, 247
   damage 235
   disorder 157
   function test 189, 192, 195, 250, 319
Lobar emphysema, congenital 48, 340, 341
Lobed placenta 373
Lobulations, structure of 373
Long bone injuries 352
Loose stools 334
Low birth weight 138, 154, 159, 204
   infant
      care of 328
      prevention of 88t
Low platelet 128
   count 134
Lower intestinal tract 331
Lower limb 38
   edema of 202
   right 333
Lower urinary tract obstruction 27, 30, 338, 342, 343
Lower uterine segment 184, 373
Low-molecular-weight heparin 213
Lumbar meningomyelocele 41f
Lung
   development 47t
      stage of 47
   disease, chronic 222
   growth, accelerate 49
   malformations 48
   maturity 201
   parenchymal malformations 47, 48
Lung-to-head ratio 111
Lupus
   anticoagulant 369
   nephritis 139, 141t
Luteal phase deficiency 369
Lymphadenopathy 245
Lymphangiomas 148
Lymphocytic choriomeningitis virus 228, 230
Lymphocytic hypophysitis 124
Lysosomal storage disorders 26

M

Macrosomia 350
Maculopapular rash 266f
Magnesium 179
    therapy 194
    toxicity 194
Magnesium sulfate 166, 331
    antenatal 179
    intravenous 180
    therapy 166, 194
    treatment 22
Malaise 245, 264, 265
Malaria 128
Malformations, congenital 35, 111t
Malrotation 79
    with midgut volvulus 345
Mandelbrot formula 96
Marijuana 149
Massive hydrocephalus 357
Maternal anemia, prevention of 181
Maternal antibody, transmission of 373
Maternal blood glucose, high 121
Maternal cardiomyopathy 156
Maternal care 360
Maternal causes 214
Maternal chorioamnionitis 172
Maternal complications 207, 222
Maternal conditions 149
Maternal disorders 214
Maternal drugs 331
Maternal endocrine
    disorders 119
    illness 119
Maternal fever 219, 266
Maternal history 366
Maternal infection 21, 108t, 214
    nonprimary 245
Maternal malperfusion 376
Maternal medical
    administration 26t
    condition 104, 105t
    history 6
    illness and fetal effects 117
Maternal medications 153
Maternal monitoring 191
Maternal morbidity 142, 366
Maternal rubella 240fc
    infection
        diagnosis of 239
        management of 241t
        management of 240
Maternal seroconversion status 235
Maternal substance abuse 149, 153
Maternal surface 376
Maternal symptoms 218, 263
Maternal syphilis 257f
    stages of 257t
Maternal systemic medical illness and fetal effect 156
Maternal treatment 253
Maternal-fetal
    medicine units 174
    transmission 240
Mean arterial pressure 7, 189
Mean corpuscular
    hemoglobin 8
    volume 8, 100
Measles 228, 282, 373

Mechanical ventilation 352
Mechanical ventilator 59, 319f
Meckel-Gruber syndrome 63
Meconium
    aspiration syndrome 200, 303, 337
    delayed passage of 340
    ileus 79, 340
    plug syndrome 331, 340
Meconium-stained liquor 21
Medical nutritional therapy 121
Medical therapy 24
Medicolegal claims, prevention of 359
Mega cisterna magna 40
Megalencephaly 44
Melatonin 181, 320
Membrane 163, 165t, 168, 172, 178, 219, 375
    prelabor rupture of 172, 175, 178, 180, 181, 200
    premature rupture of 28, 154, 172, 175, 216, 269
    rupture of 202, 219
Meningitis 148
Meningomyelocele 30, 338, 346
Mental disorders 158
Mental health medication 151
Mental illness 158
Mentzer's index 8
Mercury 148
Mesenteric cyst 83
Metabolic disorders 332
Metabolism, inborn error of 100, 216
Methimazole 122, 138
Methyl-mercury poisoning 148
Methylprednisolone 140
Microangiopathic hemolytic anemia 128, 134, 189
Microcephaly 40, 44, 240
Microcytic hypochromic anemia 129t
Micropenis 66f, 327f
Microphthalmia 240, 252
Micturating cystourethrogram 68, 343
Middle cerebral artery 13, 87, 97, 100, 105, 106, 108
    Doppler 27f
        flow 89f
    pulsatility index 14
Migration, disorders of 44
Miliary disease 272
Miller-Dieker syndrome 44
Minimally invasive autopsy 38
Miscarriage 211
    risk of 4, 138, 211t
Mitochondrial disorders 103, 110
Mitral regurgitation 58
Mitral valve dysplasia syndrome 58
Monochorionic monoamniotic 209
Monochorionic twins 206
    complications of 28
Monozygotic splitting 205
Morbidity 208
    neonatal 209
Morgagni hernia 48
Moro's reflex 154
Mortality 208
    neonatal 209
    rates
        maternal 370
        neonatal 370
Mother and newborn, rights of 355
Mother with fetal distress, management of 315
Mother's chest 309, 323
Mother's health, advice for 335

Mother's womb 372
Mother-child protection 334
Mother-infant dyad's health 355
Mother-to-child transmission 279
    prevention of 285
Mouth 254
Musculoskeletal malformations 75fc
Multicystic dysplastic kidney 63
Multidisciplinary team, role of 104
Multiorgan dysfunction syndrome 267
Multiple fetal poles 205
Multiple gestation 366
    diagnosis of 205
Multiple pregnancy 172, 204, 205, 311
    antenatal monitoring of 206
    epidemiology 204
    feeding in 209
    prevalence 204
    risk factors 204
Multiple sclerosis 137
Multiplex ligation-dependent probe amplification 110
Multisystem disease 187
Multisystem inflammatory syndrome 292
Mumps 148, 228, 282
Muscle brain 319
Musculoskeletal malformations 69, 71, 72t
    diagnosis of 74
    pathways of 69, 70
Musculoskeletal system
    embryonic development of 69
    fetal development of 70
Myalgia 245, 265
    severe 264
Myasthenia gravis 143, 144b
    effect of 143, 144
Mycobacteria growth 275
Mycobacterium tuberculosis 271, 274
Mycoplasma hominis 219
Myelomeningocele 40
    study, management of 30
Myocarditis 267

N

N-acetylcysteine 181
Nasal bone 4f
Nasopharynx invades 261
Necrotizing enterocolitis 171, 175, 209, 339
Negative predictive value 12
Neisseria gonorrhoeae 325
Neonatal abstinence syndrome 154
Neonatal asphyxia 316
Neonatal birth
    injuries 348
    trauma 348
Neonatal care 360
Neonatal chickenpox 262
Neonatal cross-sectional charts 90
Neonatal death 151
    early 215
Neonatal dengue 266
Neonatal encephalopathy 177, 317t
Neonatal gastrointestinal surgical conditions 339fc
Neonatal hearing loss, screening for 332f
Neonatal hypoxic-ischemic encephalopathy 16
Neonatal infection 252, 284
Neonatal intensive care 101
    unit 11, 14, 21, 76, 79, 90, 93, 98, 101, 105, 111, 173, 175, 184, 321, 358, 374

Neonatal lupus erythematosus 140
Neonatal management 83, 221, 281
Neonatal morbidity 142
Neonatal mortality, causes of 323
Neonatal problems 121
    mechanism of 121
Neonatal resuscitation 22, 22t, 185, 299, 300t, 317
    protocol 22
Neonatal symptomatic disease 235
Neonatal treatment 253
Neonate born, management of 303
Neonate diagnosed, management of 90
Neostigmine 144
Nerve injuries 351
Nescroft test 8
Neural tube 41f
    defects 40, 41, 111
    formation 40
Neuraminidase antigens 263
Neuraxial anesthesia 22
Neuroimaging 247, 268
Neurologic endpoints trial 179
Neurologic injury 252
Neurologic manifestations 245
Neurological disorder, pregnancy with 157
Neurometabolic disorders, pregnancy with 157
Neuromuscular disorders 201
Neuromuscular junction 143
Neuronal injury 177
Neuronal tissue, cellular hypoxia of 11
Neurophenotype presentation, primary 245
Neuroprotection 166
Neuroprotective strategies 319
Neurosyphilis 257
Neutropenia 253
Neutrophil infiltration 220
Nevirapine 281, 283
Newborn infant 228t
    treatment for 284
Next-generation sequencing 43, 62
Nicotine 153
Nipple
    cracked 334
    flat 334
Nitric oxide 49, 59
Non-bilious vomiting 340
Nonimmune hydrops fetalis 95, 98, 99t, 100, 100fc, 101t
    management of 100
    pathophysiology of 98
Noninvasive electronic fetal monitoring 17
Noninvasive fetal monitoring 10
Noninvasive prenatal test 5, 75, 109, 113
Non-nucleoside reverse transcriptase inhibitor 280
Nonpenicillin regimens 257
Nonsteroidal anti-inflammatory drugs 56, 140, 196
Non-stress test 14, 142, 189, 192, 206, 314
Nontreponemal tests 257b
Nonvertex presentation 21
Nonvigorous 303
Nuchal translucency 3, 5, 75
    measurement of 3f
Nucleated cell, total 312
Nucleic acid amplification test 274, 275, 290
Nutrients, exchange of 373
Nutritional anemia 127

O

Obstetric
    analgesia 196
    cholestasis 157
    Doppler 190
    history, previous 216
    indications 220
    management 220
        strategies 279
Occipital encephalocele 41f
Occipital osteodiastasis 349
Occipitofrontal diameter 82
Oil massage 332
Oligodendroglial death, pathogenesis of 177f
Oligohydramnios 65, 198, 200, 201
    causes of 200
    etiology of 200b
    management of 201
Omental cyst 83
Omphalocele 81, 357
Opaque fetal surface 376f
Open fetal surgery 24
Open maternal fetal therapy 25
Open neural tube defect 346f
Operation theater 59
Opiates 331
Opioid 154
Oral hypoglycemic agents 121
Oral iron, role of 129t
Oral maintenance treatment 190t
Organ specific actions 171
Organ system 317
Oropharyngeal swab 232
Orthopnea 202
Ortolani maneuver 327f
Ortolani test, positive 333
Oseltamivir 265t
Osteogenesis imperfecta 76
Osteomyelitis 349
Otitis media 264
Otoacoustic emission 332f
Overt hyperthyroidism 121
Overt hypothyroidism 121
Oxidative stress 164
Oxygen
    saturation 58
    therapy, maternal 20
Oxygenation 328
Oxytocin admin 280

P

Packed cell
    transfusion, indication of 130b
    volume 98
Packed red blood cells 96, 131
Pain 252
Parechovirus 228, 230
Parental chromosomal rearrangements 212
Parental counseling 320
Parvovirus 26, 78
    B19 148, 228
Patellar reflex, absent 194
Patent ductus arteriosus 59, 150, 151, 357
Peak systolic velocity 96, 97, 106, 108
Pelviureteric junction 68, 342
    obstruction 64

Pemphigus 144
    neonatal 144
    vulgaris 144
Penicillin 257
    therapy 257
Percutaneous shunting 27
Perinatal asphyxia 314
    antepartum risk factors for 314t
    intrapartum risk factors for 314t
    neonate with 317
    prognosis of 320
    risk factors for 314
Perinatal autopsy 367
Perinatal brain
    damage, pathophysiology of 177
    damage, risk factors for 178
    injury, antenatal neuroprotective interventions for prevention of 178
Perinatal chickenpox 262
Perinatal death, risk of 138
Perinatal monitoring 120
Perinatal mortality 200f
    rate 365
Perinatal outcomes, pathophysiology of 185fc
Perinatal pathology 144
    role of 114
Perinatal period, medicolegal issues in 358
Perinatal risk factors 299, 299t
Perinatal transmission, risk of 279
Perinatal tuberculosis 271, 273, 274t
    infection
        pathophysiology of 271
        types of 272fc
    signs of 273t
    symptoms of 273, 273t
    treatment of 276, 276t
Perineal hypospadias 327f
Periodontal disease 163
Peripartum hysterectomy 375
Periventricular leukomalacia 178f
Periviable births 170
Periviable gestations 356, 358fc
Pernicious anemia 128
Persistent bradycardia 306
Persistent pulmonary hypertension 49, 92, 93, 98, 150, 151, 339
Persistent truncus arteriosus 55
Personal protective equipment 307
Petechiae 235
Phenylketonuria 149, 151
Phosphodiesterase 22
Phrenic nerve injury 352
Phytonadione 326
Pierre Robin sequence 307
Pig-tailed shunt 25
Pituitary disorders 123
Pituitary insufficiency 124
Pituitary necrosis, post-partum 124
Placenta 188, 198, 220, 218, 310, 372, 373
    accreta 184, 185
    battledore 373
    development of 372
    diameter of 375
    examination of 374, 375
    level of 309
    marginal 373
    membranacea 374, 374f
    peripheral margin of 373
    previa 184, 184t, 312, 373
        complete 375f
    succenturiata 374, 374f

Placental abruption 315
Placental causes 214
Placental circulation, removal of 309
Placental cord pathology 220
Placental disorders 372
Placental examination 367, 372
　indications of 374*t*
Placental function 374
Placental growth factor 7, 87
Placental transfusion 301, 309
　physiology of 309
Placental viviparity 372
Placentation, abnormal 373
Plasma protein, pregnancy-associated 3, 7, 87
Platyspondyly 369*f*
Pleural effusion 28
Pneumococcal conjugate vaccines 282
Pneumococcal polysaccharide vaccine 282
Pneumococcal vaccines 282
Pneumonia 235, 245, 248, 263, 292, 337
Pneumonitis 252
Pneumothorax 307
Polio vaccines 282
Poliovirus 228
　vaccine, inactivated 282
Polyarthralgia 239
Polyarthritis 239
Polycystic kidney disease 62
Polycystic ovarian syndrome 7, 124, 213
Polyhydramnios 78, 79, 198, 201, 202, 227, 344
　approach and management 201
　complications 202
　etiology of 202*b*
　mild 202
　moderate 202
　severe 202, 202*t*
　treatment 202
Polymerase chain reaction 101, 108, 112, 238, 252-255, 281, 283, 290
Polymicrogyria 247
Polymorphonuclear leukocyte 220
Positive end expiratory 59
　pressure 59, 98
Positive predictive value 12, 98
Positive pressure ventilation 302, 304, 305, 305*fc*, 307, 318*f*
Posterior fossa, abnormalities of 40, 44
Posterior urethral valve 68, 27*f*
Postexposure prophylaxis 263
Postnatal care 331
Postnatal chickenpox 262
Postnatal evaluation 38
Postnatal examination 38
Postnatal hydronephrosis 343*fc*
Postnatal management 79, 80, 97, 317
Postpartum 214
　care 121, 195, 196, 335
Postresuscitation care 306
Precipitous delivery 348
Preconception care 195
Preconceptional prenatal diagnostic test 110
Predischarge screening 332
Prednisolone 140
Prednisone 237
Preeclampsia 3, 87, 133, 141*t*, 187, 191, 192*fc*, 193, 290, 374
　prediction of 6
　recurrent 196
　severe 173

Pregnancy 138, 200
　adrenal pathologies in 124
　and childbirth care, quality-of-care indicator of 365
　and lactation labeling rule 107
　anemia in 127, 127*t*
　associated plasma protein A 3, 5, 9, 86, 109
　contraindicated in 138
　diabetes in 119
　ectopic 373
　effect on 144, 290
　genital herpes in 254*fc*
　gestosis in 187
　high-risk 315
　hyperglycemia in 119
　hypertensive disorders of 103, 104, 187
　induced hypertension 122
　interval between 163
　loss 211, 213*t*
　management of 138, 215
　toxoplasmosis in 234*fc*
　treatment in 247
Pregnant women, testing strategy in 289
Preimplantation genetic
　diagnosis 114
　testing 114
Premature birth 267
　prevention of 164, 178, 215
Premature cellular senescence 164
Premature deliveries 211
Premature rupture of membranes, management for 181*t*
Prematurity, encephalopathy of 177
Prenatal diagnosis 240
　investigations in 70
Prenatal genetic testing 113
Prenatal neuroprotective strategies 177
Prenatal screening tests 3
Prenatal ultrasonography 66
Prepregnancy 120
Prescription drugs 154
Preterm birth 163, 204
　four direct causes of 163
　recurrent 214
Preterm delivery 211
　risk of 138
Preterm infants 263
Preterm labor 163
　diagnosis of 163
　management of 166
　progesterone in 179*t*
　signs of 202
　symptoms of 202
　treat 167
Preterm prelabor rupture 163, 168, 172, 178, 215, 219
　management of 165*t*
　of membranes
　　diagnosis of 164
　　management of 165
Primary infection, settings of 246
Prior preterm birth 163
Pritchard's regimen 179
Progesterone
　administration 215
　role of 178
　supplementation 206
Progestogen compounds prophylaxis 164
Proliferation, disorders of 44

Prophylaxis 281
　maternal 285
　neonatal 285
Propranolol 138
Propylthiouracil 122, 138
Prostaglandin
　E1 59
　release 219
Protein
　particularly interleukins 220
　S deficiency 369
Proteinuria, urine for 189
Prothrombin gene mutation 369
Prothrombin time 138
Prune belly syndrome 66
Pseudomonas 221
　infection 325
Pseudoparalysis 350
Psychiatric illness, maternal 158
Pulmonary agenesis 51
Pulmonary artery hypertension 59
Pulmonary atresia 55, 57
Pulmonary circulation, duct-dependent 60*t*
Pulmonary embolism 142
Pulmonary hypertension 139, 156, 159
Pulmonary hypoplasia 48, 51, 201
Pulmonary sequestration 51*t*
Pulmonary status 201
Pulmonary stenosis 57
Pulmonary valve 57*f*
Pulmonary vascular resistance 59
Pulmonary venolobar syndrome 52
Pulse oximetry screen 333*f*
Pump twin 208
Purpura 245
Pyelogram, intravenous 107
Pyloric stenosis, congenital hypertrophic 339-341
Pyrazinamide 276, 278
Pyridostigmine 144
Pyrimethamine 237
Pyruvate kinase deficiency 26

Q

Quality of life 357
Quintero staging 207*t*

R

Racing car sign 43
Radiation 124
Radiofrequency
　ablation 25
　identity 325
Randomized controlled trial 24, 49, 170, 179
Rapid plasma reagin 259
Rash 148, 268
Raynaud's disease 142
Raynaud's phenomenon 142
Reactive oxygen species, reduction of 181
Recurrent pregnancy loss 212, 216
　etiology of 212*f*
　treatment of 213
Recurrent prematurity 215
Red blood cell 127, 128, 130
　positive 96
Red watering eyes 264
Refractory thrombocytopenia 248
Renal abnormalities 150

Renal agenesis 63
Renal ciliopathies 63
Renal disease 196
    end-stage 62
Renal disorders 158
Renal ectopia 64
Renal failure, acute 158, 159
Renal function test 192, 319
Renal pelvic dilatation 66
Renal pelvis, anteroposterior diameter of 343
Renal transplant, women with 158
Renal tubular injury 92
Replogle catheter 79
Reproductive mode 372
Rescue therapy 166
Respiratory care 317
Respiratory conditions 340
Respiratory depression 194
Respiratory distress 303, 328, 339fc, 350
    neonatal 151
    syndrome 121, 138, 159, 170, 171, 175, 221
Respiratory efforts 303, 323
Respiratory problems 273
Respiratory syndrome coronavirus, severe acute 227, 289, 300
Resuscitation 301f, 307t
    custom-made 311
    drugs for neonatal 306t
    neonates needing immediate 311
    noninitiation of 306
Retinal dysplasia 252
Retinoblastoma 326
Retinoids 36, 149
Retinopathy of prematurity 92, 209, 222, 357
Retracted nipple 334
Rh
    alloimmunized infants 311
    incompatibility 311
    isoimmunisation, management of 27
Rhesus D-negative women 369
Rheumatoid arthritis 7, 134, 137, 142, 143, 189
    effect of pregnancy on 143
Rifampicin 276, 278
Right atrium 54, 56
Right ventricle 54, 56, 57, 60, 309
    dependent coronary circulation 60
Right ventricular
    filling 309
    outflow tract 56, 60
Ringer's lactate 316
Rotavirus 282
Routine antenatal care 11
Routine care 301
Rubella 148, 227, 228, 239, 240, 242, 282, 373
    cataract, congenital 241f
    infection 239
        acute 239
        congenital 240
        prevention of 242
    specific IgG 242
    specific IgM 242
    susceptible women 239
    syndrome, congenital 108, 240fc, 241f, 242f
    testing 240fc
    virus 239
        isolation of 242
Running nose 264

S

Sacrococcygeal teratoma 338
Saliva 232
Sapporo revised criteria 141
SARS-CoV-2 infection 289, 292
Scalp injury, types of 350t
Scarring 252
Schizencephaly 40, 44
Schizophrenia 158
Scimitar syndrome 52
Scleroderma 134, 142
Screening tests, follow-up of 109fc
Screen-positive pregnancies, management of 6
Second-trimester screening 4
Sedatives 151
Seizure 188, 253, 262, 273
    disorder 103
        maternal 104
    electrographic 318
    management 318
Selective serotonin reuptake inhibitor 56, 151
Semilobar holoprosencephaly 42f
Sensorineural hearing loss 99, 250
Sepsis 337
    bacterial 267
    development of 335
    early-onset 221, 222
Serodiscordant couples 280
Serological tests 242, 246t, 248, 267
Serum
    bilirubin 189
    biochemistry 3
    creatinine 189, 277
    electrolytes 189
    iron 310
    lactate dehydrogenase 135
    magnesium level 194, 194t
    screening 4
    uric acid 189
Severe acute respiratory syndrome coronavirus 2 230
Severe disease, prevent 264
Sex determination 368
Sexual development, disorder of 65, 65f, 68
Sexually transmitted diseases 256
Shock 317
Short rib polydactyly syndrome 76
Sick neonates and feeding protocols, management of 92
Sickle cell 128
    anemia 128
    syndromes 128
Sideroblastic anemia 129
Silver sulfadiazine 344f
Single nucleotide polymorphism 110
Single-gene disorders 43, 110
Sinusoidal pattern 19
Sjögren's syndrome 137, 142
Skeletal dysplasia 74, 75, 76fc, 201
Skeletal malformation 76
Skin 254
    eye, mouth disease 252
    lesions 252
    papillae 148
    tags 148
Skin-to-skin
    care, advantages of 324tt
    contact 323, 323f
Skull fracture 348
Small intestine, anomalies of 79
Smear, peripheral 189
Smith-Lemli-Opitz syndrome 151

Soft tissue 352
    injuries 352
Sore throat 264
Spina bifida 30, 42f, 245
    occulta 326
Spinal cord injury 352
Spine 38
    examination 326
Splenic injury 353
Splenomegaly 235
Staphylococcus aureus 221, 325
Statins 151
Stenosis 79, 340
    critical pulmonary 57f
Sternocleidomastoid injury 350
Steroids, dose of 206
Stillbirth 211, 213, 365, 365t
    causes of 214, 366
    classification of 366, 367b
    diagnosis of 214
    incidence of s 213
    investigation of 366
    prevention of 369
    previous 214t
    rate 365, 366
    recurrence of 214
    risk factors for 367b
Streptomycin 276
Stroke 196
Subdural empyema 349
Subgaleal hemorrhage, management of 349
Substance abuse 153
Sudden infant death syndrome 153, 332
Sulfadiazine 237
Superoxide dismutase 178
Supraventricular tachycardia 26
Surgery 124
Surgical conditions, spectrum of 337
Surgical management 82
Surrogacy 359
Symptomatic infant 236, 275
Symptomatic neonate 221, 245
Syncytiotrophoblast 372
Syncytium 372
Synthetic nucleoside analog 263
Syphilis 90, 148, 227, 256, 257, 259f
    burden of 256
    clinical stages of 256t
    congenital 258, 258t
    diagnosis of 257
    during pregnancy 256
    early congenital 258
    epidemiology of 256
    treatment of 257
    treponemal tests for 258
Systemic circulation, duct-dependent 59t
Systemic inflammation 177
Systemic lupus erythematosus 7, 134, 137, 139, 140, 189, 193, 213, 321, 374
    effect of 139
    flare, management of 141
    long-term risk of 140
    management of 140
Systemic sclerosis 142
Systolic blood pressure 190

T

Tachycardia 82
    maternal 219
    supraventricular 59

Tachypnea 292
Tactile stimulation 302
Talipes equinovarus 70
Tear drop sign 43
Telangiectasia 142
Temperature, airway, breathing, and circulation 347
Tenofovir disoproxil fumarate 280
Teratogenic abnormalities 70
Teratogenic agents 106t, 107
  classification of 150t
Teratogenic exposure 147
Teratogenicity 103, 105
Teratogens 147
Teratoma 338
Tetanus 373
Tetracyclines 151
Tetralogy of Fallot 55, 59, 99
Thalassemia 8, 128
  prenatal diagnosis for 8
Thanatophoric dysplasia 76
Therapeutic hypothermia 319, 319t
  mechanism of 319
Thermoregulation 317, 324, 328
Thionamides 138
Thoracic circumference 76
Thoracic malformations, congenital 47, 52
Thoracic vascular malformations 47, 48
Throat 232
Thrombocytopenia 133, 135, 138b, 139, 187, 189, 195, 235, 239, 240, 246, 257, 263, 266
  causes of 133b
  fetal 21
  gestational 133-135
  maternal 135b
  severe 133
Thrombophilia 193, 213
Thrombosis 290
Thrombotic complications 142
Thrombotic microangiopathy 134
Thrombotic thrombocytopenic purpura 134, 135
Thyroid
  abnormalities 214
  autoimmune disorders 138
  disorder 121, 149
    incidence of 121t
  dysfunction
    causes of 122t
    effects of 122t
  function test 121
  gland, enlarged 26f
Thyroidectomy 138
Thyroid-stimulating hormone 121, 122, 138
  receptor 125
Thyroxine-binding globulin 125
Tissue
  samples 236
  sealants 201
Tobacco smoking 149
Tocolysis 20, 166, 167
Tocolytic agents 167t
Toluene 148
Total anomalous pulmonary venous return 55, 59
Total body iron 310
Total parenteral nutrition 347
Toxicity 194t, 253

Toxoplasma 233, 236
  chorioretinitis 233
  gondii 233
  nucleic 236
Toxoplasma infection 234
  clinical manifestation of 233
  congenital 234-237, 237t
  etiopathogenesis of 233
  management of 234, 235t
Toxoplasmosis 90, 148, 227, 233, 234fc
  congenital 236, 236b, 237
Toxoplasmosis, rubella cytomegalovirus, herpes simplex 103, 231-233
  screening
    maternal 229
    results 229
  virus report, interpretation of 231fc
T-piece
  device 301f
  resuscitator 301f
Trachea-esophageal fistula 78, 337
Tracheal occlusion 49
Tracheoesophageal fistula 150, 340, 341, 343
Transabdominal sonography 70, 75
Transferrin saturation 310
Transient cortical blindness 188
Transient ischemic attack 142
Transient tachypnea 166, 171, 173
Transmembranous pathway 198
Transplacental intrauterine infection 292
Transplacental transmission, risk of 256
Transvaginal sonography 70, 75
Traumatic injury 358
Treponema pallidum 256, 257
Treponemal tests 257
Tricuspid
  atresia 148
  flow 4
  regurgitation 4, 60
  valve 60
Trimester screening tests, detection rates of first- and second 5t
Triple-drug regimen 280
Triplet pregnancy 311
Trisomy 3, 44, 70, 78
Trophoblastic cells 372
Troponin 319
Truncus arteriosus 55
Tuberculin skin test 274, 275
Tuberculosis 128, 271, 275, 277
  congenital 272, 276
  infection 275
  pathophysiology of 271
  postnatal 273
Tuberculous endometritis 272
Tumor 124
  necrosis factor 220
Twin
  anemia-polycythemia sequence 207, 209
  occurrence of 204
  pregnancy 205, 311
    terminologies in 204
  reversed arterial perfusion 25, 28, 30, 208
Twin-to-twin transfusion syndrome 25, 26, 28, 100, 207, 209
  management of 28, 207t

U

Ultrasonography 48, 66f, 68, 69, 70, 75, 97, 189, 378
Ultrasound 339
  biophysical profile 314, 315
Umbilical arterial blood
  normal 316
  parameters 316
Umbilical arterial cord gas 316f
Umbilical artery 207, 374
  Doppler 87, 88f
    assessment of 374
    in normal 375f
Umbilical cord 310, 337, 345f, 372, 375
  arterial gas parameters 316b
  avulsion 312
  care of 324
  clamping 309
  granuloma 325
  insertion of 373
  management 309
  milking 310
  pathology 220
  segment 310
Umbilical vein 208, 309
Umbilical venous catheter 302
Umbilical vessels 220
Undescended testes 65, 65f
Univentricular repair 60
Upper duodenal stenosis 340
Upper limbs 38
  right 333
Upper respiratory infections 269
Ureaplasma urealyticum 219
Ureter 111
  anomalies of 64
Urethra, dilated 64f
Urethral valve, posterior 62, 64, 338
Urinary bladder 111
Urinary retention 335
Urinary tract 62
  infection 64, 158, 159, 163, 342, 343
Urine 232
  dipstick 189
  frequency 334
  output 194
Urogenital system, embryology of 62
Uterine artery
  Doppler 87, 88f
  high-resistance flow in 7f
  pulsatility index 7, 87, 93
  waveform 7f
Uterine atony 202
Uterine contraction 310
Uterine hyperstimulation 19
Uterine malformations, congenital 212
Uterine overdistension 202
Uterine tube, isthmus of 373
Uteroplacental circulation 372
Uteroplacental insufficiency 200, 201
Uterus
  enlarged 202
  overdistension of 208

V

Vacuoles 372
Vaginal delivery, difficult 316

Vaginal discharge 252
Vaginal secretions 271
Valganciclovir 248, 249
Valproic acid 151
Valvular heart disease 156, 159
Varicella 148, 261, 264*fc*
    prevention 263
    rash, characteristic of 262
    symptoms 262
    syndrome, congenital 262, 262*f*, 269
    vaccine 282
    virus 261
Varicella zoster 261
    immune globulin 262, 264
    virus 230, 261
        infections 228
Vascular and cardiac changes 187
Vascular endothelial growth factor 171, 187
Velamentous insertion 373
Venereal disease research laboratory 258, 259
Venous thrombosis 142
Ventilation 300, 328
    adequate 305
    corrective measures 305*t*
    positive-pressure 299, 311
Ventricular septal defect 57, 60, 149
Ventricular system 40, 41
Ventriculomegaly 36
Vermian hypoplasia 40
Vertical transmission 244, 287

Vesicles 252
Vesicoamniotic shunting 27
Vesicoureteral reflux 64, 64*f*, 67, 68, 342
Villitis
    acute 273
    chronic 273
    of unknown etiology 377
Viral culture 248, 253
Viral hepatitis 284
Viral infection 261
    serologic diagnosis of 232
Viral sepsis, maternal 252
Viremia 261
Virus isolation 267
Visceral injuries 352
Vision 332
    problems 188
Vitamin
    B_{12} 127
        deficiency 128
    D 181
        supplementation, maternal 181
    D deficiency 122
        fetal effects of 123*t*
        maternal of 123*t*
        stage of 123
    K 326
        administration of 326
        dose of 326
Viviparity 372

Vomiting 273, 334
von Willebrand's disease 138
Vulva 202

W

Walker-Warburg syndrome 44
Warm environment 331
West Nile virus 228
Western equine encephalitis virus 228
Wharton's jelly 81

X

X-linked dominant 113
    disorder 110
X-ray, abdominal 339, 341

Z

Zidovudine 280
Zika virus 228, 230, 261, 267, 268
    infection 268
        congenital 268, 269*fc*
        syndrome, congenital 268, 269, 269*fc*
Zuspan's regimen 179
Zygosity 204, 205, 205*f*
Zygotes 372

EU GSPR Authorised Reprsentative
Logos Europe, 9 rue Nicolas Poussin
1700, La Rochelle, France
Phone: +33 (0) 6 67 93 73 78
E-mail: contact@logoseurope.eu